DOUBLE CONTRAST GASTROINTESTINAL RADIOLOGY

with Endoscopic Correlation

IGOR LAUFER, M.D.

Associate Professor of Radiology, University of Pennsylvania;
Chief, Gastrointestinal Radiology Section, Hospital of the
University of Pennsylvania, Philadelphia; Formerly Assistant
Professor of Radiology, McMaster University Medical Center,
Hamilton, Ontario, Canada

1979

W. B. SAUNDERS COMPANY / Philadelphia / London / Toronto

W. B. Saunders Company: West Washington Square
Philadelphia, PA   19105

1 St. Anne's Road
Eastbourne, East Sussex BN21 3UN, England

1 Goldthorne Avenue
Toronto, Ontario M8Z 5T9, Canada

Double Contrast Gastrointestinal Radiology with
Endoscopic Correlation

ISBN   0-7216-5734-6

Last digit is the print number: 9   8   7   6   5   4   3   2   1

To my parents, Sara and Henry Laufer,
and
my wife, Bernice

CONTRIBUTORS

IGOR LAUFER, M.D.

Chief, Gastrointestinal Radiology Section, Hospital of the University of Pennsylvania, Philadelphia; Associate Professor of Radiology, University of Pennsylvania, Philadelphia. Formerly Assistant Professor of Radiology, McMaster University Medical Center, Hamilton, Ontario.

CLIVE I. BARTRAM, M.D.

Consultant Radiologist, St. Bartholomew's and St. Mark's Hospitals, London, England.

HANS HERLINGER, M.D., F.R.C.R.

Associate Professor of Radiology, Hospital of the University of Pennsylvania, Philadelphia. Formerly Chairman of Radiology, St. James's (University) Hospital, Leeds, England; Senior Clinical Lecturer in Radiology, University of Leeds.

HERBERT Y. KRESSEL, M.D.

Assistant Professor of Radiology, Hospital of the University of Pennsylvania, Philadelphia.

MASAKAZU MARUYAMA, M.D.

Department of Internal Medicine, Cancer Institute Hospital, 1-37-1 Kami-Ikebukuro, Toshima-ku, Tokyo, Japan. Visiting Professor, University of Peru, Cayetano Heredia.

J. ODO OP DEN ORTH, M.D.

Consultant Radiologist, Department of Radiology, St. Elisabeth's of Groote Gasthuis, Haarlem, Holland.

GILES W. STEVENSON, M.D.

Associate Professor of Radiology, McMaster University Medical Center, Hamilton, Ontario.

AKIYOSHI YAMADA, M.D.

Department of Surgery, Institute of Gastroenterology, Tokyo Women's Medical College, 10 Kawada-cho Shinjuko-ku, Tokyo, Japan.

PREFACE

My purpose in writing this book is to provide radiologists with the information they need to perform and interpret double contrast examinations of the gastrointestinal tract. I believe that the techniques are applicable in all types of radiologic practice, including university and community hospitals and office practice. The emphasis is on detection of lesions rather than on differential diagnosis. It is my firm belief that most serious radiologic errors are due to nondetection of lesions. Once the lesion is detected, the diagnosis is usually easy in the gastrointestinal tract, but even when differential diagnosis is a problem the clinical approach is usually clear: treat and repeat, endoscope or operate. Clearly, if the lesion is not detected our clinical and radiologic knowledge is of no avail.

This book does not pretend to be an encyclopedic treatise on gastrointestinal radiology. It is limited to diseases as seen on double contrast studies, with emphasis on the common everyday pathology and its many variations. There are few examples of exotic pathology, which are rarely seen except at the most specialized centers. Furthermore, this is a relatively new field and many basic problems still need to be elucidated. For example, we know almost nothing of the significance of the surface patterns, such as the areae gastricae or the innominate grooves in the colon, and their alteration in disease states.

The preface to a book gives an author a rare opportunity for self-indulgent autobiography and for public acknowledgement of those to whom he is most grateful. My interest in gastrointestinal radiology had been piqued during my residency at the Beth Israel Hospital in Boston. Dr. Norman Joffe convinced me of the important contribution that individual effort, skill, and knowledge could make in gastrointestinal diagnosis. This interest was heightened by the enthusiasm and erudition of Dr. Richard Marshak's many lectures in Boston during those years. As a resident, I also recall a lecture by Dr. Roscoe Miller in which he talked about the radiologic detection of lesions in the rectum that had been missed by sigmoidoscopy. I filed that away for later reference.

I started work in 1972 in the Department of Radiology at the McMaster University Medical Center under the Chairmanship of Dr. Peter Cockshott. This first job as a gastrointestinal radiologist started on the day that the hospital was scheduled to open. Unfortunately, the fluoroscopic equipment had not yet been installed, and I was left to do some general radiology and to prepare for my role as a GI radiologist. At Peter's suggestion and gentle urging, I tried to learn about double contrast techniques. When we started clinical work, the cases were few and we had the opportunity to experiment and to develop standardized techniques. Because of my inexperience in GI radiology, particularly with double contrast techniques, progress was slow and there were many frustrations. However, Peter was always ready with suggestions, either for solutions or with the names of people who might help solve our problems.

As the techniques developed and the patient load increased, we were faced with the problem of interpretation of radiographic appearances that we had never seen before. As an example, when I first saw the normal areae gastricae I thought it was some form of minute gastric polyposis. Thanks to a unique atmosphere of interdepartmental collaboration fostered at McMaster University, it was possible for me to start doing endoscopy myself—both in the upper and lower GI tract. Since I have no recollection of negotiating this privilege myself, I must assume that this arrangement was concluded by Peter Cockshott and our gastroenterologist, Dr. John Hamilton. Needless to say, this has proved to be of critical importance in helping us understand the mucosal abnormalities seen on double contrast studies, particularly in inflammatory diseases. I also believe that improvement in our understanding of radiologic findings has helped us to become better endoscopists. Without a doubt, patients have been best served by close collaboration between radiology and endoscopy.

I spent four years at McMaster in an almost idyllic setting—a new medical school, an ultramodern building with many architectural innovations, the newest equipment, and an avant-garde philosophy of medical care and education allowing people to cross traditional departmental barriers. However, the patient volume was relatively small and the variety of pathology was limited. One day I got a call from Dr. Stanley Baum, who had recently been appointed Professor and Chairman of Radiology at the University of Pennsylvania, the oldest medical school in North America and the first university-owned hospital. I was reluctant to think about leaving Hamilton, but because of the great radiology tradition of Philadelphia and the University of Pennsylvania I consented to look at the position. I was finally convinced by the potential of the department under Stanley Baum and by the charms of Philadelphia to accept the offer. In this position, I have been able to work with a much larger volume of patients and a wider variety of pathology. I have been most fortunate to have the continued personal support of the Chairman, Stanley Baum, and to benefit from his overall efforts to make the Radiology Department a stimulating environment.

Insofar as possible, I have tried to make this book a reflection of one person's experience. However, I have asked a number of experts to contribute or participate in some of the chapters. I met Drs. Herlinger, Bartram, and Stevenson during my visit to England in 1975. Dr. Herlinger was the Director of Radiology at St. James's University Hospital in Leeds, and had spent a year as Visiting Professor in the Department of Radiology at the University of Pennsylvania. He has recently joined our full-time faculty as my colleague in the Gastrointestinal Radiology Section. Dr. Clive Bartram has the good fortune to carry on the tradition of excellence at St. Mark's Hospital for Diseases of the Colon and Rectum. We had the pleasure of working closely with him during his three months' stay in our department during 1977. Dr. Giles Stevenson came to McMaster University in 1976 and became responsible for gastrointestinal radiology and endoscopy.

During my visit to Japan in 1977, I had the honor and pleasure of meeting Professor Hikoo Shirakabe, the man most responsible for the development of double contrast radiology of the stomach. He introduced me to Drs. Akiyoshi Yamada and Masakazu Maruyama. Dr. Yamada is a surgeon at the Institute of Gastroenterology, Tokyo Women's Medical College. He has been writing about the radiologic diagnosis of early esophageal carcinoma since 1971, although many of his publications are in Japanese. Dr. Maruyama is a gastroenterologist with vast experience in the radiologic diagnosis of gastrointestinal cancer. He is a frequent Visiting Professor in South America, and in the Fall of 1978 he made his first professional visit to the United States, lecturing at the University of Pennsylvania and delivering a paper at the meeting of the Society of Gastrointestinal Radiologists.

Dr. J. Odo Op den Orth is a radiologist in Holland who has been contributing regularly to the American literature and has also been a regular contributor to the scientific exhibits at the annual meetings of the Radiological Society of North America. He has contributed important and exquisite work on many aspects of double contrast radiology in the upper gastrointestinal tract.

Dr. Herbert Y. Kressel is my colleague in the Gastrointestinal Radiology Section at the Hospital of the University of Pennsylvania. He trained in radiology and held a fellowship in gastrointestinal radiology at the University of California, San Francisco, under the chairmanship of Dr. Alexander R. Margulis. We have worked together now for one and one half years. Apart from making my work a great deal easier and more pleasant, he has brought a new analytical and theoretical approach to double contrast radiology. He has been instrumental in developing the basic concepts and general principles involved in these studies. These considerations are reflected in the content of Chapter 2, "Principles of Double Contrast Diagnosis."

I would also like to acknowledge the assistance and support of another valued colleague, Dr. Vijay K. Gohel. In addition to being an expert GI radiologist, he is Chief of the Radiology Service at our affiliated Veterans' Administration Hospital in Philadelphia. He has been instrumental in the establishment of double contrast techniques on a routine basis in that hospital, and some of the radiographs in this book come from patients studied at the VA hospital.

The radiology residents at Penn and McMaster have been most cooperative and have adopted these techniques enthusiastically. They performed many of the studies illustrated in this volume.

There are, of course, many other people and circumstances for which one feels grateful. I have always had an enthusiastic, helpful, and charming group of technologists to work with, headed by Lynn Gledhill at McMaster and Patrice Nelson at Penn. My surgical and gastroenterologic colleagues have been most helpful and receptive to our new techniques. In particular, I would like to mention Drs. John Hamilton, Ted Mullens, and Jim Lind at McMaster and a distinguished group of gastroenterologists at Penn under the leadership of Dr. Sidney Cohen, including Drs. Frank Brooks, Edward C. Raffensperger, Bruce Trotman, Roger Soloway, Gary Levine, and Bob Long. These colleagues have been invaluable in helping us understand these new radiologic techniques by providing us with encouragement and vital endoscopic information. They have contributed many of the endoscopic photographs found in Chapter 10.

I would also like to thank my secretary, Rosemary Sheehan, who labored on the manuscript through the advanced stages of pregnancy. Rochelle Fertik and Lorraine Woods also graciously provided expert assistance whenever it was requested.

Finally, a word of thanks to the staff at W. B. Saunders, including

Marie Low, Ray Kersey, Herb Powell, Lorraine Battista, and Constance Burton. They have provided constant encouragement and yet have given me free rein to develop the content and style of this book. I am particularly grateful to them for keeping the production time down to less than two years from the start of writing until publication.

Most of all, I am grateful to my fellow radiologists whose interest in my work has led to the writing of this book.

IGOR LAUFER, M.D.
Philadelphia, December 1978

CONTENTS

1

INTRODUCTION

There are three basic components of barium contrast studies in the gastrointestinal tract. These are (a) barium-filled views with compression, (b) mucosal relief, and (c) double contrast. The ideal examination technique would utilize each of these components to best advantage. However, in practice this is not feasible because optimal results in the various phases of the examination require different types of barium suspensions. Therefore, the examiner must choose a basic approach to gastrointestinal contrast studies, giving emphasis to one or two of the basic components. He will then choose materials that are appropriate to this type of study, realizing that the other phases of the examination may be compromised but are not eliminated.

CONVENTIONAL BARIUM STUDIES

Principles

The most prevalent approach to barium contrast studies of the gastrointestinal tract in the Western world places emphasis on barium-filled views with compression and mucosal relief views. We shall refer to these as "conventional barium studies." Because of the need to penetrate the opacity of the barium column, these films are exposed at a relatively high kVp. Mucosal relief films are obtained with the organ collapsed either

1

after the administration of a small volume of barium, as in the stomach, or after evacuation of the barium, as in the colon. Even here, there must be a compromise in the choice of barium suspension, since a low density barium chosen for its suitability for barium-filled compression studies will not necessarily give the optimal coating for mucosal relief views. "Air contrast" views are frequently obtained to supplement the information obtained during the earlier phases of the examination. In the upper gastrointestinal study the volume of gas that happens to be in the stomach is utilized, and on occasion adequate distension of the antrum and duodenum can be obtained. However, the quality of mucosal coating is seldom of high quality, and there is rarely sufficient distension for an adequate study of the body and fundus of the stomach. In the colon, double contrast views are frequently obtained by insufflation of air after the patient has evacuated the barium. This type of "secondary air contrast study" has many deficiencies. The type of barium used for the single contrast enema does not produce good mucosal coating. The degree of evacuation is variable, and therefore the volume of residual barium is variable. The time interval during which the patient is evacuating the barium may result in flocculation or flaking of the barium coating. In addition there is frequently flooding of the small bowel which will obscure the sigmoid loops.

Drawbacks

It is clear that the accuracy of the type of examination described above will depend primarily on the quality of the barium-filled and mucosal relief films. Several major problems are encountered in using this technique.

A. In order to obtain greater distension of the organ it is necessary to increase the volume of barium. Therefore, increasing distension results in increasing opacity, which can obscure lesions that are not caught in profile. This problem also applies to the examination of segments of the gastrointestinal tract with a wide caliber, such as the gastric fundus or the right colon.

B. Areas of the gastrointestinal tract that are not accessible for palpation cannot be examined optimally. This generally refers to areas such as the gastric fundus, the colonic flexures, and the rectum. This problem also exists in any patient in whom effective compression cannot be applied, either because of obesity, anatomic abnormalities, or local tenderness.

C. In the colon, high quality mucosal relief films are not obtained reproducibly. The degree of evacuation is variable. In some patients the entire barium enema is evacuated, leaving no mucosal relief, while in others very little is evacuated, and again no mucosal relief is seen. Even when the mucosal relief is well seen in one part of the colon, it is usually not possible to map the state of the mucosa thoroughly throughout the entire colon. This may be of particular importance in the assessment of patients with inflammatory bowel disease and in the differentiation between ulcerative and granulomatous colitis.

D. This technique depends heavily on diagnostic fluoroscopy. It relies on the keenness of the fluroscopist's powers of observation to detect a lesion, and in many cases a diagnostic conclusion is based on fluoroscopic impression. This may pose no problem if the fluoroscopist is extremely skilled and experienced. However, there is no possibility in many cases for an intelligent second opinion, since the critical information may have been fluoroscopic. This poses a particular problem in departments in which many studies are performed by residents and trainees whose fluoroscopic skills are not fully developed.

Diagnostic Accuracy

Despite these theoretical deficiences, conventional barium studies were thought to be generally quite accurate until recent years. This is understandable, since evidence of radiologic error was usually found only at surgery or autopsy when advanced lesions missed by radiologic study may have been discovered. It would be a reasonable assumption that smaller lesions were missed in many patients who did not come to surgery or autopsy. The development of fiberoptic endoscopy in the last decade has provided a valuable new tool with which to evaluate the accuracy of our contrast studies in the gastrointestinal tract. Endoscopic experience has shown that the majority of small lesions and even a disturbing number of large lesions are missed by conventional barium studies.

UPPER GASTROINTESTINAL TRACT

Several endoscopic studies have assessed the accuracy of the conventional barium examination of the stomach and duodenum.[1-5] The results are summarized in Table 1–1. Radiologic errors were made in an average of 29 per cent of patients coming to endoscopy. In 22 per cent, the radiologic error was a false negative, in which a significant lesion was not detected. For the purpose of these statistics, mucosal inflammation and erosions were not included as significant lesions. In an additional 7 per cent of patients, a lesion diagnosed radiologically could not be confirmed by endoscopy. It is likely that in some of these cases the radiologic diagnosis was correct, and the lesion may have been overlooked at endoscopy. However, it is probable that in most cases the endoscopic diagnosis was accurate. In a review of 31 conventional barium studies in which radiologic errors were made, we found that the major causes of false neg-

TABLE 1–1 RADIOLOGIC ERROR RATES WITH CONVENTIONAL BARIUM STUDY*

Series	Number of Patients	False Negative (%)	False Positive (%)	Total (%)
Cotton[2]	518	27	6	35
Papp[3]	85	18	6	24
Dellipiani[4]	137	19	5	24
Barnes et al.[5]	50	14	4	18
Laufer et al.[1]	175	11	11	22
Total	965	22	7	29

*From: Laufer, I., Gastroenterology, 71:874, 1976. Reproduced by permission.

ative errors were failure to recognize an abnormality on the film and the small size of some of the lesions. Most false positive diagnoses were due to deformity or to prominent mucosal folds which were mistaken for or which simulated pathologic lesions.[1] It seemed to us that many of these errors could be avoided by using a technique that made gross pathology more obvious, allowed for detection of smaller lesions, and resulted in better gastric distension and effacement of normal mucosal folds.

COLON

Colonoscopy has had a dramatic effect on our approach to colonic polyps. A major fringe benefit of the development of colonoscopy has been the opportunity to assess the accuracy of radiologic examination of the colon, particularly with respect to polyp detection,[6] but also with respect to inflammatory bowel disease.[7] Several studies have indicated that 40 to 50 per cent of all colonic polyps are missed on the conventional barium enema.[8, 9] These results are particularly important because of the increasing evidence that many colonic carcinomas arise in benign polypoid tumors.[10-12]

Of course it is difficult to distinguish between errors due to imperfect performance or interpretation and errors due to inherent limitations of technique. Nevertheless, it seems safe to suggest that the conventional barium enema has definite limitations in the examination of segments not accessible to palpation, such as the rectum and the colonic flexures; in the differentiation of extraneous material from true pathologic findings; and in the detection of the early changes in inflammatory bowel disease, such as mucosal granularity in ulcerative colitis and aphthoid ulcers in Crohn's disease.[13-16]

DOUBLE CONTRAST STUDIES

The accumulation of evidence regarding the deficiencies of these conventional studies caused many radiologists to reconsider their gastrointestinal radiologic techniques. This search has led to renewed interest in the development of double contrast techniques, either for routine use or to supplement the standard examination. In response to this renewed interest, new barium suspensions and other accessories have been developed to make possible an efficient, high quality double contrast examination on a routine basis.[17-23] With increasing use of these techniques, many new and confusing radiologic appearances have been seen. In this respect, fiberoptic endoscopy has been an invaluable tool for clarifying the nature and significance of these findings and for sharpening interpretative skills.

Advantages

Double contrast diagnosis depends primarily on gaseous distension and mucosal coating with a thin layer of high density barium. In theory, many of the deficiencies associated with the conventional barium study can be overcome. (a) Increasing distension is obtained without increasing opacity and therefore without loss of surface detail. Thus the wide caliber portions of the gastrointestinal tract are easily examined. (b) The segments of the gastrointestinal tract that are inaccessible to palpation are easily examined. (c) Excellent mucosal detail is achieved routinely. (d) Diagnostic fluoroscopy is minimized. The emphasis is placed on a series of routine radiographs obtained in standard projections. Fluoroscopy is used primarily for determining the correct volume of contrast media and for positioning and timing spot films. Of course if an abnormality is noticed at fluoroscopy, additional views are taken. Further opinions can usually be obtained in the absence of fluoroscopic information.

Double contrast techniques have another advantage that has not been widely appreciated. They make it much easier to distinguish between true pathology and extraneous material. This distinction is made by the use of gravity and horizontal beam films. The extraneous material almost always flows to the dependent segment with barium, leaving the air-filled segments clean. Even on recumbent view double contrast radiographs it is possible to distinguish filling defects on the elevated wall from those on the dependent wall (Chapter 2). Thus any filling defect on the elevated wall is almost certainly a true polyp, since extraneous material would be expected only on the dependent wall. Because of these factors it has frequently been possible to find small polypoid lesions in the colon even in the presence of extensive fecal residue.

Because of the interest in surface detail the radiographic exposures in a double contrast study are considerably lighter and can be exposed at a lower kV than the single contrast study. Therefore, it is usually possible to obtain high quality spot films even when using equipment capable of very low mA and kV output. The exposures are shorter and there is less scatter because there is no need to penetrate the opaque barium column.

Historical Development

DOUBLE CONTRAST ENEMA

The principles of double contrast technique were first applied to the colon in 1923 by Fischer[24] in Germany and subsequently by Weber[25] at the Mayo Clinic. Major advances in the understanding, performance, and interpretation of these studies were contributed by Welin in Malmö, Sweden, where over 70,000 such examinations have been performed.[26-30] Despite its high polyp detection rate and exquisite demonstration of minute mucosal abnormalities in neoplastic and inflammatory disease, the technique did not become popular in North America. It is likely that many radiologists tried this technique but could not reproduce the results obtained by Welin. This is probably the result of failure to obtain the same degree of colonic cleansing and failure to appreciate the need for specific types of barium suspensions, different diagnostic maneuvers, and variations in the appearance of various pathologic lesions on the double contrast films.

In the 1960's the message of the double contrast enema was taken up by Miller, who was largely responsible for the development of new apparatus, barium suspensions, and accessories.[17, 31] These developments have made it possible to perform efficiently double contrast studies of high quality. There has therefore been a renewed interest in this technique. A recent survey by Thoeni and Margulis showed that over the last decade there has been a 50 per cent increase in the utilization of the double contrast enema, although only a small minority of radiographic examinations of the colon are performed in this way.[32, 33] In particular, the double contrast enema is rarely utilized for the evaluation of patients with inflammatory bowel disease, although the method is particularly valuable in those patients.

UPPER GASTROINTESTINAL TRACT

The potential value of the double contrast technique as an alternative to the palpation method was recognized by Hampton in 1937.[34] Utilizing swallowed air and a barium suspension of creamy consistency, he showed examples of duodenal ulcers and a prepyloric carcinoma. Schatzki described the importance of en face views with air contrast for diagnosis of gastric ulcers.[35] In 1952 Ruzicka and Rigler[36] described a method for double contrast examination of the stomach. Their examination required nasogastric intubation. The quality of the coating was not excellent because of the barium suspensions available at that time.

In about 1950 a group of gastroenterologists in Japan, under the leadership of Professor Hikoo Shirakabe, were studying the pathologic morphology of intestinal tuberculosis, utilizing double contrast examination of the colon. This study led them to develop a double contrast technique for the examination of the stomach.[37] Their initial interest was in the demonstration of gastric ulcers, particularly linear ulcers that had not been demonstrated on conventional studies. This experience led them to further refinements of the technique for the radiologic diagnosis of early gastric cancer.[38] This type of examination became standard in Japan during the 1960's, and spectacular results have been achieved in both mass screening programs and the evaluation of symptomatic patients. Such patients have had a 5-year survival of 90 per cent or more.[39]

The Japanese work seemed to attract little interest in the West because of its emphasis on early gastric cancer, a disease with a much lower and declining incidence in the West. In the late 1960's and early 1970's several short papers appeared describing modifications of the Japanese technique.[18, 40, 41] The quality of mucosal coating in these early radiographs was suboptimal because of the poor effervescent agents available and the relatively poor coating produced by the barium suspensions at that time. In the early 1970's more attention was directed to technical details of the examination and in particular to the quality of the barium preparations. This led to the development of new barium suspensions which were specifically designed to produce high quality double contrast examinations of the stomach.[22] Several papers then reported that subtle pathologic lesions which had not been seen before were now being diagnosed. These included superficial gastric erosions,[42, 43] linear ulcers,[44, 45] and ulcer scars.[45, 46] Recently a report by Quizlbash and coworkers[47] suggested that an increased frequency of early gastric cancer in their hospital could be attributed at least in part to the institution of double contrast examination of the stomach.

Diagnostic Accuracy

COLON

It has been shown in several studies that the double contrast enema can be highly accurate for the detection of polypoid lesions greater than 5 mm in diameter. Ninety per cent or more of such polyps are detected on high quality double contrast enema examinations.[6, 9, 48] This type of study has also been shown to be accurate in reflecting the visual mucosal abnormalities in patients with inflammatory bowel disease.[14, 49-51]

UPPER GASTROINTESTINAL TRACT

Several studies have now compared the radiologic diagnoses utilizing double contrast technique with endoscopic findings. In these series the double contrast method has been found to be more than 90 per cent accurate.[45, 52, 53] Furthermore, we found that radiologic errors were generally predictable, in that they were usually confined to those studies that were considered to be unreliable by the examiner. The increased accuracy of these radiologic techniques has had its impact on the practice of gastrointestinal endoscopy. With increasing confidence in the radiologic diagnosis the endoscopic examination can be reserved for those patients in whom the results of radiologic study either are equivocal or demonstrate a lesion requiring confirmation or histologic diagnosis.

Drawbacks

Despite the advantages of increased resolution with double contrast studies, there are a number of significant drawbacks. For the practicing radiologist the method represents a commitment of time and energy to learn new techniques. It requires a revised concept of the relative roles of fluoroscopy and radiography in gastrointestinal diagnosis. It also requires a reorientation to interpretation of the films, since there is much more emphasis on the en face appearance of lesions than on their appearance in profile. The old familiar pathology may have different appearances, and the examiner must retrain himself to look for the more subtle lesions that are diagnosable by these techniques.

It is likely that the double contrast examinations are slightly more time-consuming than the conventional barium studies. This is particularly true during the early stages when the examiner is becoming familiar with these techniques. However, if one considers the increased yield and the fewer number of repeat examinations, we believe that the extra time is more than justified.

The technical quality of a double contrast study is highly dependent on the materials used and in particular on the quality of the barium suspension. Thus the radiologist must constantly monitor the quality of barium preparations and must be willing to try new products that might improve the quality of the study.

A high quality double contrast study can provide aesthetic pleasure approaching that of a work of art. However, a poor study, whether the fault of the examiner or the patient or both, may be not only useless but misleading.[54] It is probably true that a poor quality double contrast examination is more dangerous than a poor quality single contrast examination. Therefore, the utilization of double contrast techniques requires a commitment to the development of technical excellence.

CONCLUSION

We feel certain that the radiologist who spends the time and effort to master these techniques will be rewarded by gastrointestinal studies of increased diagnostic value and in many cases of great aesthetic quality. Our experience suggests that this combination stimulates interest in gastrointestinal radiology not only for the radiologist but also for students, technologists, and referring physicians. This can only result in greater diagnostic accuracy and an enhanced appreciation of the role of radiology in the diagnosis of gastrointestinal disorders.

REFERENCES

1. Laufer, I. Mullens, J. E., and Hamilton, J.: The diagnostic accuracy of barium studies of the stomach and duodenum—correlation with endoscopy. Radiology, *115*:569, 1975.
2. Cotton, P. B.: Fiberoptic endoscopy and the barium meal—results and implications. Br. Med. J. 2:161, 1973.
3. Papp, J. P.: Endoscopic experience in 100 consecutive cases with the Olympus GIF endoscope. Am. J. Gastroenterol., *60*:466, 1973
4. Dellipiani, A. W.: Experience with duodenofiberscopes. Scott. Med. J., *19*:7, 1974.
5. Barnes, R. J., Gear, M. W. L., and Nicol, A.: Study of dyspepsia in a general practice as assessed by endoscopy and radiology. Br. Med. J , *4*:214, 1974.
6. Williams, C. B., Hunt. R. D., and Loose, H.: Colonoscopy in the management of colon polyps. Br. J. Surg., *61*:673, 1974.
7. Colcher, H., and Nugent, F. W.: Endoscopy in inflammatory bowel disease. Gastroenterology, *69*:567, 1975
8. Wolff, W. I., Shinya, H., Geffen, A., et al.: Comparison of colonoscopy and the contrast enema in five hundred patients with colo-rectal disease. Am. J. Surg., *129*:181, 1975.
9. Thoeni, J. F., and Menuck. L.: Comparison of barium enema and colonoscopy in the detection of small colonic polyps. Radiology, *124*:631, 1977.
10. Morson, B. C.: The polyp-cancer sequence in the large bowel. Proc. R. Soc. Med., *67*:451, 1974.
11. Lane, N., Fenoglio, C. M.: The adenoma-carcinoma sequence in the stomach and colon. 1. Observations on the adenoma as precursor to ordinary large bowel carcinoma. Gastrointest. Radiol., *1*:111, 1976.
12. Wayne, J. D.: The development of carcinoma of the colon. Am. J. Gastroenterol., *67*:427, 1977.
13. Laufer, I., Hamilton, J.: The radiological differentiation between ulcerative and granulomatous colitis by double contrast radiology. Am. J. Gastroenterol., *66*:259, 1976.
14. Laufer, I., Mullens, J. E., and Hamilton, J.: Correlation of endoscopy and double-contrast radiography in the early stages of ulcerative and granulomatous colitis. Radiology, *118*:1, 1976.
15. Laufer, I.: Air contrast studies of the colon in inflammatory bowel disease. CRC Crit. Rev. Diagnost. Imaging, *9*:421, 1977.
16. Laufer, I., and Costopoulos, L.: Early lesions of Crohn's disease. Am. J. Roentgenol., *130*:307, 1978.
17. Miller, R. E.: Barium enema examination with large bore tubing and drainage. Radiology, *82*:905, 1964.
18. Gelfand D. W., and Hachiya, J.: The double contrast examination of the stomach using gas-producing granules and tablets. Radiology, *93*:1381, 1969.
19. Pochaczevski, R.: Bubbly barium: A carbonated cocktail for double contrast examinations of the stomach. Radiology, *107*:461, 1973.
20. Miller, R. E., Chernish, S. M., Skucas, J., et al.: Hypotonic roentgenography with glucagon. Am. J. Roentgenol., *121*:264. 1974
21. Laufer, I.: A simple method for routine double-contrast study of the upper gastrointestinal tract Radiology, *117*:513, 1975.

22. Gelfand D. W.: High density, low viscosity barium for fine mucosal detail on double-contrast upper gastrointestinal examinations. Am. J. Roentgenol., *130*:831, 1978.

23. Hisamichi, S., Masuda, Y., Shirane, A., et al.: Barium enema examination using a remote controlled positive and negative contrast media inflator. Radiology, *125*:533, 1977.

24. Fischer, A. W.: Über eine neue röntgenologische Untersuchungsmethode des Dickdarms: Kombination von Kontrasteinlauf and Luftaufblähung. Klin. Wochenschr., 2:1595, 1923.

25. Weber, H. M.: Roentgenologic demonstration of polypoid lesions and polyposis of large intestine. Am. J. Roentgenol., *25*:577, 1931.

26. Welin, S.: Modern trends in diagnostic roentgenology of colon. Br. J. Radiol., *31*:453, 1958.

27. Welin, S.: Advances in roentgen diagnosis of ulcerative colitis. Acta Chir. Scand., *125*:482, 1963.

28. Welin, S.: Results of the Malmö technique of colon examination. JAMA, *199*:369, 1967.

29. Welin, S., and Brahme, F.: The double contrast method in ulcerative colitis. Acta Radiol., *55*:257, 1961.

30. Welin, S., and Welin, G.: The Double Contrast Examination of the Colon. Experiences with the Welin Modification. Stuttgart, Georg Thieme Verlag, 1976.

31. Miller, R. E.: Examination of the colon. Curr. Probl. Radiol., *5*(2):3, 1975.

32. Margulis, A. R., and Goldberg, H. I.: The current state of radiologic technique in the examination of the colon: a survey. Radiol. Clin. North Am., 7:27, 1969.

33. Thoeni, R. F., and Margulis, A. R.: The state of radiographic technique in the examination of the colon: A survey. Radiology, *127*:317, 1978.

34. Hampton, A. O.: A safe method for the roentgen demonstration of bleeding duodenal ulcers. Am. J. Roentgenol., *38*:565 1937.

35. Schatzki, R., and Gary, J. E.: Face-on demonstration of ulcers in the upper stomach in a dependent position. Am. J. Roentgenol., *79*:722, 1958.

36. Ruzicka, F. F., and Rigler, L. G.: Inflation of the stomach with double contrast: roentgen study. JAMA, *145*:696, 1951.

37. Shirakabe, H.: Double Contrast Studies of the Stomach. Stuttgart, Georg Thieme Verlag, 1972.

38. Shirakabe, H., Ichikawa, H., Kumakura, K., et al.: Atlas of X-Ray Diagnosis of Early Gastric Cancer. Philadelphia, J. B. Lippincott 1966.

39. Yamada, E., Nagazato, H., Koite, A., et al.: Surgical results of early gastric cancer. Int. Surg., *59*:7, 1974.

40. Obata, W. G.: A double-contrast technique for examination of the stomach using barium sulfate with simethicone. Am. J. Roentgenol., *115*:275, 1972.

41. Scott-Harden, W. G.: Radiological investigation of peptic ulcer. Br. J. Hosp. Med., *10*:149, 1973.

42. Laufer, I., Hamilton, J., and Mullens, J. E.: Demonstration of superficial gastric erosions by double contrast radiology. Gastroenterology, *68*:387, 1975.

43. Poplack, W., Paul, R. E., Goldsmith, M., et al.: Demonstration of erosive gastritis by the double contrast technique. Radiology, *117*:519, 1975.

44. Poplack, W., Paul, R. E., Goldsmith, M., et al.: Linear and rod-shaped peptic ulcers. Radiology, *122*:317, 1977.

45. Laufer, I.: Assessment of the accuracy of double contrast gastroduodenal radiology. Gastroenterology, *71*:874 1976.

46. Gelfand, D. W.: The Japanese-style double contrast examination of the stomach. Gastrointest. Radiol., *1*:7, 1976.

47. Quizlbash, A., Harnorine, C., and Castelli, M.: Early gastric carcinoma: Value of combined use of endoscopy, air contrast x-ray films, cytology and multiple biopsy specimens, Arch. Pathol., *101*:610, 1977.

48. Laufer, I., Smith, N. C. W., and Mullens, J. E.: The radiological demonstration of colorectal polyps undetected by endoscopy. Gastroenterology, *70*:167, 1976.

49. Simpkins, K. C., and Stevenson, G. W.: The modified Malmö double-contrast enema in colitis: an assessment of its accuracy in reflecting sigmoidoscopic findings. Br. J. Radiol., *45*:486, 1972

50. Kinsey, I., Hornnes, N., and Anthonisen, P.: The radiological diagnosis of nonspecific hemorrhagic proctocolitis (hemorrhagic proctitis and ulcerative colitis). Acta Med. Scand., *176*:181, 1964.

51. Fraser, G. M., and Findlay, J. M.: The double contrast enema in ulcerative and Crohn's colitis. Clin. Radiol., *27*:103, 1976.

52. Moule, E. B., Cochrane, K. M., Sokhi, G. S., et al.: A comparative study of the diagnostic value of upper gastrointestinal endoscopy and radiology. Gut, *16*:411, 1975

53. Herlinger, H., Glanville, J. N., and Kreel, L.: An evaluation of the double contrast barium meal (DCBM) against endoscopy. Clin. Radiol., *28*:307, 1977.

54. Hartzell, H. V.: To err with air. JAMA. *187*:455, 1964.

2

PRINCIPLES OF DOUBLE CONTRAST DIAGNOSIS

HERBERT Y. KRESSEL, M.D.,
and IGOR LAUFER, M.D.

INTRODUCTION

Successful application of double contrast techniques in gastrointestinal radiology requires the development of skill both in the performance and in the interpretation of these studies. The transition from single contrast to double contrast radiology requires more than a minor adjustment in technique. Indeed, the double contrast approach requires a major reorientation to the performance and interpretation of gastrointestinal studies.

11

The purpose of this chapter is to outline the general principles in the performance and interpretation of these examinations. When properly performed, they make it possible to provide a precise translation from the radiographic abnormalities to the gross pathology, and in many cases to the microscopic pathology. Examples and illustrations will be drawn from the entire gastrointestinal tract to stress the general applicability of these principles. Their specific applications will be discussed in detail in the appropriate chapters. We would also like to stress the causes of potential error in the use of these techniques and to suggest some approaches whereby some of these errors can be avoided.

DIFFERENCES BETWEEN SINGLE AND DOUBLE CONTRAST STUDIES

In order to understand the double contrast approach to gastrointestinal radiology, it is important to clarify the basic differences between single and double contrast studies. The single contrast study concentrates on examination of the contour and lumen of the gastrointestinal tract.[1] Its most important component is the fluoroscopic study whereby the volume of barium is monitored, graded compression is applied, and in most cases a diagnostic impression is reached. The purpose of multiple radiographs is to provide complementary views of the same lesion or the same surface. In general one expects to see a lesion on all or most radiographs that incorporate the area in question. We are generally content to identify an abnormality and suggest its pathologic nature. We are usually not interested in precise three-dimensional reconstruction or localization, and in particular we are rarely concerned with differentiation between the dependent and the nondependent surfaces.

By comparison, the double contrast examination is concerned primarily with delineation of mucosal detail, and secondarily with abnormalities of the contour and lumen. Fluoroscopy is utilized primarily for monitoring of the volume of contrast materials and for accurate localization and timing of spot films. Diagnostic fluoroscopy is minimized. The mainstay of diagnosis is careful examination of multiple radiographs. The multiple radiographs taken in different projections are additive rather than complementary, since each film presents a certain proportion of the mucosal surface for diagnostic evaluation while the remainder of the mucosal surface is obscured by the high density barium. Thus the total examination requires the interpolation and integration of the information obtained from the multiple radiographs.[2] It is not surprising that some lesions may be visible on only one or two of a dozen or more films.

The adequacy of this type of study is judged by the en face appearance of the mucosal surface and not by the visibility of the contour of the bowel. Similarly, diagnostic interpretation is based largely on an analysis of the en face appearance of the mucosal surface. Accurate interpretation of these radiographic findings depends on a clear understanding of the differing appearances of structures and lesions on the dependent and nondependent surfaces. This understanding allows for an accurate translation from radiographic abnormalities to pathologic condition. It also allows for an appreciation of the limitations of each radiograph and suggests maneuvers for demonstrating suspected lesions in great detail.

Finally, these new techniques present a variety of artifactual appearances.[3] These will be illustrated in specific chapters in conjunction with the types of pathology they may simulate.

COMPONENTS OF THE DOUBLE CONTRAST EXAMINATION

Patient Preparation

Adequate cleansing of the mucosal surface throughout the gastrointestinal tract is of obvious importance, so that the barium coating will provide an accurate reflection of the mucosal surface. Residual debris will obscure the mucosal surface, and residual fluid results in dilution of the barium suspension, producing poor mucosal coating as well as artifacts because of patchy coating (Fig. 2–1).

Mucosal Coating

HIGH DENSITY BARIUM

Relatively little is known about the ingredients and additives in the various commercial barium suspensions.[4, 5] In particular, the physical and chemical properties that produce good mucosal coating are unknown. One would expect that the ideal barium suspension for double contrast studies would have low viscosity and high density. However, there are other important factors, such as the resistance of a suspension to acid, mucin, or alkali. Because of these many factors, there is no single barium suspension that produces good results throughout the gastrointestinal tract. As a result, in our barium kitchen we have a "menu" from which we choose a barium suspension best suited for the examination being performed. In general terms, the upper gastrointestinal study requires a high density (200% W/V), low viscosity barium suspension, whereas the colon examination gives best results with an intermediate density (85% W/V), higher viscosity suspension. The requirements for the small bowel examination are still different (Chapter 11).

The important point is that barium cannot be considered a homogeneous product with differences only in concentration, flavoring, and coloring. There are variations in viscosity, as well as other differences related to the addition of unspecified ingredients, that may affect the quality of mucosal coating. Therefore, the radiologist interested in performing double contrast examinations must be familiar with the properties of these suspensions and must be able to choose a product appropriate to the specific study being performed.

DISTENSION

Gaseous distension is produced by different means throughout the gastrointestinal tract. The common goal is to separate the surfaces of the viscus and to efface the mucosal folds. In some areas, such as the gastric fundus, this is difficult to achieve, but at a minimum the mucosal folds should be straightened.

The degree of gaseous distension affects the quality of mucosal coating, since increasing distension requires increasing volumes of barium to adequately wash and coat the mucosal surfaces. Inadequate distension will cause lesions to be hidden among the mucosal folds (Fig. 2–2). However, it should also be appreciated that overdistension can mask certain lesions, particularly if there is a prominent submucosal component (Fig. 2–3). Therefore, the ideal double contrast examination would be performed with three varying degrees of distension (Chapter 7). This is difficult to achieve in the routine examination. However, in the detailed evaluation of a suspected abnormality, varying the degree of distension can be very informative.

Bubble formation may be one of the undesirable side effects of gaseous distension. In an effort to counteract this problem, simethicone has been added to the barium suspensions designed for double contrast studies as well as to most of the effervescent agents. Occasionally, however, additional simethicone may be needed if bubbling is excessive.

MANEUVERS

For each examination a set of maneuvers is required to wash the barium bolus across the mucosal surface. The purpose is to remove mucus and debris from the mucosal surface and to achieve good mucosal coating. The more frequent the washing, the better the mucosal coating. The maneuvers should also be designed to avoid loss of contrast material and to avoid overlapping loops of bowel until spot films of any given segment have been obtained. If there are overlapping loops, additional spot films in different obliquities are required (Fig. 2–4). The procedure must be executed quickly to prevent both overlap and deterioration in the quality of coating.

CRITERIA OF GOOD MUCOSAL COATING

When there is good mucosal coating, the mucosal surface has a uniform grayness which fades at the edge to blend with the continuous smooth white line at the periphery, representing the profile view of the mucosa. The coating must be continuous, with no artifacts resulting from patchy coating. In the stomach, demonstration of the areae gastricae serves as an additional criterion of good coating (Fig. 2–5).[6] A similar surface pattern, the innominate grooves, may be seen in the colon (Fig. 2–6),[7] but with much less frequency.

Poor mucosal coating can be recognized by a lack of grayness to the en face appearance of the mucosa, with contrast provided only by the gas. The profile view of the mucosa may show thin, irregular, or interrupted coating (Fig. 2–1). This type of coating may be the result of incorrect choice of barium, or of improper preparation of the barium suspension, or of fluid, acid, or mucin within the bowel. In the colon such poor coating, with flaking of the barium suspension, may be seen on postevacuation films.

In the presence of poor or patchy coating, lesions are easily missed (Fig. 2–7A).[8] Therefore, in such cases the barium bolus must be washed across the area of poor coating until adequate coating is achieved (Fig. 2–7B).

Text continued on page 20

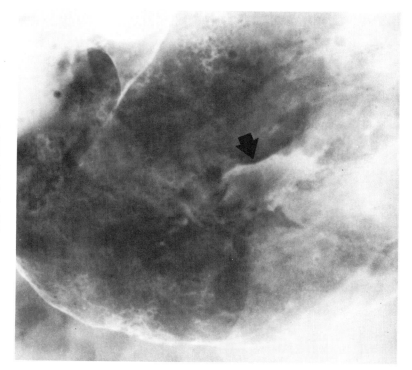

FIGURE 2–1 Patchy coating simulating an ulcer. There is poor coating owing to fluid and debris within the stomach. This has resulted in an irregular collection on the posterior wall which resembles an ulcer (*arrow*). A repeat study with good mucosal coating showed no abnormality.

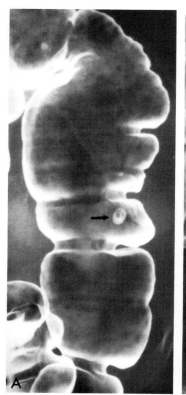

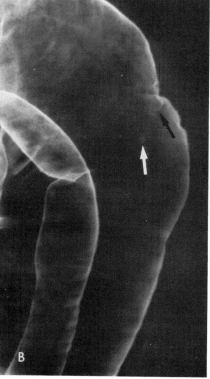

FIGURE 2–2 The value of varying degrees of distension.

A. With moderate distension the small diverticulum in the descending colon is clearly seen (*arrow*). The adjacent polyp is seen only with difficulty.

B. With further distension the polypoid lesion is seen more clearly (*black arrow*), while the diverticulum is faintly seen (*white arrow*).

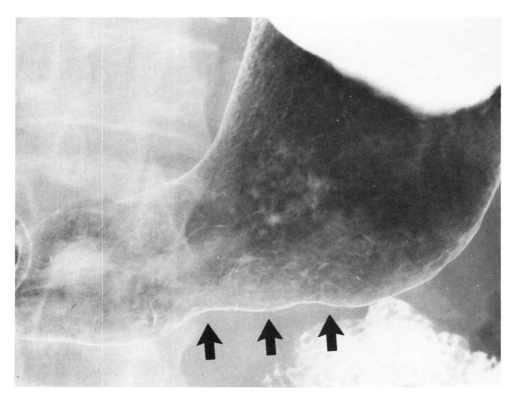

A. With considerable gastric distension there is only a suggestion of nondistensibility along the greater curvature (*arrows*). In addition, a few faint white lines are seen in the proximal portion of the antrum, but these are very difficult to evaluate and their significance is uncertain.

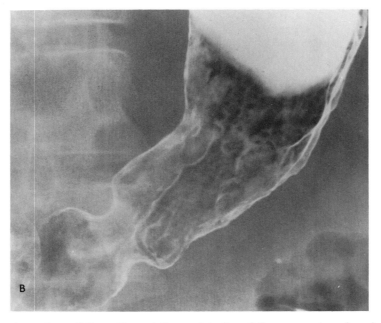

B. With the stomach partially collapsed the nodularity of the mucosal surface is seen much more clearly. These findings were the result of a scirrhous adenocarcinoma of the stomach.

FIGURE 2–3 Risks of overdistension.

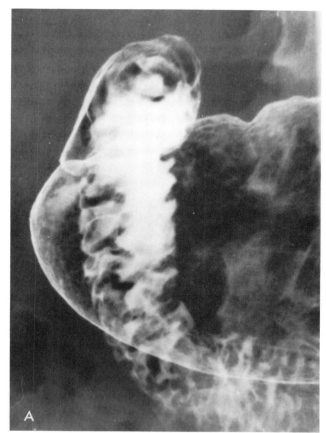

FIGURE 2–4 The importance of projection.

A. In the supine projection the duodenum overlaps the distal antrum and pylorus.

B. In the left posterior oblique projection this area is clearly seen, and the small lesser curvature ulcer is identified (*arrow*).

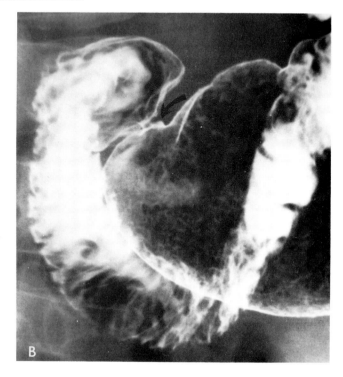

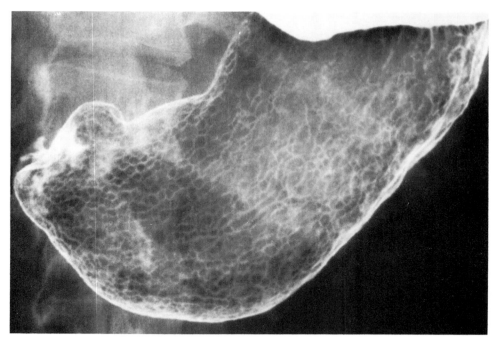

FIGURE 2–5 The areae gastricae. The fine reticular appearance of the normal surface pattern of the stomach is seen throughout the antrum and body.

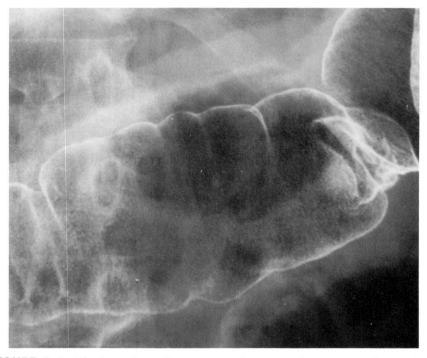

FIGURE 2–6 The innominate lines representing the surface pattern of the colon.

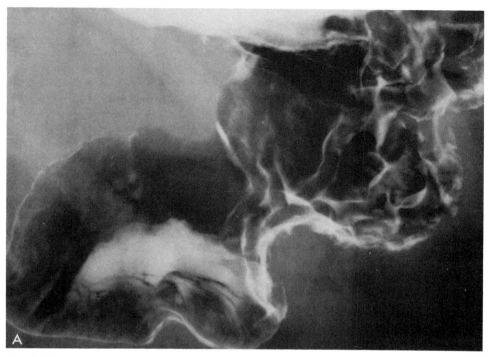

A. With poor mucosal coating no definite abnormality can be identified in the stomach.

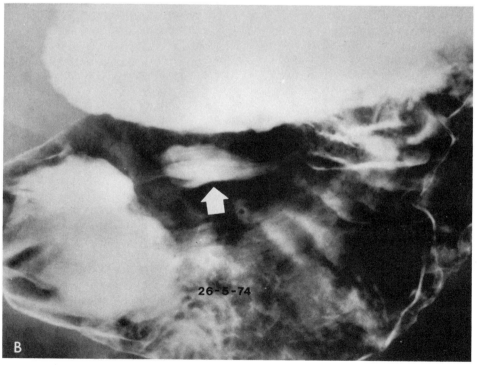

B. With improved coating a large ulcer on the posterior wall near the lesser curvature is clearly identified (*arrows*). See also Plate 24. (*From:* Laufer, I.: Radiology, 117:513, 1975.[8] Reproduced by permission.)

FIGURE 2–7 The hazards of poor mucosal coating.

Compression

The compression study is not as critical in the double contrast study as it is in the single contrast. Nevertheless, in some cases a lesion may be seen only on the compression spot films, while in others it may be appreciated and defined more easily on the compression radiograph. This is particularly true for polypoid lesions (Fig. 2–11). Therefore, it must be emphasized that compression spot films are a routine and indispensable component of the complete double contrast examination.

Relaxant Drugs

There is no doubt that the use of relaxant drugs results in a higher quality double contrast examination. In the examination of the colon it has the additional advantage of decreasing patient discomfort.[9, 10] However, the use of an injectable drug presents a slight nuisance and delay in the examination as well as a small increase in cost. With the use of glucagon there are virtually no side effects except for the remote possibility of a hypersensitivity reaction. However, glucagon in the upper gastrointestinal tract may delay filling of the duodenum, which may prolong the examination. It must be appreciated that the various organs differ in their sensitivity to glucagon. The upper gastrointestinal tract is very sensitive to glucagon in doses as low as 0.05 mg, whereas in the colon we believe that a dose of at least 1 mg is required to be effective.

At the present time we tend to use intravenous glucagon 0.10 mg routinely for our upper gastrointestinal studies. We do not use a relaxant drug for the double contrast enema unless we encounter severe patient discomfort, spasm, or persistent stricture. Occasionally we require a relaxant drug for the examination of the esophagus. For this purpose we use Pro-Banthine 15 to 30 mg intravenously, since glucagon is ineffective in abolishing esophageal peristalsis.[11]

Radiographic Technique

Attention to radiographic technical details is of utmost importance, since surface detail can easily be obscured by faulty technique. Theoretically, the smaller the focal spot size, the better the resolution on the films. However, in practice we have been able to obtain more than satisfactory studies with focal spot sizes as large as 1.2 and 2.0 mm provided that the exposure is short enough. The mA should be set as high as possible to obtain the shortest possible exposure. We have been able to obtain satisfactory studies of most patients with equipment capable of providing only 200 mA. The short exposure time is particularly important in the examination of the upper gastrointestinal tract where motion is more prominent.

For the demonstration of surface detail a low kV would be desirable. However, this lengthens the exposure and may result in a film that shows too much contrast, such that a small area of the film is well exposed while the rest is poorly exposed. The exposure is particularly sensitive to the position of the phototimer cell. We have used approximately 105 kV for our films to shorten the exposure and to provide greater latitude. With the shorter exposure times possible with the rare earth screens, it should be possible to use a lower kV.

Endoscopic and Pathologic Correlation

With the use of double contrast techniques many unfamiliar appearances will be encountered. There is not yet a large body of literature to help the radiologist in such cases. We have relied heavily on endoscopic and pathologic correlation for clarification of the nature and significance of new radiologic findings.[12-14] It is important for the radiologist to actually see the specimen or to look through the endoscope to appreciate the mucosal surface, rather than to rely on a written report. By recognizing the normal appearances and their variations throughout the gastrointestinal tract as well as the gross pathologic appearances of various types of surface abnormalities he will come to appreciate the limitations and confidence limits of endoscopic and pathologic diagnosis. With the development of technical and interpretative skills, the radiologist can help the endoscopist and pathologist to appreciate more subtle anatomic and pathologic details.

We consider constant endoscopic and pathologic correlation an indispensable tool in the development of technical and interpretative skills in gastrointestinal radiology. For this reason we have included a chapter devoted to the correlation of double contrast radiographs with endoscopic or pathologic photographs (Chapter 10).

ESSENTIALS OF INTERPRETATION

Elements of the Double Contrast Image

In general terms, there are three elements contributing to each double contrast image. These are the dependent surface, the nondependent surface, and the barium pool (Fig. 2–8). The specific surface that is in the dependent or nondependent position is determined by the position of the patient. The barium pool will be found in the most dependent segment.

The dependent surface is lined by a layer of barium. The radiographic sequence is generally such that as much barium as possible is removed from this surface before the radiograph is exposed. However, in some cases there may be a small puddle of barium on the dependent surface, particularly if the surface has any undulations. The nondependent surface has a thinner coating of barium, and there is no barium pool or puddle since any free barium would tend to fall off. The barium pool is discussed in detail later in this chapter.

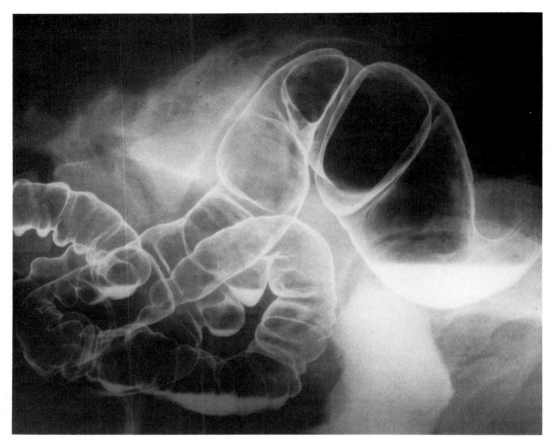

FIGURE 2–8 Components of the double contrast image. Cross-table lateral view of the rectum and sigmoid with the patient prone. Dependent and nondependent surfaces can be identified. There are barium pools in the distal rectum and sigmoid in addition to smaller barium puddles throughout the sigmoid colon.

Anterior Versus Posterior Wall Structures

Because of the differences in barium coating of the dependent and nondependent surfaces, anatomic structures on the anterior and posterior walls have somewhat differing appearances. These differences are illustrated in Figures 2–9 and 2–10. For purposes of this discussion we will assume that the patient is in the supine position, and therefore the posterior surface is dependent and the anterior surface is nondependent. A rugal fold on the posterior wall of the stomach appears as a radiolucent defect in the barium puddle on the posterior wall. However, a rugal fold on the anterior wall appears as two thin white lines, as the x-ray beam is attenuated by barium coating on the side of the fold. There is obviously no barium pool or puddle on the anterior surface. Thus the anterior wall fold is "etched in white." On the supine radiograph in Figure 2–10 it is possible to distinguish between posterior wall and anterior wall folds. Similar reasoning applies to all protrusions, whether they are normal folds or polypoid lesions. On the dependent surface they appear as a radiolucent filling defect, whereas on the nondependent surface the margin of the lesion is "etched in white" (Fig. 2–11).

With these high density barium suspensions, drops of barium are frequently seen hanging from protrusions on the nondependent surface (Fig. 2–12A). This has been termed the "stalactite phenomenon" by Op den Orth.[15] An appreciation of the differences between dependent and nondependent wall structures makes it easy to recognize these stalactites and to differentiate them from ulcers. They are always seen in relation to a protrusion on the nondependent surface (Fig. 2–12B), and therefore they could not possibly represent ulcers. Furthermore, the presence of the stalactite indicates that there is a protrusion on the nondependent surface. This may be either a normal fold or a polypoid lesion.

Text continued on page 27

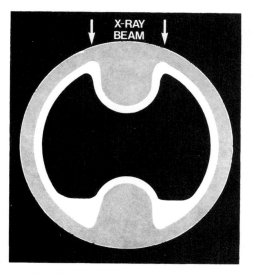
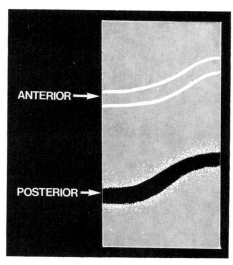

FIGURE 2–9 *A* and *B*   Diagrammatic representation of the appearances of a rugal fold on the anterior and posterior wall of the stomach.

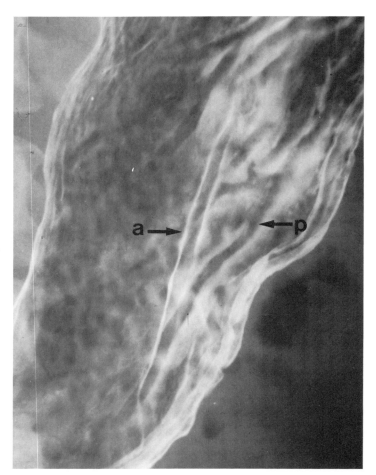

FIGURE 2–10   Supine view double contrast radiograph, showing the distinction between anterior (*a*) and posterior (*p*) wall rugal folds.

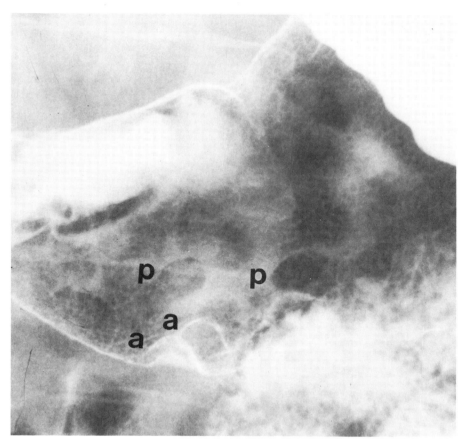

A. On the supine view double contrast radiograph the anterior wall polyps (*a*) are etched in white, while the posterior wall polyps (*p*) are seen as radiolucent filling defects.

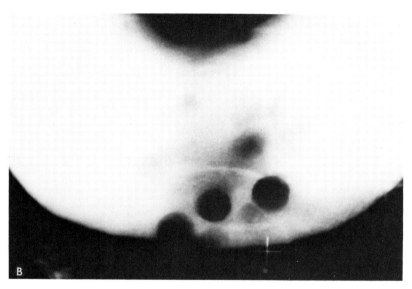

B. The compression study shows the polyps to good advantage, but it is not possible to distinguish between the anterior and posterior wall lesions.

FIGURE 2–11 Anterior and posterior wall polyps.

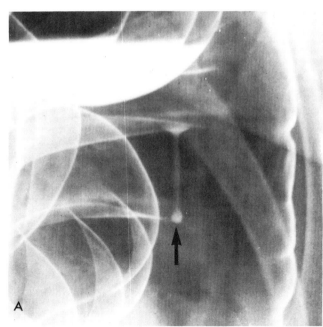

FIGURE 2–12 The stalactite phenomenon.

A. A film of the colon in the upright position shows a long droplet of barium hanging from a haustral fold.

B. Sigmoid polyp with a stalactite. There is a polypoid lesion in the sigmoid colon. The lesion is etched in white and is therefore on the nondependent surface. The central density represents a hanging droplet or stalactite.

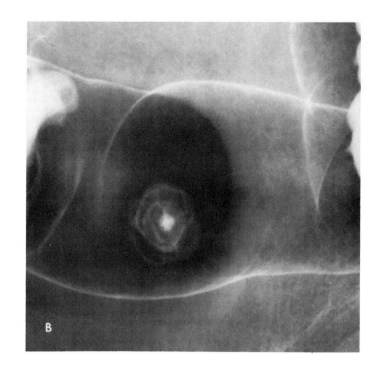

Basic Roentgen Pathology

Two basic types of pathologic processes are encountered in the gastrointestinal tract. These are protruded lesions, such as polyps, inflammatory swellings, or malignant tumors, and depressed lesions, such as ulcers and diverticula. The basic roentgen manifestations of these types of lesions are similar throughout the gastrointestinal tract.

PROTRUDED LESIONS

The basic appearance of a polypoid lesion on the anterior or posterior wall has been described earlier. A polyp on the dependent surface appears as a radiolucent filling defect, whereas a polyp on the nondependent surface is "etched in white" (Fig. 2–11) and may produce a ring shadow (Figs. 2–13B and 2–21A). Several additional features of polypoid lesions are frequently seen. The "bowler hat sign" indicates that the filling defect forms an acute angle with the bowel wall.[16] This sign is illustrated and explained diagrammatically in Figure 2–13. It consists basically of a ring, representing the barium in the angle between the polyp and the bowel wall, and a curvilinear density, representing the dome of the polyp. When the two densities are caught at a particular oblique angle, the bowler hat sign is produced. At other angles differing appearances are produced, and when seen en face, only a single ring shadow is visible (Fig. 2–13).

The demonstration that a filling defect has a stalk is also conclusive proof that it is a true polypoid lesion. The stalk may be seen in profile, but it may also be seen end-on through the head of the polyp, producing the "Mexican hat sign" (Fig. 2–14).[16] These two signs are helpful in the distinction between true polyps and extraneous material. In addition, if a protruding lesion can be demonstrated to be on the nondependent surface either because it is etched in white or because it is associated with a stalactite, it almost certainly represents a true polypoid lesion, since extraneous material would usually be expected only on the dependent surface. However, in some cases fecal residue may be adherent to the nondependent surface and cannot be differentiated from a true polyp.

The appearance of a protrusion is determined not only by its location but also by its shape, and in particular by the configuration of its margins. Figure 2–15 illustrates diagrammatically various types of polypoid lesions. It can be seen that if a polypoid lesion on the anterior wall has gradually sloping margins, it probably will not be seen on the supine radiograph because there is no abrupt edge to be seen tangentially. A similar lesion on the dependent wall may be visualized, but may seem smaller than it actually is because the peripheral portion of the lesion may be obscured by the dense barium. A plaque-like lesion may be very difficult to detect on the nondependent surface if its elevation is very slight. In addition, if the edge is tapered (Fig. 2–16A and B) or if one of the edges is on a curved surface, that edge may not be seen and the entire plaque-like lesion may be manifest only as a single line (Fig. 2–16C and D).

Annular lesions can be recognized as contour defects on double contrast studies, just as on the single contrast examination. In addition, they can be recognized end-on when seen through overlapping loops of bowel (Fig. 2–17). The irregularity and nodularity of the lumen are clearly apparent and can be confirmed by the appropriate oblique projection.

Text continued on page 33

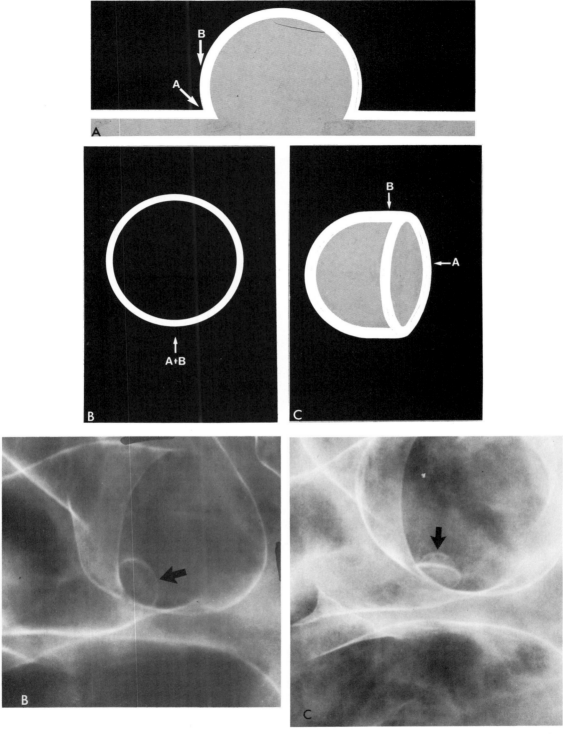

FIGURE 2–13 The bowler hat sign.

A. Diagrammatic representation of the bowler hat sign.
B. With the dome of the polyp and its base overlapping, a ring shadow is produced.
C. A typical bowler hat sign resulting from a sigmoid polyp.

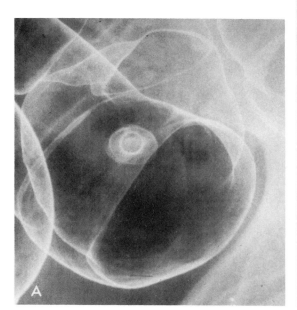
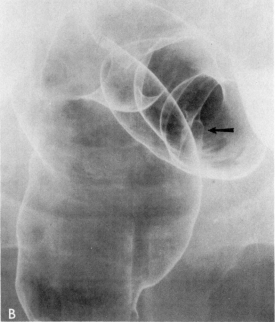

FIGURE 2-14 The Mexican hat sign.

A. With the patient supine, the pedunuclated polyp is seen hanging from the anterior wall. The central ring represents the stalk seen end-on, while the outer ring represents the head of the polyp.

B. With the patient in the upright position, the polyp and its stalk are clearly seen (*arrow*).

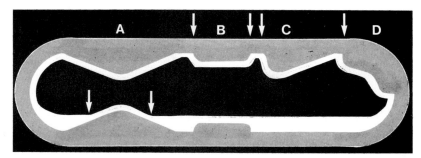

FIGURE 2-15 Diagrammatic representation of the effect of the shape of the polyp on its roentgen appearance.

A. A polypoid lesion with sloping edges on the nondependent surface will probably not be seen on the radiograph in the supine position because no edge will be visible tangentially. A similar lesion on the dependent surface will be detected, although it will appear to be smaller than its true size because the peripheral portion of the lesion may be obscured by barium.

B. A flat plaque-like lesion on the nondependent surface will produce a very fine white etching which may be difficult to detect. A similar lesion on the dependent surface may be obscured by the barium pool, but will be seen if the barium pool is thinned out.

C. A polypoid lesion with a sloping margin may be seen as only a single line representing the nonsloping edge. See Figure 2-16*A* and *B*.

D. A plaque-like lesion on a curved surface. Only the edge of the lesion tangential to the x-ray beam will be seen. See Figure 2-16*C* and *D*.

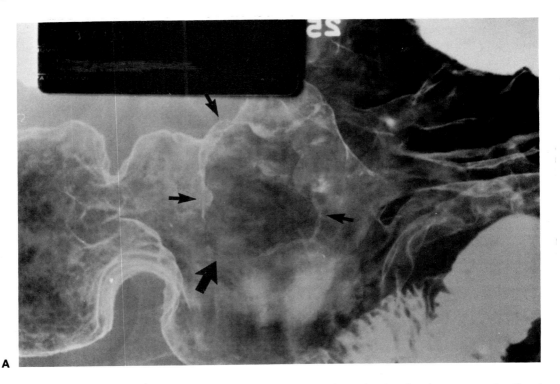

A

A. The supine view double contrast radiograph shows an irregular ring density representing the ulcer on the anterior wall (*small arrows*). The distal margin of the lesion is ill defined (*large arrow*) because of its sloping margin.

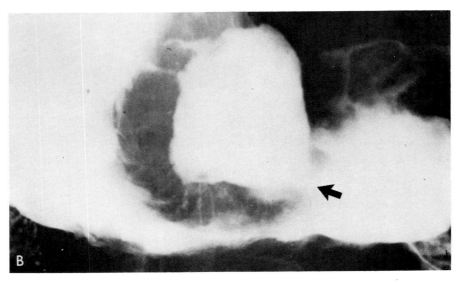

B. A film taken in the prone position shows the large ulcer, filled with barium, and the core of tumor tissue surrounding it except at its distal edge (*arrow*) where the tumor mass becomes less prominent.

FIGURE 2–16 Ulcerated, plaque-like carcinoma on the anterior wall.

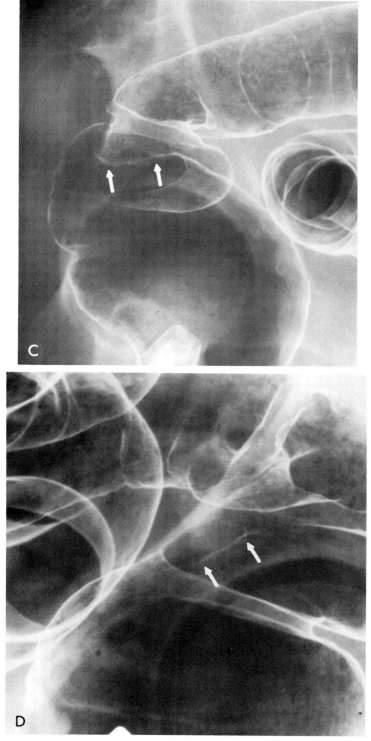

FIGURE 2–16 *Continued.*

C and *D*.   Plaque-like rectal carcinoma. Since the tumor is on a curved surface, only one of its edges is seen tangentially as a straight white line *(arrows)*.

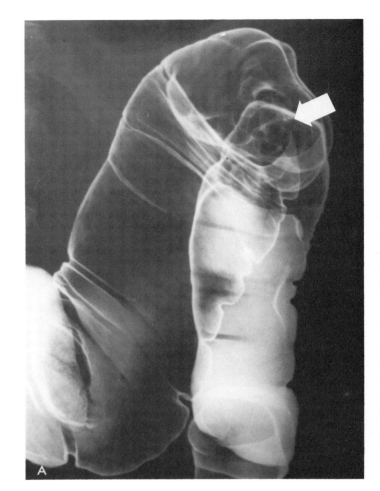

FIGURE 2–17 Annular carcinoma seen en face and in profile.

A. The irregularity of the lumen seen end-on (*arrow*) is the result of an annular carcinoma.

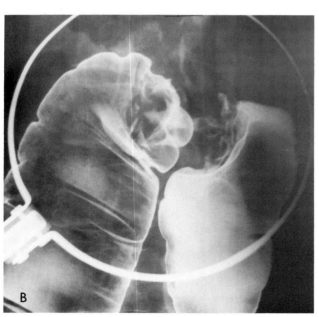

B. This is confirmed on the appropriate oblique projection.

Submucosal lesions (Fig. 2–18) form a right angle with the bowel wall and stretch the overlying mucosa. Therefore, they have a very smooth surface in profile and very sharp margins en face. In addition, mucosal folds may appear to fade out as they approach the lesion (Fig. 2–18 *C*).

Extrinsic masses (Fig. 2–19) may be seen in profile or en face as an ill-defined radiolucency. When viewed in an oblique projection, only a white line representing one edge of the extrinsic mass may be seen (Fig. 2–19*C*). Because of the marked gastric distension, the stomach may appear to surround an extrinsic mass, which may simulate an intramural lesion (Fig. 2–19*D*).[17]

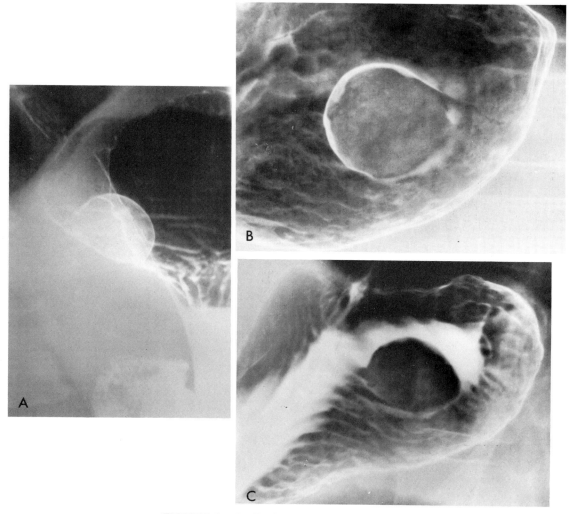

FIGURE 2–18 Typical submucosal lesion.

A. The profile view shows the right angle with the gastric wall and the smooth mucosal surface.
B. En face view shows the very abrupt, well-defined edge of the tumor.
C. Another projection shows mucosal folds fading out at the edge of the lesion.

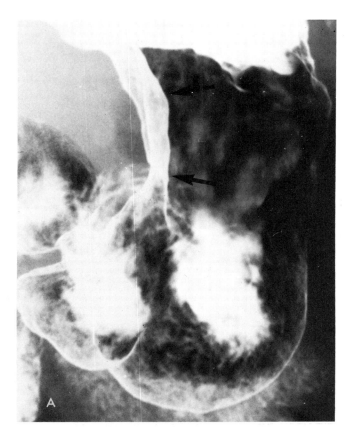

FIGURE 2-19 Extrinsic mass due to carcinoma of the pancreas.

A. Lateral view, showing extrinsic compression on the posterior wall of the stomach (*arrows*).

B. Frontal view showing an ill-defined radiolucency caused by the retrogastric mass.

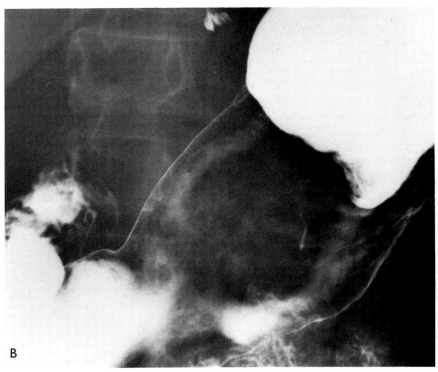

Illustratiion continued on opposite page

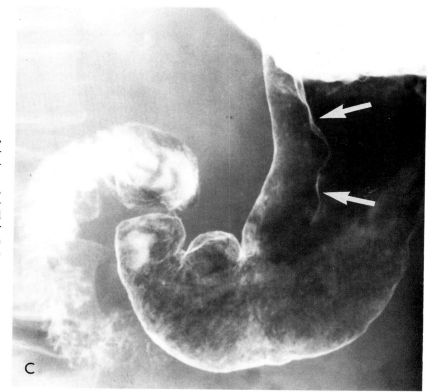

FIGURE 2–19 *Continued*

C. Oblique projection, showing a curving line representing the edge of the retrogastric mass (*arrows*).

D. In another patient, there is a prominent impression owing to an enlarged caudate lobe of the liver (*arrow*). The appearance simulates an intramural gastric lesion.

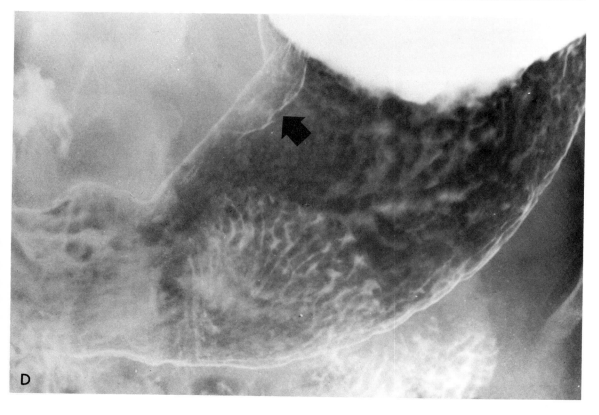

DEPRESSED LESIONS

An ulcer crater on the dependent surface is easily recognized by the familiar barium collection. If there are radiating folds, these will also have the characteristics of dependent wall structures, i.e., they will be radiolucent filling defects (Fig. 2–20A). However, if the ulcer crater is shallow the barium may escape, leaving only a ring shadow. This can be considered to be the appearance of an empty crater, with a ring shadow due to coating of the base and sides of the ulcer crater (Fig. 2–20B and C). An empty ulcer crater on the nondependent wall will also produce a ring shadow (Fig. 2–20D).

To summarize, a ring shadow may represent several different types of pathology. It may represent a polypoid lesion on the nondependent surface (Fig. 2–21A). With careful analysis of the radiographs, it is usually possible to determine whether the ring shadow is due to a protrusion or a depression. A depressed lesion has a sharp outer border and fades to the inside (Fig. 2–20B), whereas a protruded lesion has a sharp inner border and fades to the outside (Figs. 2–11A and 2–21A).[16] In addition, turning the patient to view the lesion in profile can demonstrate conclusively whether the lesion projects into the lumen or beyond the mucosal surface. Similar reasoning applies to the differentiation between a diverticulum and a polyp (Fig. 2–21C).

A ring shadow may also be caused by several types of depressed lesions, such as an empty diverticulum (Fig. 2–21C) or an empty ulcer crater on either the dependent (Fig. 2–20B) or nondependent surface (Fig. 2–20D). It may also be the result of a filling defect, such as a blood clot within an ulcer crater (Fig. 2–21B, Plate 21). For further evaluation of a ring shadow the patient can be turned to demonstrate the lesion in profile. Attempts should also be made to wash the lesion with barium to demonstrate its appearance in the barium pool.

Occasionally a double ring shadow may be seen (Fig. 2–22), which usually indicates a lesion on the nondependent surface. It may indicate an ulcer, with the inner ring representing the neck and the outer ring the base (Fig. 2–22A and B), or it may indicate an ulcerated protruded lesion, with the inner ring representing the ulcer and the outer ring representing the edge of the protrusion (Fig. 2–27).

Text continued on page 40.

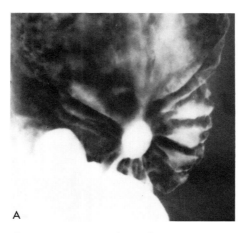

A

FIGURE 2–20 *See legend on opposite page*

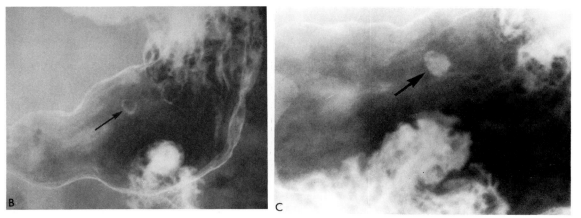

FIGURE 2-20 *A.* Gastric ulcer on the posterior wall. The ulcer crater is filled with barium, and the radiating folds are seen as radiolucent filling defects within the barium puddle.

B. A shallow posterior wall ulcer with an empty crater. The ring shadow is the result of coating of the sides of the ulcer crater. (*From:* Laufer, I., Radiology, *117*:513, 1975.[8] Reproduced by permission.)

C. With further manipulation of the barium pool the ulcer crater can be filled with barium (*arrow*).

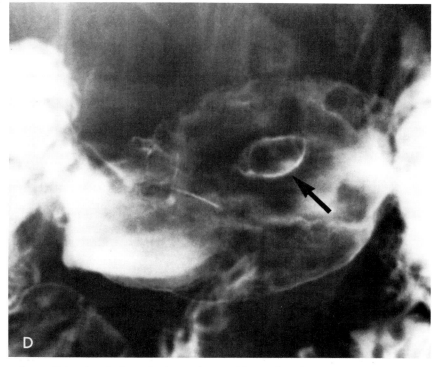

D. Anterior wall duodenal ulcer. In the supine position a ring shadow can be seen in the center of the duodenal cap. This could be filled only in the prone position, indicating that it is an ulcer on the anterior wall.

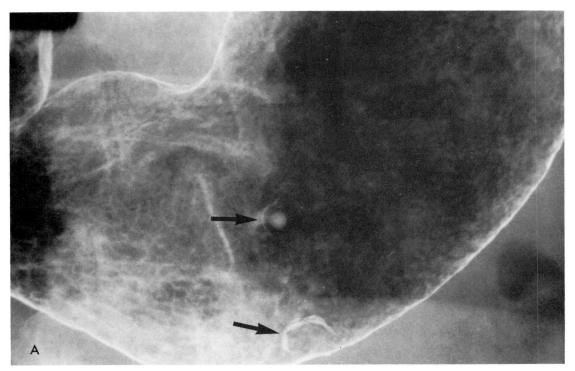

A. Ring shadows due to anterior wall polyps (*arrows*). The central polyp also exhibits the stalactite phenomenon.

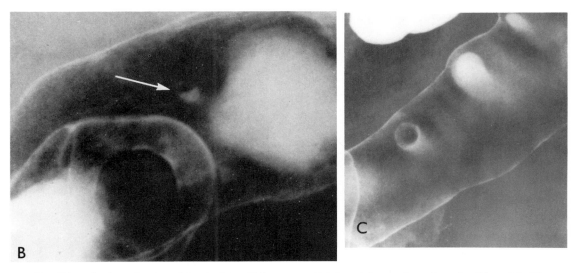

B. Ring shadow due to a blood clot within a superficial gastric erosion. See also Plate 21. (*From:* Laufer, I., Hamilton, J., and Mullens, J. E.: Gastroenterology, *68*:387, 1975.[18] Reproduced by permission.)

C. Ring shadow due to a diverticulum. Superiorly, there are barium-filled diverticula.

FIGURE 2–21

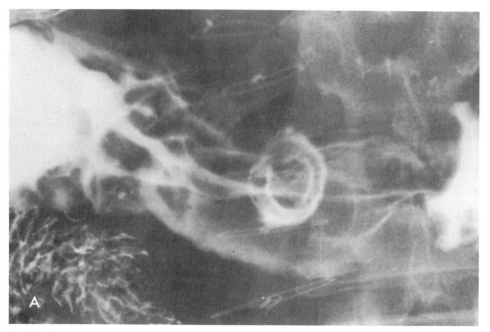

A. In the prone position, a double ring is seen. The inner ring represents the neck of the ulcer, while the outer ring represents the outer margins of the ulcer crater where it is wider in diameter.

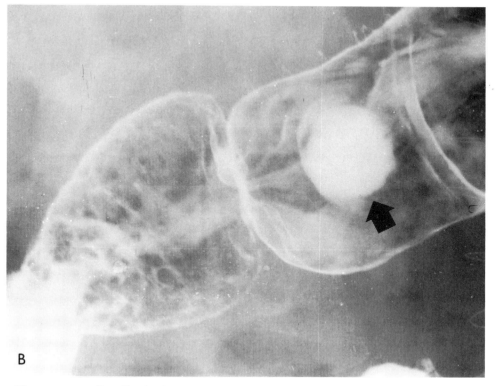

B. The corresponding film in the supine position confirms that the ulcer crater is on the posterior wall.

FIGURE   2–22 Double ring shadow due to an ulcer.

The Barium Pool

The barium pool is the bolus of free barium that is not adherent to the mucosal surface. The major portion of the bolus, which we shall call the barium pool, is found in the most dependent segment of the bowel. In addition, small "puddles" may be found in any segment where there are minor depressions (Fig. 2–8). The barium pool is of critical importance, since it is used to wash and coat the mucosal surface and to fill any depressed lesions. It can also be used to demonstrate posterior wall protrusions more clearly (Fig. 2–23). Indeed the entire double contrast examination rests on skillful manipulation of the barium pool. Nevertheless, the barium pool or puddle can lead to serious error in several different ways (Fig. 2–24). A dependent wall protrusion may not be seen because it is covered over by the barium pool (Fig. 2–25). However, even a small barium puddle may obscure or veil the fine white etching of a relatively large polypoid lesion on the nondependent surface. This principle is illustrated in Figure 2–26. In the supine position a large polypoid tumor on the posterior wall of the rectum is clearly seen as a filling defect in the barium pool on the posterior wall. However, in the prone position with the barium pool on the anterior wall, the delicate white etching of this polypoid lesion is entirely obscured. The lateral view confirms the posterior wall location of this lesion and shows the barium pool.

In addition, a barium pool may collect in an overlapping structure and obscure a pathologic lesion (Fig. 2–4). Some of the problems associated with the barium pool can be avoided by compression, as illustrated in Figure 2–27. A lesion on the nondependent surface may be seen only faintly. However, with compression it is immersed in the barium pool and is clearly seen as a radiolucent filling defect.

Thus a barium pool or puddle may be either a blessing or a curse. It improves mucosal coating; it may fill an ulcer crater on the dependent surface, and it helps to demonstrate dependent wall protrusions. On the other hand, it can obscure lesions on both the dependent and nondependent surfaces. Therefore, in many cases one may wish to take spot films with a small barium puddle and additional spot films with the puddle removed. An understanding of the potential value as well as the hazards of the barium pool is an important step in mastering double contrast techniques.

Text continued on page 45

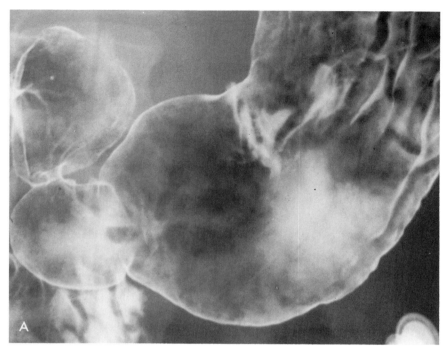

A. Radiating folds to an ulcer scar faintly seen because of the absence of a barium pool.

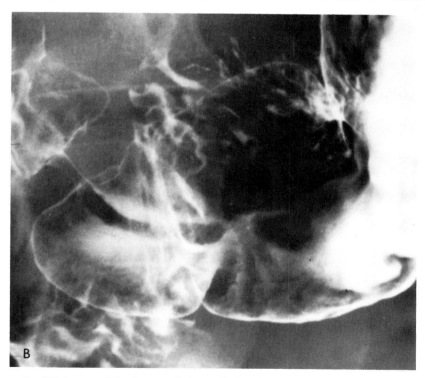

B. With a small barium pool the radiating folds are seen more clearly.

FIGURE 2-23 Value of the barium puddle for demonstration of posterior wall lesions.

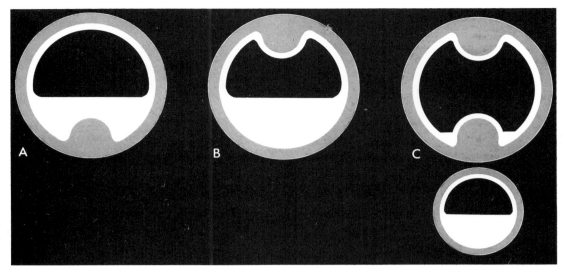

FIGURE 2–24 Diagrammatic representation of the hazards of the barium pool.

A. Barium pool obscures the lesion on the dependent surface. See Figure 2–25.

B. The barium pool obscures the fine white etching of the lesion on the nondependent surface. See Figure 2–26.

C. The barium pool in the overlapping loop of bowel may obscure a lesion on either the dependent or the nondependent surface. See Figure 2–4.

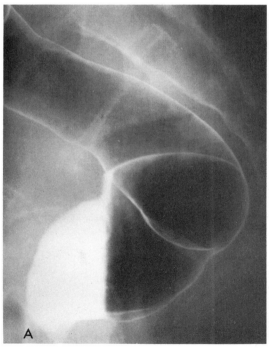

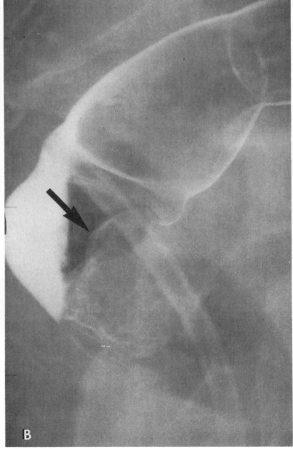

FIGURE 2–25

A. The barium pool on the anterior wall of the rectum obscures a large polypoid tumor.

B. With the patient prone, the barium pool has shifted to the posterior wall and the polypoid tumor is clearly seen.

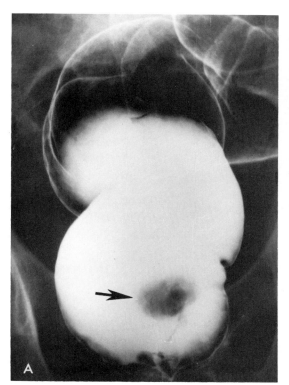

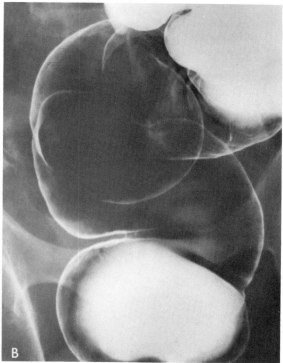

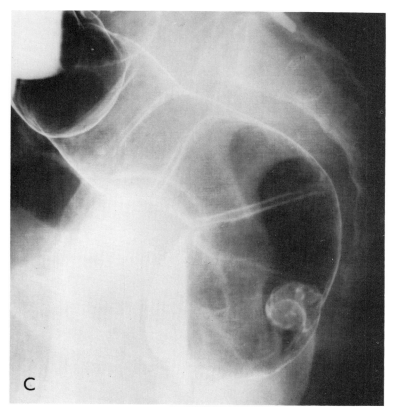

FIGURE 2–26

A. A film taken in the supine position shows a large filling defect in the rectum. This must be on the posterior wall.

B. In the prone position no abnormality can be detected because the barium pool on the anterior wall obscures the fine white etching of the polypoid tumor on the posterior surface.

C. A cross-table lateral film confirms the posterior wall location of the early polypoid carcinoma and shows the barium pool on the anterior wall.

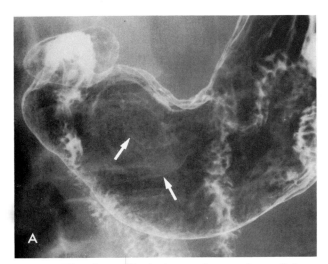

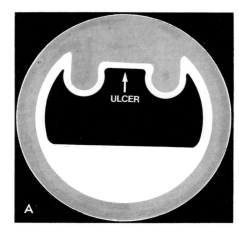

A. The plaque-like lesion on the anterior wall (*large arrows*) and the central ulcer (*small arrows*) are faintly seen.

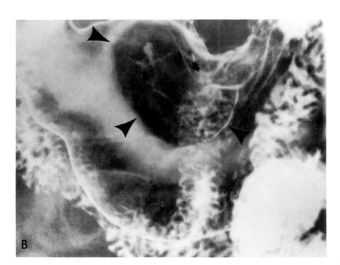

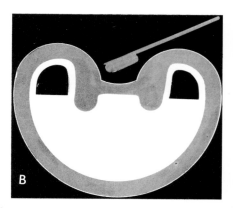

B. With compression the tumor is pushed into the barium pool, causing a radiolucent filling defect and making the tumor (*large arrows*) and the ulcer (*small arrows*) more apparent.

FIGURE 2–27 Value of compression in anterior wall lesions.

ARTIFACTS

In addition to becoming familiar with a new array of normal and pathologic appearances, the radiologist starting to use double contrast techniques must also learn to recognize a variety of artifacts that may be peculiar to double contrast techniques.[3] The causes of these artifacts are listed in Table 2–1. Many artifacts can be attributed to the high viscosity of the barium suspension and to the variations in mucosal coating. Some of these artifacts, such as patchy coating (Fig. 2–1) and the stalactite phenomenon (Fig. 2–12), have already been mentioned. Some barium suspensions may cause precipitation or flaking which may simulate diffuse mucosal ulceration (Fig. 2–28). In many cases these artifacts can be avoided by the choice of an appropriate barium suspension. However, in some patients with excessive fluid and debris they may be unavoidable.

In some patients there is insufficient gas to separate the anterior and posterior walls. The point of adhesion or adherence between the anterior and posterior walls may produce an irregular outline which may simulate an ulcer or polypoid lesion (Fig. 2–29).[8] With further distension of the area, the artifact disappears. We have termed this a "kissing" artifact.

The segment of the gastrointestinal tract outlined by double contrast becomes transparent. Therefore, opacities overlying any segment can be clearly seen and may simulate an intrinsic lesion. These opacities may be normal skeletal structures (Fig. 2–30); calcified structures, such as lymph nodes, uterine fibroids, phleboliths, or diverticula; or contrast-filled structures, such as diverticula or lymph nodes.

Extraneous material in the lumen must be differentiated from polypoid lesions in both single and double contrast techniques. However, with double contrast techniques there are additional artifacts, such as gas bubbles and undissolved effervescent pills or granules (Fig. 2–31), that must be recognized.

Text continued on page 49

TABLE 2–1 CAUSES OF DOUBLE CONTRAST ARTIFACTS

Barium-Related
High viscosity—stalactite phenomenon[15]
Patchy coating
Precipitation and flaking
"Kissing" artifact

See-Through Effect
Normal anatomic structures
Calcified structures
Contrast-filled structures

Extraneous or Foreign Material
Gas bubbles
Effervescent agent
Adherent fecal material
Others—mineral oil, Telepaque

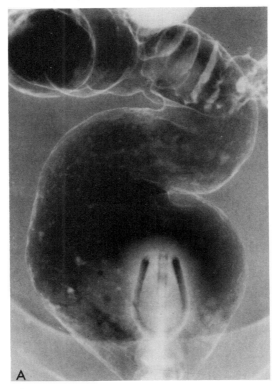

A. Barium precipitation, simulating inflammatory bowel disease.

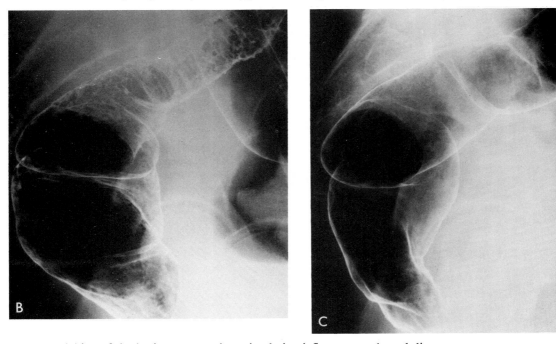

B. Flaking of the barium suspension, simulating inflammatory bowel disease.
C. In the same patient, a film taken 10 minutes before shows a perfectly normal mucosal surface.
(*From* Laufer, I.: CRC Crit. Rev. Diagnostic Imaging.[19] Reproduced by permission.)

FIGURE 2–28 Artifacts due to poor barium suspensions.

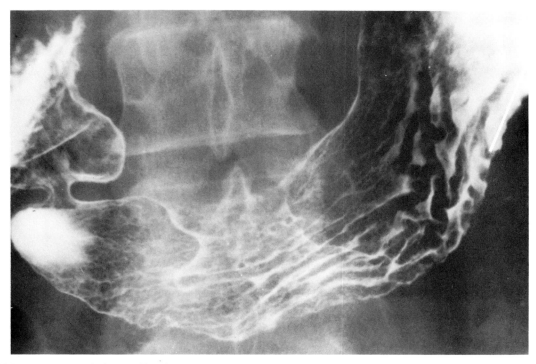

FIGURE 2–29 Kissing artifact in the antrum due to adherence of the anterior and posterior wall of the stomach.

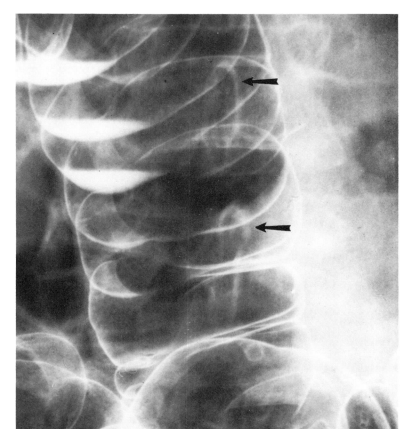

FIGURE 2–30 Spinous processes seen through the gas-filled colon may simulate polypoid lesions.

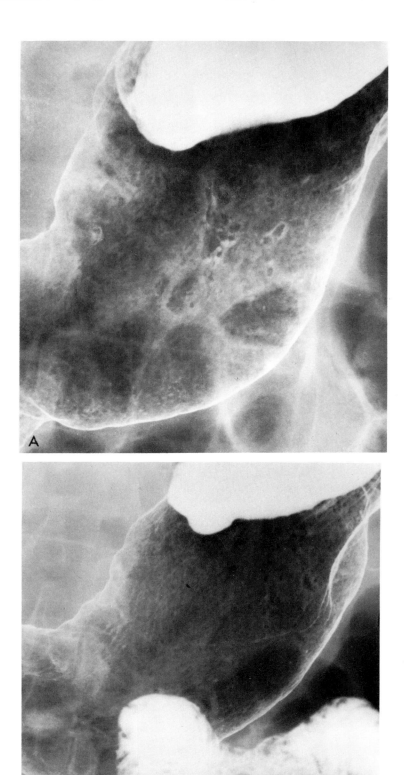

FIGURE 2–31 *A* and *B*   The early film from a double contrast study shows small filling defects in the stomach (*A*). These are due to undissolved effervescent agent. A later film shows that the filling defects are no longer present (*B*).

**TABLE 2–2 PATHOLOGIC CONDITIONS THAT MAY BE
SIMULATED BY ARTIFACTS**

Diffuse Superficial Ulceration
Barium precipitation
Flaking
Debris

Discrete Ulceration
Colonic or duodenal diverticulum
Patchy coating
Stalactite phenomenon
"Kissing" artifact

Polypoid Lesion
See-through effect
Extraneous material
"Kissing" artifact

Table 2–2 lists the various types of pathologic conditions that may be simulated by artifacts. Some of these artifacts are discussed in further detail in the specific chapters under the lesions they simulate.

SUMMARY

The use of double contrast techniques requires an understanding of the basic differences in approach between single and double contrast studies of the gastrointestinal tract. The transition from one approach to the other demands a major reorientation to the performance and interpretation of gastrointestinal radiologic studies. It also requires an understanding of the elements that combine to form the double contrast image — the dependent wall, the nondependent wall, and the barium pool. Great attention must be paid to the quality of mucosal coating as a criterion of the adequacy of the study. Materials such as barium suspensions, which are designed for double contrast studies, must be used. Although gaseous distension is generally desirable, it is important to understand the value of varying the degree of distension to best demonstrate certain types of lesions. Management of the barium pool is a critical aspect of double contrast technique. The examiner must be aware of the potential hazards posed by the barium pool as well as of its uses.

Interpretation of these studies requires a clear understanding of the difference in appearances between structures and lesions on the dependent and nondependent walls. The examiner should aim at a precise translation from the radiologic findings to the gross pathologic features of the lesion. He must concentrate on a basic analysis of the lines, points, and shadows on the film. Endoscopic and pathologic correlation should be viewed as an extension of the radiologic examination whereby the radiologist can improve the quality of his studies and the precision of his interpretation.

Figures 2–32 to 39 illustrate additional examples of the application of these principles to the performance and interpretation of double contrast studies.

Text continued on page 58

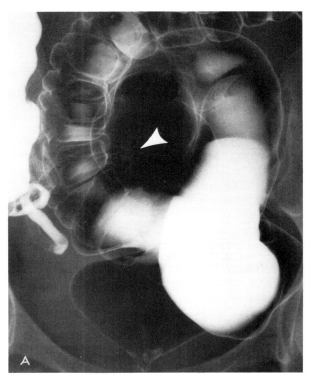

A. Frontal view with overexposure. An abnormality on the right lateral aspect of the sigmoid can only be suspected.

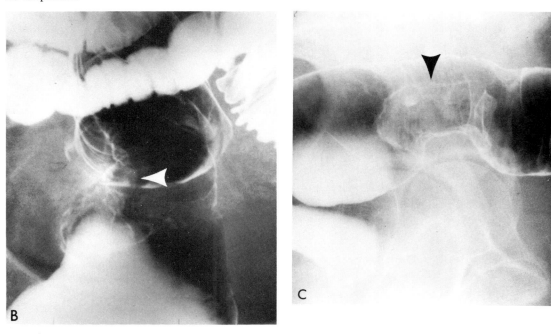

B. With a lighter exposure the irregular, plaque-like lesion on the right lateral wall of the sigmoid is clearly seen.

C. Left lateral projection in which the plaque-like lesion on the nondependent surface is etched in white. See also Plate 94.

FIGURE 2–32 Dangers of incorrect exposure.

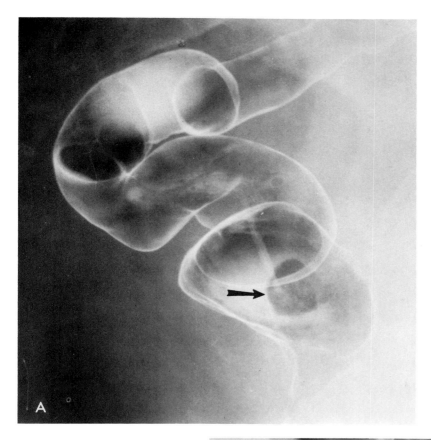

FIGURE 2–33 *A* and *B*   Left lateral view of the rectum (*A*) shows a rounded filling defect in the barium puddle. Therefore, the polypoid lesion must be on the dependent surface, i.e., the left lateral wall of the rectum. This is confirmed in the frontal projection (*B*).

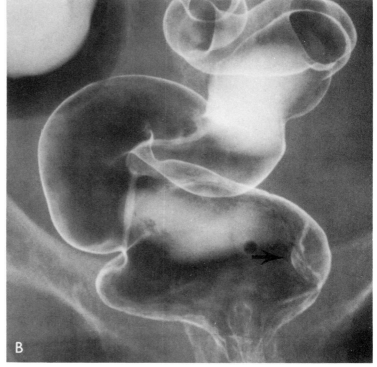

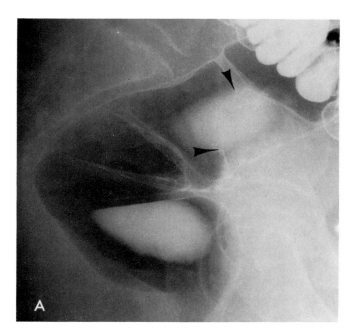

FIGURE 2–34

A. In the left lateral projection the fine white etching (*arrowheads*) is almost obscured by a small barium puddle. Because of the etched outline of the lesion, it must be on the nondependent, i.e., right lateral, wall.

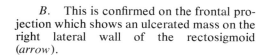

B. This is confirmed on the frontal projection which shows an ulcerated mass on the right lateral wall of the rectosigmoid (*arrow*).

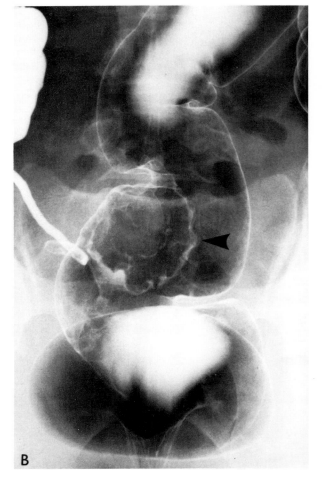

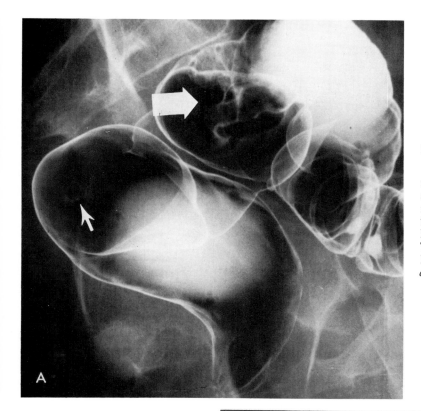

FIGURE 2–35

A. Oblique view of the rectosigmoid is suggestive of an abnormality at the rectosigmoid junction. The abnormality is seen through overlapping loops of bowel (*large arrow*). There is also a small polypoid lesion in the rectum (*small arrow*).

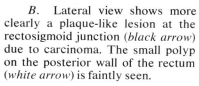

B. Lateral view shows more clearly a plaque-like lesion at the rectosigmoid junction (*black arrow*) due to carcinoma. The small polyp on the posterior wall of the rectum (*white arrow*) is faintly seen.

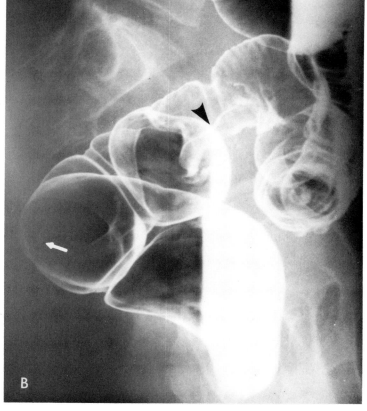

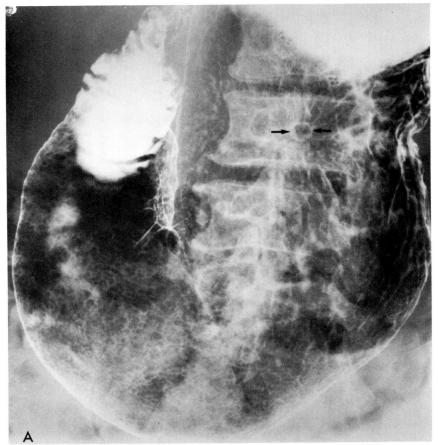

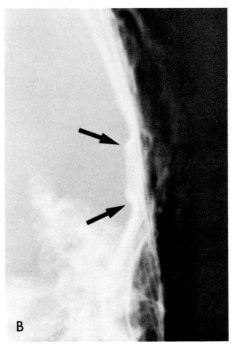

FIGURE 2–36

A. Double contrast view of the stomach in right posterior oblique projection. A ring shadow (*arrows*) is seen on the dependent surface, i.e., the lesser curvature. Since this represents an empty crater, it is likely that the ulcer is very shallow.

B. This is confirmed on the tangential view of the broad, shallow crater (*arrows*). (Courtesy of Hans Herlinger, M.D., Leeds, England.)

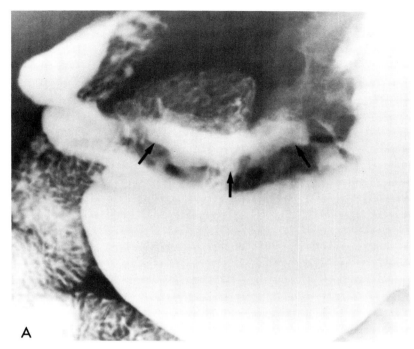

A. Conventional view of the lesser curvature ulcer (*arrows*) and the surrounding rim of tumor tissue.

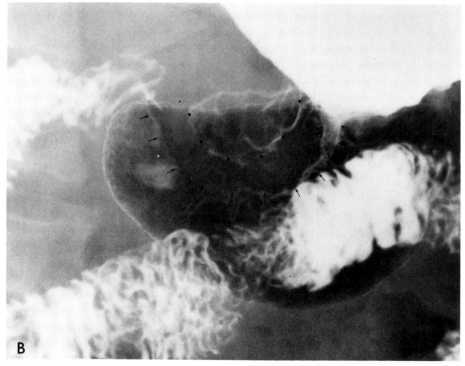

B. The double contrast view shows the rim of tumor tissue (*arrows*) and the outline of the ulcer (*dots*). Note the absence of the areae gastricae over the tumor tissue. (Courtesy of Hans Herlinger, M.D., Leeds, England.)

FIGURE 2–37 Carman's meniscus sign seen on conventional study and with double contrast.

FIGURE 2–38 Stalactite phenomenon pointing to a polypoid lesion.

 A. Prone position. There is a ring shadow (*arrow*) with a central radiodensity, representing the stalactite phenomenon. This indicates that the ring shadow must be due to a protruded lesion on the nondependent, i.e., posterior, surface of the hiatal hernia.
 B. Another view confirms the presence of a small polypoid lesion.
 C. Steep right posterior oblique projection, with the hiatal hernia reduced back into the stomach. The polypoid lesion is seen to lie posteriorly.

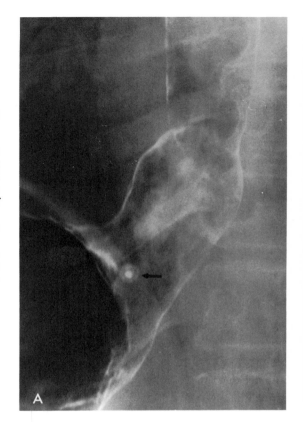

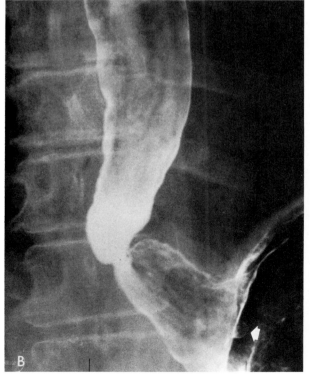

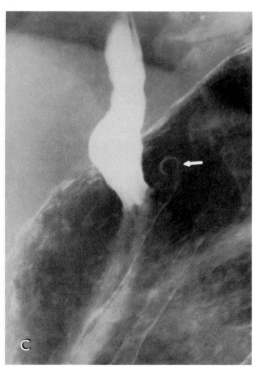

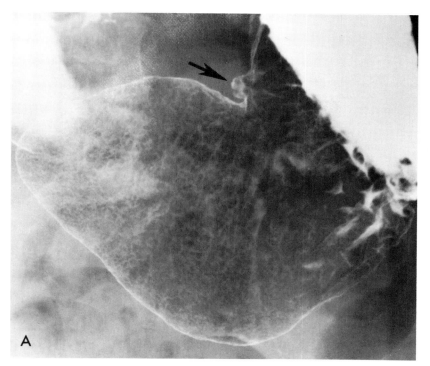

A. Supine view double contrast radiograph shows a lesser curvature ulcer (*arrow*). The surrounding folds are not well seen.

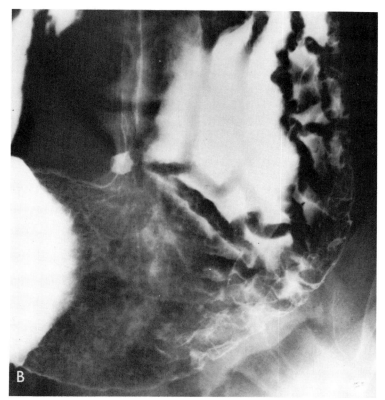

B. In a slight RPO projection the ulcer crater is filled with barium, and the surrounding mucosal folds are seen much more clearly.

FIGURE 2–39 The value of the barium puddle for demonstration of posterior wall structures.

REFERENCES

1. James, W. B.: Double contrast radiology in the gastrointestinal tract. Clin. Gastroenterol., *7*:397, 1978.
2. Shirakabe, H.: Double Contrast Studies of the Stomach. Stuttgart, Georg-Thieme Verlag, 1972.
3. Gohel, V. K., Kressel, H. Y., and Laufer, I.: Double contrast artifacts. Gastrointest. Radiol., *3*:139, 1978.
4. Miller, R. E., and Skucas, J.: Gastrointestinal agents. *In*: Miller, R. E., and Skucas, J. (eds.): Radiographic Contrast Agents. Baltimore, University Park Press, 1977, pp. 3–167.
5. Miller, R. E.: Barium sulfate as a contrast medium. *In*: Margulis, A. R., and Burhenne, H. J. (eds.): Alimentary Tract Roentgenology. 2nd ed. St. Louis, C. V. Mosby, 1973.
6. Mackintosh, C. E., and Kreel, L.: Anatomy and radiology of the areae gastricae. Gut, *18*:855, 1977.
7. Matsuura, K., Nakata, H., Takeda, N., et al.: Innominate lines of the colon. Radiology, *123*:581, 1977.
8. Laufer, I.: A simple method for routine double contrast study of the upper gastrointestinal tract. Radiology, *117*:513, 1975.
9. Miller, R. E., Chernish, S. M., Skukas, J., et al.: Hypotonic roentgenography with glucagon. Am. J. Roentgenol., *121*:264, 1974.
10. Meeroff, J. C., Jorgens, J., and Isenberg, J. I.: The effect of glucagon on barium enema examination. Radiology, *115*:5, 1975.
11. Hogan, W. J., Dodds, W. J., Hoke, S. E., et al.: The effect of glucagon on esophageal motor function. Gastroenterology, *69*:160, 1975.
12. Laufer, I., Mullens, J. E., and Hamilton, J.: The diagnostic accuracy of barium studies of the stomach and duodenum — correlation with endoscopy. Radiology, *115*:569, 1975.
13. Laufer, I., Mullens, J. E., and Hamilton, J.: Correlation of endoscopy and double contrast radiography in the early stages of ulcerative and granulomatous colitis. Radiology, *118*:1, 1976.
14. Laufer, I., Smith, N. C. W., and Mullens, J. E.: The radiologic demonstration of colorectal polyps undetected by endoscopy. Gastroenterology, *70*:167, 1976.
15. Op den Orth, J. O., and Ploem, S.: The stalactite phenomenon in double contrast studies of the stomach. Radiology, *117*:523, 1975.
16. Youker, J. E., and Welin, S.: Differentiation of true polypoid tumors of the colon from extraneous material: A new roentgen sign. Radiology, *84*:610 1965.
17. Battle, W. M., Laufer, I., Moldofsky, P. J., et al.: Anomalous liver lobulation as a cause of perigastric masses. Am. J. Dig. Dis., in press.
18. Laufer, I., Hamilton, J., and Mullens, J. E.: Demonstration of superficial gastric erosions by double contrast radiography. Gastroenterology, *68*:387, 1975.
19. Laufer, I.: Air contrast studies of the colon in inflammatory bowel disease. CRC Crit. Rev. Diagnost. Imaging, *9*:421, 1977.

3

UPPER GASTROINTESTINAL TRACT: TECHNICAL ASPECTS

BASIC REQUIREMENTS
    Gaseous Distension
    Mucosal Coating
    Maneuvers
    Attention to Technical Details

OPTIONS
    Patient Preparation
    Hypotonic Agents

THE ROUTINE EXAMINATION
    Materials
    Procedures
    Variations

BASIC REQUIREMENTS

A limited double contrast study is frequently obtained during the course of the conventional upper gastrointestinal examination. By using the gas that happens to be in the stomach, one can perform a double contrast examination of the antrum and duodenal cap. However, the quality of this part of the examination is unreliable because of the variability in the volume of gas within the stomach and the relatively poor mucosal coating produced by the barium suspensions used for the conventional study. Certainly, good double contrast views of the body and fundus of the stomach and duodenal loop are rarely achieved with this technique.

The formal double contrast examination is designed to produce a thin coating of high density barium on the mucosal surface and to distend the viscus such that the normal mucosal folds are straightened or effaced. The effects of gravity are then utilized to demonstrate each part of the organ and each surface in profile and en face. It should be emphasized that double contrast techniques place much greater emphasis on the appearance of the mucosa en face than in profile.

As indicated by Miller.[1] the term double contrast examination is applied to several different types of studies. Nevertheless, a number of basic elements form the fundamental requirements for an adequate double contrast examination.[2] These are (1) gaseous distension, (2) good mucosal coating, (3) a set of maneuvers to insure unobscured double contrast views of all areas of the upper gastrointestinal tract, and (4) attention to technical details.

Gaseous Distension

The stomach should be distended just to the point at which the normal rugal folds are effaced. If distension is inadequate, tortuous mucosal folds may hide small lesions, or barium caught between the folds may simulate an ulcer. If the stomach is overdistended, it becomes very difficult to coat the surface, and some abnormal folds, such as those radiating toward a gastric ulcer or an ulcer scar, may be obliterated (Chapter 2). In addition, gastric varices may be obliterated by overdistension.

The various methods of introducing gas into the stomach have been reviewed by James.[3] It is important that the effervescent agent liberate the gas quickly and not interfere with the barium coating of the mucosal surface. The ideal method of distending the stomach is nasogastric intubation.[4-6] This provides a reliable and controllable method of gastric distension. Clearly, this technique would meet with considerable patient resistance if applied on a routine basis. Therefore, most examiners now use effervescent tablets, granules, or powder which release carbon dioxide on contact with the fluid in the stomach.[7-10]

Several other techniques of introducing gas into the stomach have been described. O'Reilly and coworkers used two separate barium suspensions, one containing sodium bicarbonate and the other sodium citrate. These interact in the stomach and release CO_2. Pochaczewski[12] and Op den Orth[13] use a "bubbly barium" administered through a soda water dispenser. These techniques have the disadvantage that the volume of gas liberated depends on the volume of barium administered, and ideally one should be able to control the volume of gas independently of the volume of barium. A Japanese product, Baritop (Sakai Chemical Industries, Osaka Japan), is marketed specifically for double contrast examination of the stomach. This barium suspension is supposed to release carbon dioxide in the stomach. It has been shown that the volume of gas released is inadequate, probably because the evolution of gas is much too slow.[14] Another drawback of this product is that the volume of gas depends specifically on the volume of barium. Scott-Harden[15, 16] uses Schweppes tonic water as a source of carbon dioxide. Its disadvantage is that a large volume of liquid must be administered to achieve gaseous distension. This liquid also has a deleterious effect on the quality of the mucosal coating. Mohammed and Hegedüs[17] recommend drinking through a perforated straw to introduce air into the stomach, a method described by Amplatz in 1958.[18] While this may be successful in some patients, it tends to be unreliable, and the volume of air and barium cannot be controlled independently.

Obata[19] has emphasized the importance of using an antifoaming agent, such as simethicone, to disperse bubbles. Some effervescent agents contain simethicone in the preparation, and with these products additional simethicone may not be necessary. The role of antifoaming agents in double contrast studies has been reviewed by Bagnall and colleagues.[20]

Mucosal Coating

Good mucosal coating is achieved by washing a high density barium suspension across the mucosal surface. Therefore, the quality of the coating depends on the properties of the barium suspension, the volume of barium and air in the stomach, the frequency of washing, and the presence of secretions. The greater the volume of barium, the better the mucosal coating. However, if there is too much barium only a small portion of the organ can be seen in double contrast. As the volume of gas increases, the volume of barium may be increased, and indeed must be increased to achieve good mucosal coating. The patient must be turned through 360 degrees in order to wash the barium suspension across all surfaces of the stomach. If the stomach contains excess mucus or secretions, additional turning may be necessary. In the absence of good mucosal coating, small or even large lesions may be missed. In addition, uneven mucosal coating may simulate lesions (Chapter 2).

The properties of the barium suspension are very important. Several recent papers have discussed some of the physical and chemical properties of various barium sulfate suspensions in relation to their suitability for double contrast studies. It is clear that there are marked differences between the various commercial preparations with respect to viscosity,[21, 22] quality of mucosal coating in clinical studies,[22] and resistance to precipitation by gastric acid and mucin.[22, 23] Moreover, Roberts and coworkers[24] have shown that in vitro tests are not useful in predicting the clinical performance of a barium suspension.

Thus it is clear that the choice of barium suspension may be a critical determinant of the quality of the double contrast study. The quality of mucosal coating can be judged by the frequency of visualization of the areae gastricae (Fig. 3–1 *D*).[25] In our studies this varied from 10 per cent of studies with Micropaque and Barosperse to approximately 50 per cent with Baritop and E-Z-HD. With the use of hypotonic agents, better results are achieved.[22] We prefer a high density barium (200% W/V) of moderate viscosity.[26] Such bariums have only recently become available on the North American market (E-Z-HD, E-Z-EM Co., Westbury, N. Y., and HD 200, Lafayette Pharmacal, Lafayette, Ind.). Op den Orth[13] prefers a lower density barium (82.5% W/V) because the very high density barium compromises the compression and single contrast aspects of the examination.

The presence of fluid within the stomach certainly interferes with the quality of mucosal coating. Again, the properties of the barium suspension may be important, since some suspensions are easily precipitated on contact with acid while others are very resistant to acid. In such cases additional barium should be given, and the patient should be turned through several rotations to wash the barium across the surface of the stomach. If adequate coating is still not achieved, the stomach can be filled with a dilute barium suspension for a conventional study, or the examination can be repeated at a later date with a nasogastric tube for aspiration of the fluid from the stomach.

Although barium sulfate is the universal contrast medium used in double contrast studies of the gastrointestinal tract, experimental work has been performed with other substances. Goldberg and associates[27] obtained excellent double contrast views of the esophagus in cats, utilizing tantalum powder. Dodds and coworkers[28] have also obtained double contrast views of the stomach in cats using this material. Heitz[29] has used barium titanate for gastrointestinal studies. This compound was believed to produce superior mucosal coating, particularly in the pharynx and esophagus. However, it appears that barium titanate has not been used in formal double contrast examinations of the upper gastrointestinal tract.

Maneuvers

A set of maneuvers must be designed to coat all surfaces of the esophagus, stomach, and duodenum, and to produce unobscured double contrast views of each area. Thus the stomach must be examined before it is overlapped by the barium-filled duodenum and small bowel. The examination must be performed quickly to avoid overlapping small bowel and deterioration of the mucosal coating with time. Therefore, fluoroscopy is done primarily to determine the volume of the barium and gas, to insure adequate mucosal coating, and to accurately position and time spot films. Diagnostic fluoroscopy is de-emphasized, since the method depends primarily on the production of high quality spot films. Nevertheless, if an abnormality is noted or suspected at fluoroscopy, it is investigated with additional spot films. The set of maneuvers should incorporate compression fluoroscopy, since some small polypoid lesions and some small ulcers may be more obvious on compression (Chapter 2, Figs. 2–11 and 2–27). This is particularly true of lesions on the anterior wall of the stomach. Our routine consists solely of fluoroscopic spot films. We believe that the accurate timing, collimation, and positioning possible with spot films outweigh the potential advantages of superior geometry achievable with overhead radiographs.

Attention to Technical Details

There are many technical details that must be attended to obsessively and persistently in order to achieve consistently good double contrast studies. The preparation of the barium is critical. Barium and water must be weighed carefully in the preparation of the suspension. Most of the high density bariums settle quickly, and must therefore be stirred very vigorously immediately before use. We prefer to expose our spot films at approximately 100 kVp, although lower kVp can be used with the rare earth intensifying screens. The density settings on the phototimer must generally be lower than those used on conventional barium studies in order not to wash out the surface detail.

OPTIONS

Patient Preparation

Our patients are prepared for study simply by an overnight fast. Hunt[7] has emphasized the desirability of a clear stomach for optimal mucosal coating. He therefore uses an elaborate preparation to insure that the stomach is free of fluid.

The patient must arrive in the department at least 1½ hours prior to the time of the study. After being given three tablets of metoclopramide, one tablet every half hour, he is instructed to lie on the right side. Metoclopramide enhances gastroduodenal motor activity[30] and therefore helps to empty the stomach of secretions, particularly with the patient on the right side. In principle, this preparation appears to be sensible, corresponding to a laxative to clean the colon. However, this procedure would make great demands on the space available in most radiology departments and has not gained popularity. In addition, metoclopramide is not available in the United States at this time.

Hypotonic Agents

Various authors have advocated the use of hypotonic agents either routinely or selectively. Pro-Banthine has been used in the past,[31] but because of its anticholinergic side effects has been largely supplanted by glucagon. Recently it has been suggested that Pro-Banthine in a reduced dosage of 5 to 10 mg can be given intravenously with immediate and satisfactory hypotonia and minimal side effects.[32] Glucagon has been used at a dosage ranging from 0.25 to 1.0 mg intravenously.[33-36] We have found that even 0.05 to 0.10 mg produces adequate hypotonia in most patients. The intravenous injection is effective in 45 seconds, while intramuscular injections require larger doses and need approximately 15 minutes to take effect.[37, 38]

Glucagon has virtually no side effects except in the occasional patient who has a vasovagal reaction to the sight of the needle. Its only contraindications are pheochromocytoma, insulinoma, and brittle diabetes. Because glucagon does not relax the pylorus one may encounter delayed emptying of the stomach when it is used. When the relaxant effect wears off, a period of hyperperistalsis in the small bowel ensues. Therefore, a small bowel follow-through study can still be performed.

Buscopan is an anticholinergic agent that has been used in double contrast studies of the stomach and duodenum.[7, 8] This agent produces very effective, short-lived hypotonia. It has the additional advantage of relaxing the pylorus, and its use therefore results in excellent examinations of the duodenum. Buscopan appears to be free of the major side effects of Pro-Banthine, although blurred vision is still a frequent complaint. The small bowel transit time is markedly prolonged with Buscopan, such that a small bowel study becomes impractical. Buscopan is not available in the United States.

There is no doubt that the routine use of a hypotonic agent by injection improves the quality of the examination. However, it does prolong the examination and increases its risk (minimally) and its complexity. As

TABLE 3–1 INDICATIONS FOR HYPOTONIA

1. Elderly patients
2. Previous gastroduodenal surgery
3. Follow-up of gastric lesion
4. Evaluation of duodenal loop
5. Esophageal varices

the examiner acquires experience in the use of these techniques, we believe that hypotonic agents, such as glucagon, can be used selectively. Our indications for its use are outlined in Table 3–1. With elderly patients who move slowly, the time required to move them from side to side may result in loss of the barium and gas into the small bowel. With glucagon the pylorus tends to remain closed, and the barium and gas are trapped in the stomach for a short period. In patients with previous pyloroplasty or gastroenterostomy the duodenum and small bowel are also immobilized by glucagon, and excellent views of the surgical site can be achieved (see Chapter 8).

Patients being followed for gastric lesions, such as the healing of a gastric ulcer, are best examined with 1.0 mg of glucagon to insure the best possible views of the stomach. Because this dose will frequently preclude adequate examination of the duodenum, when the primary interest is in the duodenal loop the glucagon should be given after the barium has entered the duodenum. It has been shown by Liu[39] and Novak[40] that esophageal aperistalsis induced by Pro-Banthine greatly improves the detectability of esophageal varices. Since it has been demonstrated that glucagon does not inhibit esophageal peristalsis,[41] it would be preferable to use Pro-Banthine or Buscopan in these cases.

Glucagon can also be administered at any time during the routine examination if it is seen that gastric or duodenal hypermotility interferes with the quality of the study. We generally recommend that examiners starting to learn this technique routinely utilize glucagon 0.10 mg intravenously until they feel comfortable with the examination and are able to do it quickly. This very small dose should be diluted to 0.25 cc with sterile water for the injection.

THE ROUTINE EXAMINATION

Described in the following section is our routine examination of the upper GI tract in all patients referred for a gastrointestinal series. Of course, the routine can be altered as dictated by the indications for the examination or by findings as the examination proceeds.

Materials

A. Barium E-Z-HD, 200% W/V (E-Z-EM Co., Westbury, N.Y.)

B. Effervescent agent: Unik-Zoru granules (Unik Medical Labs, Montreal, Que.). This preparation has simethicone incorporated within it and therefore requires no additional antifoaming agent. Since this product is not available in the United States, we have used E-Z-Gas (E-Z-EM

Co.) and Sparkles (Lafayette Pharmacal, Lafayette, Ind.). With Sparkles, additonal simethicone is required.

C.   Antifoaming agent: simethicone in the form of Mylicon (Upjohn) or Medical Antifoam C (Dow Chemical Co.).

Procedure

We have modified this procedure only slightly since our earlier descriptions.[9, 42]

A.   An intravenous injection of 0.05 to 0.10 mg of glucagon may be given intravenously as a matter of routine. For the indications outlined in Table 3–1, a larger dose of 0.25 to 1.0 mg may be administered.

B.   The patient stands erect and swallows the effervescent agent followed by 10 cc of water (containing 0.6 ml of simethicone if necessary).

C.   The patient turns slightly to the left and takes two gulps of barium quickly. Double contrast views of the esophagus are obtained (Fig. 3–1A).

D.   The patient turns to face the table, which is brought to the horizontal position. In the prone oblique position* the patient drinks additional barium to a total of 100 to 120 ml. At the same time, barium-filled views of the esophagus are obtained in the RAO (right anterior oblique) projection (Fig. 3–1B).

E.   The patient turns onto the left side and then onto the back. The quality of mucosal coating is checked fluoroscopically, and if it is inadequate the patient turns through another 360 degrees and returns to the supine position. A frontal film of the stomach is obtained, providing a double contrast view of the distal half of the stomach (Fig. 3–1C).

F.   The patient turns to the right almost 360 degrees into the LPO (left posterior oblique) position for another spot film of the distal stomach and pylorus (Fig. 3–1D).

G.   The patient turns onto the right side for a right lateral projection, giving a double contrast view of the fundus and an assessment of the retrogastric area (Fig. 3–1E).

H.   At this time, barium-filled views of the duodenum can usually be obtained. Compression can be applied by having the patient lie on a sponge or inflatable balloon (Fig. 3–1F).

I.   Double contrast views of the duodenum are obtained in the LPO position (Fig. 3–1G), and then the patient is turned further toward the stomach for a double contrast view of the descending duodenum in the prone or slightly LAO position (Fig. 3–1H).

J.   The table is brought to the semiupright position, and the patient is turned to the right for an en face view of the lesser curvature (Fig. 3–1I). He is turned further until the barium runs out of the fundus, and then returned slightly back to the left for an RPO (right posterior oblique) view of the fundus, cardia, and high lesser curve en face (Fig. 3–1J).

K.   The table is brought to the upright position. An upright spot film, slightly LPO, shows the lesser curve with double contrast view of the fundus (Fig. 3–1K). At this time, compression fluoroscopy is also performed.

*Positions labeled with respect to the table top.

Text continued on page 72

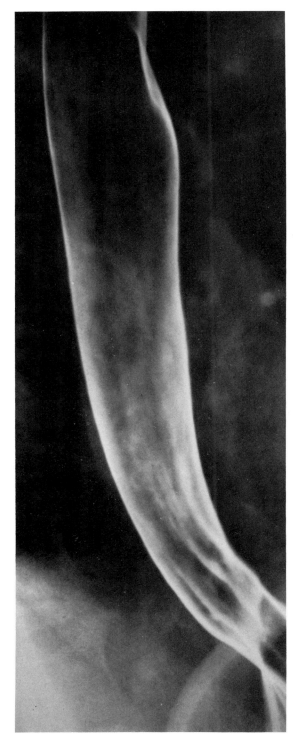

A

FIGURE 3–1 Normal routine series.

 A. Upright, double contrast of the esophagus, slightly LPO.

 B. Barium-filled esophagus, prone RAO.

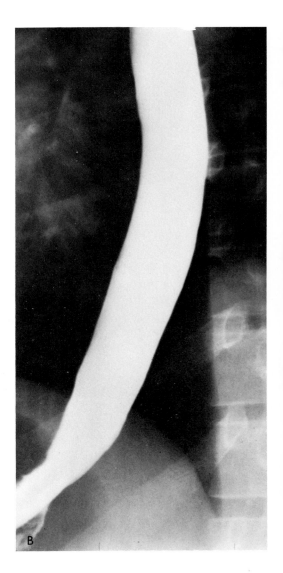

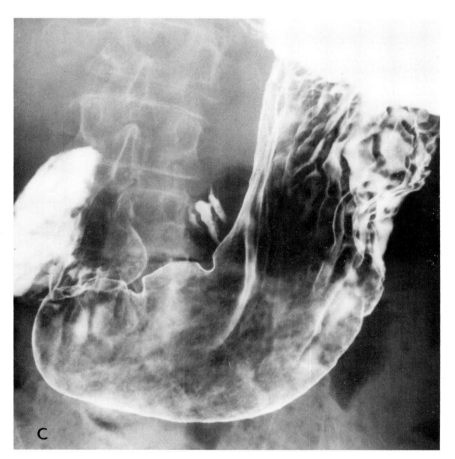

C. Supine view.

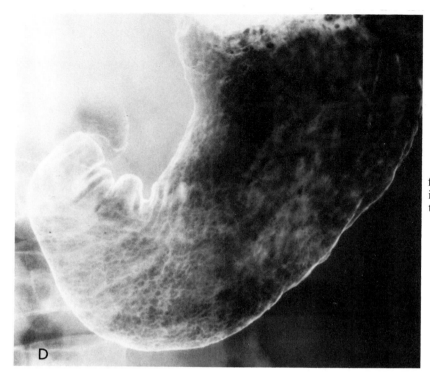

D. LPO. Note the fine, reticular appearance in the antrum representing the areae gastricae.

E. Right lateral view.

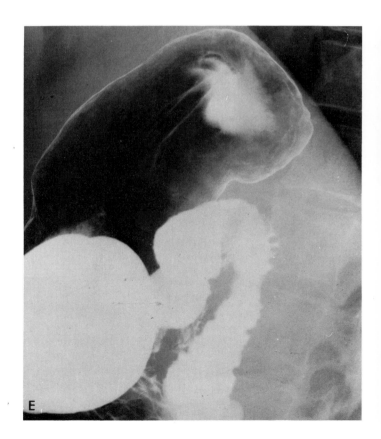

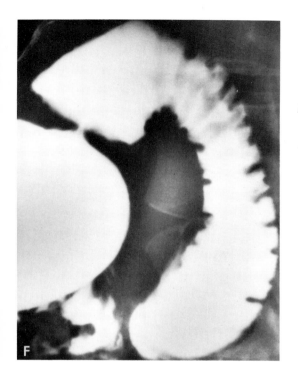

F. Barium-filled duodenum, RAO.

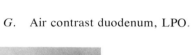

G. Air contrast duodenum, LPO.

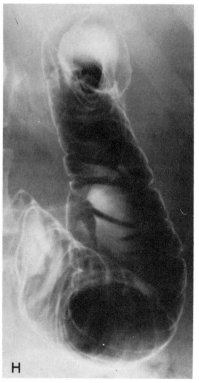

H. Descending duodenum, semi-prone LAO.

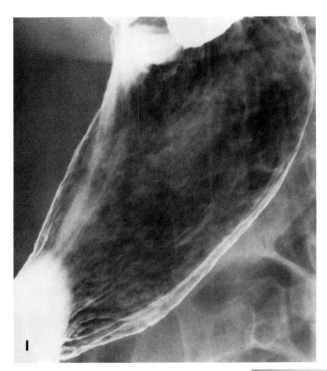

I. Slight RPO, en face view of lesser curvature of body.

J. Steep RPO, en face view of high lesser curvature, cardia, and fundus. (*From* Glass, G. B. J. (ed.): Progress in Gastroenterology. New York, Grune & Stratton, 1977.[45] Reproduced by permission.)

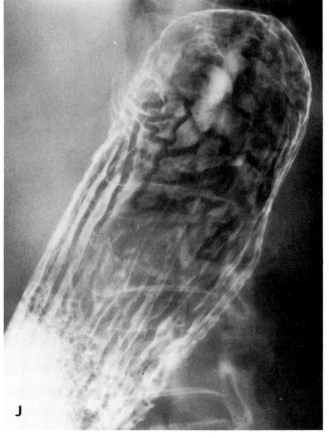

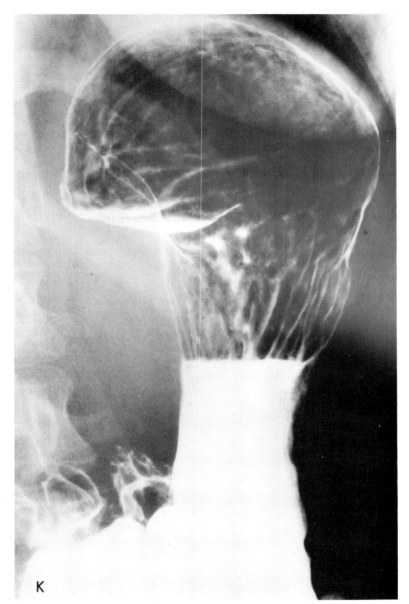

K. Upright, slightly LPO. (*From:* Laufer, I.: Radiology., *117*:513, 1975.[9] Reproduced by permission.)

TABLE 3–2 SUMMARY OF FILMING SEQUENCE

View	Purpose
Upright, LPO	Double contrast, esophagus
Prone, RAO	Barium-filled esophagus
Supine	Double contrast, distal half of stomach
LPO	Double contrast, distal stomach and pylorus
Right lateral	Double contrast, fundus, retrogastric area, barium-filled duodenum
LPO and prone	Double contrast, duodenum
RPO	Lesser curve, en face
RPO, Steeper	Cardia and fundus
Semi-upright, RPO	Fundus, cardia, high lesser curve
Upright, LPO	Lesser curve, double contrast fundus, compression study

The filming sequence and the purpose of each film are summarized in Table 3–2. The examination takes a total of 5 to 6 minutes, with 2 to 3 minutes of fluoroscopy. Ten spot films are used, and no overhead views are taken routinely. If a detailed study of the esophagus is necessary, it is performed at the end of the examination.

Variations

It should be noted that a double contrast study of the anterior wall of the stomach is not included routinely. Although such a study is probably worthwhile in Japan, where the incidence of gastric carcinoma is high, it has been demonstrated by Goldsmith and colleagues[43] that the routine double contrast study of the anterior wall of the stomach has a very low yield. In a consecutive series of 1500 cases they found 105 gastric ulcers, and only 4 of these were on the anterior wall. Only two ulcers could be seen exclusively on anterior wall views. All eleven carcinomas in their series were detectable on posterior wall views. Therefore, we recommend that the double contrast study of the anterior wall be performed on those patients either with suspicious findings on the routine study or with a very high index of suspicion of a gastric lesion.

Double contrast views of the anterior wall should be obtained with a small volume of barium (40 to 50 ml). With the patient in the prone position there will be a thin layer of barium along the anterior surface of the stomach, and the rugal pattern of the anterior wall can be seen (Fig. 3–2A). Double contrast views of the anterior wall of the antrum are obtained by tilting the table head-down while the patient raises his right side to allow barium to drain into the body and fundus (Fig. 3–2B). Double contrast views of the anterior wall of the body and fundus are obtained by elevating the head of the table until the area in question is distended with gas (Fig. 3–2C). A profile view of the anterior wall can be obtained by turning the patient into the left lateral position (Fig. 3–2D). In this position a good view of the duodenum is frequently obtained through the gas-filled stomach. On rare occasions we have used a horizontal beam with the patient supine in order to show the anterior wall.

Anterior wall views of the duodenum may also be helpful. Starting in the LPO position for double contrast views of the duodenum, the patient turns onto the left side into the prone position. This will cause barium to coat the anterior surface of the duodenum, and gas will be trapped in the descending duodenum. An inflatable balloon or pad may be used to displace the barium-filled antrum if it overlaps the duodenum. Only in this position can the minor duodenal papilla (orifice of the duct of Santorini) be identified, since it is an anterior wall structure (Chapter 9).

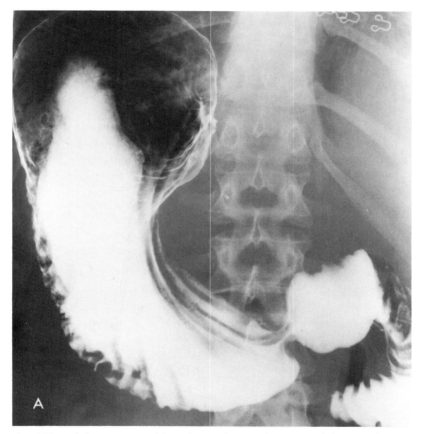

A. Film of the prone position shows the rugal pattern of the anterior wall.

FIGURE 3–2 Examination of the anterior wall.

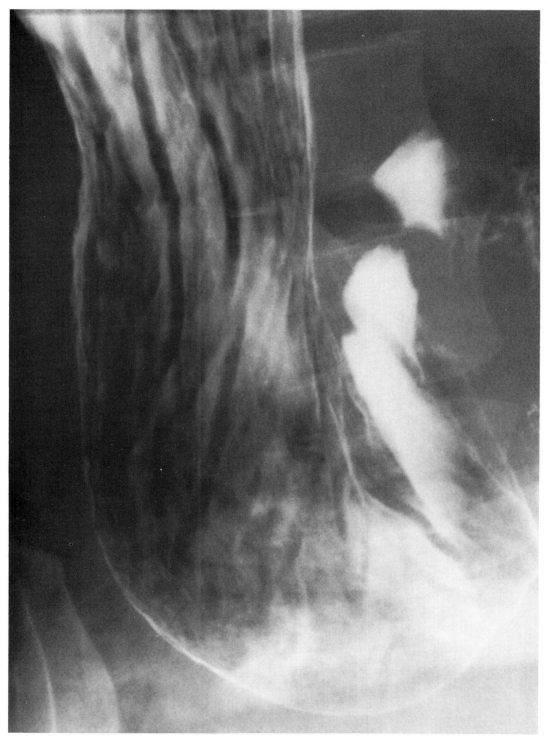

B.   Double contrast. Anterior wall of the antrum and body, LAO, with table tilted 20 to 30 degrees head down.

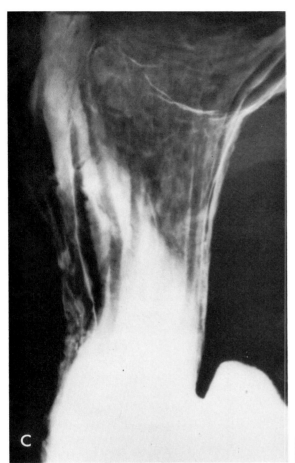

C. Double contrast. Body of the stomach.

D. Profile view of the anterior wall of the antrum in the left lateral position. Note also the good demonstration of the pylorus and duodenum in this projection.

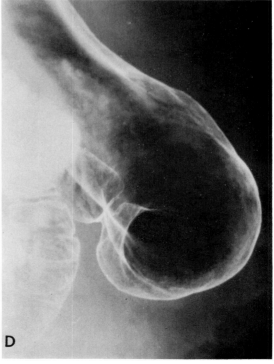

REFERENCES

1. Miller, R. E.: The air contrast stomach examination: An overview. Radiology, *117*:743, 1975.
2. Saxton, H. M.: Radiology now: Starting the double contrast barium meal. Br. J. Radiol. *50*:610, 1977.
3. James, W. B., McCreath, G., Sutherland, G. R., et al.: Double contrast barium meal examination — a comparison of techniques for introducing gas. Clin. Radiol., *27*:99, 1976.
4. Shirakabe, H.: Double Contrast Studies of the Stomach. Stuttgart, Georg Thieme Verlag, 1972.
5. Solanke, T. F., Kumakura, K., Maruyama, M., et al.: Double-contrast method for the evaluation of gastric lesions. Gut, *10*:436, 1969.
6. Kawai, K., Takada, H., Takekoshi, T., et al.: Double contrast radiograph on routine examination of the stomach. Am. J. Gastroenterol., *53*:147, 1970.
7. Hunt, J. H., and Anderson, I.F.: Double contrast upper gastrointestinal studies. Clin. Radiol., *27*:87, 1976.
8. Kreel, L., Herlinger, H., and Glanville, J.: Technique of the double contrast barium meal with examples of correlation with endoscopy. Clin. Radiol., *24*:307, 1973.
9. Laufer, I.: A simple method for routine double contrast study of the upper gastrointestinal tract. Radiology, *117*:513, 1975.
10. Goldstein, H. M.: Double contrast gastrography. Am J. Dig. Dis., *21*:797, 1976.
11. O'Reilly, G. V. A., and Bryan, G.: Double contrast barium meal — a simplification. Br. J. Radiol., *47*:482, 1974.
12. Pochaczevski, R.: Bubbly barium: A carbonated cocktail for double contrast examinations of the stomach. Radiology, *107*:461, 1973.
13. Op den Orth, J. O., and Ploem, S.: The standard biphasic-contrast gastric series. Radiology, *122*:530, 1977.
14. Ziervogel, M. A., McCreath, G. T., Weir, R., et al.: A comparison of two barium sulfate preparations — Baritop 100 and Micropaque. Clin. Radiol. *24*:302, 1973.
15. Scott-Harden, W. G.: Radiological investigation of peptic ulcer. Br. J. Hosp. Med., *10*:149, 1970.
16. Scott-Harden, W. G.: Evaluation of double contrast gastro-duodenal radiology. Br. J. Radiol., *46*:153, 1973.
17. Mohammed, S. H., and Hegedüs, V.: Double contrast examination of the stomach. Acta Radiol., *18*:249, 1976.
18. Amplatz, K.: A new and simple approach to air-contrast studies of the stomach and duodenum. Radiology, *70*:392, 1958.
19. Obata, W. G.: A double contrast technique for examination of the stomach using barium sulfate with simethicone. Am. J. Roentgenol., *115*:275, 1972.
20. Bagnall, R. D., Galloway, R. W., and Annis, J. A. D. : Double contrast preparations: an in vitro study of some antifoaming agents. Br. J. Radiol., *50*:546, 1977.
21. Cumberland, D. C.: Optimum viscosity of barium suspension for use in the double contrast barium meal. Gastrointest. Radiol., *2*:169, 1977.
22. Laufer, I., and Stein, G. E.: The physico-chemical properties of barium suspensions used in double contrast studies of the stomach. Paper presented at the annual meeting of the Association of University Radiologists. Kansas City, May 1977.
23. Roberts, G. M., Roberts, E. E., Davies, R. L., et al.: Observations on the behaviour of barium sulphate suspensions in gastric secretion. Br. J. Radiol., *50*:468, 1977.
24. Roberts, G. M., Roberts, E. E., Davies, R. L., et al.: In vivo and in vitro assessment of barium sulphate. Br. J. Radiol., *50*:541, 1977.
25. Kreel, L., Herlinger, H., Sandin, B., et al.: A technique for the in vitro testing of barium preparations. Radiography, *40*:51, 1974.
26. Gelfand, D. W.: High density, low viscosity barium for fine mucosal detail on double-contrast upper gastrointestinal examinations. Am. J. Roentgenol., *130*:831, 1978.
27. Goldberg, H. I., Dodds, W. J., and Genis, E. H.: Experimental esophagitis: Findings after insufflation of tantalum powder. Am. J. Roentgenol., *110*:228, 1970.
28. Dodds, W. J., Goldberg, H. I., Kohatsu, S., et al.: Insufflation of tantalum powder into the stomach. Invest. Radiol., *5*:30, 1970.
29. Heitz, F., Weber, A., Rosinsky, Th., et al.: Application du titanate de baryum à la mucographie gastrique. J. Radiol., Electrol Med. Nucl., *55*:169, 1974.
30. Kreel, L.: The use of oral metoclopramide in the barium meal and follow-through examination. Br. J. Radiol. *43*:31, 1970.
31. Gelfand, D. W., and Hachiya, J.: The double contrast examination of the stomach using gas-producing granules and tablets. Radiology, *93*:1381, 1969.
32. Merlo, R. B., Stone, M., Baugus, P., et al.: The use of Pro-Banthine to induce gastrointestinal hypotonia. Radiology, *127*:61, 1978.

33. Kreel, L.: Pharmaco-radiology in barium examinations with special reference to glucagon. Br. J. Radiol., *48*:691, 1975.
34. Miller, R. E., Chernish, S. M., Skucas, J., et al.: Hypotonic roentgenography with glucagon. Am. J. Roentgenol., *121*:264, 1974.
35. Gelfand, D. W.: The double contrast upper gastrointestinal examination in the Japanese-style. An experience with 2000 examinations. Am. J. Gastroenterol., *63*:216, 1975.
36. Gelfand, D. W.: The Japanese-style double contrast examination of the stomach. Gastrointest. Radiol., *1*:7, 1976.
37. Miller, R. E., Chernish, S. M., Brunelle, R. L., et al.: Dose response to intramuscular glucagon during hypotonic radiography. Radiology, *127*:49, 1978.
38. Miller, R. E., Chernish, S. M., Brunelle, R. L., et al.: Double-blind radiographic study of dose response to intravenous glucagon for hypotonic duodenography. Radiology, *127*:55, 1978.
39. Liu, C.: Visualization of esophageal varices by Buscopan. Am. J. Roentgenol., *121*:232, 1974.
40. Novak, D.: Hypotonic esophagography using propantheline bromide. Forstschr. Rontgenstr., *123*:409, 1975.
41. Hogan, W. J., Dodds, W. J., Hoke, S. E., et al.: Effect of glucagon on esophageal motor function. Gastroenterology, *69*:160, 1975.
42. Laufer, I., Mullens, J. E., and Hamilton, J.: The diagnostic accuracy of barium studies of the stomach and duodenum — correlation with endoscopy. Radiology, *115*:569, 1975.
43. Goldsmith, M. R., Paul, R. E., Jr., Poplack, W. E., et al.: Evaluation of routine double contrast views of the anterior wall of the stomach. Am. J. Roentgenol., *126*:1159, 1976.
44. Mackintosh, C. E., and Kreel, L.: Anatomy and radiology of the areae gastricae. Gut, *18*:855, 1977.
45. Laufer, I.: Double contrast radiology in the diagnosis of gastrointestinal cancer. *In*: Glass, G. B. J. (ed.): Progress in Gastroenterology. Vol. 3., New York, Grune & Stratton, 1977, pp. 643–669.

4

ESOPHAGUS

TECHNIQUE

NORMAL APPEARANCES

ARTIFACTS

INFLAMMATORY DISORDERS
    Peptic Esophagitis
    Infections
        Monilial Esophagitis
        Viral Esophagitis
    Other Types of Esophagitis
    Differential Diagnosis of Esophagitis

TECHNIQUE

We obtain our routine double contrast films of the esophagus at the beginning of the examination. The patient is upright and slightly LPO. Immediately after ingesting the effervescent agent, he gulps the high density barium suspension. The degree of obliquity is just sufficient to project the esophagus free of the spine. Spot films in rapid succession of the upper and lower esophagus (Fig. 4–1*A* and *B*) will frequently provide excellent double contrast views of the distended esophagus. After the patient takes two swallows of barium we proceed to examine the esophagus in the prone oblique projection. Even in this position, double contrast views of the esophagus can be obtained, particularly if the lower esophageal sphincter is incompetent (Fig. 4–2). If these simple maneuvers are not sufficient to produce satisfactory double contrast views, we complete the examination of the stomach and duodenum and return to the esophageal examination at the end of the study. At that time several maneuvers may be attempted to improve the quality of the esophageal examination. The patient may be asked to pinch his nose with his right hand while gulping barium. An additional dose of effervescent agent can be given, followed immediately by the barium suspension.[1, 2] Skucas[3] has stressed the value of administering separate acidic and basic solutions in the form of Seidlitz (PurePac Pharmaceutical Co., Elizabeth, N. J.). This starts to effervesce in the esophagus, and when followed immediately by the barium, good double contrast views can be obtained. Simethicone should be added to the acid solution to prevent bubble formation.

Goldstein and Dodd[4] have suggested a modification of the technique described by Brombart.[5] The patient swallows a mouthful of barium and immediately thereafter a mouthful of water or mineral oil. The barium will coat the mucosa, and the translucent fluid will distend the esophagus. In order for this procedure to be successful a barium suspension with higher viscosity should be used, and it appears that the best results have been obtained with Lafayette HD-85, a barium suspension intended primarily for double contrast colon examinations. A similar procedure has been described by Wiljasslo.[6]

If these maneuvers are not successful, excellent double contrast views can be obtained by direct injection of barium and air through a tube in the esophagus.[7] Paralysis of the esophagus by a relaxant drug will further facilitate the examination. As mentioned in Chaper 3, Buscopan and Pro-Banthine are both effective in abolishing esophageal peristalsis.[8] In Japan another drug, Coliopan (Eisai Co, Ltd., Bunkyo-ku, Tokyo), is available. This is also an anticholinergic agent which produces very effective relaxation throughout the GI tract with minimal side effects. Hogan and coworkers[9] have shown that glucagon relaxes the lower esophageal sphincter, but does not affect esophageal peristalsis. Therefore, this drug cannot be used to induce esophageal relaxation.

Most of the recent work on double contrast esophagography has employed high density barium sulfate suspensions. Heitz and colleagues[10] have worked with barium titanate and found that it adheres well to esophageal mucosa, although formal double contrast studies have not been attempted. Experimental work has also been done with tantalum powder and tantalum paste for esophagography.[11, 12] Tantalum has the desirable properties of radiodensity, adherence to mucosa, and nontoxicity. Excellent double contrast views have been obtained in normal cats and in cats with experimentally induced esophagitis.[13] Unfortunately, the tantalum must be deposited as an aerosol through a tube, and it has been difficult to obtain consistently uniform coating in humans.

Double contrast views of the esophagus can be obtained easily in most patients who are able to stand and swallow the effervescent agent and the barium. With patients unable to stand, one may have to resort to techniques involving esophageal intubation. In the presence of a tight esophageal stricture it may not be possible to get double contrast views unless gas is regurgitated from the stomach into the esophagus.

NORMAL APPEARANCES

The fully distended normal esophagus has a completely flattened, smooth mucosal surface both en face and in profile (Fig. 4–1). At the distal end a typical "arch-shaped shadow" is seen at the junction of the esophagus and the stomach (Fig. 4–1B). In the cervical esophagus a small indentation is frequently seen on the anterior wall. This is believed to represent a venous plexus[15] (Fig. 4–3) and should not be mistaken for an esophageal web (Fig. 4–4). In the middle third of the esophagus, typical indentations due to the aortic arch and left main bronchus may be seen

(Fig. 4–5). In patients with a small hiatal hernia one may see an irregular line, representing the transition between gastric and esophageal mucosa. This is almost certainly the squamocolumnar junction, or "Z line" (Fig. 4–6).

As the esophagus collapses the mucosal folds become visible as longitudinal, exquisitely straight and narrow folds (Fig. 4–7). In some patients we have seen transverse folds, usually in the midesophagus (Fig. 4–8).[16] This finding has been described as a normal feature of the feline esophagus,[11] and we believe that it is also a normal feature of the human esophagus, probably caused by contraction of the muscularis mucosae, which runs in a longitudinal band. Therefore, as it contracts it could throw the mucosa into thin transverse folds which may resemble a herringbone pattern. In some patients these transverse folds are seen transiently during gastroesophageal reflux and disappear moments later (Fig. 4–9). Most patients who have had endoscopy have not shown definite evidence of esophagitis. However, it is possible that contraction of the muscularis mucosae could represent the earliest stage of a motor abnormality in the esophagus, which might be idiopathic or a response to mild esophagitis. In the barium-filled esophagus these transverse folds may produce fine marginal irregularities which should not be mistaken for diffuse superficial ulceration. These thin, delicate, transverse folds should also be distinguished from the broad transverse bands seen in patients with diffuse esophageal spasm or tertiary contractions (Fig. 4–10).

Text continued on page 87

FIGURE 4–1 Normal esophagus, upright.

A. Normal appearance of the thoracic esophagus. Note that the esophageal contour is very smooth and the mucosal folds have been totally effaced.

B. The distal esophagus and typical arch-shaped configuration at the gastroesophageal angle (*arrow*).

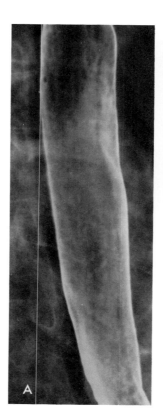
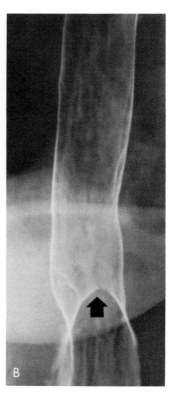

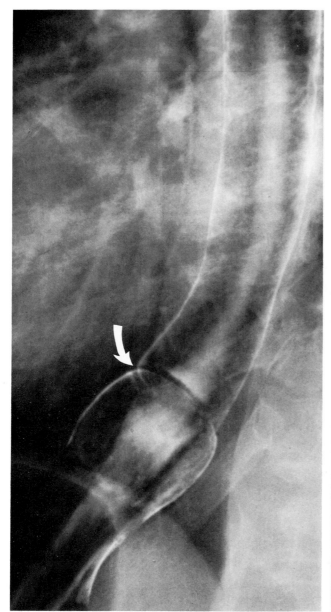

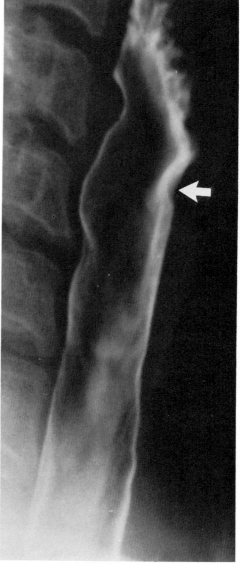

FIGURE 4–2 Prone oblique position. Double contrast view of the hiatus hernia, lower esophageal ring (*arrow*), and esophagus.

FIGURE 4–3 Normal cervical esophagus with venous indentation (*arrow*). There is slight posterior impression as well from a cervical osteophyte.

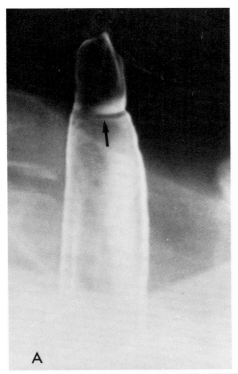

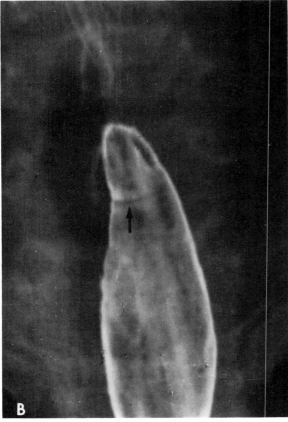

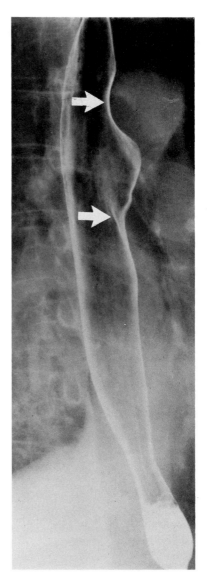

FIGURE 4–5 Normal impressions due to the aortic arch and left main bronchus.

FIGURE 4–4 *A* and *B* Cervical esophageal web seen in the lateral (*A*) and frontal (*B*) projections.

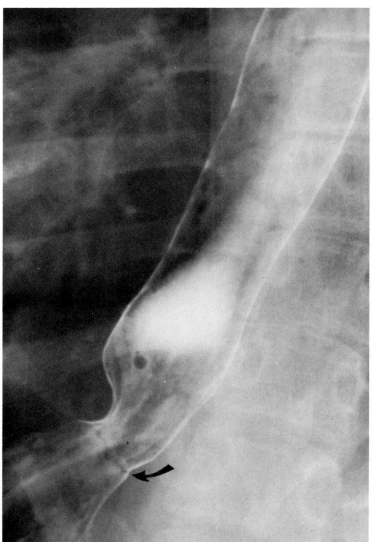

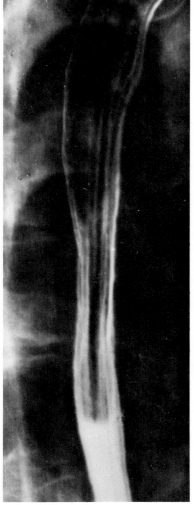

FIGURE 4–6 Zigzag radiolucent line (*arrow*), probably representing the squamocolumnar junction.

FIGURE 4–7 Normal longitudinal folds in a partially collapsed esophagus.

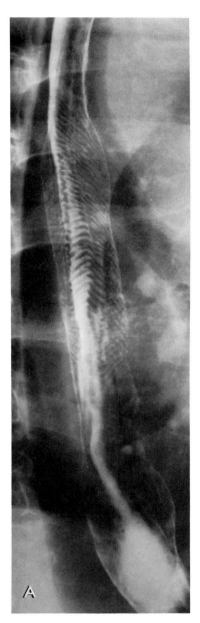

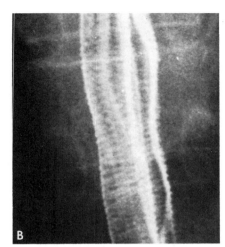

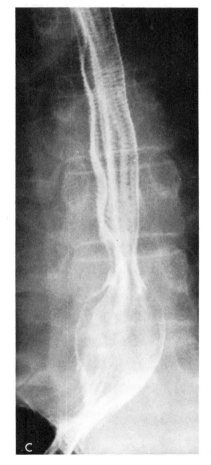

FIGURE 4–8 *A to C* Three examples of transverse folds in the esophagus. These folds are thought to be due to contraction of the muscularis mucosae. (*From*: Gohel, V. K., Edell, S. M., and Laufer, I.: Radiology, *128*:303, 1978.[16] Reproduced by permission.)

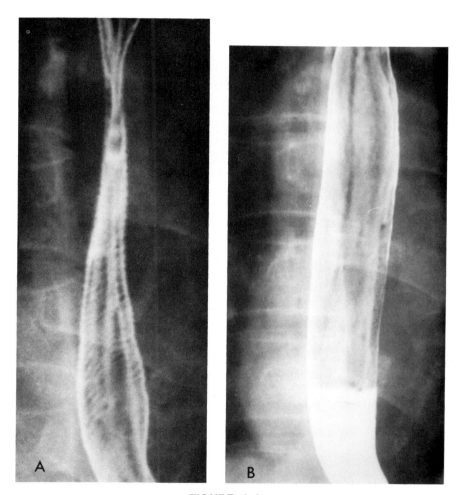

FIGURE 4–9

A. Transverse folds in the mid- and distal esophagus.
B. Moments later the folds are no longer seen.

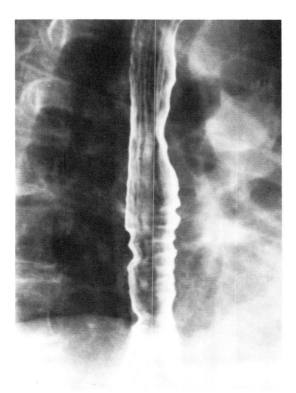

FIGURE 4–10   Transverse bands due to contraction of the muscularis propria. These bands are thicker than the transverse folds in Figures 4–8 and 4–9.

ARTIFACTS

Double contrast studies of the esophagus may produce several artifacts that may simulate disease.[17]

1. *Localized noncoating* of a segment of the esophagus may suggest the presence of a tumor (Fig. 4–11*A*). However, with additional barium the apparent abnormality disappears (Fig. 4–11*B*).

2. *Undissolved effervescent agent* may be seen transiently in the normal esophagus (Fig. 4–12), or more persistently in the presence of esophageal obstruction. This appearance should not be mistaken for the nodular mucosa of monilial esophagitis (Fig. 4–44*B*).

3. *Gas bubbles* are usually easily recognized. However, occasionally the bubbles are small and diffusely distributed (Fig. 4–13), and may simulate tiny mucosal nodules, as seen in moniliasis (Fig. 4–35), or superficial spreading carcinoma (Fig. 5–11).

4. *Barium precipitates may be seen as small white dots on the mucosal surface* (Fig. 4–14). These can be distinguished from erosions by the absence of edema, marginal irregularities, or associated motor abnormalities. This problem can be avoided by choosing a suitable barium suspension that is known not to precipitate at the high concentrations used in double contrast studies and by insuring that the suspension is prepared accurately and suspended thoroughly.

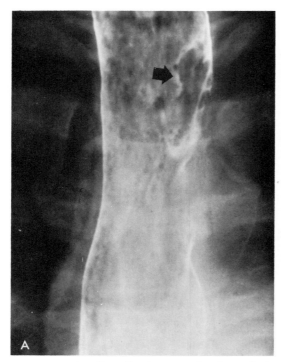

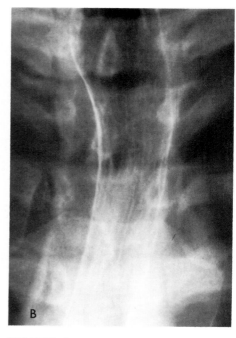

FIGURE 4–11

A. Localized noncoating (*arrow*) simulating carcinoma.
B. Further study with improved coating shows that the area is normal.

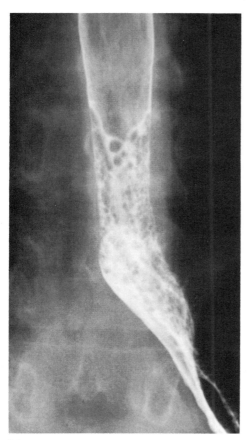

FIGURE 4–12 Undissolved effervescent granules in the distal esophagus.

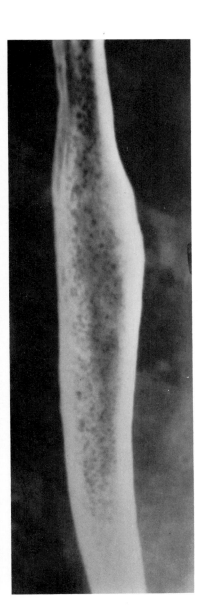

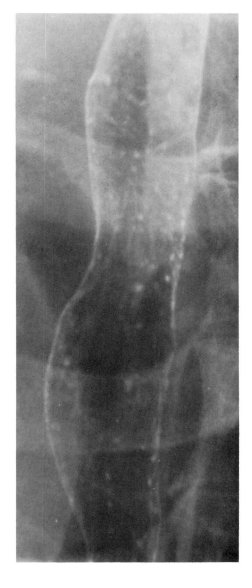

FIGURE 4–13 Gas bubbles throughout the esophagus simulating diffuse mucosal nodularity.

FIGURE 4–14 Barium precipitation.

INFLAMMATORY DISORDERS

Peptic Esophagitis

Peptic esophagitis secondary to gastroesophageal reflux is by far the most common inflammatory condition in the esophagus. Although the conventional barium swallow may show a hiatal hernia and gastroesophageal reflux, it is believed that this study does not permit an accurate assessment of esophageal mucosa for the presence of esophagitis.[18] It is generally conceded that the early morphologic changes of esophagitis are not demonstrable radiologically.[19] For this reason, the acid barium swallow was developed in an attempt to induce functional disturbances by allowing acid to come in contact with inflamed esophageal mucosa.[20, 21] The early radiographic signs of esophagitis include thickening of esophageal folds, limitation of distensibility, irregularity of the esophageal margin, and disturbance of motility. However, these findings are difficult to evaluate and are frequently found only in patients with severe disease. In many cases of esophagitis, the barium swallow either is normal or shows only indirect evidence of esophagitis. Simeone and coworkers[22] have described several cases of severe esophagitis in which the only demonstrable abnormality was the absence of peristalsis. Even in patients with advanced changes owing to esophagitis, the barium swallow may be misleading. A deep ulcer may be overlooked if it is not projected in profile, and the length of a stricture may be overestimated if the distal segment is not fully distended.

Goldberg and colleagues[14] induced an experimental form of esophagitis in cats by the infusion of acid and pepsin into the esophagus. They were able to obtain a double contrast effect by insufflation of tantalum. This technique enabled them to demonstrate some of the subtle abnormalities in the early stages of esophagitis, such as widening of the longitudinal folds, minor irregularities of contour, segmental narrowing, and ulceration. Barium esophagrams in these cats failed to demonstrate most of these changes. In some cases only luminal narrowing was demonstrated.

Most patients with reflux esophagitis have an associated sliding hiatal hernia. The double contrast method can show the hernia and associated rings (Fig. 4–15). It is likely that the gastric distension produced by the gas is a provocative factor in the production of hiatal hernias. In any case, these are not considered to be significant in the absence of either gastroesophageal reflux or evidence of esophagitis.

Several authors have noted that prominent folds around the cardia and within a hiatal hernia may be an indication of gastroesophageal reflux.[3, 23] In particular, Bleshman and coworkers[23] have noted that there is frequently a prominent mucosal fold extending to the gastroesophageal junction, with a polypoid protuberance at its end. We have also seen this appearance several times in patients with symptoms of gastroesophageal reflux. This polypoid fold may be seen either in the hernial sac (Fig. 4–16A) or in the stomach when the hernia is reduced (Fig. 4–16B).

The double contrast method allows for detailed examination of the esophageal mucosa. The mucosal changes of early reflux esophagitis can be detected and correspond closely to the endoscopic features. Several authors have described the endoscopic staging of reflux esophagitis.[18, 24, 25]

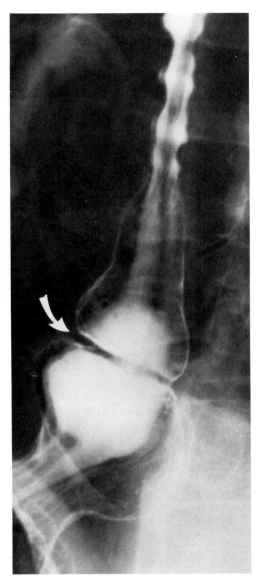

FIGURE 4–15 Hiatal hernia, lower esophageal ring (*arrow*), and tertiary contractions in the esophagus. Prone position.

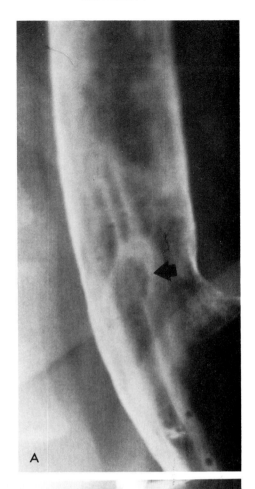

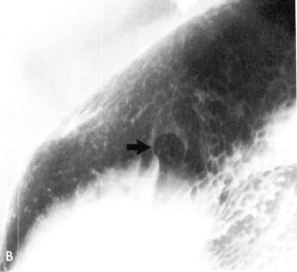

FIGURE 4–16 Polypoid esophagogastric fold and reflux esophagitis.

A. There is a prominent gastric mucosal fold extending into the distal esophagus. The tip of the fold has a polypoid protuberance (*arrow*).

B. With the esophagus collapsed the polypoid fold is seen within the stomach (*arrow*).

The earliest form of esophagitis that can be recognized with confidence consists of superficial ulceration or erosion, usually extending proximally from the gastroesophageal junction. These can be recognized radiographically as streaks or dots of barium seen against the flat mucosa in the region of the gastroesophageal junction or distal esophagus (Figs. 4–17 to 4–19). They are easiest to detect en face, but occasionally they may be seen in profile (Fig. 4–18). Frequently the superficial ulcers have a linear configuration, and there may be fine radiating folds with slight retraction of the wall of the esophagus (Fig. 4–19). In some patients this superficial erosive esophagitis may become quite widespread and extend into the midesophagus (Fig. 4–20). With healing of the superficial ulcers, endoscopy may show small white nodular areas on the mucosa, representing scarring. Radiographically this finding may be manifest as localized eccentric areas of diminished distensibility (Figs. 4–21 and 4–22). In some patients a distortion of the normal transverse fold pattern can be seen, as illustrated in Figure 4–23. The interruption of the folds is due to ulceration with scarring. There is also decreased distensibility of the distal esophagus, with superficial ulceration. With chronic disease, the mucosa may become finely nodular (Fig. 4–24) and with more extensive involvement a coarse granular appearance (Fig. 4–25) is seen, similar to that of the colon in chronic ulcerative colitis.

With further progression in the severity of the disease, deeper ulcers may develop (Figs. 4–25 to 4–27, Plate 6). These ulcers are frequently found in relation to a columnar-lined or Barrett's esophagus, although the ulcer may be found in either gastric or esophageal mucosa.[26] Even these deeper ulcers may have a linear appearance (Fig. 4–28, Plate 7). Healing of these ulcers may result in a peptic stricture which typically will demonstrate tapered margins and a smooth mucosal surface (Fig. 4–29). In other patients scarring results in the formation of multiple outpouchings in the region of the gastroesophageal junction (Fig. 4–30). These severe changes of reflux esophagitis are particularly likely to develop in patients with scleroderma involving the esophagus. Incompetence of the lower esophageal sphincter results in gastroesophageal reflux. Because of the poor esophageal motility the refluxed acid has a prolonged contact time with esophageal mucosa, resulting in severe reflux esophagitis (Fig. 4–31). The late changes in scleroderma involving the esophagus are due to smooth muscle atrophy and severe reflux esophagitis with stricture. This condition can usually be distinguished from achalasia by the presence of a hiatal hernia in scleroderma and its absence in patients with achalasia.

Barrett's esophagus should be suspected in any patient presenting with an esophageal stricture or ulcer.[27] In most cases there will be evidence of a stricture as well as ulceration (Fig. 4–32). However, in some cases only a smooth tapered stricture will be seen (Fig. 4–33). It is likely that Barrett's esophagus is a premalignant condition, with an increased incidence of adenocarcinoma in the columnar-lined esophagus (Fig. 4–34).[28]

Text continued on page 106

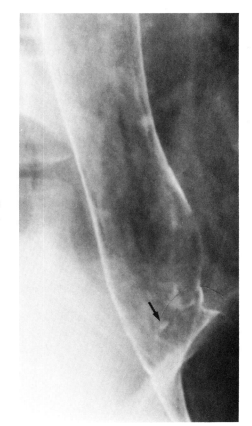

FIGURE 4–17 Superficial ulcer in the distal esophagus (*arrow*) due to reflux esophagitis. Confirmed by endoscopy. (Courtesy of Marc P. Banner, M.D., Philadelphia.)

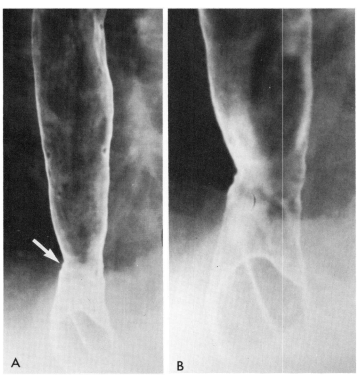

A

B

FIGURE 4–18 *A* and *B* Profile view of a shallow ulcer (*arrow*) just above the gastroesophageal junction. Note the associated slight narrowing and retraction due to scarring. Endoscopic proof.

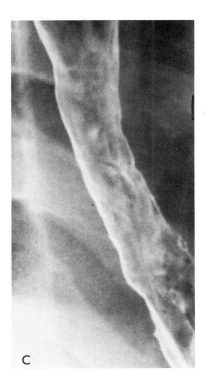

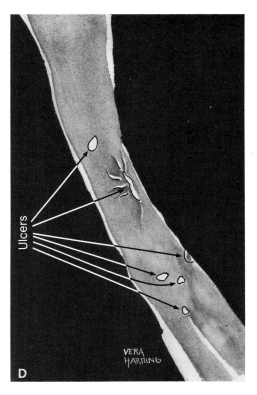

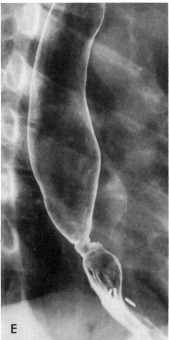

FIGURE 4–18 *C* and *D* Young man with heartburn and hematemesis. There are multiple superficial ulcers in the mid- and distal esophagus *(arrows)*. See also Plate 5.

E. Following antireflux surgery there is a recurrent hernia and a stricture at the gastroesophageal junction. The erosive esophagitis has healed.

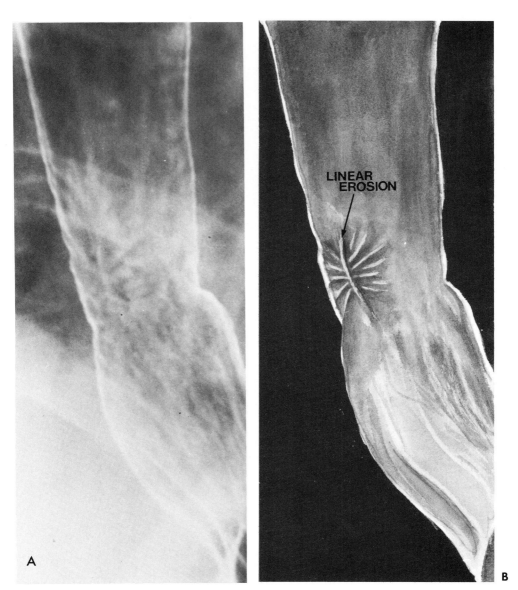

FIGURE 4–19 *A* and *B*   Linear erosion in the distal esophagus with retraction and radiating folds. Endoscopic proof. (Courtesy of Marc P. Banner, M.D., Philadelphia.)

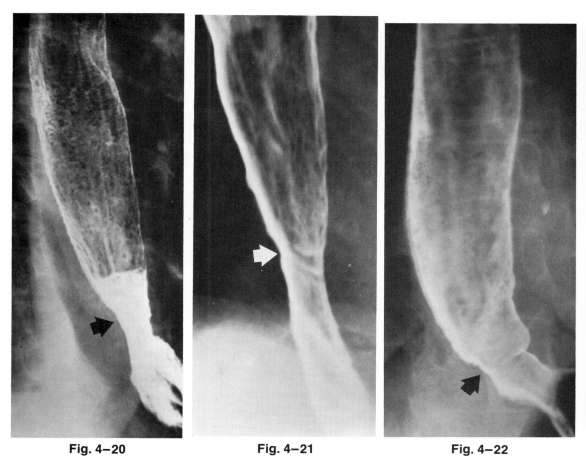

Fig. 4–20   Fig. 4–21   Fig. 4–22

FIGURE 4–20 Diffuse superficial ulceration in the esophagus with slight narrowing at the gastroesophageal junction (*arrow*). (Courtesy of Henry I. Goldberg, M.D., San Francisco.)

FIGURE 4–21 Narrowing of the distal esophagus due to scarring from reflux esophagitis (*arrow*).

FIGURE 4–22 Asymmetric flattening due to scarring (*arrow*).

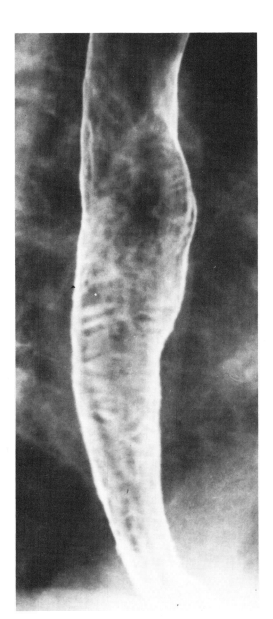 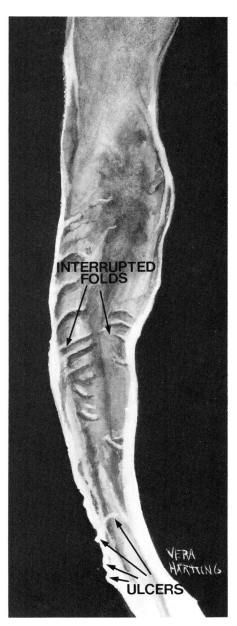

FIGURE 4–23 Chronic reflux esophagitis. There is moderate narrowing of the distal esophagus, with superficial ulceration along the right lateral wall. More proximal to this there are many abnormal, interrupted folds owing to mucosal scarring and superficial ulceration.

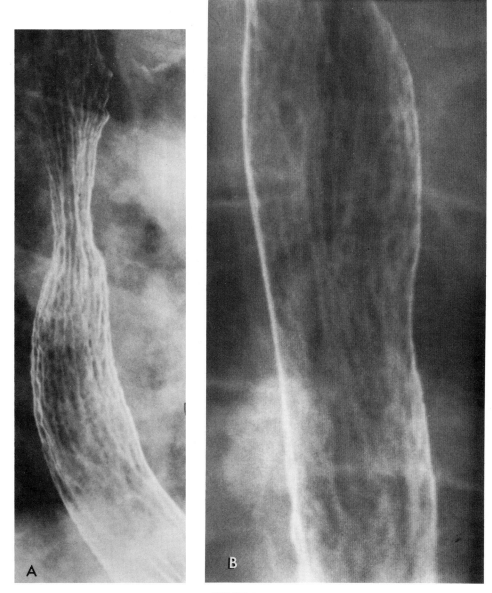

FIGURE 4–24

A. Mucosal granularity due to chronic reflux esophagitis.
B. Fine mucosal nodularity due to reflux esophagitis.

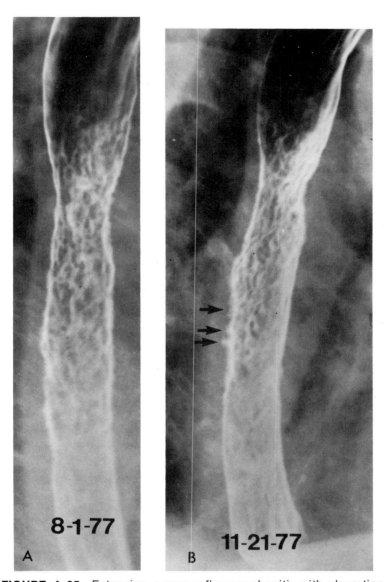

FIGURE 4–25 Extensive, severe reflux esophagitis with ulceration.

A. There is coarse granularity of the esophageal mucosa. Although the appearance may be suggestive of moniliasis, endoscopy showed that it was due to severe gastroesophageal reflux.

B. Repeat examination 3 ½ months later showed similar findings, and in addition several small ulcers (*arrows*).

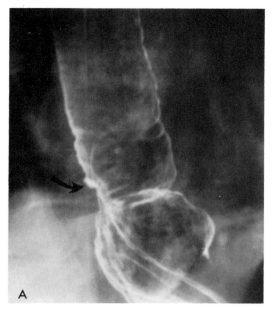

A. Seen in profile.

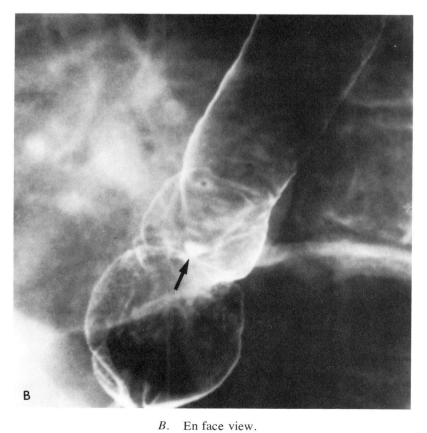

B. En face view.

FIGURE 4–26 Peptic ulcer of the esophagus. See Plate 8.

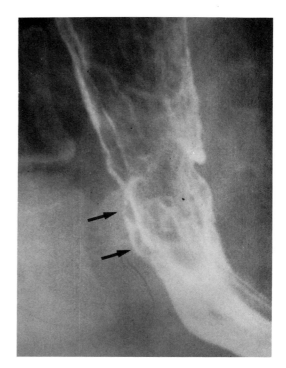

FIGURE 4–27 Broad peptic ulcer due to severe reflux esophagitis.

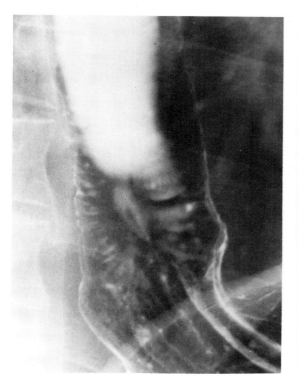

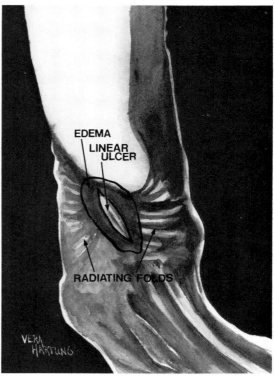

FIGURE 4–28 Linear ulcer in the distal esophagus. Note the ulcer crater, surrounding edema, and radiating folds. See also Plate 7.

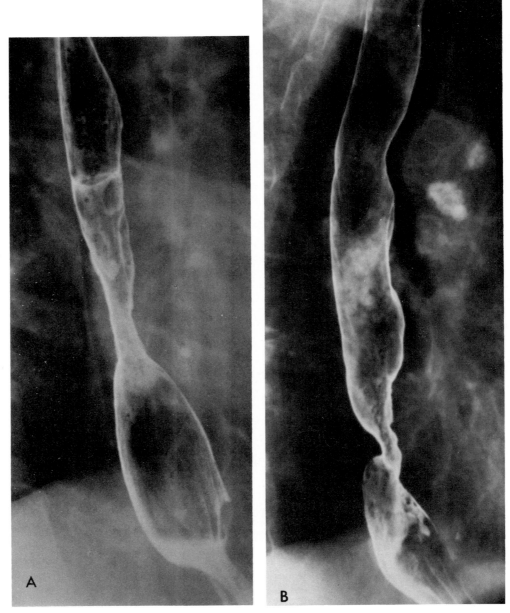

FIGURE 4–29 Stricture

A. Typical peptic esophageal stricture due to reflux.
B. Eccentric peptic stricture with ulceration due to reflux.

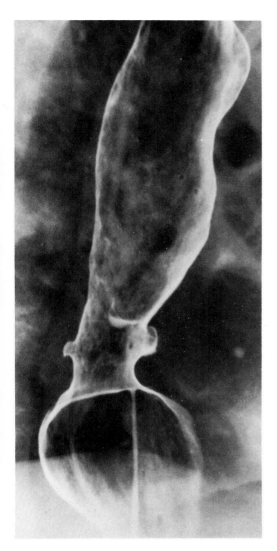

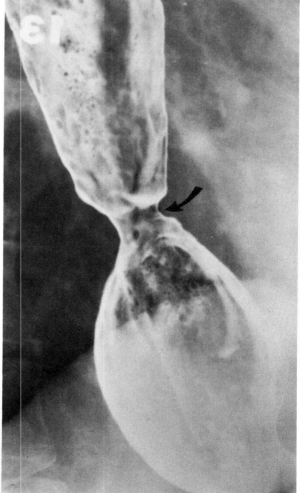

FIGURE 4–30 Sacculations of the distal esophagus due to scarring.

FIGURE 4–31 Hiatus hernia with peptic stricture (*arrow*) in a patient with scleroderma.

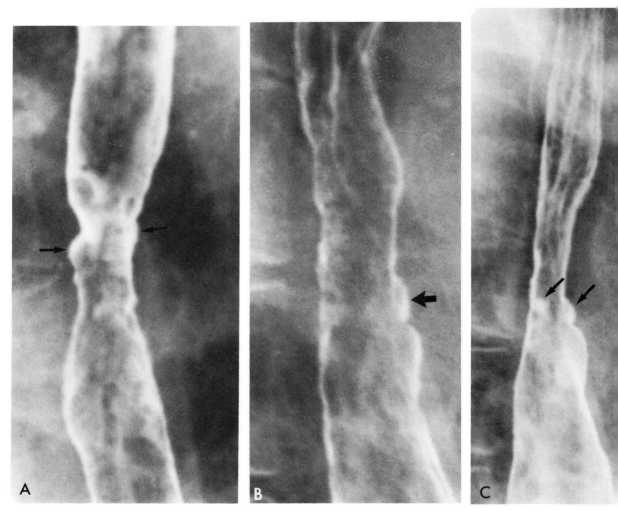

FIGURE 4–32 *A* to *C* Three examples of Barrett's esophagus with narrowing and ulceration (*arrows*). (Courtesy of Marc P. Banner, M.D., Philadelphia.)

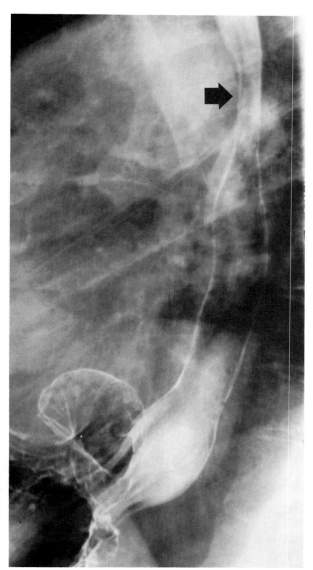

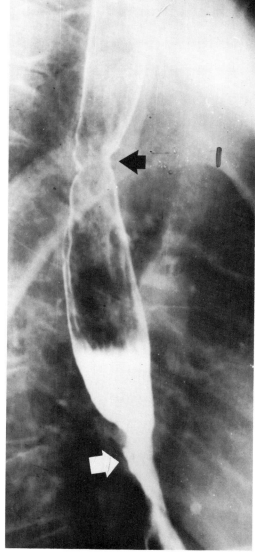

FIGURE 4–33 Barrett's esophagus with smooth stricture (*arrow*) in the upper esophagus. There had been a previous attempt at fundoplication to prevent gastroesophageal reflux. (Courtesy of Herbert Y. Kressel, M.D., Philadelphia.)

FIGURE 4–34 Adenocarcinoma and Barrett's esophagus. There is a stricture in the midesophagus (*black arrow*) as a result of Barrett's esophagus. In the distal portion of the columnar-lined esophagus there is an irregular, ulcerated area (*white arrows*) representing adenocarcinoma. (Courtesy of Robert E. Koehler, M.D., St. Louis.)

Infections

MONILIAL ESOPHAGITIS

Monilial esophagitis is by far the most common infection of the esophagus. This used to be generally considered a complication found in debilitated patients with conditions that predispose to monilial infection. These conditions include immunosuppression owing to malignant disease or chemotherapy, broad spectrum antibiotics, diabetes, and hypocalcemia.[29, 30] It was considered a rarity to find monilial esophagitis in patients with no predisposing cause.[31, 32] However, Holt[33] found that 3 of his 13 patients had no predisposing condition. A recent review by Kodsi and coworkers[34] of their endoscopic experience revealed a remarkably high incidence of monilia in the esophagus. This was found in 6 per cent of 1435 patients coming to endoscopy, although in the vast majority of cases there were only minimal manifestations of moniliasis, primarily white plaques on the mucosa. This study was also remarkable because 50 per cent of the patients with moniliasis had no symptoms referable to the esophagus, and only 12 per cent had a predisposing condition. It is therefore clear that a mild degree of monilial esophagitis is a very common condition and is not restricted to patients with predisposing illnesses.

The radiologic features of monilial esophagitis were first described by Andren and Theander,[35] and the subject has been reviewed by several authors.[31, 32, 36, 37] With moderately severe infection the mucosa has an irregular granular surface, with nodules of varying sizes representing the pseudomembrane. Cobblestoning of the mucosa may be seen in the early stages, as a result of mucosal inflammation and edema,[38] and with more extensive ulceration and pseudomembrane formation.[39] In advanced disease the mucosa has a shaggy, ulcerated appearance. Guyer[31] has reported one patient with moniliasis complicating achalasia in whom there were discrete deep esophageal ulcers.

The appearances of moniliasis on double contrast study of the esophagus correspond closely to the endoscopic and pathologic descriptions.[39, 40] In the earliest stages, tiny nodular filling defects measuring 1 to 2 mm in diameter may be seen on the esophageal mucosa (Figs. 4–35 and 4–36). These correspond to the small white plaques seen at endoscopy. In some patients these plaques have a linear orientation (Fig. 4–37). The mucosa then becomes inflamed and edematous, and a cobblestoned mucosa may be seen (Fig. 4–38)[38] Discrete shallow ulcers may develop in the inflamed mucosa (Fig. 4–39). With progression of the infection, the ulcers become covered with necrotic debris which develops into a pseudomembrane. At this time the esophageal mucosa has a coarse granular surface, similar to the colonic mucosa in chronic ulcerative colitis (Figs. 4–40 and 4–41). Motility disturbances are seen in many patients with moderately severe disease.[21, 37] With treatment of the infection, motility returns to normal.

Moniliasis may also present as polypoid lesions in the esophagus or assume other unusual appearances, such as esophageal stricture.[42] We have seen several patients with chronic or transient esophageal obstruction who developed monilial infection.[43] One of these patients had a transient paralysis of the esophagus following a Belsey antireflux operation (Fig. 4–43). Patients with chronic esophageal obstruction due to scleroderma or achalasia may exhibit unusual appearances as a result of moniliasis. These may consist of a fine lacy appearance (Fig. 4–44A), diffuse fine nodularity (Fig. 4–43), or large polypoid folds (Fig. 4–45) which return to normal after treatment with Mycostatin.

Text continued on page 115

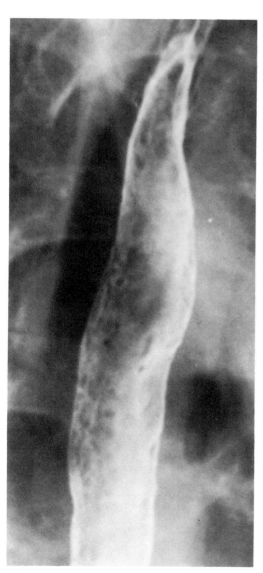 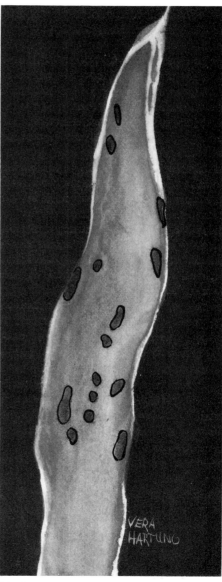

FIGURE 4–35 Early changes of monilial esophagitis with tiny mucosal plaques due to exudate on the esophageal mucosa.

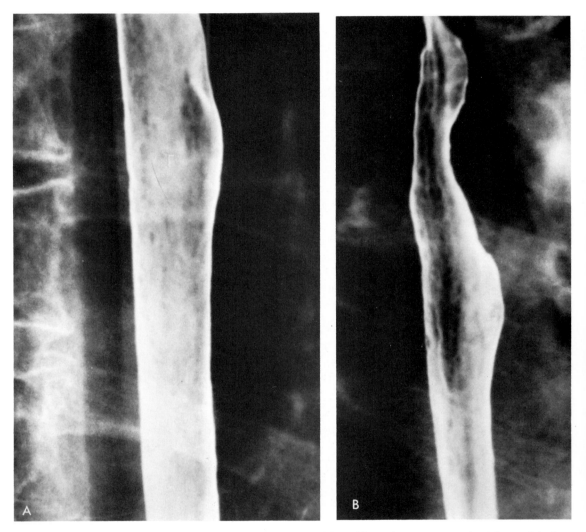

FIGURE 4–36 *A* and *B* Asymptomatic monilial esophagitis. This patient was examined for weight loss which was subsequently found to be due to carcinoma of the pancreas. There are tiny mucosal nodules throughout the proximal esophagus. Endoscopy confirmed that these were due to monilial exudates. The patient denied any symptoms referable to the esophagus. (Courtesy of Henry I. Goldberg, M.D., San Francisco.)

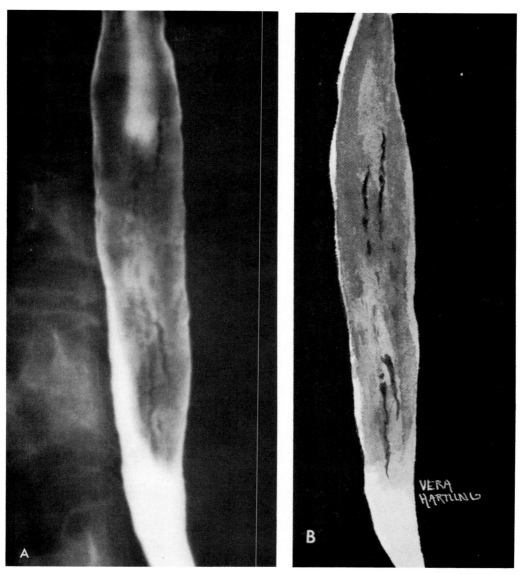

FIGURE 4–37 *A* and *B*   Linear plaques due to monilial esophagitis. Transplant patient with dysphagia. Long, thin filling defects are seen in the midesophagus. Endoscopy confirmed that these were due to monilia. See Plate 10.

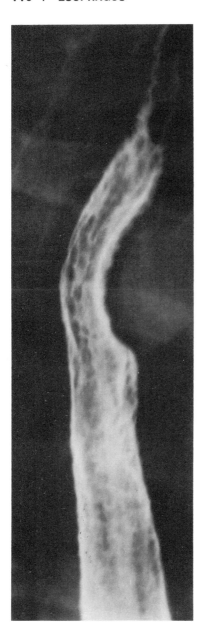

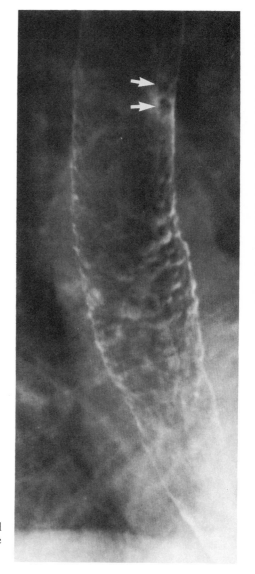

FIGURE 4–38 Cobblestoned mucosa due to monilial esophagitis.

FIGURE 4–39 Diffuse superficial ulceration in the distal esophagus due to monilial esophagitis. More proximally there are several plaques (*arrows*).

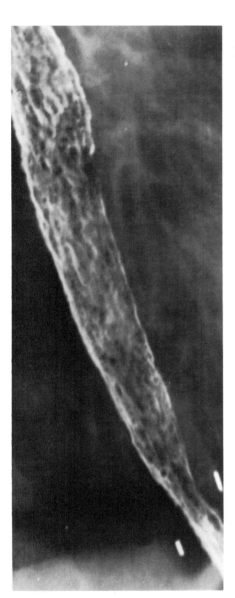

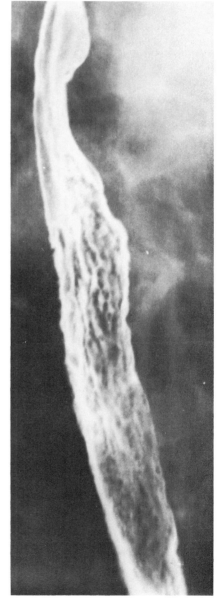

FIGURE 4–40 Extensive monilial esophagitis with coarse granular mucosa and diffuse narrowing.

FIGURE 4–41 Severe monilial esophagitis with extensive linear plaque formation in the midesophagus.

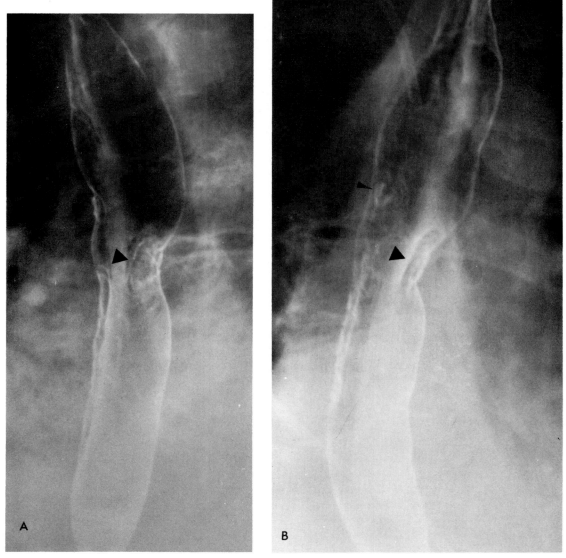

FIGURE 4–42 *A* and *B* There is a polypoid plaque in the midesophagus (*large arrow*) in addition to ulceration (*small arrow*). These findings were due to monilial esophagitis.

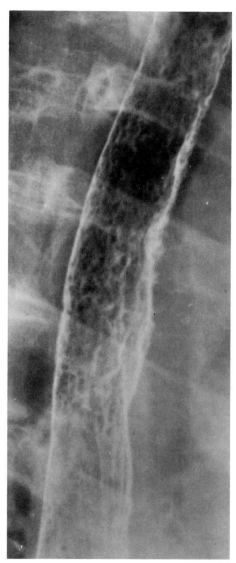

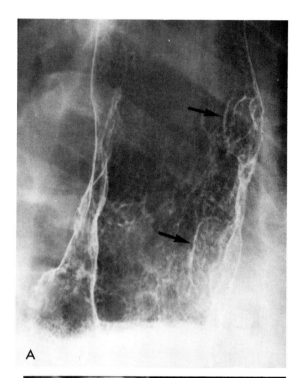

FIGURE 4–43 Monilial esophagitis following a Belsey antireflux operation. Note the coarse granular mucosa in the proximal esophagus.

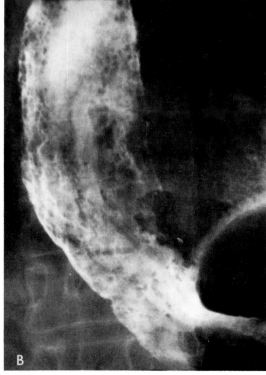

FIGURE 4–44 Chronic monilial infection in achalasia.

A. There is a lacy appearance of the mucosal surface with large plaques *(arrows).*

B. Fine nodularity of the mucosa due to monilial infection in a patient with scleroderma. Note the dilated esophagus and patulous lower esophageal sphincter.

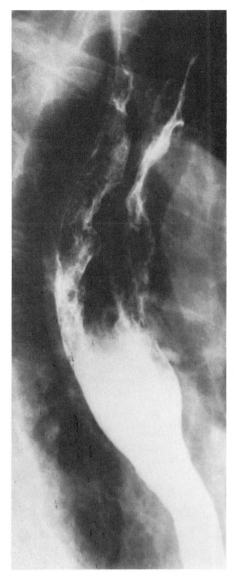

FIGURE 4–45 Chronic monilial eso-phagitis in a patient with achalasia and chronic mucocutaneous candidiasis. Monilial infection in this patient is manifest by very thickened polypoid folds. The appearance returned to normal after treatment with Mycostatin.

FIGURE 4–46 Herpes esophagitis. There are linear plaques throughout the esophagus. Biopsy confirmed that this was due to herpes simplex infection. (Courtesy of Joe Skucas, M.D., Rochester. Reproduced by permission of American Journal of Roentgenology.[44])

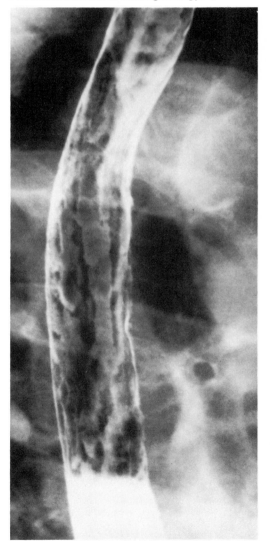

VIRAL ESOPHAGITIS

Although moniliasis is certainly the most common opportunistic infection in the esophagus, several recent reports have documented the occurrence of esophagitis caused by herpes simplex virus[44, 45] and cytomegalovirus.[46] The radiographic features in these patients appear to be indistinguishable from those of monilial esophagitis and are characterized by plaque-like filling defects (Figs 4-46 and 4-47), blistering (Fig. 4-48)

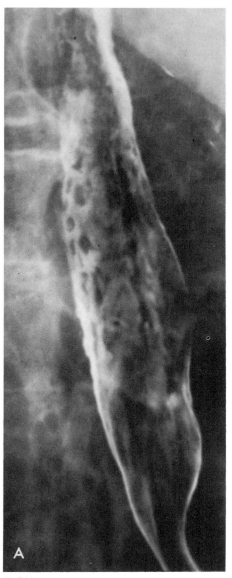
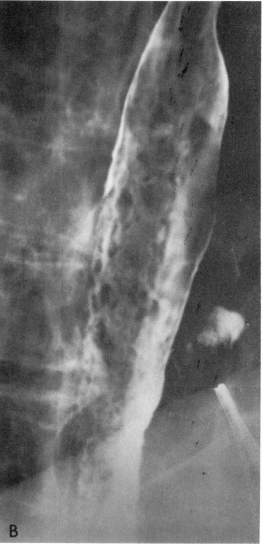

FIGURE 4–47 *A* and *B* Multiple nodular filling defects in the esophagus due to herpes simplex esophagitis. This elderly woman with carcinoma of the sigmoid had no esophageal symptoms except for hematemesis. Biopsies and cultures confirmed that this was due to herpes simplex esophagitis. The appearance returned to almost normal 1 week later with no specific treatment.

and superficial ulceration (Fig. 4–49). We have also seen a number of patients with minimal esophageal symptoms, but with definite radiologic evidence of esophagitis which resolves in a week with no specific treatment (Fig. 4–50). It is likely that these represent viral infections, some of which may be due to herpes simplex infections.

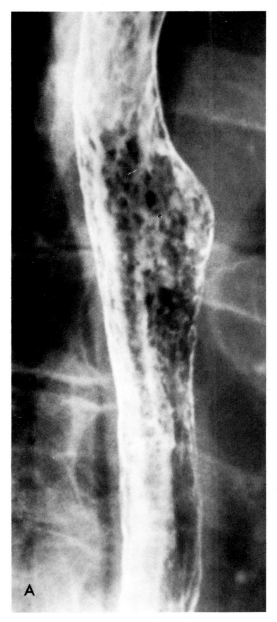 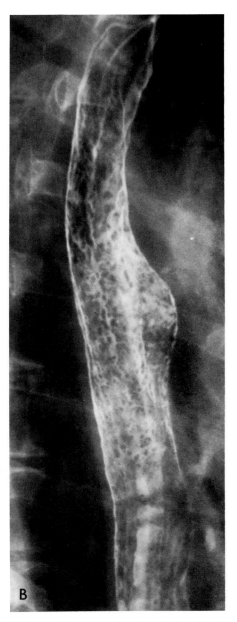

FIGURE 4–48 *A* and *B*   Probable herpes esophagitis. This middle-aged woman developed dysphagia while receiving radiation therapy for carcinoma of the thyroid. The mucosal surface of the esophagus appears blistered. The appearance returned to almost normal 1 week later with no specific treatment. Most probably this condition was due to herpes esophagitis.

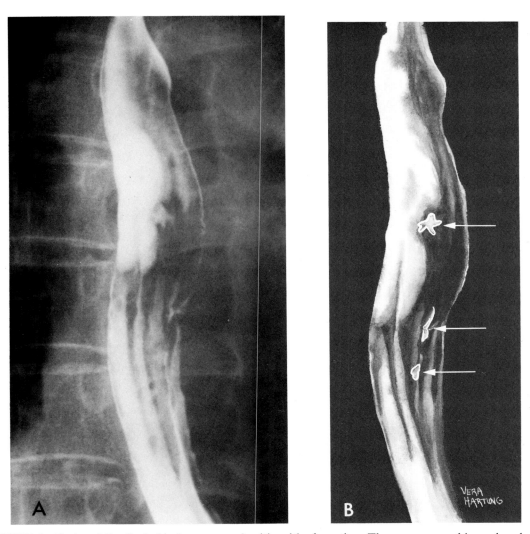

FIGURE 4–49 *A* and *B*   Probable herpes esophagitis with ulceration. There are several irregular ulcers (*arrows*) in the esophagus. The findings were confirmed on additional views. This patient had acute leukemia with herpetic lesions in the mouth.

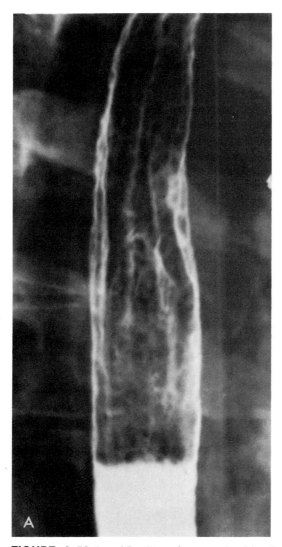
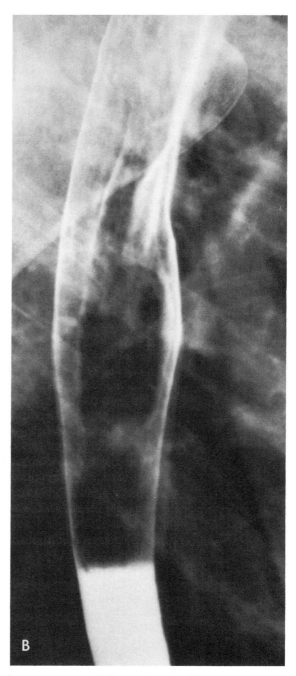

FIGURE 4-50 *A* and *B*   Transient esophagitis of unknown cause. Middle-aged male with dyspepsia. The initial study (*A*) shows changes of esophagitis in the midesophagus. One week later (*B*), with no specific treatment, the appearance has reverted to normal. This probably represents a transient esophagitis, perhaps secondary to viral infection.

Other Types of Esophagitis

Several other types of inflammatory processes may involve the esophagus.

Nasogastric Intubation. Patients with prolonged nasogastric intubation may develop a long stricture in the distal esophagus (Fig. 4–51). This probably represents a severe form of reflux esophagitis[47, 48] induced by the tube. The prolonged presence of a nasogastric tube predisposes to gastroesophageal reflux. A particularly severe form of esophagitis develops in patients who have had previous gastric surgery. There is reflux of bile into the stomach, and if gastroesophageal reflux is present the bile refluxes into the esophagus as well. This is very irritating to the esophageal mucosa and incites a severe inflammatory reaction which may go on to stricture.

Lye Ingestion. Long strictures with ulceration may also be seen in patients who have ingested lye (Fig. 4–52). Long-standing lye stricture appears to predispose to the development of esophageal carcinoma.[49] Therefore, any mucosal irregularity in a chronic lye stricture should raise the possibility of carcinoma (Fig. 4–53).

Radiation Therapy. Radiation therapy to the chest or mediastinum may cause acute esophagitis when the dose to the esophagus approaches 5000 to 6000 rads. Rarely, irradiation of a normal esophagus may progress to stricture (Fig. 4–54).[50] Radiation stricture is frequently seen following successful treatment of esophageal carcinoma (Fig. 5–24).

Other. Other inflammatory diseases, such as Crohn's disease[51] and bullous pemphigoid, may also involve the esophagus.[52]

Differential Diagnosis of Esophagitis

Nodularity. Mucosal nodularity may be a feature of chronic reflux esophagitis or opportunistic infection. However, it may also be seen in other conditions, such as leukoplakia, acanthosis nigricans, and superficial spreading carcinoma (Fig. 4–55A).[53] Rarely, an advanced carcinoma may present as diffuse mocosal nodularity (Fig. 4–55B).

Ulceration. Mucosal ulceration may be simulated by the profile appearance of transverse folds, described on page 81 (Fig. 4–8). Scarring due to ulceration may produce outpouchings at the gastroesophageal junction which may be mistaken for ulcers (Fig. 4–30). Intramural pseudodiverticulosis (Fig. 4–56) is another cause of barium projections, which must be differentiated from ulceration.[54] The pseudodiverticula have a narrow neck, and there is no apparent inflammatory reaction. Although this condition has been associated with monilial infection, we have also found it in association with severe reflux esophagitis in the absence of monilia. We believe that this probably represents a nonspecific sequela of severe esophagitis.

Abnormal Mucosal Folds. Thickened and tortuous folds in chronic esophagitis must be distinguished from esophageal varices (Fig. 4–57 A to D). Varices are best demonstrated with the esophagus at rest, with the aid of an anticholinergic drug.[55] Varicoid carcinoma may also present as enlarged tortuous folds (Fig. 4–58).[56]

Text continued on page 127

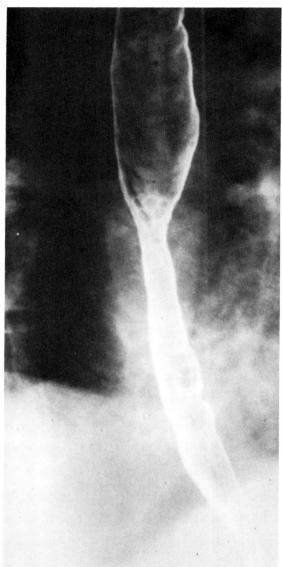

FIGURE 4–51 Long stricture of the distal esophagus secondary to prolonged nasogastric intubation.

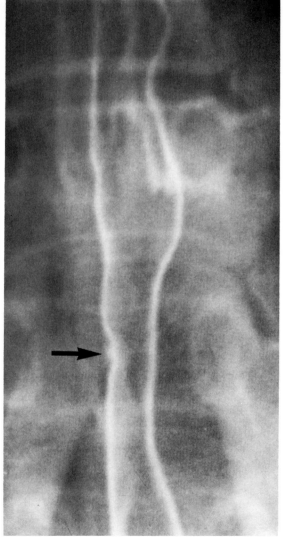

FIGURE 4–52 Long stricture with ulceration (*arrow*) secondary to lye ingestion.

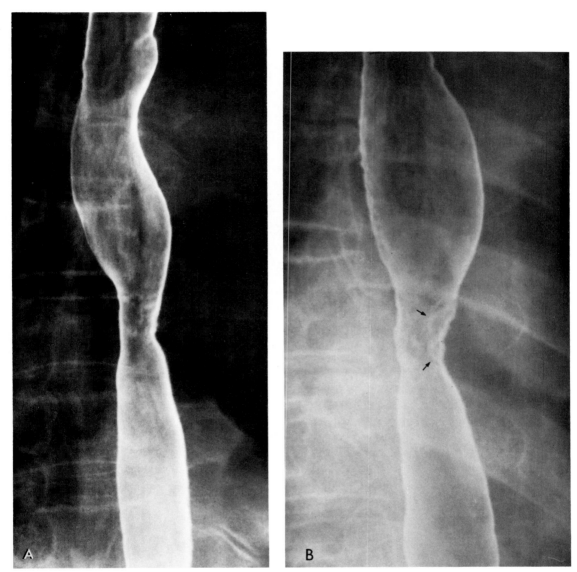

FIGURE 4–53 Carcinoma developing at the site of a lye stricture. This 70-year-old man had sustained a lye burn at the age of 4.

A. Smooth narrowing in the midesophagus compatible with lye stricture.

B. Mucosal nodularity at the site of stricture suggests the possibility of carcinoma. Cytologic findings showed squamous carcinoma, but the patient refused surgery.

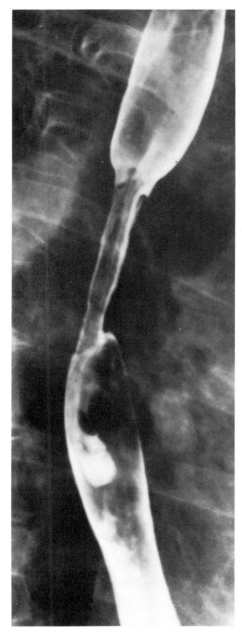

FIGURE 4–54 Radiation stricture. (Courtesy of Harvey M. Goldstein, M.D., Houston, Texas. Reproduced by permission of Gastrointestinal Radiology.[4])

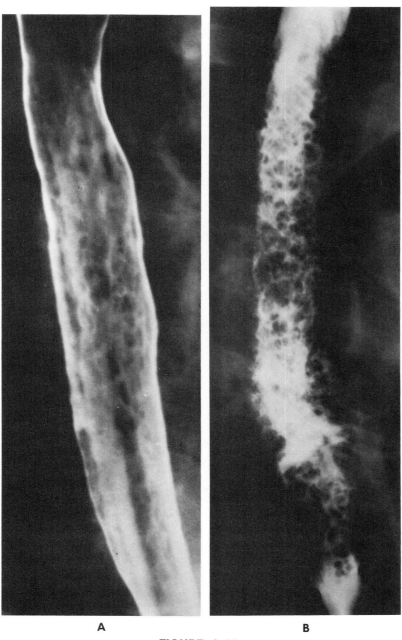

A   B

FIGURE 4–55

A. Diffuse mucosal nodularity due to superficial spreading carcinoma of the esophagus. (Courtesy of A. Yamada, M.D., Tokyo.)

B. Diffuse mucosal nodularity due to advanced esophageal carcinoma (Courtesy of Hans Herlinger, M.D., Leeds, England.)

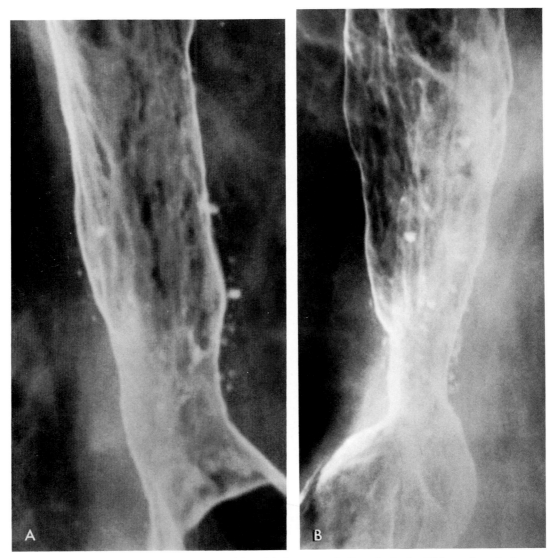

FIGURE 4–56 *A* and *B*   Chronic esophagitis with intramural diverticulosis. This patient had severe gastroesophageal reflux, and esophagitis is manifest by thickened folds in the distal esophagus. The multiple outpouchings seen in profile and en face represent intramural diverticula.

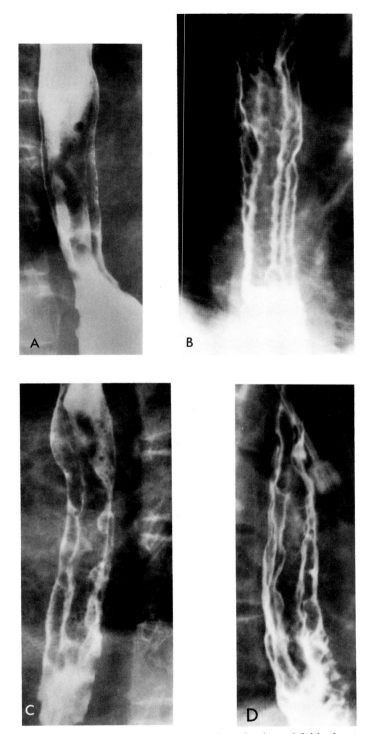

FIGURE 4–57 *A* to *D*   Esophageal varices. Four examples of enlarged folds due to esophageal varices show how these might mimic the enlarged folds in patients with esophagitis.

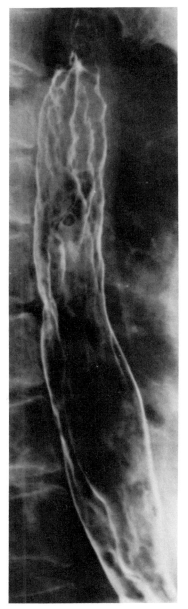

FIGURE 4–58 Varicoid carcinoma. The enlarged, tortuous folds simulate the appearances of varices and enlarged folds in esophagitis. This was a superficial esophageal carcinoma. (Courtesy of A. Yamada, M.D., Tokyo.)

REFERENCES

1. Friedenfelt, H.: A double-contrast method for the roentgen examination of esophageal strictures. Acta Radiol., *46*:499, 1956.
2. Skucas, J., and Schrank, W. W.: The routine air-contrast examination of the esophagus. Radiology, *115*:482, 1975.
3. Skucas, J.: The routine double-contrast examination of the esophagus. CRC Crit. Rev. Radiol., in press.
4. Goldstein, H. M., and Dodd, G. D.: Double-contrast examination of the esophagus. Gastrointest. Radiol., *1*:3, 1976.
5. Brombart, M.: Roentgenology of the esophagus. In: Margulis, A. R., and Burhenne, H. J. (eds.): Alimentary Tract Roentgenology. 2nd ed. St. Louis, C. V. Mosby, 1973, pp. 347–460.
6. Wiljasslo, M., and Rissanen, P.: A new double contrast method in esophageal roentgenology. Ann. Med. Intern. Fenn., *55*:77, 1966.
7. Suzuki, H., Kobayashi, S., Endo, M., et al.: Diagnosis of early esophageal cancer. Surgery, *71*:99, 1971.
8. Novak, D.: Hypotonic esophagography using propanthelin bromide (Pro-Banthine). Fortschr. Geb. Roentgenstr. Nuklearmed., *123*(5):409, 1975.
9. Hogan, W. J., Dodds, W. J., Hoke, S. E., el al.: Effect of glucagon on esophageal motor function. Gastroenterology, *69*:160, 1975.
10. Heitz, F., Weber, A., Rosinsky, Th., et al.: Application du titanate de baryum à la mucographie gastrique. J. Radiol., *55*:169, 1974.
11. Dodds, W. J., McGloughlin, P. S., and Goldberg, H. I.: Esophageal roentgenography using tantalum paste. Radiology, *102*:204, 1972.
12. Esguerra, A., and Segura, J.: Tantalum esophagography: A preliminary clinical evaluation. Radiology, *97*:181, 1970.
13. Nadel, J. A., Dodds, W. J., Goldberg, H. I., et al.: Insufflation of powdered tantalum in the esophagus: New esophagographic technique. Invest. Radiol., *4*:57, 1969.
14. Goldberg, H. I., Dodds, W. J., and Jenis, E. H.: Experimental esophagitis: Findings after insufflation of tantalum powder. Am. J. Roentgenol., 110:228, 1970.
15. Friedland, G. W., and Filly, R.: The post-cricoid impression masquerading as an esophageal tumor. Am. J. Dig. Dis., *20*:287, 1975.
16. Gohel, V. K., Edell, S. M., Laufer, I., et al. Transverse folds in the esophagus. Radiology, *128*:303, 1978.
17. Gohel, V. K., Kressel, H. Y., and Laufer, I.: Double-contrast artifacts. Gastrointest. Radiol., *3*:139, 1978.
18. Behar, J.: Reflux esophagitis: Pathogenesis, diagnosis and management. Arch. Intern. Med., *136*:560, 1976.
19. Wolf, B. S.: Roentgenology of the esophagogastric region. *In*: Margulis, A. R., Burhenne, H. J., (eds.); Alimentary Tract Roentgenology. 2nd ed. St. Louis, C. V. Mosby, 1973, pp. 500–552.
20. Donner, M. W., Silbiger, M. L., Hookman, P., et al.: Acid barium swallows in the radiographic evaluation of clinical esophagitis. Radiology, *87*:220, 1966.
21. McCall, I. W., Davies, E. R., and Delahunty, J. E.: The acid-barium test as an index of intermittent gastroesophageal reflux. Br. J. Radiol., *46*:578, 1973.
22. Simeone, J. F., Burrell, M., Toffler, R., et al.: Aperistalsis and esophagitis. Radiology, *123*:9, 1977.
23. Bleshman, M. H., Banner, M. P., Johnson, R. C., et al.: Inflammatory esophagogastric polyp and fold. Radiology, *128*:589, 1978.
24. Kobayashi, S. and Kasugai, T.: Endoscopic and biopsy criteria for the diagnosis of esophagitis with a fiberoptic esophagoscope. Am. J. Dig. Dis., *19*:345, 1974.
25. Rasmussen, C. W.: A new endoscopic classification of chronic esophagitis. Am. J. Gastroenterol., *65*:409, 1976.
26. Wolf, B. S., Marshak, R. H., and Som, M. L.: Peptic esophagitis and peptic ulceration of the esophagus. Am. J. Roentgenol., 79:741, 1958.
27. Robbins, A. H., Hermos, J. A., and Schimmel, E. M.: The columnar-lined esophagus — analysis of 26 cases. Radiology, *123*:1, 1977.
28. Naef, A. E., Savary, M., and Ozzello, L.: Columnar-lined lower esophagus: An acquired lesion with malignant predisposition. J. Thorac. Cardiovasc. Surg., *70*:826, 1975.
29. Eras, P., Goldstein, M. J., and Sherlock, P.: Candida infection of the gastrointestinal tract. Medicine, *51*:367, 1972.
30. Jensen, K. B., Stenderup, A., Thomsen, J. B., et al.: Esophageal moniliasis in malignant neoplastic disease. Acta Med. Scand., *175*:456, 1964.
31. Guyer, P. B., Brunton, F. J., and Rooke, H. W.: Candidiasis of the esophagus. Br. J. Radiol., *44*:131, 1971.

32. Scheft, D. J., and Shrago, G.: Esophageal moniliasis: the spectrum of the disease. JAMA, *213*:1859, 1970.
33. Holt, J. M.: Candida infection of the esophagus. Gut, *9*:227, 1968.
34. Kodsi, B. E., Wickremesinghe, P. C., Kozinn, P. J., et al.: Candida esophagitis: a prospective study of 27 cases. Gastroenterology, *71*:715, 1976.
35. Andren, L., and Theander, G.: Roentgenographic appearances of esophageal moniliasis. Acta Radiol., *46*:571, 1956.
36. Lewicki, A. M., and Moore, J. P.: Esophageal moniliasis. A review of common and less frequent characteristics. Am. J. Roentgenol., *125*:218, 1975.
37. Athey, P. A., Goldstein, H. M., and Dodd, G. D.: Radiologic spectrum of opportunistic infections of the upper gastrointestinal tract. Am. J. Roentgenol., *129*:419, 1977.
38. Goldberg, H. I., and Dodds, W. J.: Cobblestone esophagus due to monilial infection. Am. J. Roentgenol., *104*:608, 1968.
39. Kaufman, S. A., Scheff, S., and Levine, G.: Esophageal moniliasis. Radiology, *75*:726, 1960.
40. Gonzalez, G.: Esophageal moniliasis. Am. J. Roentgenol., *113*:233, 1971.
41. Ho, C. S., Cullin, J. B., and Gray, R. R.: An unusual manifestation of esophageal moniliasis. Radiology, *123*:287, 1977.
42. Ott, D. J., and Gelfand, D. W.: Esophageal stricture secondary to candidiasis. Gastrointest. Radiol. *2*:323, 1978.
43. Gefter, W., Gohel, V. K., Edell, S. M., et al.: Monilial infection in the obstructed esophagus. In preparation.
44. Skucas, J., Schrank, W. W., Meyers, P. C., et al.: Herpes esophagitis: a case studied by air contrast esophagography. Am. J. Roentgenol., *128*:497, 1977.
45. Meyers, C., Durkin, M. G. and Love, L.: Radiographic findings in herpetic esophagitis. Radiology, *119*:21, 1976
46. Toghill, P. J.: Cytomegalovirus esophagitis. Br. Med. J., *2*:294, 1972.
47. Graham, J., Barnes, J., and Rubenstein, A. S.: The naso-gastric tube as a cause of esophagitis and stricture. Am. J. Surg. *98*:116, 1959.
48. Nagler, R., and Spiro, H. M.: Persistent gastro-esophageal reflux induced during prolonged gastric intubation. N. Engl. J. Med., *269*:495, 1963.
49. Lansing, P., Ferrante, W., and Ochsner, J.,: Carcinoma of the esophagus at the site of lye stricture. Am. J. Surg., *118*:108, 1969.
50. Goldstein, H. M., Rogers, L. F., Fletcher, G. H., et al.: Radiological manifestations of radiation-induced injury to the normal upper gastrointestinal tract. Radiology, *117*:135, 1975.
51. Cynn, W. S., Chon, H. K., Gureghian, P. A., et al.: Crohn's disease of the esophagus. Am. J. Roentgenol., *125*:359, 1975.
52. Person, J. R., and Rogers, R. S.: Bullous and cicatricial pemphigoid. Clinical, histopathologic and immunopathologic correlations. Mayo Clin. Proc., *52*:54, 1977.
53. Itai, Y., Kogure, T., Okuyama, Y., et al.: Diffuse finely nodular lesions of the esophagus. Am. J. Roentgenol., *128*:563, 1977.
54. Fromkes, J., Thomas, F. B., Mekhjian, H., et al.: Esophageal intramural pseudodiverticulosis. Am. J. Dig. Dis., *22*:690, 1977.
55. Cockerill, E. M., Miller, R. E., Chernish, S. M., et al.: Optimal visualisation of esophageal varices. Am. J. Roentgenol., *126*:512, 1976.
56. Lawson, T. L., Dodds, W. J., and Sheft, D. J.: Carcinoma of the esophagus simulating varices. Am. J. Roentgenol., *107*:83, 1969.
57. Rohrmann, C. A., Jr., and Kidd, R.: Chronic mucocutaneous candidiasis: Radiologic abnormalities in the esophagus. Am. J. Roentgenol., *130*:473, 1978.

5

TUMORS OF THE ESOPHAGUS

IGOR LAUFER, M.D., AND AKIYOSHI YAMADA, M.D.

BENIGN TUMORS

MALIGNANT TUMORS
    Early Diagnosis
    Advanced Cancer
    Other Malignant Tumors
    Posttreatment Studies

BENIGN TUMORS

Benign tumors are relatively uncommon in the esophagus.[1] The majority of benign esophageal tumors are intramural lesions, primarily leiomyomas. These tumors stretch and efface the overlying mucosa, resulting in a very smooth surface (Fig. 5–1). They are also characterized by their position in a right angle or obtuse angle with the wall of the esophagus (Fig. 5–2). As with other locations in the gastrointestinal tract, application of the "spheroid sign" will also indicate the intramural location of the lesion.[2] These tumors are frequently asymptomatic, although patients may present with upper gastrointestinal bleeding when central ulceration occurs (Fig. 5–3). Intramural lesions may also be produced by dilated cystic glands in the lower esophagus, a condition that has been termed esophagitis cystica (Fig. 5–4A).[3]

Benign epithelial tumors, such as papillomas, are uncommon.[4] They are frequently very small and difficult to demonstrate. Rarely, they may be multiple (Fig. 5–4B).[5] Inflammatory[6] and fibrovascular[7] polyps are also found in the esophagus. These may have a typical pedunculated appearance. Pedunculated polyps resulting from lipomas have also been reported.[8]

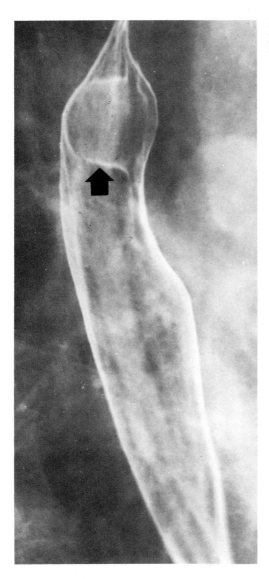

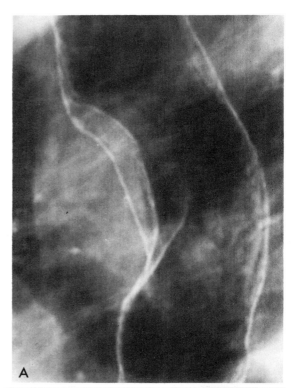

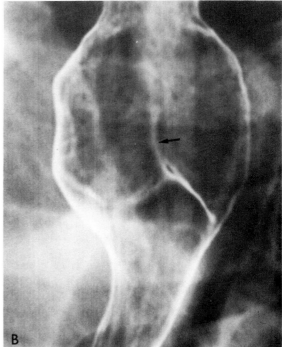

FIGURE 5–1 Typical submucosal tumor in the proximal esophagus, demonstrating smooth, stretched mucosa over the tumor.

FIGURE 5–2 Esophageal leiomyoma.

A. Lateral view shows the typical right angle between the tumor and the mucosal surface.

B. En face view shows widening of the esophageal lumen and a smooth mucosal surface with a central furrow *(arrow)*. Courtesy of Marc P. Banner, M.D., Philadelphia.)

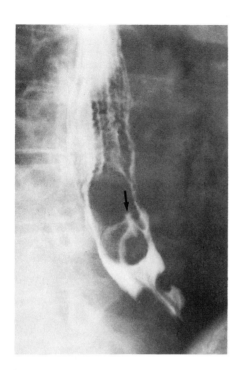

FIGURE 5–3 Submucosal tumor with ulceration *(arrow)*.

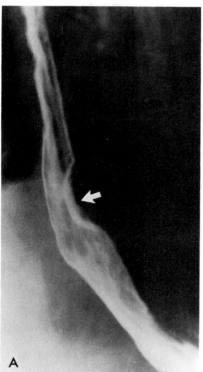

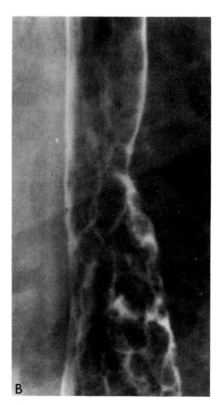

FIGURE 5–4 Other benign tumors.

A.   Submucosal mass in the distal esophagus due to dilated cystic glands.

B.   Multiple small filling defects in the distal esophagus due to esophageal papillomatosis. See also Plate 12.

MALIGNANT TUMORS

Early Diagnosis

Patients with carcinoma of the esophagus usually present with extensive tumor. Rarely, patients with small esophageal carcinomas present with dysphagia. Koehler and coworkers[9] reported nine such patients. The lesion was missed on the initial radiologic study in four of these patients, resulting in diagnostic and therapeutic delays of between 9 and 22 months. In a related study, Moss and associates[10] found that 35 per cent of small esophageal carcinomas had been missed on the initial esophagogram. They found that increasing sensitivity to subtle abnormalities decreases the frequency of false negative results, but increases the frequency of false positive diagnoses of esophageal cancer.

The early findings in esophageal carcinoma may be very subtle.[9, 11, 12] Double contrast views must be obtained in multiple projections to detect and confirm the presence of the lesion. Squamous carcinoma may start as a flat sessile polyp (Fig. 5–5), or as a plaque along one wall of the esophagus (Fig. 5–6). Many lesions have a small central ulcer (Figs. 5–7 to 5–9). A localized area of wall stiffness is the most difficult sign to detect.[10] This finding may be present in early esophageal cancer (Fig. 5–6) as well as in benign conditions, such as peptic esophagitis (Fig. 4–22). In some cases an abnormality may be suspected only on the screening examination (Fig. 5–10*A*). Detailed examination with intubation and hypotonia may be necessary to confirm and define the lesion (Fig. 5–10*B*). Superficial spreading carcinoma is a rare form of esophageal malignancy. This type of lesion appears as multiple tiny mucosal elevations which give the mucosal surface a reticular appearance (Fig. 5–11). This appearance may simulate moniliasis, leukoplakia, or acanthosis nigricans.[13]

In some patients, polypoid tumors may become quite large but remain confined to the submucosa (Figs. 5–12 and 5–13). The double contrast study may also reveal evidence of superficial spread (Fig. 5–9) as well as metastatic (Fig. 5–9) or multiple lesions (Fig. 5–14).

Although the radiologic study may define the size and surface features of a carcinoma, it may be difficult to assess the depth of invasion. Regrettably, in many small lesions invasion of the serosa or lymph node metastasis has already occurred, and in such patients the prognosis is poor despite the small size of the tumor. At present, considerable work is being done in the Department of Surgery of the Tokyo Women's Medical College to evaluate the radiologic criteria for resectability in esophageal carcinoma and to determine whether prognosis can be predicted from the radiologic features.

Text continued on page 141

FIGURE 5–5   Early cancer presenting as a sessile polyp. (Courtesy of Harvey Goldstein, M. D., Houston, Texas. Reproduced by permission of Gastrointestinal Radiology.[31]

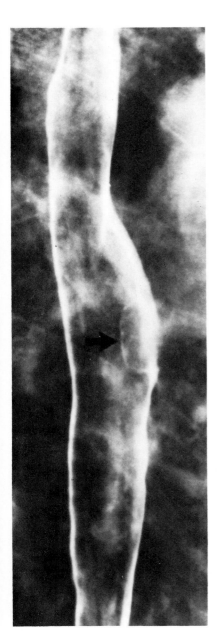

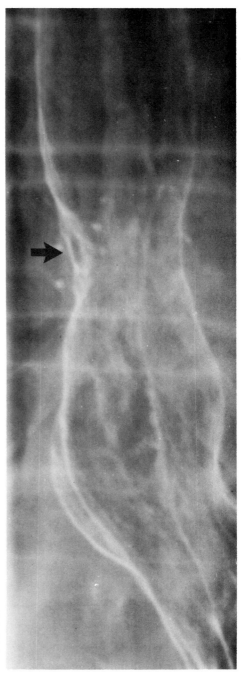

FIGURE 5–6   Small carcinoma in an asymptomatic patient. There is a plaque-like lesion along the right lateral wall just above the gastroesophageal junction. This was confirmed to be squamous cell carcinoma in a patient with a history of smoking and drinking. There are also small opacities owing to contrast from a previous myelogram.

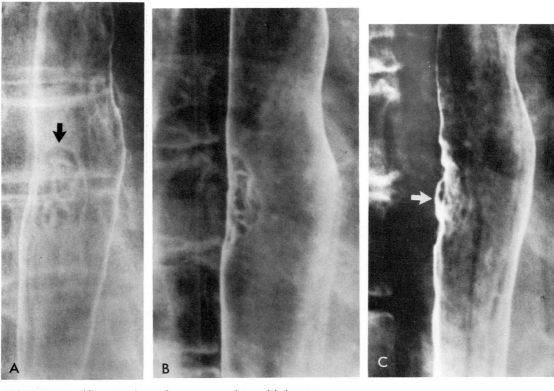

FIGURE 5–7 Ulcerated carcinoma seen in multiple projections.

A. En face view shows a filling defect in the esophagus, with an irregular surface.

B. Oblique view shows the polypoid nature of the lesion.

C. A steeper oblique view shows the shallow central ulcer *(arrow)*.

This was a squamous carcinoma with invasion limited to the submucosa, although there was invasion of the blood vessels.

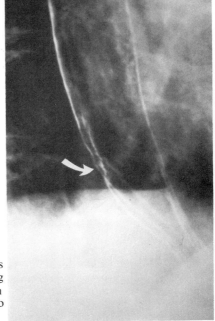

FIGURE 5–8 Flat carcinoma with minimal ulceration. There is slight thickening of the folds in the distal esophagus extending toward an irregularity of the mucosal surface caused by ulceration *(arrow)*. This was a squamous carcinoma with invasion limited to the muscularis mucosa.

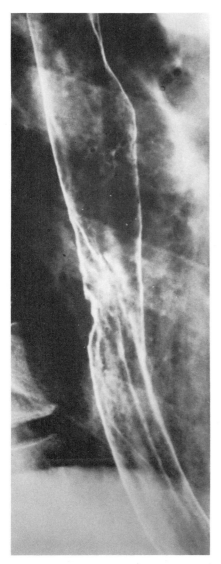 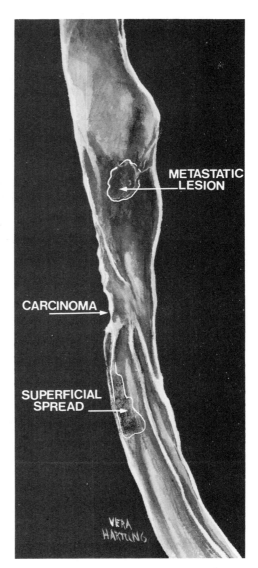

FIGURE 5–9 Ulcerated carcinoma with a proximal metastasis and superficial spread distally. In the midthoracic esophagus there is a mass lesion with central ulceration. Extending distally there is an area of granular mucosa, representing superficial spreading carcinoma. A discrete nodule is faintly seen just proximal to the main lesion. This represents a metastatic lesion. This was squamous carcinoma with invasion limited to the submucosa, but with blood vessel, lymphatic, and lymph node metastases.

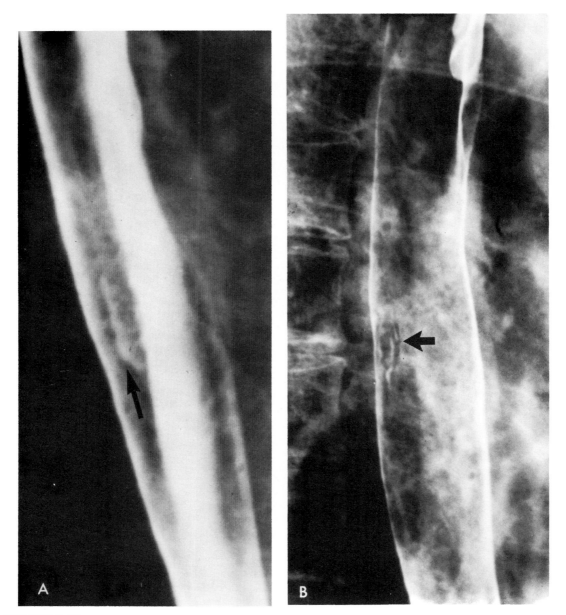

FIGURE 5–10

A. The screening examination shows only a linear collection of barium *(arrow)*.

B. The detailed examination shows more clearly an area of abnormal mucosa representing a superficial, ulcerated carcinoma. Invasion was limited to the submucosa.

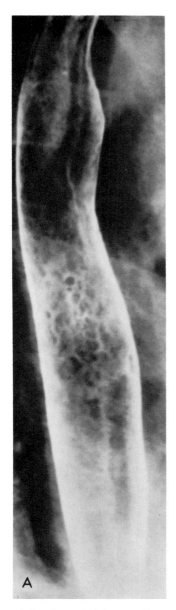
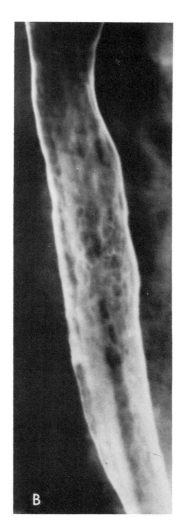

FIGURE 5–11 *A* and B   Superficial spreading carcinoma of the esophagus. The mucosa has a coarse granular appearance owing to tiny mucosal elevations. A lesion such as this may have differing appearances with varying degrees of distension. Therefore, multiple films should be obtained with varying degrees of distension. Invasion was limited to the muscularis mucosa.

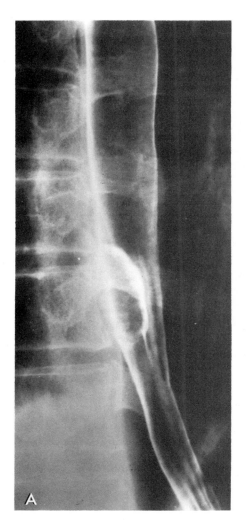

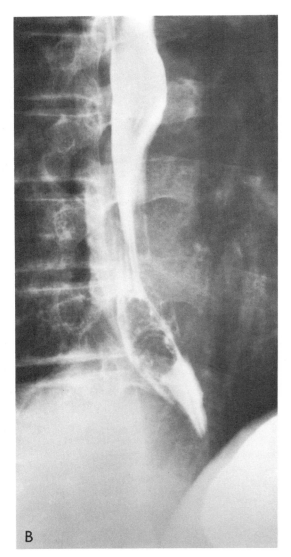

FIGURE 5–12 Polypoid carcinoma with invasion confined to the submucosa.

    A.   The appearance of the polypoid tumor in the distended esophagus.

    B.   The collapsed esophagus also shows the polypoid nature of the tumor.

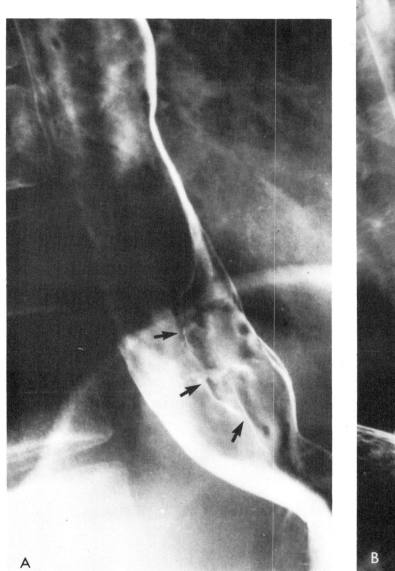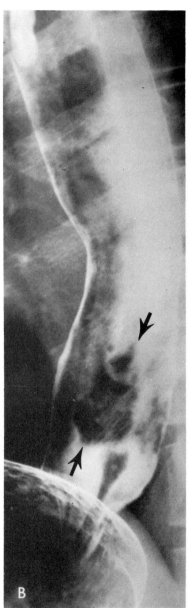

FIGURE 5–13 Early polypoid carcinoma.

A. In the upright position a large polypoid tumor *(arrows)* is seen arising from the anterior wall of the distal esophagus.

B. In the prone position the tumor is seen en face. Invasion was limited to the submucosa, but there were lymphatic and lymph node metastases, and the patient died 19 months later.

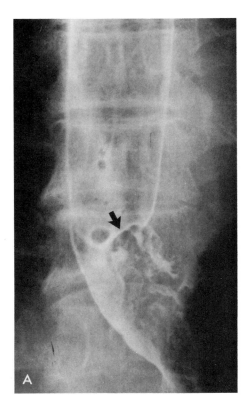

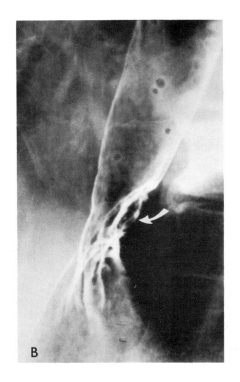

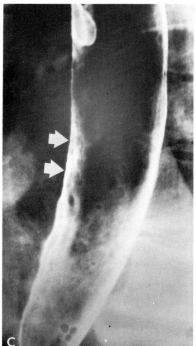

FIGURE 5–14 Multiple superficial esophageal carcinomas.

A and *B.* There is an obvious polypoid tumor with ulceration near the gastroesophageal junction, seen in frontal *(A)* and RPO *(B)* projections. Invasion was limited to the submucosa, but there was lymph node metastasis.

C. There is slight irregularity and granularity *(arrows)* in the midesophagus. This was a carcinoma limited to the muscularis mucosa. This lesion was recognized only in retrospect following surgery on the lower esophageal tumor. The prognosis in patients with multiple esophageal carcinomas is very poor. This patient died 2 years and 5 months following surgery because of recurrent carcinoma.

Advanced Cancer

Despite the fact that the vast majority of patients with esophageal carcinoma present with extensive disease, 8 to 10 per cent of the carcinomas are missed on the initial esophagram, while another 15 per cent are diagnosed as something other than carcinoma.[14, 15] There are three basic patterns to the gross appearance of esophageal carcinoma — polypoid (Fig. 5–15A), infiltrating (Fig. 5–15B), and ulcerating (Fig. 5–15C). Combinations of these three basic patterns are frequently seen (Fig. 5–16A and B). Occasionally the tumor may present primarily as enlarged tortuous folds and may resemble varices (Figs. 5–17 and 5–18). This has been termed varicoid carcinoma.[16, 17] This type of tumor can be distinguished from esophageal varices by the rigidity of the esophagus and the unchanging appearance of the enlarged folds. In addition, the mid- or proximal esophagus may be involved without involvement of the distal end.

In any patient with a lower esophageal lesion or with dysphagia and a normal appearance in the esophagus, the gastric fundus and cardia must also be examined. Most adenocarcinomas involving the distal esophagus are actually gastric carcinomas extending into the distal esophagus. Examination of the stomach may show the true origin of the tumor as well as the extent of gastric involvement. In addition, symptoms of dysphagia are frequently due to tumors arising at or around the gastric cardia and may be apparent only on examination of the stomach (Fig. 5–19).

Double contrast esophagography should be performed not only in patients with esophageal symptoms but also in the routine screening of asymptomatic patients who are at high risk for esophageal carcinoma. The predisposing factors include the combination of alcoholism and smoking, Plummer-Vinson symdrome, lye stricture (Fig. 5–20A),[18] Barrett's esophagus (Fig. 5–20B),[19] carcinoma of the head and neck,[20] celiac disease (Fig. 5–15A),[21, 22] and tylosis.[23]

A special problem is posed by the increased incidence of carcinoma in patients with achalasia.[24] Because of the partial obstruction with retention of fluid and food the carcinoma may be difficult to detect. Patients with long-standing achalasia should have regular esophagrams to facilitate the early detection of carcinoma. Esophageal lavage should be used if necessary to cleanse the esophagus prior to radiologic study. Under these conditions, in patients with partial esophageal obstruction and absence of peristalsis a good double contrast esophagogram is easily obtained (Fig. 5–20C). The tumor in patients with achalasia usually arises in the middle third of the esophagus and is a bulky, polypoid, squamous cell carcinoma. We have also seen one example of a carcinosarcoma arising in a patient with achalasia.[25]

Once a lesion has been detected radiologically, its presence and nature will usually be confirmed at esophagoscopy. However, there is great variability in the accuracy of the histologic and cytologic diagnosis of carcinoma. Edwards[26] reported that 50 per cent of the initial biopsy findings in patients with esophageal carcinoma failed to reveal evidence of a tumor. By contrast, Roesch[27] found that the combination of histologic and cytologic studies was 100 per cent accurate in the diagnosis of carcinoma. In most institutions the results are intermediate, and negative biopsy results should not exclude the diagnosis of carcinoma in the presence of a highly suggestive radiologic appearance. In some cases repeated radiologic studies, biopsies, or surgery may be necessary to establish the diagnosis.

Text continued on page 148

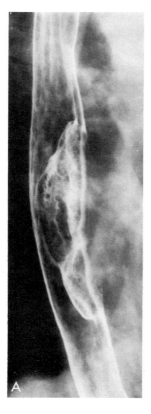

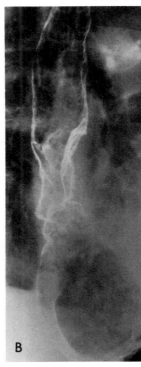

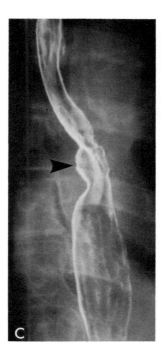

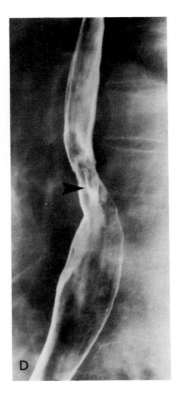

FIGURE 5–15 Basic radiographic patterns of advanced esophageal carcinoma.

A. Polypoid tumor in a patient with malabsorption owing to nontropical sprue (see Plate 14). From: Collins, S. M., Hamilton, J. D., Lewis, T. D., et al.: Radiology, *123*:603, 1978[21]

B. Infiltrating carcinoma.

C. and *D.* Ulcerating carcinoma. There is an ulcer in the distal esophagus *(arrows)* with relatively little mass effect. The ulcer is seen in profile *(C)* and en face *(D)*.

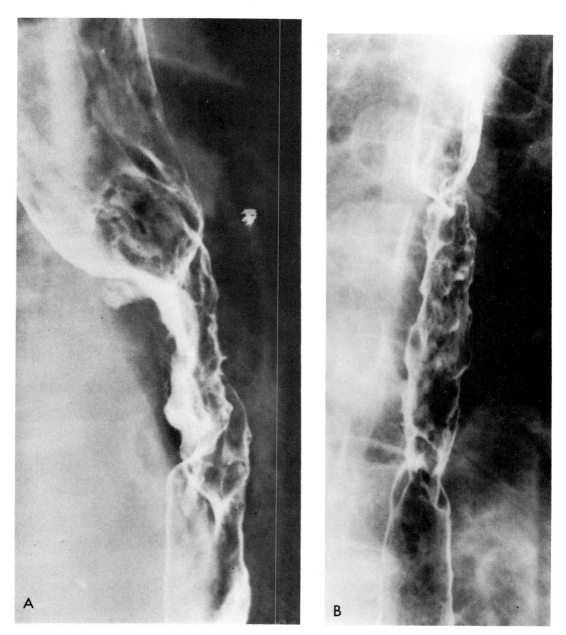

FIGURE 5–16 Mixed radiographic patterns in advanced esophageal carcinoma.

      A. Polypoid, infiltrating, and ulcerating carcinoma.
      B. Infiltrating carcinoma with ulceration.

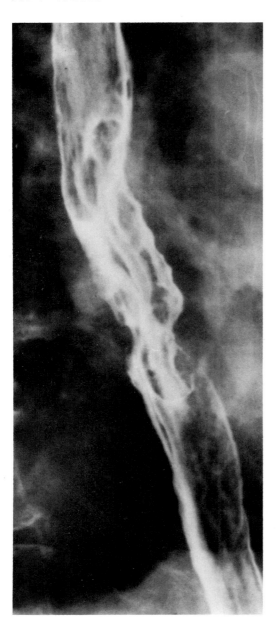

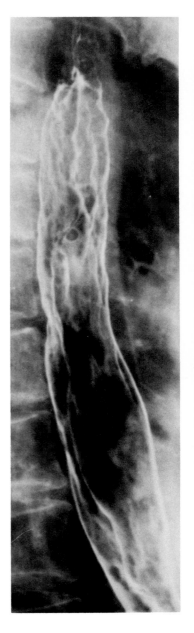

FIGURE 5–17 Varicoid carcinoma with enlarged folds in the midesophagus which could be mistaken for esophageal varices.

FIGURE 5–18 There are prominent scalloped folds throughout the esophagus. The appearance is very suggestive of varices. In this case it was due to diffuse superficial carcinoma.

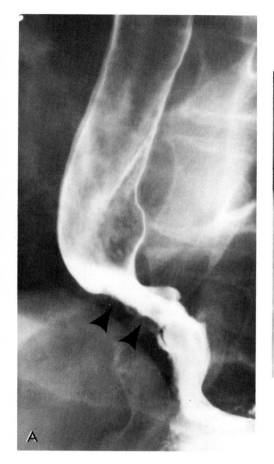

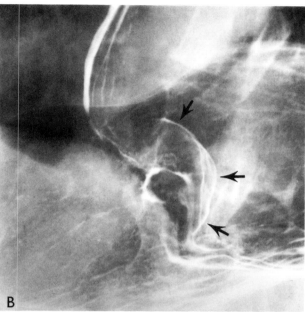

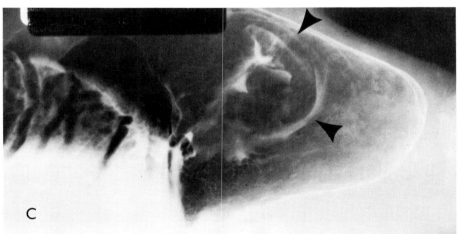

FIGURE 5–19 Carcinoma at the cardia, causing dysphagia.

A. Upright view of the esophagus shows minimal irregularity along the very distal esophagus.
B. RPO projection, showing the surface of a plaque-like tumor at the cardia.
C. Double contrast view of the cardia and fundus in lateral projection shows a plaque-like filling defect *(arrows)* around the cardia resulting from adenocarcinoma. There are small areas of ulceration within the tumor.

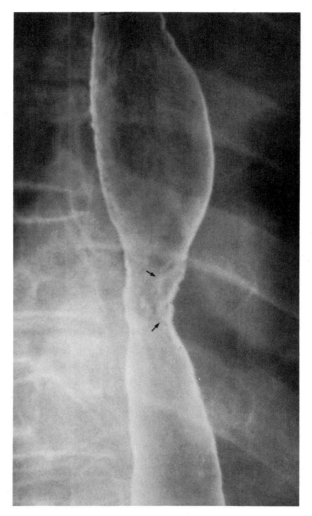

A

FIGURE 5–20 Carcinoma developing in patients with predisposing conditions.

A. Carcinoma in a patient with a lye stricture. This is a 74-year-old man who ingested lye at the age of 4 years and thereafter had minimal dysphagia for solids. He developed a sudden increase in the degree of dysphagia. The double contrast study shows mild narrowing owing to the lye stricture. There are also small plaquelike mucosal lesions and superficial ulcers. Endoscopy showed mucosal friability and superficial ulceration. Cytologic findings showed squamous carcinoma.

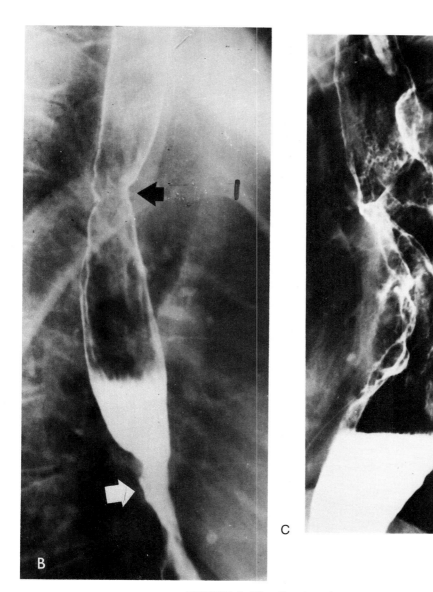

FIGURE 5–20 *Continued*

B. Carcinoma in a patient with Barrett's esophagus. There is an area of narrowing in the mid-esophagus, typical of Barrett's esophagus. In the distal portion of the columnar-lined esophagus there is irregular narrowing and ulceration owing to adenocarcinoma. (Courtesy of Robert E. Koehler, M.D., St. Louis.)

C. Extensive polypoid carcinoma in a patient with achalasia.

Other Malignant Tumors

A variety of other malignant tumors may involve the esophagus. Leiomyosarcomas tend to be larger than leiomyomas, but may otherwise be indistinguishable from them (Fig. 5–21). Carcinosarcoma, a rare form of esophageal malignancy, presents as a bulky polypoid lesion which may be pedunculated Fig. 5–22A and B). It frequently attains a very large size,

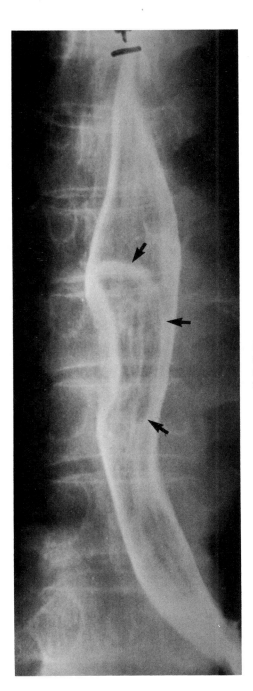

FIGURE 5–21 Leiomyosarcoma of the esophagus. There is a large intramural tumor in the midesophagus. The appearance is indistinguishable from that of other submucosal tumors.

but despite this it is relatively nonaggressive and carries a much better prognosis than squamous carcinoma.[28] Bulky polypoid tumors may also be due to primary melanosarcoma of the esophagus (Fig. 5–23).[20] Lymphoma may also involve the esophagus, usually by direct extension from the stomach.[30]

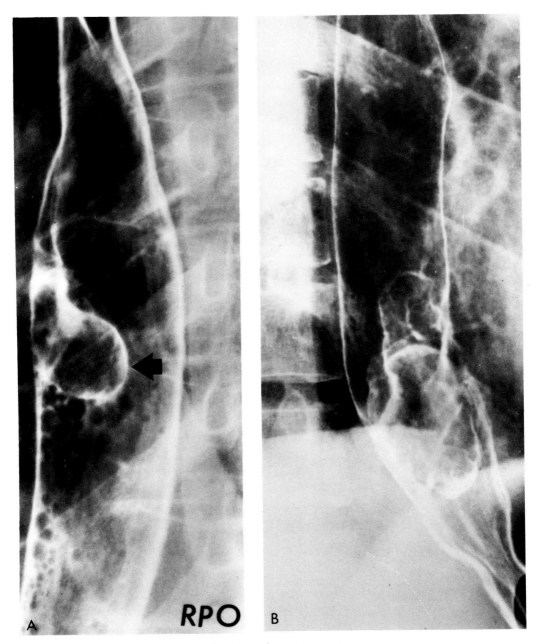

FIGURE 5–22 Carcinosarcoma.

A. There is a small polypoid tumor in the midesophagus owing to carcinosarcoma. (Courtesy of Harvey Goldstein, M.D., Houston, Texas. Reproduced by permission of Gastrointestinal Radiology.[31]

B. There is a bulky, multilobulated polypoid tumor in the distal esophagus owing to carcinosarcoma.

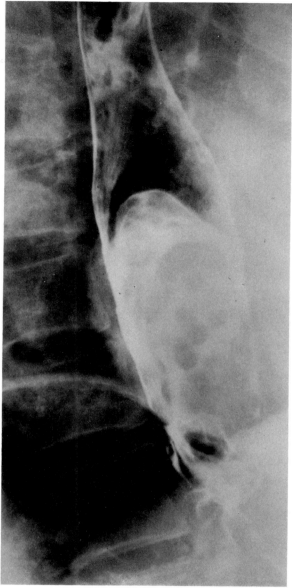

FIGURE 5–23 Melanosarcoma. There is a very large mass lesion with multiple polypoid excrescences in the distal esophagus, resulting from melanosarcoma of the esophagus.

Posttreatment Studies

Double contrast studies can also be performed following treatment of esophageal tumor, either by radiation therapy or by surgery. The primary tumor often responds dramatically to radiotherapy (Figs. 5–24 and 5–25), although the disease invariably recurs or spreads widely. Double contrast views can also be obtained following esophagogastric anastomosis to show the normal anatomy (Fig. 5–26A) as well as the pathologic conditions at the anastomosis (Fig. 5–26B).

FIGURE 5–24

 A. Esophageal carcinoma with extensive ulceration.
 B. After radiotherapy there is a smooth stricutre, with only one area of ulceration along the left lateral wall *(arrow).*

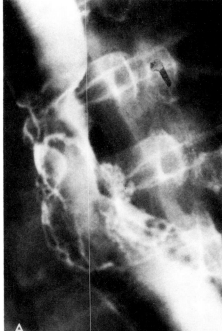
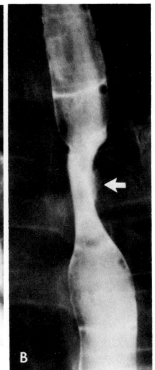

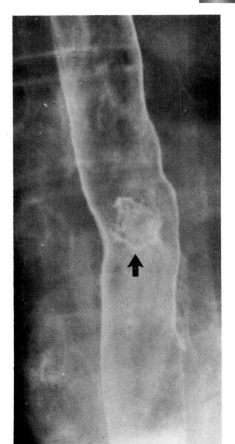

FIGURE 5–25 Following radiation therapy of an extensive esophageal carcinoma there is only a small residual polypoid lesion.

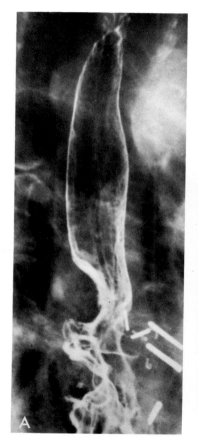
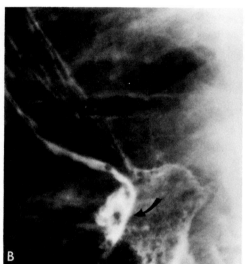

FIGURE 5–26   Appearances following esophagogastric anastomosis.

A.   Normal postoperative appearance.
B.   Anastomotic ulcer *(arrow)* following esophagogastrectomy for esophageal papillomatosis (Fig. 5–4*B*).

Figures 5–7 to 5–14, 5–18, 5–20C, 5–21, 5–22B and 5–23 are from the Tokyo Women's Medical College.

REFERENCES

1. Attah, E. B., and Hajdu, S. I.: Benign and malignant tumors of the esophagus at autopsy. J. Thorac. Cardiovasc. Surg., *55*:396, 1968.
2. Stein, L. A., and Margulis, A. R.: The spheroid sign. A new sign for accurate differentiation of intramural from extramural masses. Am. J. Roentgenol., *123*:420, 1975.
3. Farman, J., Rosen, Y., Dallenmand, S., et al.: Esophagitis cystica: lower esophageal retention cysts. Am. J. Roentgenol., *128*:495, 1977.
4. Kostianen, S. Teppi, L., and Irkkula, L.: Papilloma of the esophagus. Report of a case. Scand. J. Thorac. Cardiovasc. Surg., *7*:95, 1973.
5. Benisch, B. M., and Mantell, C.: Multiple squamous papillomas of the esophagus. Arch. Otolaryngol., *100*:379, 1974.
6. LiVolsi, V. A., and Perzin, K. H.: Inflammatory pseudotumors (inflammatory fibrous polyps) of the esophagus. A clinico-pathologic study. Am. J. Dig. Dis., *20*:475, 1975.
7. Burrell, M., and Toffler, R.: Fibrovascular polyps of the esophagus. Am. J. Dig. Dis., *18*:174, 1973.
8. Liliequist, B., and Wiberg, A.: Pedunculated tumors of the esophagus. Two cases of lipoma. Acta Radiol., *15*:383, 1974.
9. Koehler, R. E., Moss, A. A., and Margulis, A. R.: Early radiographic manifestations of carcinoma of the esophagus. Radiology, *119*:1, 1976.
10. Moss, A. A., Koehler, R. E., and Margulis, A. R.: Initial accuracy of esophagograms in detection of small esophageal carcinoma. Am. J. Roentgenol., *127*:909, 1976.
11. Yamada, A., Kobayashi, S., Kawai, B., et al.: Study on x-ray findings of early oesophageal cancer. Austral Radiol., *16*:238, 1972.
12. Itai, Y., Kogure, T., Okuyama, Y., et al.: Superficial esophageal carcinoma. Radiology, *126*:597, 1978.
13. Itai, Y., Kogure, T., Okuyama, Y., et al.: Diffuse finely nodular lesion of the esophagus. Am. J. Roentgenol., *128*:563, 1977.
14. Appelqvist, P.: Carcinoma of the esophagus and gastric cardia: A retrospective study based on statistical and clinical material from Finland. Acta Chir. Scand. (Suppl.), *430*:1, 1972.
15. Bruni, H. C., and Nelson, R. S.: Carcinoma of the esophagus and cardia: Diagnostic evaluation in 113 cases. J. Thorac. Cardiovasc. Surg., *70*:367, 1975.
16. Silver, T. M., and Goldstein, H. M.: Varicoid carcinoma of the esophagus Am. J. Dig. Dis., *19*:56, 1974.
17. Lawson, T. L., Dodds, W. J., and Sheft, D. J.: Carcinoma of the esophagus simulating varices. Am. J. Roentgenol., *107*:83, 1969.
18. Wynder, E. L., and Mabuchi, K.: Cancer of the gastrointestinal tract: etiological and environmental factors. JAMA, *226*:1546, 1973.
19. Naef, A., Savary, M., and Ozzello, L.: Columnar-lined lower esophagus — an acquired lesion with malignant predisposition. J. Thorac. Cardiovasc. Surg., *70*:826, 1975.
20. Burdette, W. J., and Jesse, R.: Carcinoma of the cervical esophagus. J. Thorac. Cardiovasc. Surg., *63*:41, 1972.
21. Collins, S. M., Hamilton, J. D., Lewis, T. D., et al.: Small-bowel malabsorption and gastrointestinal malignancy. Radiology, *123*:603, 1978.
22. Harris, O. D., Cooke, W. T., Thompson, H., et al.: Malignancy in adult celiac disease and idiopathic steatorrhea. Am. J. Med., *42*:899, 1967.
23. Harper, P. S., Harper, R. M. J., and Howel-Evans, A. W.,: Carcinoma of the esophagus with tylosis. Quart. J. Med., *34*:317, 1970.
24. Carter, R., and Brewer, L.: Achalasia and esophageal carcinoma: Studies in early diagnosis for improved surgical management. Am. J. Sur., *130*:114, 1975.
25. Laufer, I.: Tumors of the esophagus. *In*: Haskins, M. E., and Teplick, S. G. (eds.): Surgical Radiology. Philadelphia, W. B. Saunders, in press.
26. Edwards, D. A. W.: Carcinoma of the esophagus and fundus. Postgrad. Med. J., *50*:223, 1974.
27. Roesch, W.: Carcinoma of the esophagus and cardia-endoscopy. Postgrad. Med. J., *50*:227, 1974.
28. Kenneweg, D. J., and Cimmino, C. V.: Carcinosarcoma of the esophagus. Am. J. Roentgenol., *101*:482, 1967.
29. Saibil, E., and Palayew, M. J.: Primary malignant melanoma of the esophagus. Am. J. Gastroenterol., *61*:63, 1974.
30. Carnovale, R. L., Goldstein, H. M., Zornoza, J., et al.: Radiologic manifestations of esophageal lymphoma. Am. J. Roentgenol., *128*:751, 1977.
31. Goldstein, H. M., and Dodd, G. D.: Double-contrast examination of the esophagus. Gastrointest. Radiol., *1*:3, 1976.

6

STOMACH

NORMAL APPEARANCES

The normal appearance of the stomach is familiar to all physicians. However, with the double contrast method, additional details of anatomic structure and surface detail become apparent. These include (1) the surface pattern, (2) the cardia, and (3) compression by adjacent structures.

155

Surface Pattern

Whereas conventional barium examinations of the stomach rely heavily on analysis of the rugal fold pattern, in double contrast studies we prefer to have the normal rugal folds effaced. Abnormal folds, such as those associated with a healing gastric ulcer or an early gastric carcinoma, tend to be stiffer than normal and therefore to resist effacement. They may become particularly prominent when the surrounding normal folds are flattened. When good mucosal coating and adequate distension have been achieved, the surface pattern or areae gastricae can be seen (Fig. 6–1).[1, 2] The frequency of visualization of the surface pattern depends to a large extent on the type of barium being used and can be enhanced by the use of hypotonic agents.[3] This surface pattern is easier to appreciate on radiographs than at endoscopy. Presumably the mucous coating of the stomach makes it difficult to appreciate the small hills and valleys of the gastric mucosa. However, this appearance can be demonstrated by scattering dye, such as methylene blue, on the mucosal surface (Plate 16). The surface of the stomach is particularly well demonstrated on scanning electron micrographs (Fig. 6–2).

The surface pattern is seen most frequently in the antrum, although in some patients it may also be seen in the proximal body and fundus (Fig. 6–1D). In some patients the surface pattern may have an unusually coarse appearance (Fig. 6–3). We feel that this probably represents a form of superficial gastritis, but there have been no controlled correlative studies between the radiologic and histologic appearances to document the significance of variations in the surface pattern.

We have noted that in some young women the areae gastricae may become prominent and rounded, resulting in a coarse nodular surface (Fig. 6–4 and Plate 17). Biopsy findings in several such patients have shown only nonspecific inflammation. In other cases the biopsies have shown intestinal metaplasia. The clinical significance of these findings in young patients is as yet undetermined. Tim and coworkers[4] have described a similar appearance caused by benign lymphoid hyperplasia of the gastric antrum. In any case this seems to be a benign form of mucosal inflammation of uncertain significance. Certainly, mucosal lesions may be demonstrated even in the absence of the areae gastricae. However, for the present we try to demonstrate this surface pattern on our films in order to be confident that we have good mucosal coating. In the future, with refinements in technical and interpretative skills, minor variations in the surface pattern may be helpful in the diagnosis of gastritis and early gastric cancer.[5]

Text continued on page 160

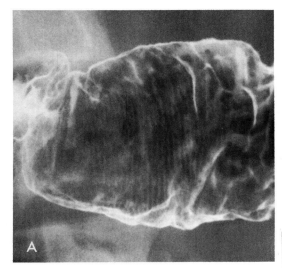

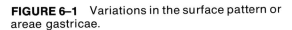

FIGURE 6–1 Variations in the surface pattern or areae gastricae.

A. A prominent transverse pattern in the antrum. This has also been called gastric striae.

B. Fine surface pattern throughout the stomach.

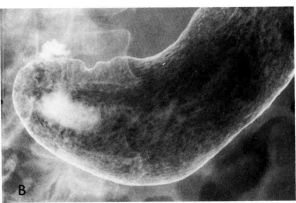

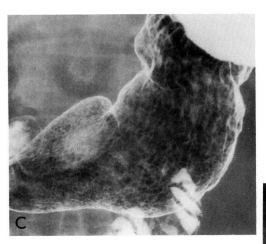

C. Coarse surface pattern.

D. Areae gastricae in the fundus.

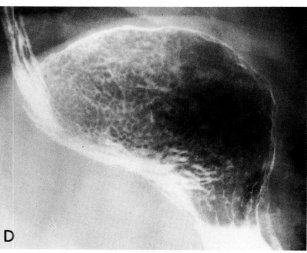

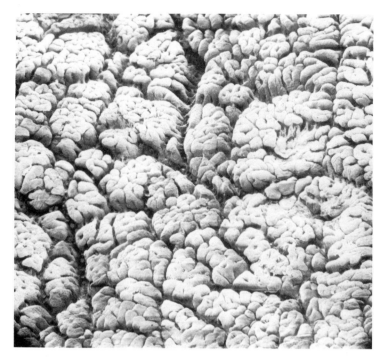

FIGURE 6–2 Scanning electron micrograph showing the surface pattern of the stomach (× 24). The gastric sulci account for the reticular appearance seen on radiographs. The little black dots represent the openings of the gastric pits. (Courtesy of Drs. G. D. Dodd, J. D. Anderson, and H. M. Goldstein, Houston, Texas.)

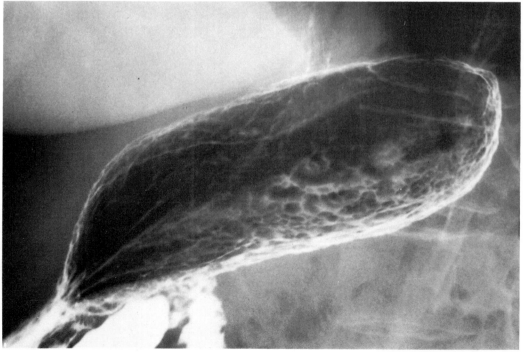

FIGURE 6–3 Coarse polypoid surface pattern in the fundus. The significance of this pattern is unknown.

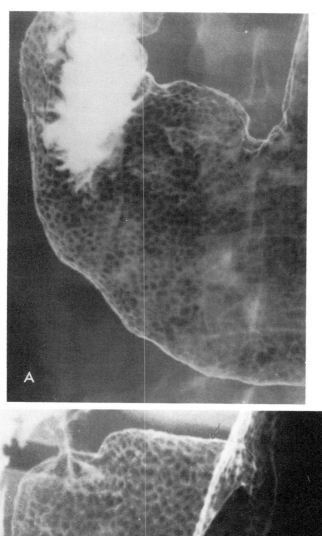

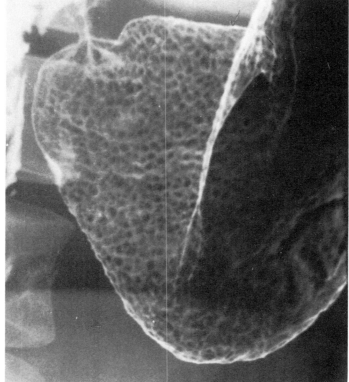

FIGURE 6–4

A and *B*.   Micronodular appearance of the surface pattern in 2 patients. We have noted this appearance in young women with vague epigastric pain. In *(A)* biopsy results showed intestinal metaplasia. See also Plates 17 and 18.

Cardia

The cardia and fundus are particularly well demonstrated by the double contrast technique (Fig. 6–5). There is considerable variation in the appearance of the cardia, particularly when seen en face. Cimmino[6] has described the sign of the "burnous" as the typical appearance of the cardia when seen en face. This consists of a hood with folds streaming away from it (Fig. 6–5B). Demonstration of this anatomic landmark provides good evidence that the cardia is normal. However, this is just one of the several appearances of a normal cardia.

In an analysis of over 200 examinations, we found 3 basic radiographic appearances of the cardia, as illustrated in Figure 6–5.[7] The differences can be explained by the laxity of ligaments around the cardia and by the presence or absence of a hiatal hernia.

The type I cardia has three components (Fig. 6–5A): a rounded soft tissue mass, three or four short radiating folds, and long gastric rugae. In these patients the ligaments are tight, and there is no tendency toward herniation. As the stomach expands around the gastroesophageal junction the distal esophagus is left pouting into the stomach. Therefore, the soft tissue mass represents the invaginated esophagus, and the radiating folds represent the termination of esophageal mucosal folds. An identical appearance can be produced in a resected stomach by invaginating the esophagus into the stomach.

In the type II cardia there is more laxity of the ligaments anchoring the cardia. The radiographic appearance consists of short, very fine folds radiating toward the esophageal orifice, as seen in Figure 6–5B. There is no filling defect due to a soft tissue mass because the distal esophagus is no longer invaginated into the stomach. However, the termination of the esophageal folds is still seen as fine radiating lines.

In the type III cardia there is further laxity of the ligaments such that part of the cardia may be herniated. The fine radiating folds are no longer seen. There is instead a crescentic line caused by the residual angle between the esophagus and stomach (Fig. 6–5C). Gastric rugae are also seen streaming away from the cardia. This appearance corresponds most closely to the sign of the burnous.[5]

In the presence of an obvious hiatal hernia there is no identifiable cardiac structure within the stomach, but gastric rugae may be seen streaming toward the hernia (Fig. 6–6).

Thorough familiarity with the range of appearances of the cardia is necessary in order to avoid mistaking the normal appearance for a pathologic lesion and to recognize some of the subtle abnormalities in this region. These include an ulcer adjacent to the cardia (Fig. 6–7A) which may be mistaken for the esophageal orifice; carcinoma of the cardia (Fig. 6–7B), in which the normal structures around the cardia are completely distorted; and gastric varices (Fig. 6–7C and D), in which the normal cardiac folds are enlarged and scalloped.

Text continued on page 164

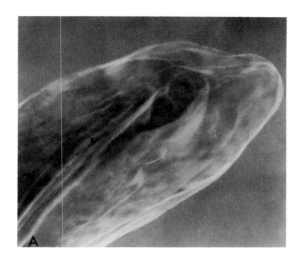

FIGURE 6–5 The gastric cardia and its variations.

A. Type I. There is a rounded filling defect, radiating folds, and gastric rugae streaming away from the cardia.

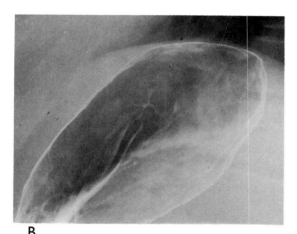

B. Type II. There is a crescentic fold *(arrow)* with gastric rugae streaming away from it.

C. Type III. There are fine radiating folds towards a central point, representing the esophageal orifice.

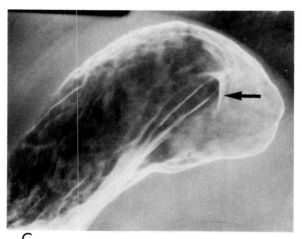

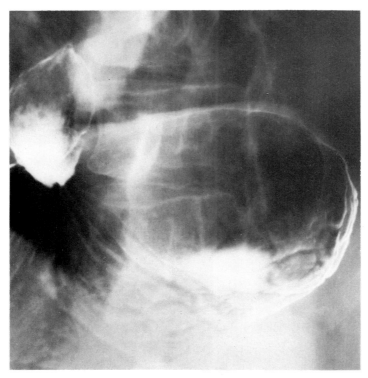

FIGURE 6–6 There is an obvious hiatal hernia. Thefore, there is no identifiable cardiac structure within the stomach, but gastric rugae are seen streaming toward the hernia.

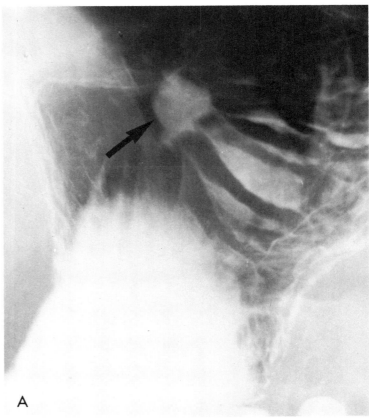

FIGURE 6–7 Abnormalities around the cardia.

A. Gastric ulcer. There is a large barium collection. The radiating folds are much longer and more prominent than the radiating folds related to the normal cardia.

A

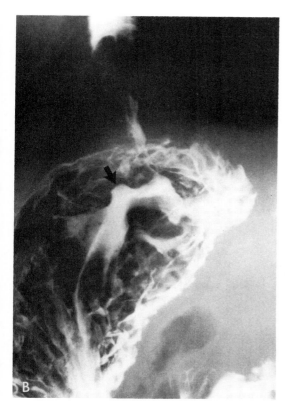

FIGURE 6–7 *Continued*

B. Carcinoma of the cardia. There is a small ulcer *(arrow)* adjacent to the cardia, with no evidence of the normal cardiac structures. The tumor extends into the distal esophagus.

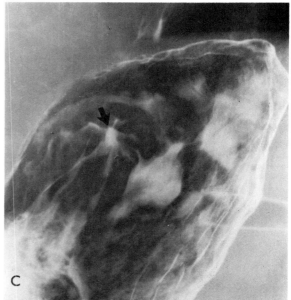

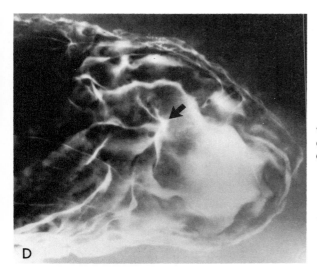

C and *D.* Two examples of gastric varices with enlargement and lobulation of the folds adjacent to the cardia. The esophageal orifice is indicated by an arrow.

Extrinsic Impressions

The double contrast examination results in considerable distension of the stomach, particularly with a hypotonic drug. As a result, normal neighboring structures may produce an impression on the distended stomach. In the lateral view one frequently sees compression of the posterior wall by the normal retrogastric structures (Fig. 6–8A). This compression may become very prominent in thin patients (Fig. 6–8B). Impressions caused by the normal liver are usually quite subtle. However, hepatomegaly and anomalous lobulation of the liver may cause localized compression, which may simulate an intramural gastric lesion (Fig. 2–19D) or a retrogastric mass (Fig. 6–61).[8]

In normal patients, impressions of the spleen and splenic flexure of the colon may also be seen. Abnormal retrogastric impressions can be recognized as an extrinsic mass effect when seen in profile, as a double contour when seen through the air-filled stomach, or as an ill-defined translucency when seen en face (Fig. 2–19).

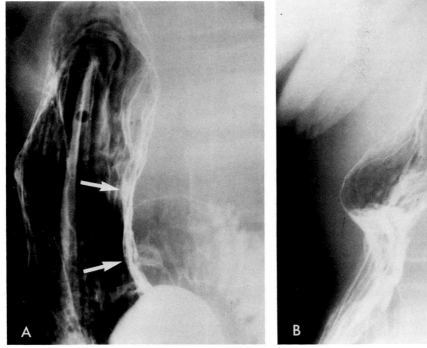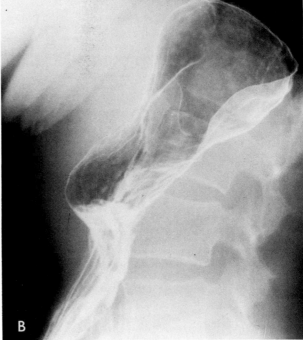

FIGURE 6–8 Normal retrogastric impressions.

A. In the usual case there is a subtle impression on the posterior wall of the stomach *(arrows)* by normal retrogastric structures.

B. In some thin patients these impressions may become very prominent, but are still normal.

Mucosal Folds

In the routine study the rugal folds in the antrum should be completely effaced. Persistence of the folds despite adequate distension is almost always due to antral gastritis. Other causes, such as an arteriovenous malformation, may be encountered rarely (Plate 34).[9]

The rugal folds in the body and fundus may present a particularly confusing appearance (Fig. 6–9A). It may not be possible to efface these folds completely, but with sufficient distension it should be possible to show that they are straight and normal (Fig. 6–9B). Nevertheless, in some cases one may not be able to distinguish normal large folds from those infiltrated by tumor (Fig. 6–10).

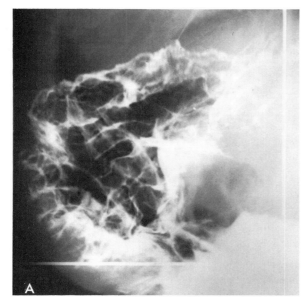

FIGURE 6–9 Importance of distension in the evaluation of large gastric folds.

A.   A right lateral view shows markedly thickened folds in the proximal portion of the stomach, suggesting diffuse infiltration by tumor.

B.   With further distension the folds are seen to straighten, and there is no evidence of tumor.

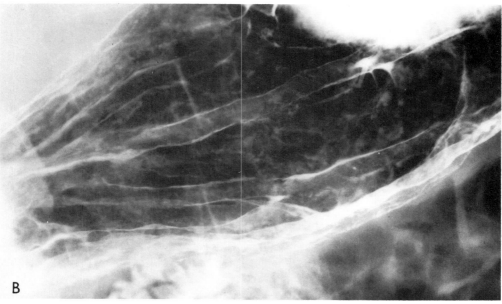

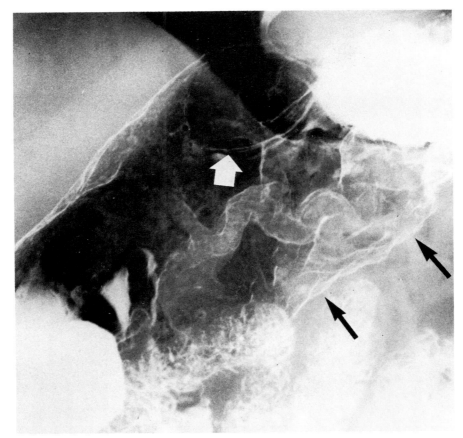

FIGURE 6–10 Localized fold enlargement due to carcinoma. There is a polypoid tumor at the cardia *(white arrow)*. In addition, there is localized enlargement and tortuosity of gastric rugae associated with a plaque-like lesion along the greater curvature *(black arrows)*. *(From:* Kressel, H. Y., et al.: Radiology, *129*:451, 1978.)

ARTIFACTS

The general nature of double contrast artifacts has been discussed in Chapter 2.[10] The most common artifacts encountered in the stomach will be illustrated later. The "kissing" artifact is seen particularly frequently in the stomach and should not be mistaken for a polypoid or ulcerated lesion (Fig. 6–11).

EROSIVE GASTRITIS

An erosion is defined as an epithelial defect that does not penetrate beyond the muscularis mucosae. These lesions are very frequently found at endoscopy. In our review of 267 patients referred for gastroduodenoscopy, erosions were present in 11.2 per cent. In approximately 50 per cent of these cases there were causative factors, such as analgesics, eth-

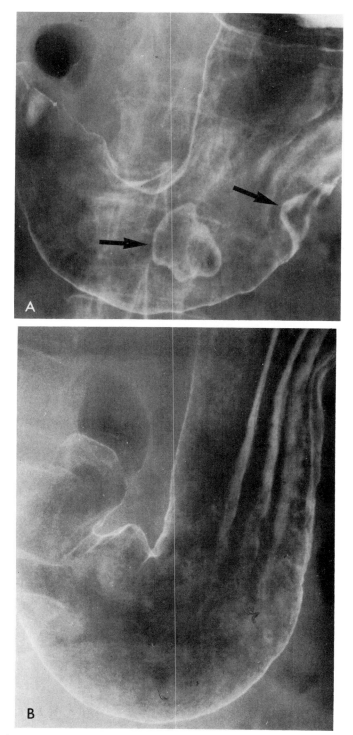

FIGURE 6–11 Kissing artifacts simulating a gastric lesion.

A. In the supine position, the anterior and posterior walls are adherent *(arrows)*. The resulting artifacts may simulate a polypoid or ulcerated lesion.

B. With further distension the walls are separated, and these artifacts disappear. (*From*: Laufer, I.: Radiology, *117*:513, 1975.[32] Reproduced by permission.)

anol, or anti-inflammatory agents. In the other 50 per cent there were no known predisposing causes. Less than 20 per cent of patients with erosions presented with gastrointestinal bleeding.[11]

Despite the frequency with which erosions are seen at endoscopy, they have only rarely been demonstrated on single contrast studies,[12-17] with the notable exception of the studies of Frik and Hesse,[18] who found erosions in 2 per cent of all upper gastrointestinal studies.

Utilizing double contrast techniques, we have found erosions in 2 per cent of our studies.[19] Other authors have reported an incidence of erosive gastritis ranging from 0.5 per cent[20] to 1.7 per cent.[21] However, in their most recent experience, Op den Orth and Dekker[22] reported that erosions were found in over 10 per cent of 500 patients examined.

Gastric erosions present two basic radiographic appearances. The most common appearance is the *varioliform erosion,*[23] which presents as a small target lesion with a central collection of barium representing the erosion and the surrounding radiolucent halo representing the elevated mucosa (Fig. 6–12). These lesions are almost always multiple, although occasionally a single erosion may be seen (Fig. 6–13A). In some patients the mucosal folds are thickened (Fig. 6–13B). The antrum is virtually always involved, although extension into the fundus may be seen rarely. In some patients, erosive gastritis may be manifest only by nodularity or scalloping of prominent antral folds (Fig. 6–14). Depending on the quality of mucosal coating, the erosion itself may not be seen or may be seen only on one of several films. Scalloped folds may also be the result of healing of erosions (Fig. 6–14B). It has been shown by Walk[24] that gastric erosions are a cause of polypoid lesions in the elderly. In some patients, erosions may persist for years even in the absence of clinical symptoms.[25, 26]

The *incomplete erosion* is an epithelial defect without elevation of the surrounding mucosa.[23] This is much more difficult to detect radiologically and may be diagnosed by the reproducible demonstration of linear streaks or dots of barium (Fig. 6–15A). In some cases recognition may be aided by slight deformity or flattening along the greater curvature (Fig. 6–15B).

In the absence of gastrointestinal hemorrhage, the clinical significance of erosive gastritis is unclear. Most patients with this condition present with vague dyspepsia or ulcerlike symptoms which are frequently indistinguishable from those found in patients with normal upper gastrointestinal studies. With increasing radiologic recognition of erosive gastritis, it may be possible to establish the clinical significance of this condition.

There are a few conditions that may be manifested as erosive gastritis. In some patients, erosive gastritis may be a manifestation of the early stages of Crohn's disease involving the stomach (Fig. 6–16).[27, 28] This will be discussed in more detail in Chapter 16. Severe erosive gastritis has also been reported in opportunistic viral infection due to cytomegalovirus[29] and herpes simplex virus[30] in immunosuppressed patients.

Most commonly, gastric erosions must be differentiated from barium precipitates.[10] The latter are very sharp, crisp, and well defined (Fig. 6–17). They do not have a radiolucent halo, and when seen in profile they appear as small lumps of barium sitting on the mucosal surface, rather than as small projections of barium.

Text continued on page 174

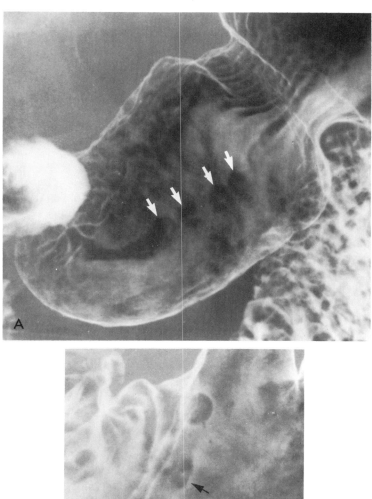

FIGURE 6–12 *A* to *D*   Four examples of varioliform erosions characterized by central barium collections surrounded by a radiolucent halo. (Figure 6–12*D* from Laufer, I., Mullens, J. E., and Hamilton, J.: Radiology, *115*:569, 1975.[88] Reproduced by permission.)

Illustration continued on the following page.

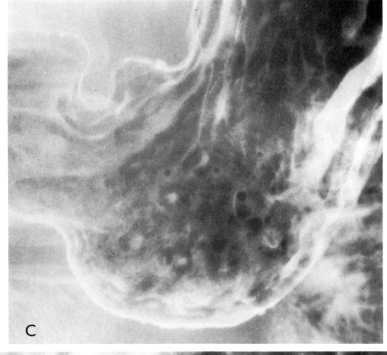

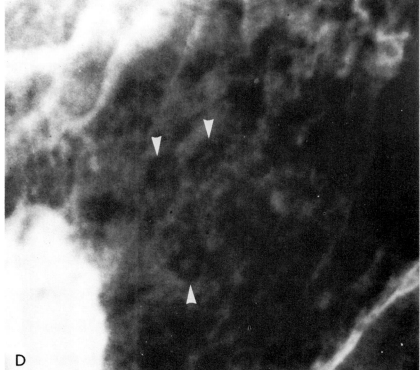

FIGURE 6–12 *Continued*

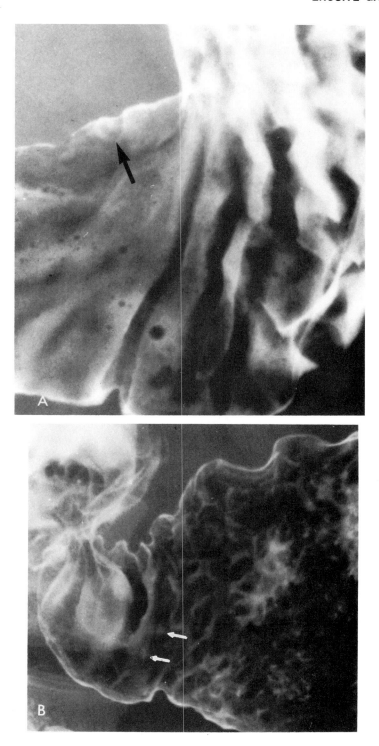

FIGURE 6–13

A. Solitary gastric erosion *(arrow)*. Confirmed by endoscopy. .
B. Multiple superficial gastric erosions in the antrum *(arrows)* associated with thickening of the antral folds.

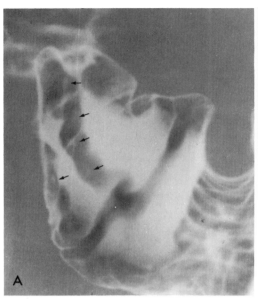

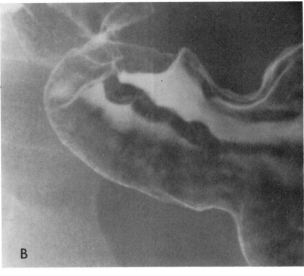

FIGURE 6–14

   A.   Scalloping of the antral folds owing to erosive gastritis. The erosions *(arrows)* are faintly seen on the crest of the rugal fold.

   B.   Residual scalloped antral fold following healing of the erosions.

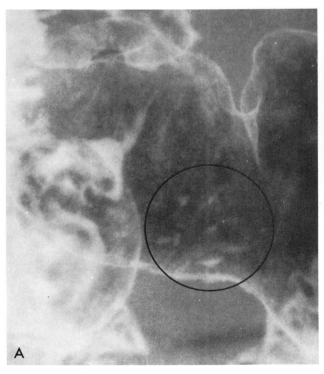

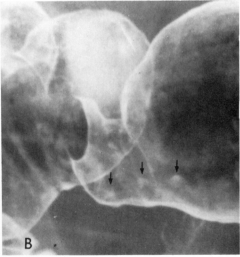

FIGURE 6–15   Incomplete erosions.

   A.   In the antrum there are several rounded and linear collections of barium which were reproduced on multiple films. Endoscopy confirmed that these were incomplete erosions. See Plate 20.

   B.   Small barium collections along the greater curvature of the antrum, representing incomplete erosions. There is also some associated flattening and deformity of the greater curvature.

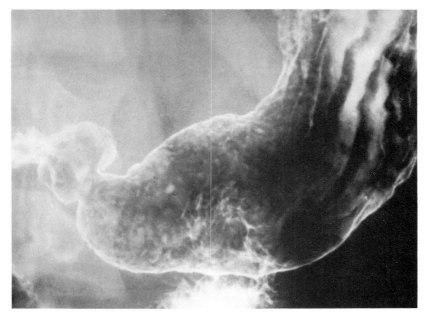

FIGURE 6–16 Erosive gastritis due to Crohn's disease. The distal portion of stomach is studded with superficial gastric erosions. There is also a duodenal ulcer. This patient had changes typical of Crohn's disease in the terminal ileum. Endoscopy confirmed the presence of superficial gastric erosions and biopsy results showed noncaseating granulomata (Plate 75). (*From*: Laufer, I., Trueman, T., and De Sa, D.: Br. J. Radiol., *49*:726, 1976.[27] Reproduced by permission.)

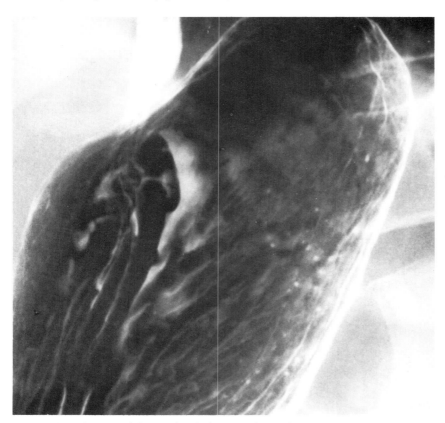

FIGURE 6–17 Small barium precipitates simulating gastric erosions. However, the precipitates are very sharp and distinct, and there is no surrounding radiolucent halo.

GASTRIC ULCERS

The double contrast examination of the stomach was developed for the detection of early gastric cancer in Japan. However, its ability to detect small ulcers and evaluate their features in great detail makes it particularly valuable in North America. Although deformity of the mucosal surface or gastric wall may be helpful in locating a gastric ulcer, the ulcer crater itself must be demonstrated in order to make a definitive diagnosis. The ulcer crater should be demonstrated both in profile and en face.[31] The en face appearance is particularly helpful in evaluating the surrounding gastric mucosa in the differentiation between benign and malignant ulcers.

Technical Points

MUCOSAL COATING

In the search for gastric ulcers it is critical that adequate mucosal coating be achieved. In the absence of adequate coating, small (Fig. 6–18) and even very large ulcers can easily be overlooked (Fig. 2–7).

DISTENSION

Uneffaced mucosal folds may hide a small ulcer, and small collections of barium may get trapped between folds. Therefore, the stomach must be distended sufficiently to efface normal mucosal folds. This will demonstrate the ulcer crater and will also highlight any abnormal folds or areas of diminished distensibility in relation to the ulcer (Fig. 6–19).

POSITIONING

An adequate number of views must be obtained to show each area of the stomach clearly. This is particularly important when a peristaltic wave may conceal a small lesion or when overlapping loops of small bowel may obscure surface detail (Fig. 6–20). In addition, the duodenal cap may overlap the distal antrum and pyloric channel. Small degrees of rotation may bring a lesion into view (Fig. 2–4). Gastric ulcers are commonly found high on the lesser curvature.[33] They may be difficult to detect in profile because of the prominent rugal folds that are normally found in this area. Thus the en face view, with the patient turned to the right and barium drained out of the fundus, is particularly important for the evaluation of this area (Fig. 6–21).

COMPRESSION STUDY

Compression study may show some ulcers that have not been shown on double contrast views, particularly if the mucosal coating is inadequate or if there is active gastric peristalsis.

Text continued on page 179

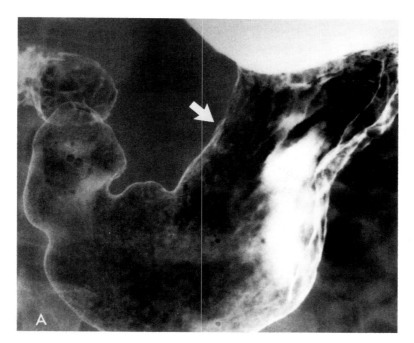

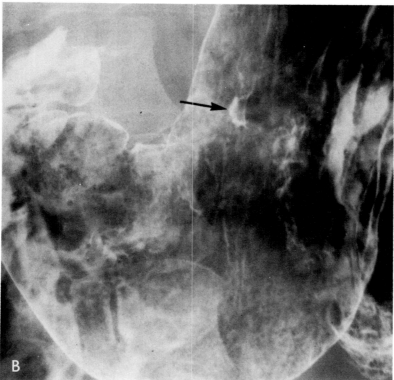

FIGURE 6–18 Danger of poor coating.

A. Supine view double contrast radiograph of the stomach. No definite abnormality is seen, but there is an area of incomplete coating near the lesser curvature *(arrow)*.

B. With improvement in the coating, the semilunar shadow of an ulcer crater is clearly seen (see also Plate 25).

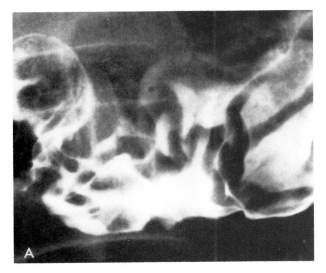

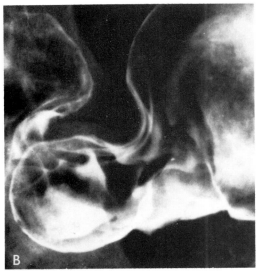

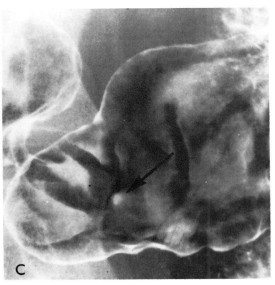

FIGURE 6–19 The importance of gaseous distension.

A. With the antrum collapsed, no diagnosis is possible.

B. With partial distension of the antrum, the ulcer crater is recognizable only in retrospect.

C. With adequate distension, the small ulcer crater *(arrow)* and its radiating folds are clearly seen. See also Plate 22. (*From*: Laufer, I., Mullens, J. E., and Hamilton, J.: Radiology, *115*:569, 1975.[88] Reproduced by permission.)

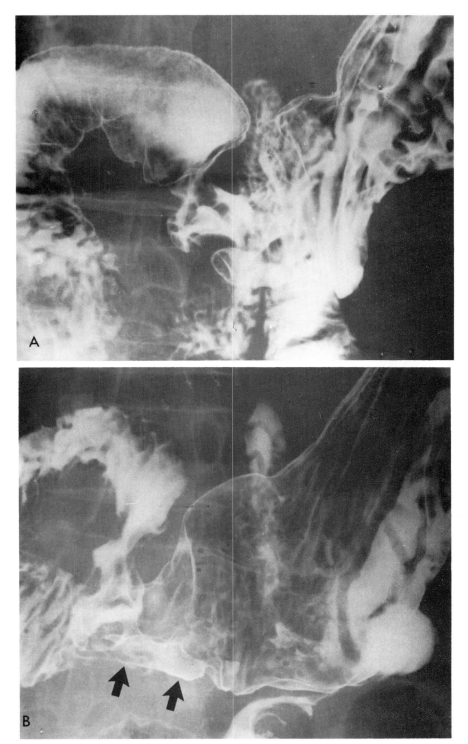

FIGURE 6–20 Importance of projection.

A. Small bowel loops overlap the greater curvature of the stomach in the LPO projection.
B. In the supine projection the overlapping loops are removed, and the large greater curvature ulcer
(arrows) is clearly seen.

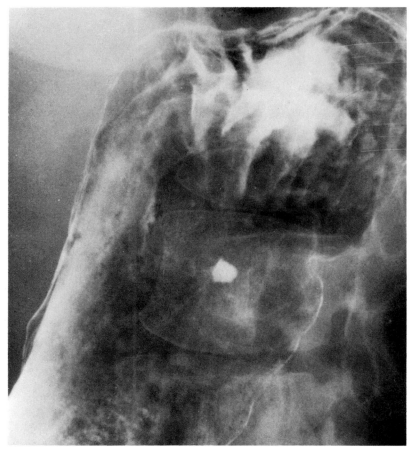

FIGURE 6–21 High lesser curvature ulcer seen en face in the right posterior oblique projection.

Recognition of Gastric Ulcers

On conventional barium studies, the presence of gastric ulcer may be suggested by secondary signs, such as abnormal mucosal folds, edema, or spasm. However, definitive diagnosis requires the demonstration of a barium collection representing the ulcer niche. Ideally, this should be demonstrated in profile and en face.

The appearance of a gastric ulcer on double contrast study will vary according to whether it is on the dependent or on the nondependent wall of the stomach (Chapter 2). An ulcer crater on the dependent wall may collect a pool of barium, resulting in the conventional appearance of an ulcer crater (Fig. 6–22). However, if the ulcer crater is very shallow it may be coated with only a thin layer of barium. This will result in a ring shadow (Fig. 6–23A). If the patient is rotated to wash the barium across the surface of the ulcer, the crater can frequently be filled (Fig. 6–23B and C).

An ulcer crater on the nondependent wall of the stomach will lose its barium pool, but may remain coated. If the ulcer margins are abrupt it will be seen as a ring shadow, which can be confirmed to represent an ulcer by a profile view, or by turning the patient 180 degrees, or by compression (Fig. 6–24). In some cases, in which the base of the ulcer is broader than its neck, a double ring shadow may be seen (Fig. 6–25).

Therefore, one must learn to recognize a ring shadow as an important sign of an ulcer. The ring shadow may be the result of (a) a shallow, dependent wall ulcer that is coated with barium; (b) an ulcer on the nondependent wall coated with barium, or (c) a dependent wall ulcer with a filling defect, such as a blood clot, in its base.

An ulcer crater may have several other appearances. When an ulcer crater is seen not quite tangentially, it may be manifest only as a crescentic (Fig. 6–26) or semilunar line (Fig. 6–18B). By turning the patient under fluoroscopic control this can usually be demonstrated to represent a projecting ulcer crater. In a few patients, particularly those who are unable to turn through 360 degrees, a large ulcer crater may be manifest only as a collection of air before the entry of barium (Fig. 6–27).

While it is important to be able to recognize a gastric ulcer, it is also important to be aware of the peculiar double contrast artifacts that may simulate a gastric ulcer.[10] These have been discussed in detail in Chapter 2, and include the stalactite phenomenon (Fig. 6–28); the see-through effect, whereby colonic or small bowel diverticula may mimic the ring shadow of a gastric ulcer (Fig. 6–29); and patchy coating due to mucus in the stomach, which may simulate an irregular superficial ulcer (Fig. 2–1). Normal anatomic structures may also simulate an ulcer. Radiating folds are seen as part of the normal cardia complex.[7] If the cardia is slightly open it may collect a drop of barium, and the appearance may be very suggestive of a gastric ulcer (Fig. 6–5A). The normal pylorus may also be seen on end, particularly in the right posterior oblique projection. The pyloric canal may be seen as a ring shadow with radiating folds (Fig. 6–30), or there may be a drop of barium trapped in the pyloric channel. In both cases, it may resemble a shallow ulcer.

Text continued on page 186

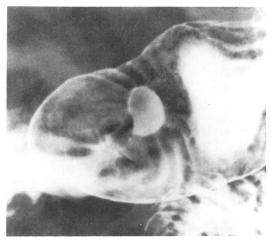

FIGURE 6–22 An ulcer crater on the posterior wall of the antrum with a barium collection and radiating folds.

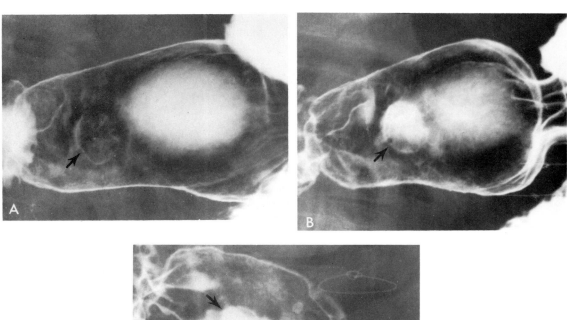

FIGURE 6–23 Varying degrees of filling of a posterior wall ulcer crater.

A. An empty crater with a ring shadow due to coating of the sides of the ulcer.
B. Partial filling of the crater.
C. Complete filling of the crater, indicated by the opacity of the barium collection.

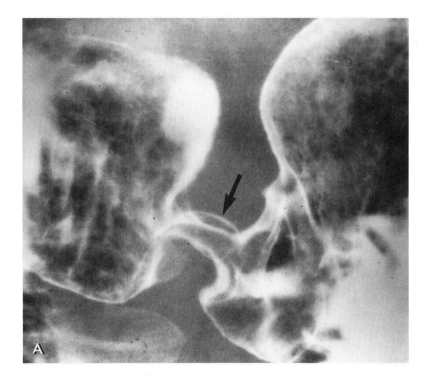

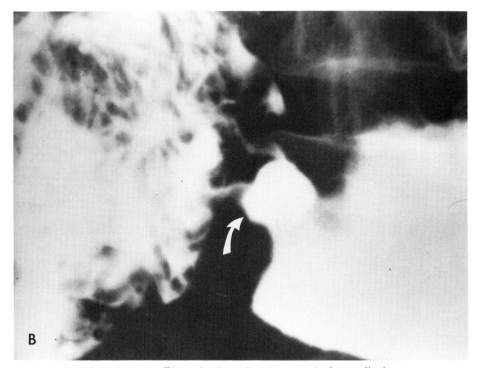

FIGURE 6–24 Ring shadow due to an anterior wall ulcer.

A. In the supine position a ring shadow *(arrow)* is seen in the pyloric channel.
B. With the patient in the prone position the anterior wall ulcer crater fills with barium *(arrow)*.

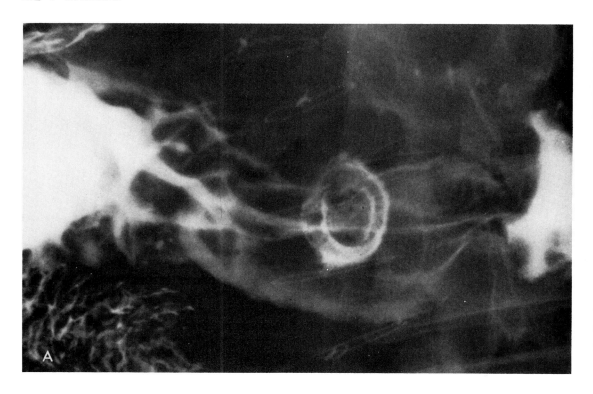

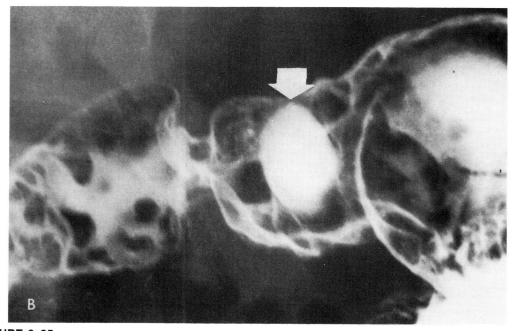

FIGURE 6–25

A. Double ring shadow due to an empty ulcer crater on the posterior wall. The patient is in the prone position.

B. A radiograph taken in the supine position confirms the presence of a posterior wall crater.

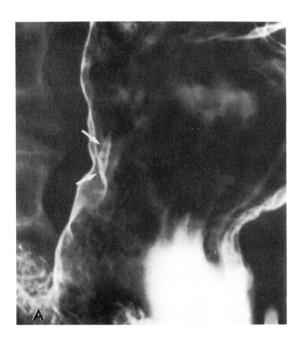

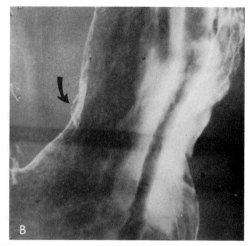

FIGURE 6–26

A. An ulcer crater, not quite seen in profile, is represented by a crescentic line *(arrows)*.

B. With slight rotation the projecting ulcer is seen.

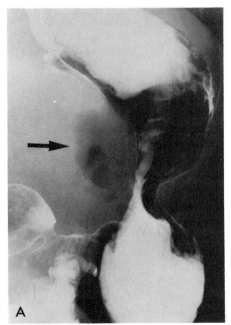

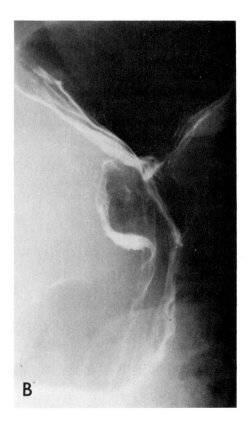

FIGURE 6–27 *A* and *B*. An early film from the upper gastrointestinal study *(A)* shows a large air collection adjacent to the lesser curvature. This represents a large ulcer crater which is coated with barium on the subsequent film *(B)*.

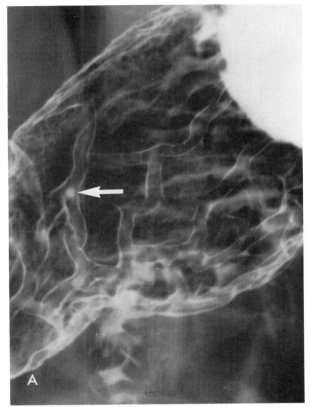

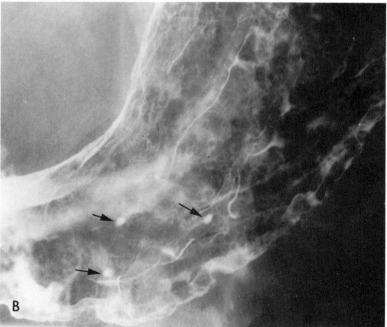

FIGURE 6–28 Stalactite phenomenon.

    A. There is a small rounded density overlying an anterior wall fold. This represents a hanging droplet or stalactite.

    B. Multiple stalactites.

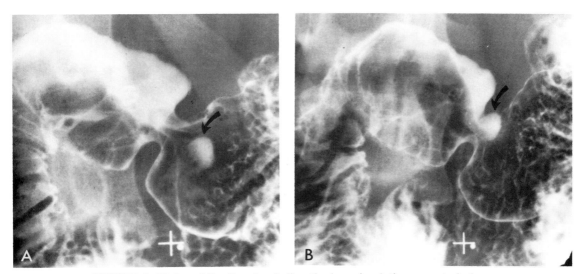

FIGURE 6–29 *A* and *B*   Duodenal diverticulum simulating an antral ulcer.

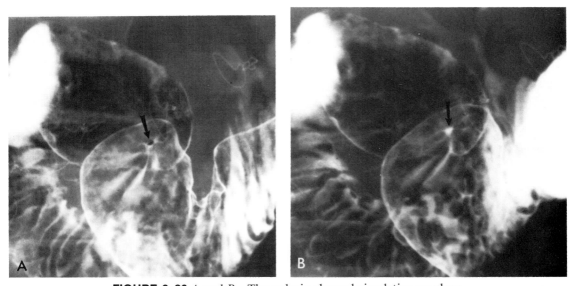

FIGURE 6–30 *A* and *B*   The pyloric channel simulating an ulcer.

Features of Gastric Ulcers

SHAPE

Radiologists are accustomed to looking for a circular collection of barium representing an ulcer crater. However, utilizing double contrast techniques, linear (Fig. 6–31) and rod-shaped ulcers (Fig. 6–32A) can be demonstrated.[19, 34] These are often seen in the healing phase of larger ulcers. Ulcer craters may also have other unusual forms, such as rectangular (Fig. 6–32B), irregular and serpiginous (Fig. 6–32C), or flame-shaped (Fig. 6–33). Their only importance is that the radiologist should be aware that barium collections of unusual shape may represent ulcer craters.

SIZE

Gastric ulcers may be of any size, and it is now accepted that the size of the ulcer has no relationship to the presence of carcinoma.[35] The majority of gastric ulcers are under 5 mm in diameter. Figures 6–34 to 6–36 illustrate a variety of small gastric ulcers.

LOCATION

Benign gastric ulcers are most commonly found along the lesser curvature of the stomach or on its posterior wall. However, benign gastric ulcers may be found almost anywhere,[36, 37] although they are exceedingly rare in the fundus. Younger patients tend to have ulcers in the distal part of the stomach (Fig. 6–37), while in older patients ulcers tend to occur high on the lesser curvature (Fig. 6–38).[38, 39] Stevenson found that over 50 per cent of the gastric ulcers in his series were in the mid- or upper body of the stomach.[33] Clearly, the distribution of ulcers is influenced by the age of the patients being studied.

Greater curvature ulcers are becoming more common with increasing use of anti-inflammatory agents, such as acetylsalicylic acid and steroids. These ulcers produce considerable deformity and frequently appear to lie within the confines of the stomach wall (Fig. 6–39).[40] Patients taking aspirin frequently have multiple greater curvature antral ulcers (Fig. 6–40), or erosive gastritis in addition to an ulcer (Fig. 6–41). When these greater curvature ulcers heal they leave considerable deformity, with outpouchings that may be mistaken for active ulcers (Fig. 6–42A). However, careful study of the mucosa en face will show that these appearances are the result of radiating folds and scarring (Fig. 6–42B). Greater curvature ulcers also have a tendency to penetrate deeply and to progress to gastrocolic fistulae (Plates 28 and 29).[41]

Benign gastric ulcers are virtually never seen along the greater curvature in the proximal half of the stomach. Therefore, any ulcer occurring in this area should be considered to be malignant (Fig. 6–43). Gastric ulcers may also be found within hiatal hernias. They are most commonly seen adjacent to the gastroesophageal junction or at the point of compression of the hernial sac by the esophageal hiatus (Fig. 6–44).[42]

Text continued on page 201

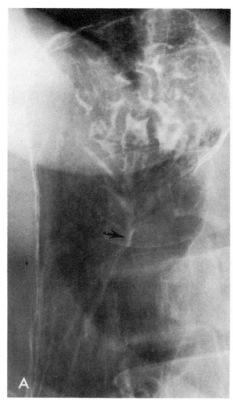

FIGURE 6–31 *A* and *B*   Two examples of linear gastric ulcers. (Figure 6–31 *A* from Laufer, I.: Gastroenterology, *71*:874, 1976.[19] Reproduced by permission. Figure 6–31*B* courtesy of Hans Herlinger, M. D., Leeds, England.)

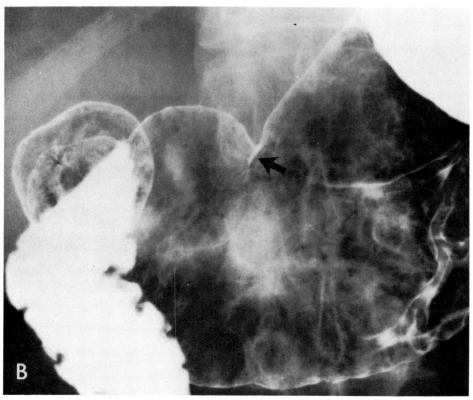

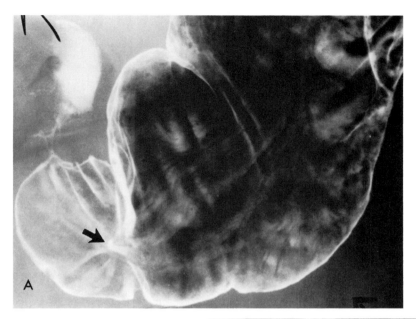

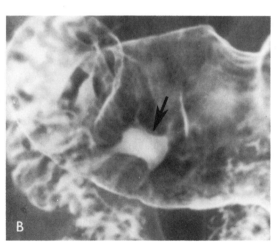

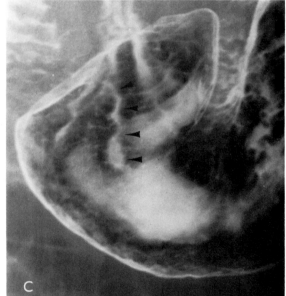

FIGURE 6–32

A. Rod-shaped antral ulcer *(arrow)*.
B. Rectangular antral ulcer.
C. Serpiginous antral ulcer.

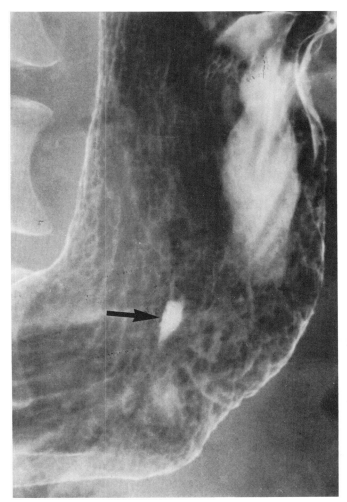

FIGURE 6–33 Flame-shaped posterior wall ulcer. Note that there is slight retraction along the greater curvature owing to scarring. In addition, the surface pattern or areae gastricae extends right to the margin of the ulcer crater. These are all features of a benign gastric ulcer. (*From*: Laufer, I.: Gastroenterology, *71*: 874, 1976.[19] Reproduced by permission.)

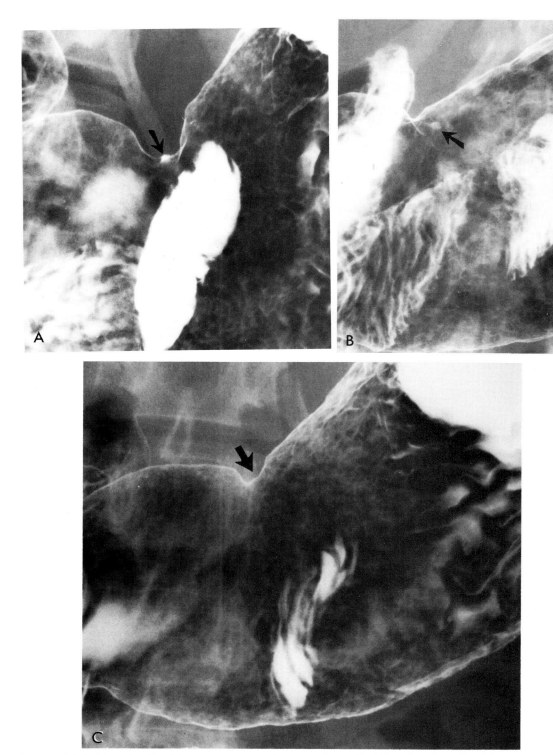

FIGURE 6–34 *A* to *C*   Small lesser curvature ulcer seen in profile *(A)* and en face *(B)*. After healing of the ulcer there is a short, flat scar along the lesser curvature *(C)*

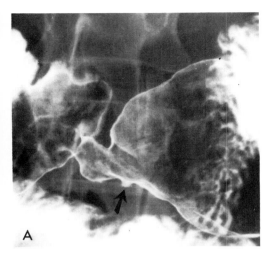

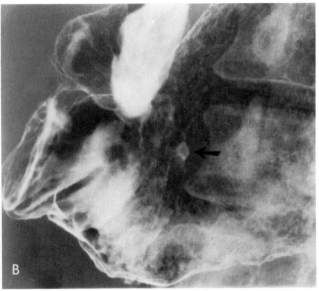

FIGURE 6–35 A variety of small gastric ulcers.

A. Antral ulcer on the greater curvature.

B. Posterior wall antral ulcer.

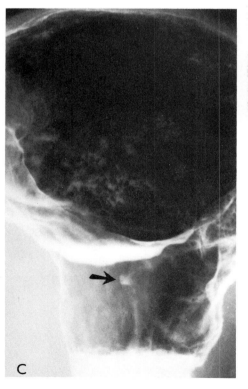

C. Posterior wall ulcer high in the body of the stomach.

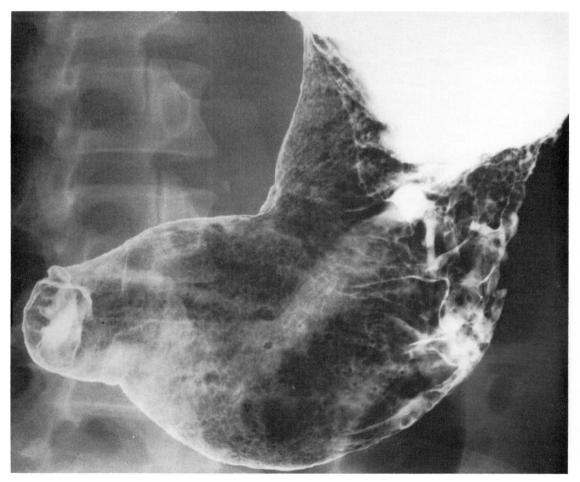

FIGURE 6–36 A broad, shallow ulcer along the lesser curvature at the angle of the stomach.

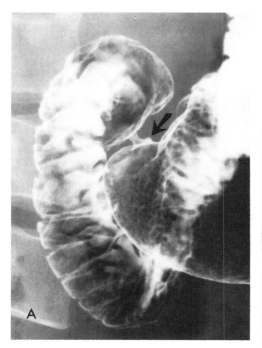

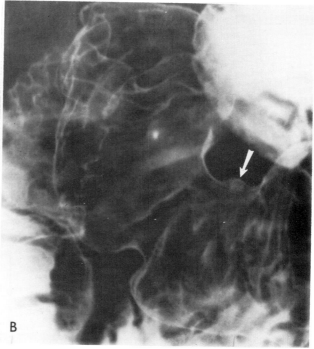

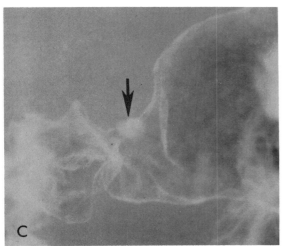

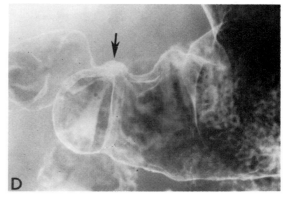

FIGURE 6–37 *A* to *D* A variety of antral ulcers in young patients.

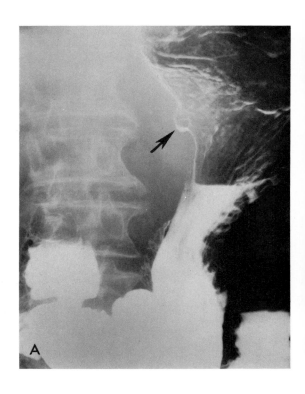

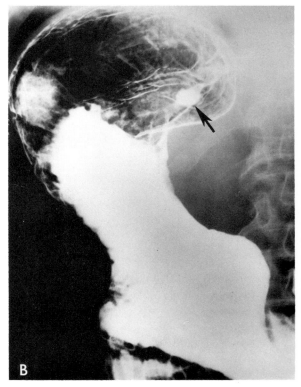

FIGURE 6–38 *A* and *B*   High lesser curvature ulcer seen in profile *(A)* and en face in the prone position *(B)*. This is the so-called geriatric ulcer.

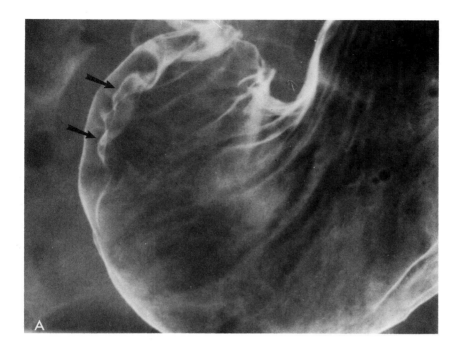

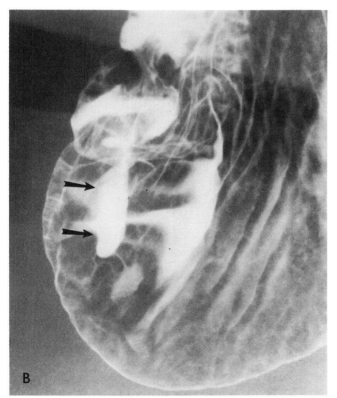

FIGURE 6–39 Greater curvature ulcer due to acetylsalicylic acid.

A. Air contrast view of the ulcer crater in the distal antrum along the greater curvature. The ulcer crater appears to lie within the stomach.

B. The ulcer crater filled with barium.

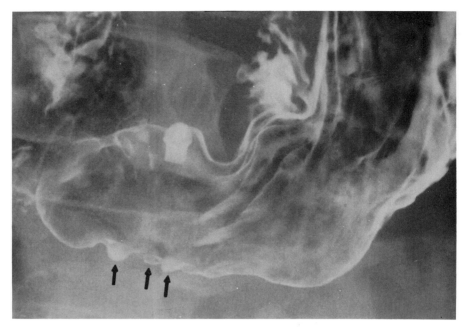

FIGURE 6–40 Multiple greater curvature antral ulcers due to acetylsalicylic acid.

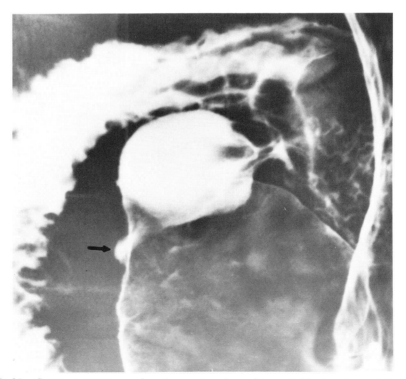

FIGURE 6–41 Greater curvature ulcer *(arrow)* and erosive gastritis due to acetylsalicylic acid.

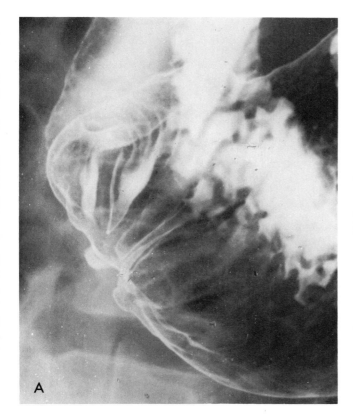

FIGURE 6–42 Multiple ulcer scars along the greater curvature.

A. There are several outpouchings along the greater curvature associated with radiating folds. These outpouchings could be mistaken for gastric ulcers.

B. In a steeper oblique projection it is apparent that there are two ulcer scars *(arrows)* associated with radiating folds. The outpouchings are due to scarring and do not represent active ulcers.

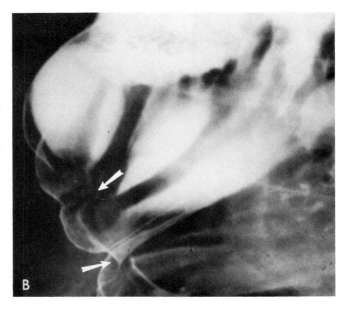

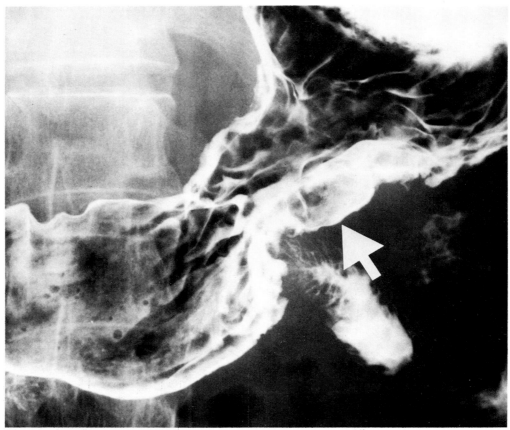

FIGURE 6–43 Malignant ulcer on the greater curvature of the body of the stomach. This is associated with nondistensibility of the midportion of the stomach with circumferential infiltration. Greater curvature ulcers in the proximal half of the stomach are almost always malignant.

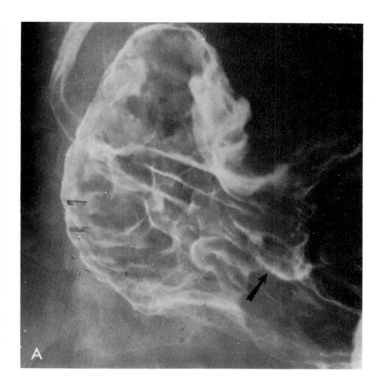

FIGURE 6–44

A. Ring shadow due to an ulcer in a hiatus hernia.

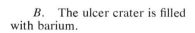
B. The ulcer crater is filled with barium.

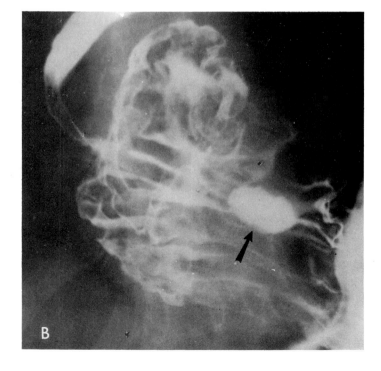

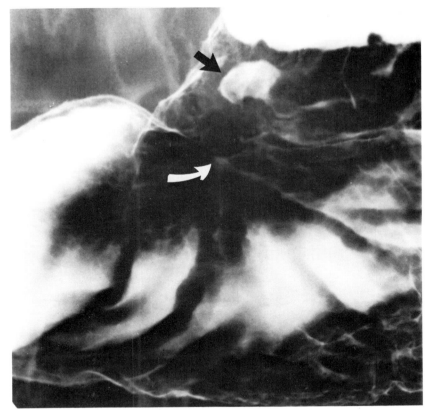

FIGURE 6–45 Two gastric ulcers. One of the ulcers is quite large, while the second is very small.

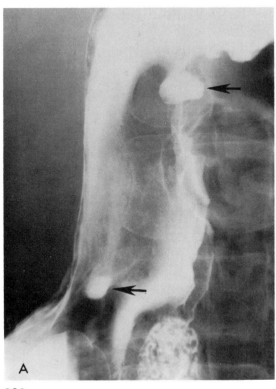

FIGURE 6–46 Multiple gastric ulcers.

A. Acute phase.
B. Healing phase.

MULTIPLE ULCERS

The frequency of multiple gastric ulcers based on conventional single contrast barium studies has ranged from 2.3 per cent[43] to 8 per cent.[44] However, data based on autopsy or surgical specimens indicate a much higher incidence of multiple ulcers, ranging from 17 per cent[45] to 23.6 per cent.[46] Thus it seems clear that the conventional barium study has underestimated the frequency of multiple gastric ulcers. This may be of some importance, since Taxin and coworkers[47] have shown that multiplicity of ulcers is not in itself a sign of benignity. In their series of 29 patients with multiple ulcers, 20 per cent had a malignant lesion. They pointed out that each ulcer must be assessed separately for evidence of malignancy. Bloom and colleagues[48] used double contrast techniques and found multiple ulcers in 23.4 per cent of all patients who had either an ulcer or an ulcer scar. These findings approximate much more closely the results found at autopsy or surgery, and suggest that the double contrast method results in a more accurate detection rate for ulcers.

As mentioned previously, multiple ulcers are frequently seen in patients taking aspirin (Fig. 6–40), although they may also be seen in patients taking no medications (Fig. 6–45). There is frequently a marked discrepancy between the size of the ulcers. The second ulcer may be very small indeed (Fig. 6–46).

Healing of Gastric Ulcers

The radiologic assessment of healing in gastric ulcers is important not only in evaluating therapy but also in detecting malignancy. The progression of ulcer healing has been described by Keller and coworkers.[49] The acute ulcer may have a mound of edema simulating a mass (Fig. 6–47A). With the onset of healing, the mound subsides and the ulcer crater decreases in size and depth. Radiating folds appear, usually extending to the edge of the ulcer crater (Figs. 6–47B and 6–48). This phase may be associated with slight retraction and stiffening of the wall of the stomach.

In some cases the retraction becomes very pronounced and results in an hourglass or stenotic stomach (Fig. 6–49). The ulcer crater may disappear, leaving a patch of bald or granular mucosa (Fig. 6–48D). The ulcer scar may evolve over a period of 2 to 3 years, eventually returning completely to normal, or the radiating folds may persist. A small, central, epithelialized pit may persist at the convergence of the folds in some patients (Fig. 6–50). In some cases this may be a linear depression whose appearance is indistinguishable from that of an active ulcer except it remains unchanged over several months (Fig. 6–51). Scarring may be particularly marked, with ulcers along the greater curvature. This may result in some unusual or picturesque scars (Fig. 6–52).

Complete radiologic healing has been considered a reliable sign of the benign nature of a gastric ulcer. It is certainly true that complete healing is extremely rare in a malignant ulcer.[50] Sakita and coworkers[51] have shown that 71 per cent of ulcerated early gastric cancer showed significant healing, but only one case went on to complete healing. Kagan and Steckel[52] have also reported complete healing of a large ulcer in an area of carcinoma. This healing was confirmed by endoscopy. Similarly, in the Veterans' Administration Hospital Cooperative Study on gastric ulcer Kirsh[53] found four patients with apparent radiologic healing of gastric ulcers that turned out to be malignant. However, in all of these cases there were residual deformities in the surrounding gastric mucosa, which should raise the possibility of underlying carcinoma. This may be manifested by nodularity of the ulcer scar or by irregularity, clubbing, or amputation of the radiating folds. The diagnosis of malignancy in gastric ulcers will be considered further in the next section and in Chapter 7.

Role of Gastroscopy

The role of gastroscopy in gastric ulcer remains controversial and has defied standardization.[54] We agree with Weinstein[55] that early gastroscopy is not necessary in every patient with a radiologically benign gastric ulcer. Rather, we recommend endoscopy in the following circumstances: (a) if the radiologic findings on the initial study are not typical of a benign ulcer; (b) if healing of the ulcer does not progress at the expected rate; (c) if the ulcer crater heals but the mucosa has a nodular surface or any other suspicious features that might indicate an underlying early gastric cancer; or (d) if a technically adequate radiologic examination of the ulcer or ulcer scar cannot be performed. Utilizing such an approach, no cancers should be missed, and at worst a diagnostic delay of a few weeks would occur in the occasional patient.

Text continued on page 208

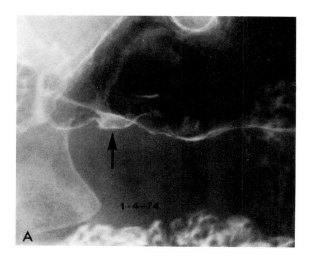

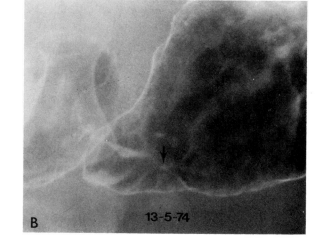

FIGURE 6–47 Healing of a greater curvature ulcer.

A. Acute ulcer. See also Plate 23.

B. Six weeks later there is a tiny residual ulcer *(arrow)* with radiating folds.

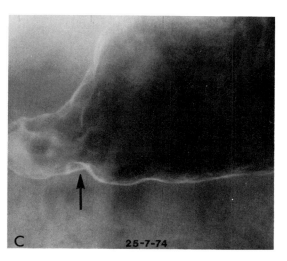

C. Two months later there is an ulcer scar with no residual ulcer crater.

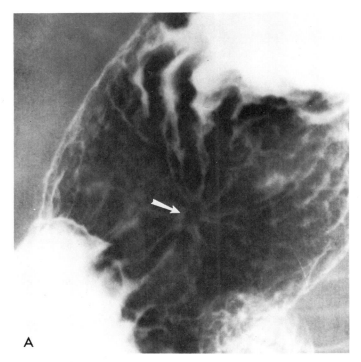

A

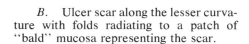

FIGURE 6–48 A variety of ulcer scars.

A. Healing ulcer with radiating folds to a central radiolucency *(arrow),* representing a very shallow, almost completely healed ulcer.

B. Ulcer scar along the lesser curvature with folds radiating to a patch of "bald" mucosa representing the scar.

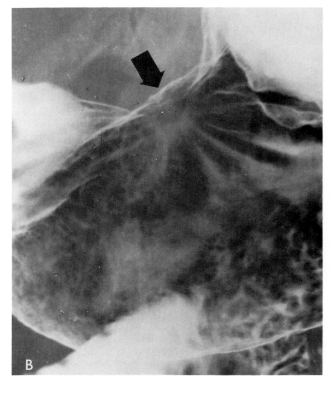

B

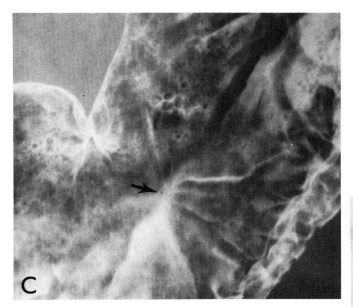

C. Radiating folds to an ulcer scar on the posterior wall of the body of the stomach.

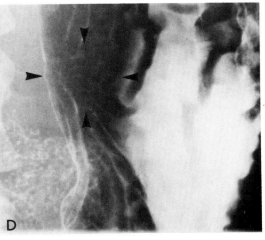

D. An ulcer scar near the lesser curvature of the body of the stomach. There are smooth radiating folds that stop short of a patch of granular mucosa, representing the ulcer crater. (*From*: Laufer, I.: Radiology, *117*:513, 1975[32] Reproduced by permission.)

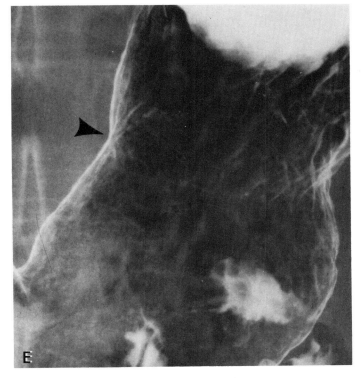

E. Ulcer scar high on the lesser curvature with slight retraction *(arrow)* and radiating folds.

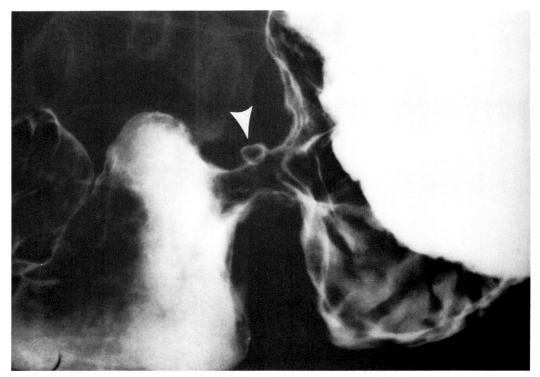

FIGURE 6–49   Hourglass deformity of the stomach due to a healing ulcer *(arrow)*.

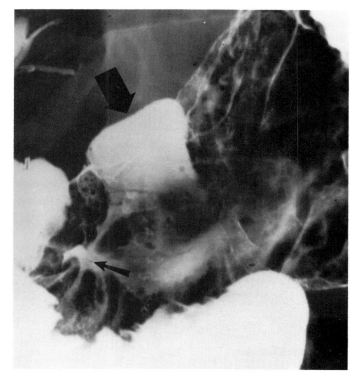

FIGURE 6–50   An ulcer scar *(small arrow)* with radiating folds and a central, epithelialized pit that resembles an active ulcer crater. The large arrow indicates the site of a cystogastrostomy.

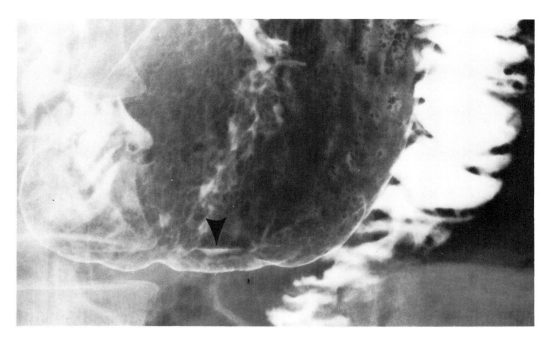

FIGURE 6–51   Linear ulcer scar. There is a linear collection near the greater curvature *(arrow)*. This is associated with slight retraction proximally and distally. At endoscopy, this represented an epithelialized ulcer scar.

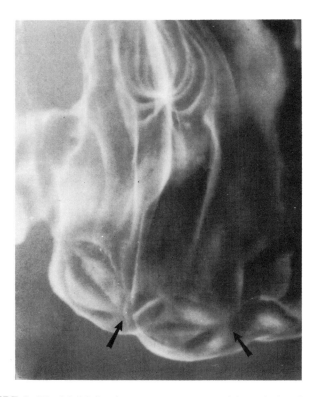

FIGURE 6–52   Multiple ulcer scars *(arrows)* with radiating folds and retraction.

BENIGN TUMORS

Mucosal Polyps

Benign gastric polyps are generally considered to be uncommon lesions.[56] However, in routine double contrast studies of the stomach, we have found gastric polyps in 2 per cent of all studies. Since most gastric polyps are known to be very small lesions, it is likely that most are being overlooked on conventional barium studies.

A gastric polyp on the dependent wall of the stomach may be seen as a negative filling defect in the thin layer of barium (Fig. 6–53). If the lesion is on the anterior wall or nondependent surface of the stomach, it may be etched in white against the intraluminal gas (Fig. 6–54). If the polyp is pedunculated, its stalk may be seen en face overlying the head of the polyp, producing the "Mexican hat" appearance (Fig. 6–54). Frequently a stalactite will hang down from the anterior wall polyp. When this hanging droplet is seen en face, it may resemble ulceration within the polypoid lesion (Fig. 6–55). If this is observed for a period of time it will be seen to disappear as the droplet falls off. In addition, if compression studies are performed no ulcer is demonstrated.

The vast majority of polypoid lesions in the stomach are hyperplastic polyps.[57] These are usually small lesions, under 1 cm in diameter, and are found in patients with chronic gastritis. They are frequently multiple (Fig. 6–56), with gradation in size from slightly heaped-up mucosa to well-defined polyps with a stalk. These polyps appear to be particularly frequent in patients with pernicious anemia.[58] Malignant transformation of these polyps is extremely rare, but there is a significant incidence of associated carcinoma. It appears that both the hyperplastic polyp and the carcinoma are related to the underlying chronic atrophic gastritis.[57, 59]

Adenomatous polyps tend to be larger and have a much higher incidence of malignant transformation.[57, 59, 60] The incidence of carcinoma is related to polyp size, and becomes significant when the polyp reaches a diameter of 2 cm. (Fig. 6–57). There is also a high incidence of coexisting carcinoma in the remainder of the stomach. Thus it is clear that any stomach found to contain single or multiple polyps must be examined carefully for the possibility of a coexisting carcinoma.[56]

Gastric involvement in the polyposis syndromes is discussed in Chapter 14.

Text continued on page 212

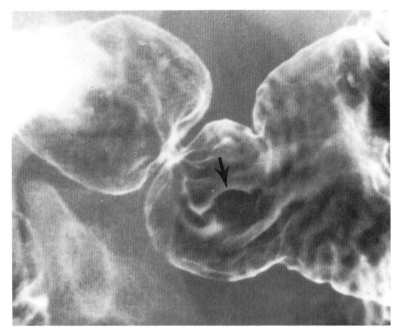

FIGURE 6–53 Antral polyp on the posterior wall seen as a radiolucent filling defect.

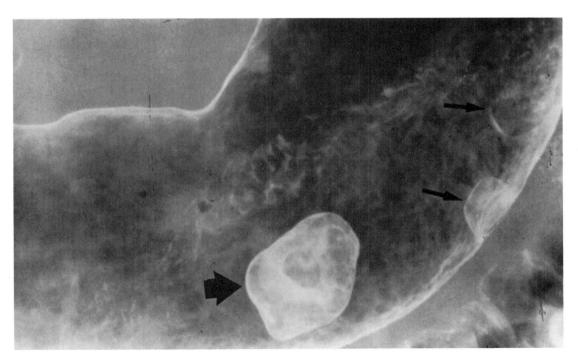

FIGURE 6–54 Multiple anterior wall polyps. The largest polyp exhibits the Mexican hat sign, with the central lucency representing the stalk of the polyp.

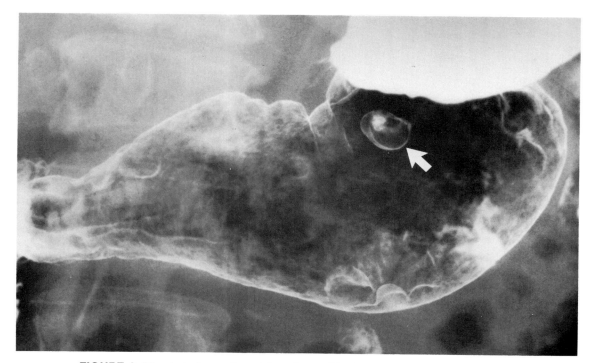

FIGURE 6–55 Anterior wall gastric polyps with the stalactite phenomen *(arrow)*.

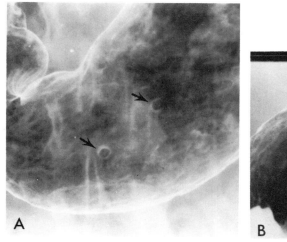

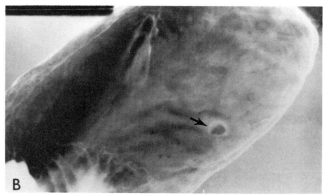

FIGURE 6–56 *A* and *B* Multiple small hyperplastic polyps.

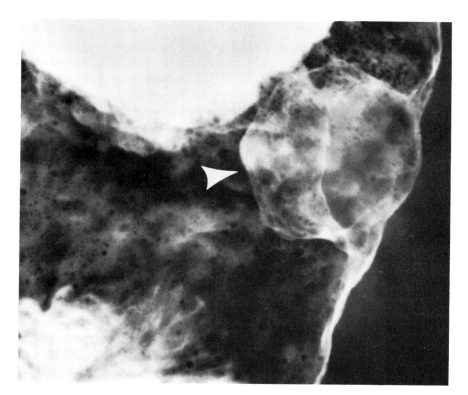

FIGURE 6–57   Adenomatous polyp with carcinoma. The large polyp along the greater curvature measured 3.5 cm in diameter. It was largely an adenomatous polyp with a focus of carcinoma in its center.

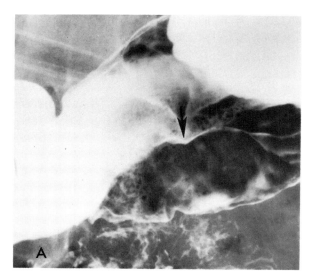

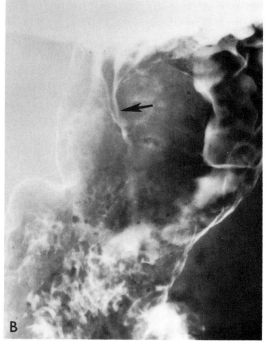

FIGURE 6–58 *A* and *B*   Gastric lipoma in a patient with neurofibromatosis. The tumor, seen in profile *(A)* and en face *(B)*, has a central furrow *(arrow)*.

Submucosal Tumors

Leiomyoma is by far the commonest submucosal tumor in the stomach. Neurofibromas and lipomas are seen less frequently. Even in patients with generalized neurofibromatosis, the most common gastric tumor is a leiomyoma or lipoma rather than a neurofibroma (Fig. 6–58).[61] A submucosal tumor can be recognized by the right angle that it forms with the gastric wall and by its smooth margin and surface (Fig. 6–59). When seen en face, the mucosal folds tend to fade out as they approach the tumor (Fig. 2–18). These lesions vary in size from growths of several millimeters to enormous tumors. The growth may be primarily exogastric and they have a tendency to ulcerate and cause gastrointestinal bleeding. In general the various submucosal tumors are indistinguishable from each other on radiologic grounds, except that a lipoma may change in shape, providing a clue to the specific diagnosis. Malignancy is usually suggested only by the larger size of a submucosal tumor or by extensive ulcerations (Fig. 6–60).

Several types of lesions may mimic submucosal tumors. Pancreatic rests may produce a submucosal mass, usually in the distal portion of the stomach. Approximately half of these lesions have a small central barium collection, and the overall appearance may suggest an ulcerating submucosal tumor.[62]

An acute antral ulcer with a large mound of edema may also simulate an intramural lesion. In such cases there will be a more gradual transition between the edematous mound and the normal adjacent gastric mucosa.[63] In some patients, extrinsic compression of the stomach by normal or enlarged liver, spleen, pancreas, or kidney may not be distinguishable from an exophytic submucosal tumor (Fig. 6–61). In such patients, additional investigation, such as ultrasound, isotope scans, computerized tomography (CT) scans, or angiography may be useful.

Text continued on page 216

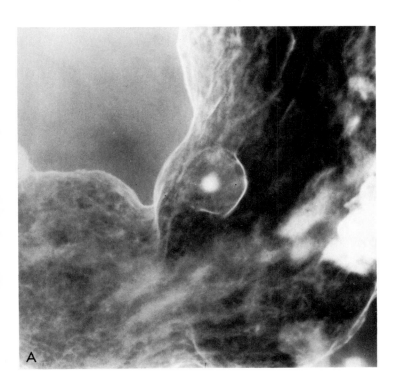

FIGURE 6-59
   A.   Anterior wall leiomyoma with stalactite phenomenon.

B.   An oblique projection confirms the anterior wall location of the tumor and its submucosal characteristics.

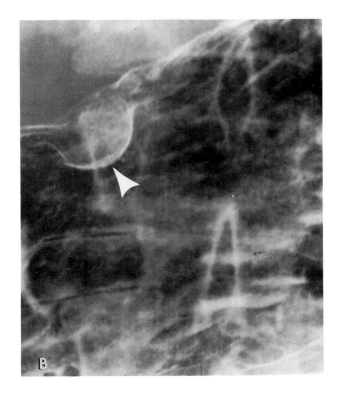

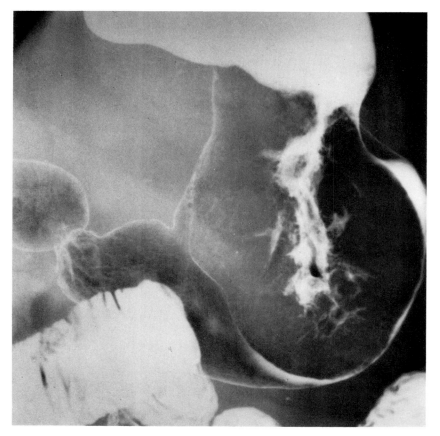

FIGURE 6–60   Large leiomyosarcoma on the posterior wall of the stomach with a large, irregular ulceration. (Courtesy of Hans Herlinger, M.D., Leeds, England.)

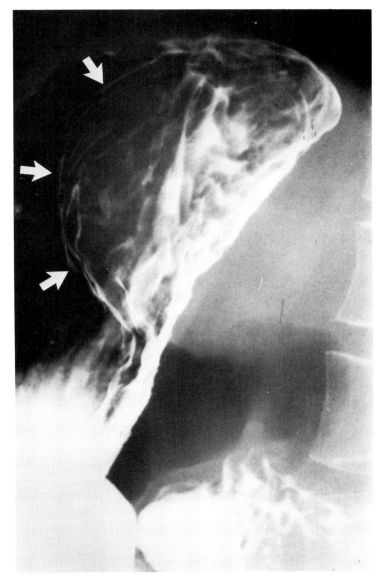

FIGURE 6–61 Extrinsic compression on the posterior aspect of the stomach by a pancreatic pseudocyst. This type of compression may be difficult to distinguish from an exophytic intramural tumor.

MALIGNANT TUMORS

Carcinoma

ADVANCED TUMORS

Most patients with carcinoma of the stomach present with advanced tumors. Grossly, these can usually be classified as infiltrative, polypoid, ulcerative, plaque-like or large fold type, based on their most prominent feature (Figs. 6–62 to 6–66). Cooley[64] has summarized the literature regarding the accuracy of the conventional barium meal in the diagnosis of gastric cancer. He concluded that despite the advanced stage of many of these lesions, approximately 10 per cent of gastric carcinomas were missed on the initial barium study, and an additional 15 per cent were misdiagnosed as benign lesions. Several studies have shown that infiltrating tumors and tumors involving the proximal part of the stomach are most likely to be missed.[65, 66] These are precisely the lesions that require accurate radiologic diagnosis, since they frequently yield negative endoscopic biopsy and cytologic results.[67] In the detection of advanced gastric cancer the double contrast technique is particularly valuable for the demonstration of infiltrating lesions (Fig. 6–67) and for the examination of the proximal portion of the stomach.

Localized areas of rigidity or decreased distensibility are accentuated by the gastric distension achieved during the double contrast study (Fig. 6–67). Indeed, the greater the degree of distension the more apparent localized areas of rigidity may become. However, it must be remembered that overdistension may obscure some of the surface details of the lesion which are better seen in the less distended state (Fig. 2–3). The important feature is that gastric distension can be achieved without obscuring surface detail by large volumes of barium. In some patients, very thick mucosal folds may simulate the appearance of a tumor. With adequate gastric distension, the folds may be straightened out to present a normal appearance (Fig. 6–68).

The proximal portion of the stomach is notoriously difficult to examine by conventional barium study. Even large lesions around the cardia or in the fundus may be missed (Fig. 6–69A).[68] With the addition of gas, these lesions become obvious (Fig. 6–69B, Plate 39). With careful attention to the region of the cardia, even small tumors can be detected (Fig. 6–70A).[69] These patients frequently present with dysphagia. In some patients, carcinoma involving the fundus or cardia presents with a radiologic picture in the esophagus indistinguishable for that of achalasia.[70] However, careful examination of the region of the cardia and fundus will invariably demonstrate the primary gastric carcinoma (Fig. 6–63). The achalasia-like picture is due to submucosal spread of tumor along the esophagus.

The radiologic diagnosis of recurrent gastric carcinoma and primary gastric stump carcinoma is considered in detail in Chapter 8.

Text continued on page 226

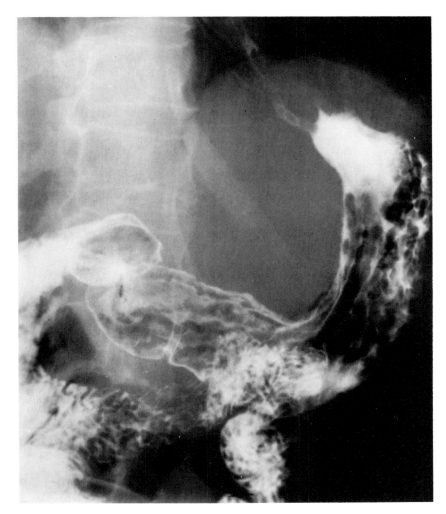

FIGURE 6–62   Scirrhous carcinoma involving the whole stomach. There was also involvement of the distal esophagus, producing a picture indistinguishable from that of achalasia. The patient presented with dysphagia.

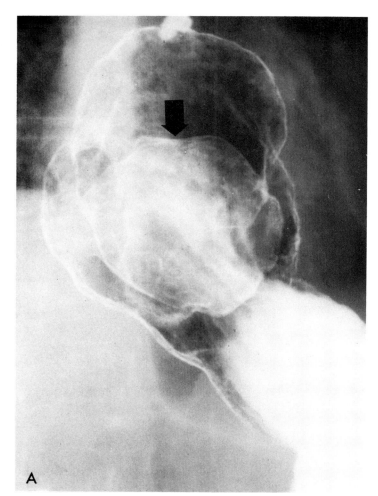

A

FIGURE 6–63 Polypoid carcinoma.

A. Large polypoid carcinoma in a hiatus hernia.

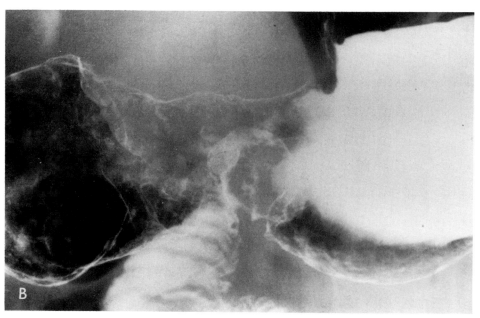

B

B. Right posterior oblique projection, showing an annular polypoid carcinoma involving the midportion of the stomach.

218

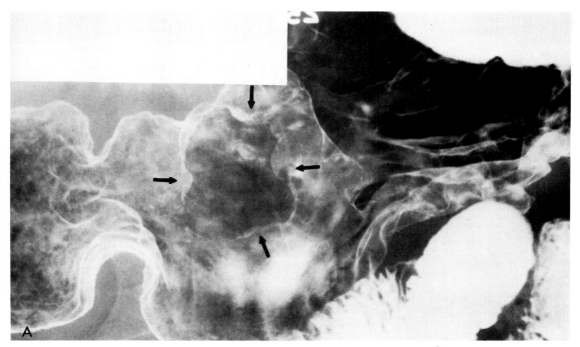

A. In the supine position only an irregular ring shadow is seen *(arrows)*.

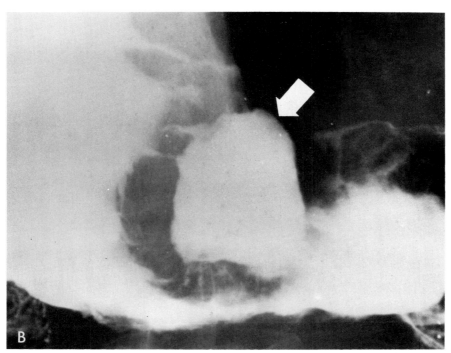

B. In the prone position the large ulcer *(arrow)* and the surrounding rim of tumor tissue are clearly seen.

FIGURE 6–64 Ulcerated carcinoma on the anterior wall.

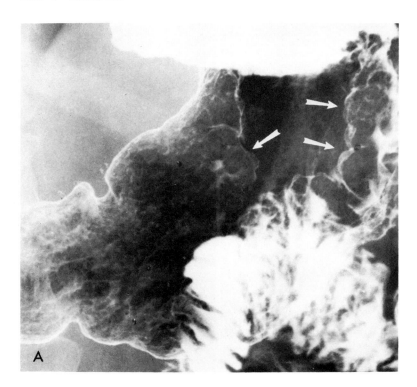

A

FIGURE 6–65

A. Scirrhous carcinoma presenting as large, lobulated mucosal folds.

B. Close-up view shows the disorganization of the folds in the body of the stomach.

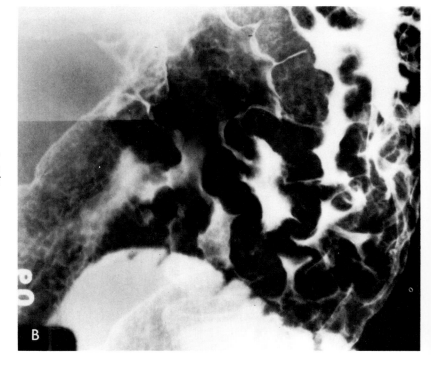

B

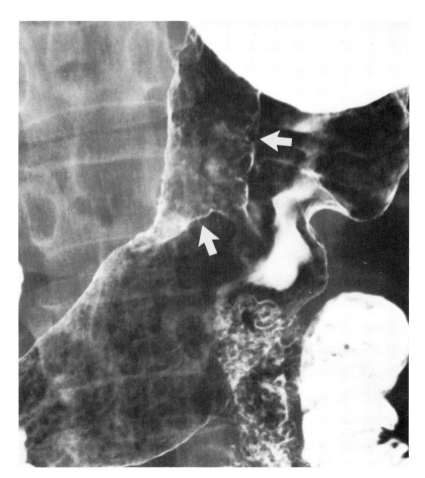

FIGURE 6-66   Plaque-like carcinoma high along the lesser curvature of the stomach.

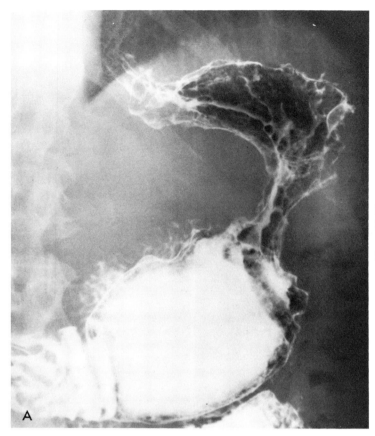

FIGURE 6–67 Additional examples of infiltrating carcinoma.

  A. Tumor involving the proximal half of the stomach.

  B. Diffuse infiltration of the entire stomach, with a broad ulcer crater along the lesser curvature *(arrow).* See also Plate 37.

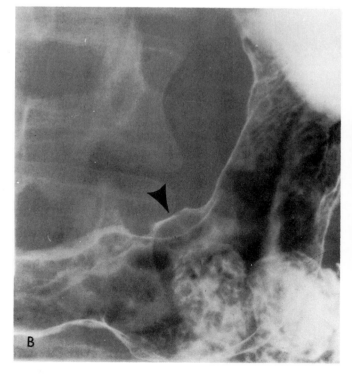

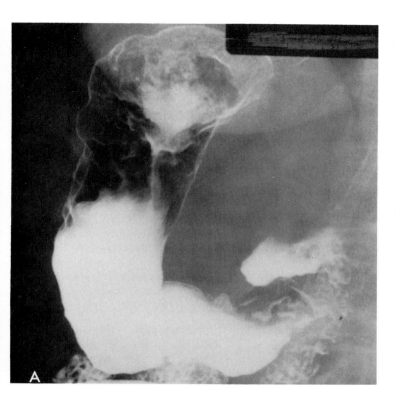

FIGURE 6–68

A. Thick folds in the proximal portion of the stomach, raising the possibility of tumor.

B. With adequate gaseous distension the folds are effaced, ruling out the possibility of tumor.

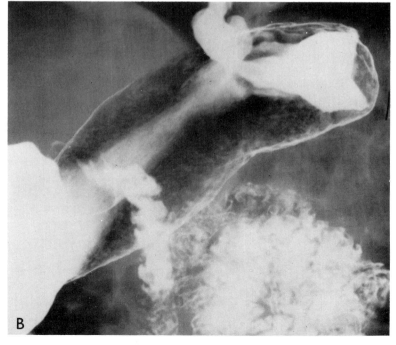

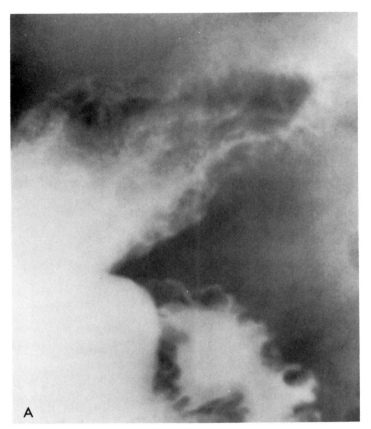

FIGURE 6–69 Ulcerated carcinoma at the cardia.

A. Without gaseous distension the tumor is not seen.

B. With distension the large ulcer *(arrows)* adjacent to the cardia is clearly seen. See Plate 39. (*From*: Glass, G. B. J. (ed.): Progress in Gastroenterology. Vol. 3. New York, Grune & Stratton, 1977. Reproduced by permission.)

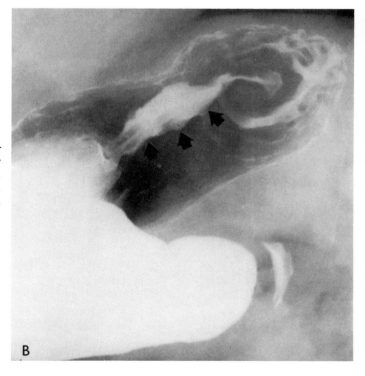

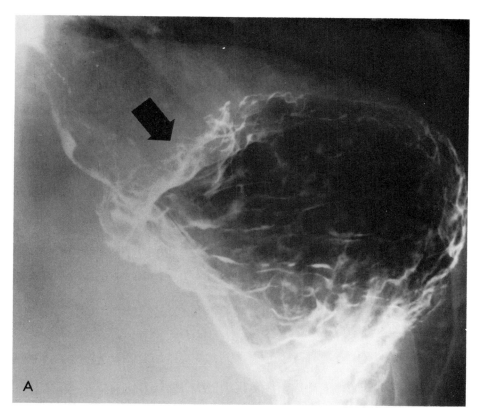

A. Film in upright position, showing localized infiltration of the medial aspect of the fundus as a result of tumor.

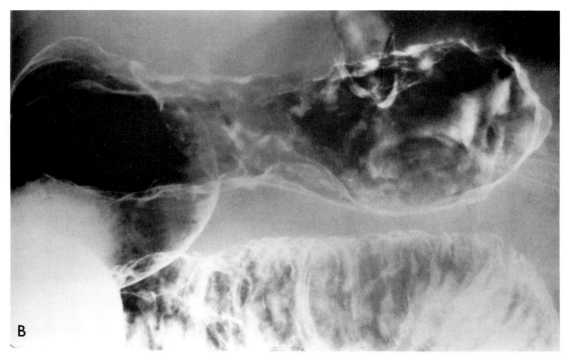

B. Right lateral projection showing involvement of the fundus and proximal body of the stomach by infiltrating tumor.

FIGURE 6–70 Two examples of carcinoma involving the cardia and fundus.

MALIGNANT VERSUS BENIGN ULCERS

The double contrast study is helpful in the differential diagnosis of benign and malignant gastric ulcers. The typical distinguishing features of a benign ulcer on conventional barium study have been well described and are well known.[71-73] These include: projection beyond the contour of the stomach, radiating folds to the edge of the ulcer, intact surrounding mucosa, Hampton line, and absence of filling defects. Nevertheless, in many cases the presence or absence of these signs cannot be determined. The double contrast method facilitates the detection of malignant changes by allowing the most detailed study of the surrounding mucosa in the search for evidence of mass, mucosal destruction, nodularity, or rigidity (Figs. 6–71 to 6–74). In a benign ulcer the normal surface pattern or areae gastricae can frequently be seen extending to the edge of the ulcer crater (Fig. 6–33). By contrast, in a malignant lesion the surface pattern may be distorted or may stop short of the ulcer crater (Fig. 6–75).

Radiating folds are associated with the healing stages of a gastric ulcer. In benign lesions the folds are thin, straight, and uniform. They are often best seen in relation to a healing ulcer or an ulcer scar (Fig. 6–48). However, malignant ulcers also may have radiating folds. In these cases the folds are irregular and nodular, and may stop well short of the ulcer crater (Figs. 6–72 and 6–74). The tips of the folds may be fused, clubbed, or amputated (Chapter 7) (Fig. 7–9).[74]

Many patients with benign gastric ulcers will have some features that may raise the possibility of carcinoma (Fig. 6–75). This is particularly true in patients with acute or active gastric ulcers in which the inflamed mucosa surrounding the ulcer may be nodular or disorganized. Such patients may be reexamined after two weeks of medical treatment. Once the inflammatory reaction subsides, the mucosa surrounding the ulcer crater has a much more benign appearance. Alternatively, these patients may be evaluated by endoscopy with biopsies and brushings for cytology. In some institutions these techniques are very accurate for the detection of carcinoma.[75] However, in many institutions a significant number of carcinomas are missed by biopsies and cytologic examination. Segal and coworkers[76] have reported negative results in 30 per cent of patients with malignant lesions. Therefore, if a lesion is highly suggestive of malignancy on radiologic grounds, negative endoscopic or cytologic findings should not be taken as definitive evidence of its benign nature. Additional follow-up studies should be performed at frequent intervals, and if the lesion does not resolve surgical resection may be necessary.

Because of the subtlety of detail visible with the double contrast technique, it is probably true that the possibility of malignancy is raised in many benign gastric ulcers. The value of the double contrast method and the specific radiologic signs of benignity or malignancy using this technique have not yet been evaluated outside Japan. Therefore, until further experience provides this information, it seems prudent to err on the side of caution by suggesting the possibility of early carcinoma in benign lesions rather than calling lesions with uncertain findings benign.

Text continued on page 230

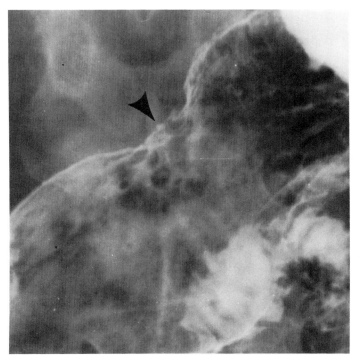

FIGURE 6–71   Early gastric cancer with an ulcer along the lesser curvature *(arrow)*. There is nodularity of the mucosa surrounding the ulcer crater.

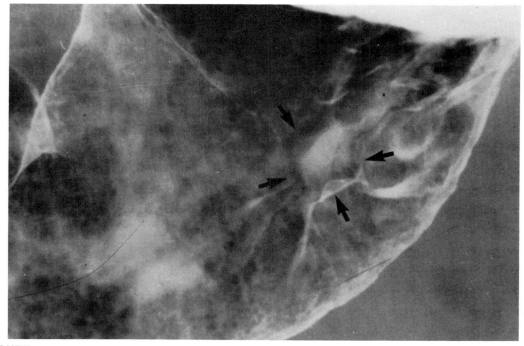

FIGURE 6–72   Ulcerated gastric carcinoma. The radiating folds are nodular and irregular. There is a shallow ulcer *(arrows)* with a tumor nodule in its wall. See Plate 40. (Courtesy of Frederick M. Kelvin, M.D., Durham, North Carolina. *From*: Glass, G. B. J. (ed.): Progress in Gastroenterology. Vol. 3. New York, Grune & Stratton, 1977. Reproduced by permission.)

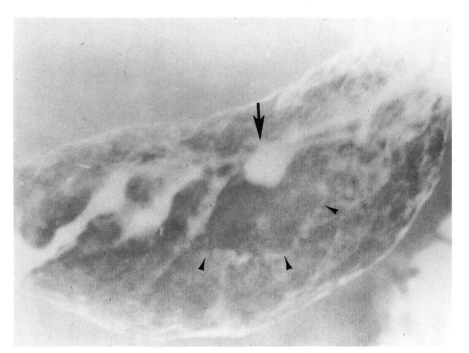

FIGURE 6–73 Early gastric cancer with an ulcer *(large arrow)*, interruption of the normal mucosal surface *(small arrows)*, and nodularity of the mucosa distal to the ulcer.

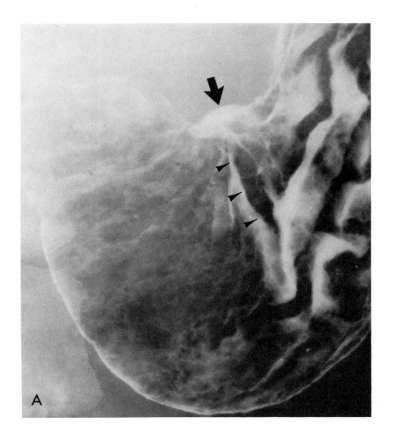

FIGURE 6–74

A. Early gastric cancer with a lesser curvature ulcer *(arrow)*. The surrounding mucosal folds are disorganized and slightly lobulated, and taper as they approach the ulcer *(small arrows)*. *(From:* Glass, G. B. J. (ed.): Progress in Gastroenterology. New York, Grune & Stratton, 1977. Reproduced by permission.)

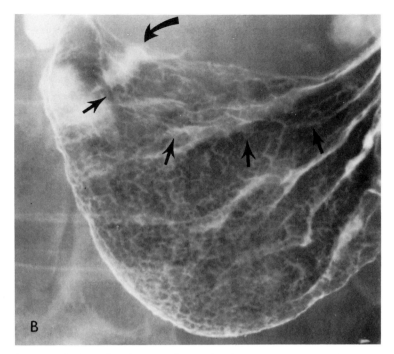

FIGURE 6–74 *Continued B.* Carcinoma along the lesser curvature of the antrum. The areae gastricae are distorted in the region of the tumor *(short arrows)*. The distal portion is ulcerated *(large arrow)*.

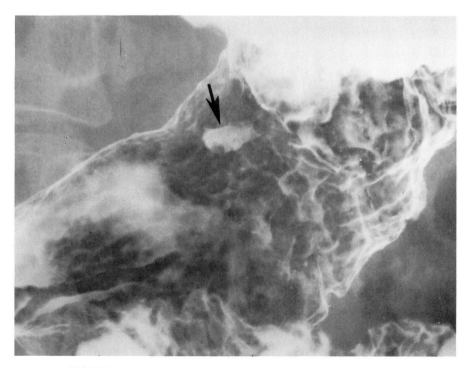

FIGURE 6–75 Benign ulcer with a malignant appearance.

There is a 1 cm ulcer crater near the lesser curvature, with a mass effect. The surrounding mucosa has a nodular appearance, suggestive of malignancy. This ulcer developed in a patient taking phenylbutazone. Endoscopy and biopsy showed no evidence of malignancy. Phenylbutazone was stopped and 1 month later, endoscopy showed complete healing of the ulcer with no evidence of tumor.

Lymphoma

The stomach may be involved primarily, as the sole site of lymphoma, or it may be involved secondarily, in patients with diffuse lymphoma. Lymphomatous involvement of the stomach is usually due to lymphosarcoma or reticulum cell sarcoma, and rarely to Hodgkin's disease. The gross pathologic and radiologic features of gastric lymphoma are extremely variable and are usually categorized as infiltrative, ulcerative, or polypoid (Figs. 6–76 to 6–79)[77-79]. In most cases the radiographic appearance cannot be distinguished from that of carcinoma. However, the combination of enlarged rigid mucosal folds in a stomach that retains normal distensibility appears to be highly suggestive of lymphoma. These tumors are also more apt to extend across the pylorus into the duodenal bulb.[80]

In most cases the radiologist will be able to accomplish no more than suggest the presence of malignancy within the stomach. Accurate radiologic diagnosis is of particular importance in these cases, since the endoscopic appearance may be inconclusive. Endoscopic biopsies and cytologic findings have a much lower accuracy than in gastric carcinoma.[81]

In any patient with the radiologic findings of a malignant tumor in the stomach, histologic diagnosis should be obtained because of the possibility of gastric lymphoma. Specific therapy with radiation and chemotherapy is available for this disease, and the prognosis is certainly more favorable than that for gastric carcinoma.[82]

Metastatic Disease

Metastatic lesions to the stomach are often manifest as submucosal tumors (Fig. 6–80). They frequently ulcerate (Fig. 6–81A) and may produce a typical "bull's-eye" or "target" lesion (Fig. 6–81B).[83] Such lesions are seen most typically in metastatic melanoma,[84] but may also be seen in metastatic adenocarcinoma and lymphoma.[85] Metastatic disease from breast carcinoma tends to result in a scirrhous reaction which may be indistinguishable from a primary linitis plastica gastric carcinoma (Fig. 6–82).[86]

Text continued on page 237

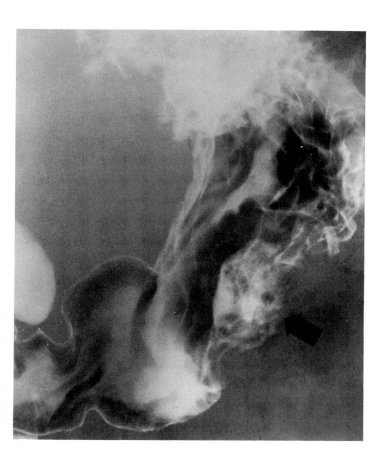

FIGURE 6-76 Ulcerated mass *(arrow)* along the greater curvature as a result of gastric lymphoma.

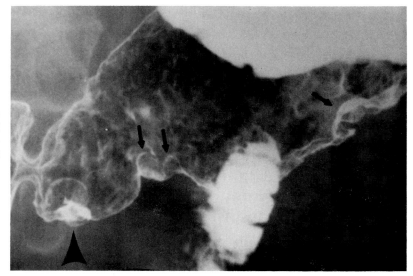

FIGURE 6-77 Multiple submucosal masses *(small arrows)* due to gastric lymphoma. The most distal mass is ulcerated *(large arrow)*.

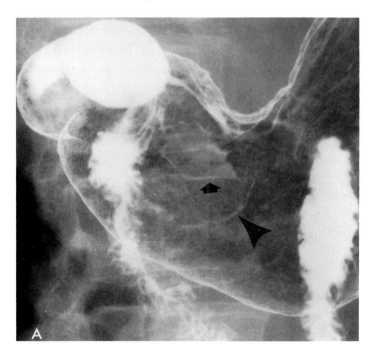

FIGURE 6–78 Ulcerated plaque on the anterior wall due to gastric lymphoma.

A. The film in the supine position shows the faint outline of a plaque on the anterior wall *(large arrows)* with a central ulcer *(small arrow)*.

B. The compression study confirms the presence of a protruded lesion with a central ulcer *(arrow)*.

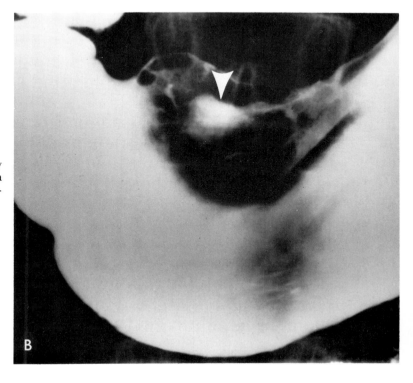

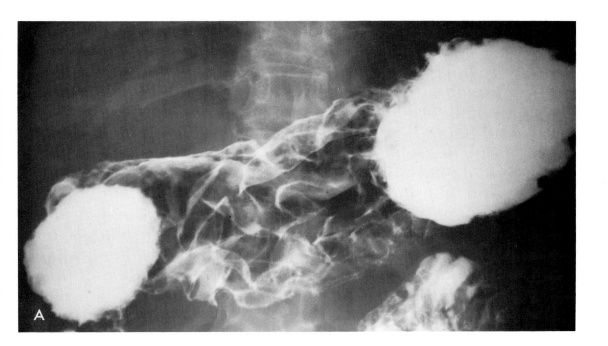

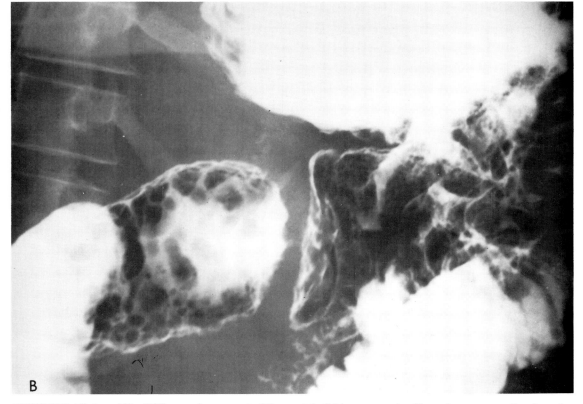

FIGURE 6–79 *A* and *B*   Diffuse enlargement of the gastric folds as a result of lymphoma extending into the duodenal bulb. (Courtesy of A. Megibow, M.D., and Patricia Redmond, M.D., New York.)

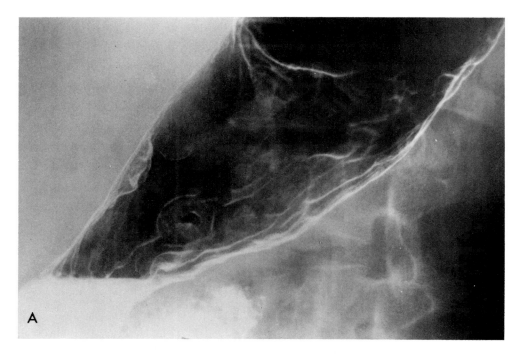

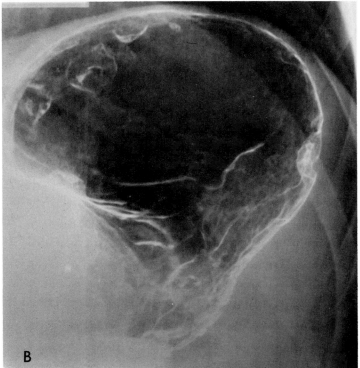

FIGURE 6–80 *A* and *B* Multiple submucosal nodules due to metastatic melanoma. (Courtesy of Herbert Y. Kressel, M.D., Philadelphia.)

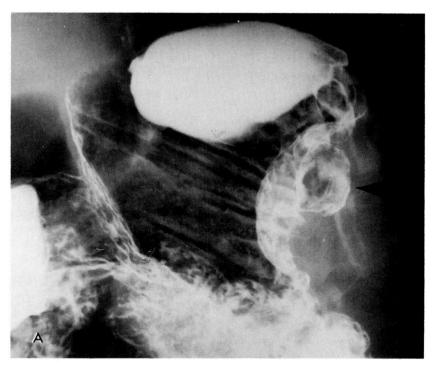

A. Ulcerated submucosal metastasis along the greater curvature of the stomach in a patient who had undergone a colectomy for carcinoma of the splenic flexure 3 years previously.

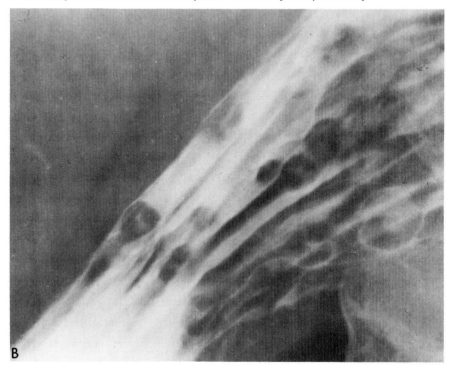

B. Multiple target lesions representing ulcerated metastases from an adenocarcinoma, primary site unknown. See also Plate 43.

FIGURE 6–81 Ulcerated metastatic disease.

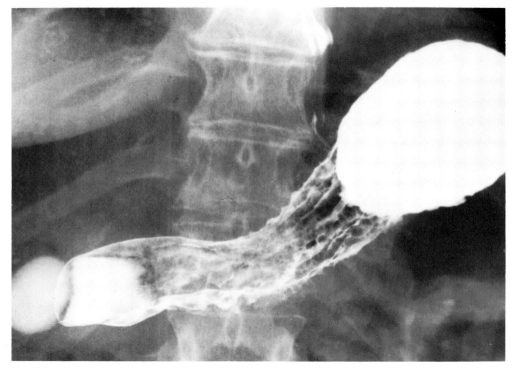

FIGURE 6–82 Linitis plastica due to metastatic carcinoma from the breast. Note the absent left breast shadow.

REFERENCES

1. Kreel, L.: Recent advances in gastroduodenal radiology: The surface patterns of the stomach. Proc. R. Soc. Med., *68*:111, 1975.
2. Mackintosh, C. E., and Kreel, L.: Anatomy and radiology of the areae gastricae. Gut, *18*:855, 1977.
3. Laufer, I., and Stein, G. E.: The clinical and physico-chemical properties of barium suspensions for use in double contrast studies of the stomach. Paper presented at the Annual Meeting of the Association of University Radiologists, Kansas City, May 1977.
4. Tim, L. O., Bank, S., Marks, I. N., et al.: Benign lymphoid hyperplasia of the gastric antrum—another case of "état mammelonné." Br. J. Radiol., *50*:29, 1977.
5. Koga, M., Nakata, H., and Kuyonari, H.: Minute mucosal patterns in gastric carcinoma. Magnification radiography on resected gastric specimens. Radiology, *120*:199, 1976.
6. Cimmino, C. V.: Sign of the burnous in the stomach. Radiology, *75*:722, 1960.
7. Grossman, R., Herlinger, H., Laufer, I., et al.: The gastric cardia and its variations on double contrast study. In preparation.
8. Battle, W., Trotman, B., Moldofsky, P., et al.: Anomalous liver lobulation as a cause of perigastric masses. Am. J. Dig. Dis., in press.
9. Lewis, T. D., Laufer, I., and Goodacre, R. L.: Arteriovenous malformation of the stomach. Radiologic and endoscopic features. Am. J. Dig. Dis., *23*:467, 1978.
10. Gohel, V. K., Kressel, H. Y., and Laufer, I.: Double-contrast artifacts. Gastrointest. Radiol., *3*:139, 1978.
11. Laufer, I., Hamilton, J., and Mullens, J. E.: Demonstration of superficial gastric erosions by double contrast radiography. Gastroenterology, *68*:387, 1975.
12. Cummack, D. H.: Gastro-intestinal X-ray Diagnosis: A Descriptive Atlas. Edinburgh, E & S Livingstone, 1969, p. 64.
13. Yamagata, S., and Ishikawa, M.: Endoscopic camera correlation. *In*: Margulis, A. R., and Burhenne, H. J. (eds.): Alimentary Tract Roentgenology. St. Louis, C. V. Mosby, 1973, pp. 1450–1462.
14. Roesch, W., and Ottenjann, R.: Gastric erosions. Endoscopy, *2*:93, 1970.
15. Abel, W.: Die roentgendiagnose der gastritis erosiva. Fortschr. Geb. Roentgenstr. Nuklearmed., *80*:39, 1954.
16. Frik, W.: Stomach. *In*: Vol 5. Schinz, H. R., and Baensch, W. E. (eds.): Roentgen Diagnosis. New York, Grune & Stratton, 1967, pp. 148–150.
17. Henning, N., and Schatzki, R.: Gastrophotographisches und roentgenologisches bild der gastritis ulcerosa. Fortschr. Geb. Roentgenstr. Nuklearmed., *48*:177, 1933.
18. Frik, W., and Hesse, R.: Die roentgenologische Darstellung von Magenerosionen. Dtsch. Med. Wochenschr., *81*:1119, 1956.
19. Laufer, I.: An assessment of the accuracy of double contrast gastroduodenal radiology. Gastroenterology, *71*:874, 1976.
20. Poplack, W., Paul, R. E., Goldsmith, M., et al.: Demonstration of erosive gastritis by the double contrast technique. Radiology, *117*:519, 1975.
21. Op den Orth, J. O., and Dekker, W.: Gastric erosions: radiological and endoscopic aspects. Radiol. Clin., *45*:88, 1976.
22. Op den Orth, J. O., and Dekker, W.: Gastric polyps or erosions. Am. J. Roentgenol., *128*:357, 1977.
23. Demling, L., Ottenjann, R., and Elster, K.: Endoscopy and biopsy of the esophagus and stomach. Philadelphia, W. B. Saunders, 1972, pp. 86–88.
24. Walk, L.: Polyps caused by gastric erosions. Radiologe, *15*:354, 1975.
25. Walk, L.: Long-term prognosis of idiopathic gastric erosions. Radiologe, *15*:356, 1975.
26. McAdam, W. A. F., Morgan, A. G., Jackson, A., et al.: Multiple persisting idiopathic gastric erosions. Gut, *16*:410, 1975.
27. Laufer, I., Trueman, T., deSa, D.: Multiple superficial gastric erosions due to Crohn's disease of the stomach — radiologic and endoscopic diagnosis. Br. J. Radiol., *49*:726, 1976.
28. Stevenson, G. W., Hyland, J., Somers, S., et al.: Gastroduodenal lesions in Crohn's disease. In preparation.
29. Freeman, H. J., Shnitka, T. K., Piercey, J. R. A., et al.: Cytomegalovirus infection of the gastrointestinal tract in a patient with late onset immunodeficiency syndrome. Gastroenterology, *73*:1397, 1977.
30. Hawiler, W., and Goldberg, H. I.: Gastroesophageal involvement in herpes simplex. Gastroenterology, *70*:775, 1976.
31. Schatzki, R., and Gary, J. E.: Face-on demonstration of ulcers in the upper stomach in a dependent position. Am. J. Roentgenol., *79*:772, 1958.
32. Laufer, I.: A simple method for routine double contrast study of the upper gastrointestinal tract. Radiology, *117*:513, 1975.

33. Stevenson, G. W.: The distribution of gastric ulcers: Double contrast barium meal and endoscopy findings. Clin. Radiol., *28*:617, 1977.
34. Poplack, W., Paul, R. E., Goldsmith, M., et al.: Linear and rod-shaped peptic ulcers. Radiology, *122*:319, 1977.
35. Boudreau, R. P., Harvey, J. P., and Robins, S. L.: Anatomic study of benign and malignant gastric ulcerations. JAMA, *147*:374, 1951.
36. Niwayama, G., and Terplan, K.: A study of peptic ulcer based on necropsy records. Gastroenterology, *36*:409, 1959.
37. Sun, D. C. H., and Stempien, S. J.: The Veterans' Administration Cooperative Study on Gastric Ulcer. Site and size of the ulcer as determinants of outcome. Gastroenterology, *61*:576, 1971.
38. Sheppard, M. C., Holmes, G. K. T., and Cockel, R.: Clinical picture of peptic ulceration diagnosed endoscopically. Gut, *18*:524, 1977.
39. Amberg, J. R., and Zboralske, F. F.: Gastric ulcers after seventy. Am. J. Roentgenol., *96*:393, 1966.
40. Zboralske, F. F., Stargardter, F. L., and Harell, G. S.: Profile roentgenographic features of benign greater curvature ulcers. Radiology, *127*:63, 1978.
41. Laufer, I., Thornly, G. D., and Stolberg, H.: Gastrocolic fistula as a complication of benign gastric ulcer. Radiology, *119*:7, 1976.
42. Hocking, B. V., and Alp, M. H.: Gastric ulceration within hiatus hernia. Med. J. Aust., *2*:207, 1976.
43. Smith, F. H., Boles, R. S., Jr., and Jordon, S. M.: Problem of gastric ulcers reviewed. JAMA, *153*:1505, 1953.
44. Welch, C. E., and Allen, A. W.: Gastric ulcer: study of Massachusetts General Hospital cases during the 10 year period 1938–1947. N. Engl. J. Med., *240*:277, 1949.
45. Valdez-Dapena, A., and Stein, G.: Morphologic Pathology of the Alimentary Canal. Philadelphia, W. B. Saunders, 1970.
46. Portis, S. A., and Jaffee, R. H.: Study of peptic ulcer based on necropsy records. JAMA, *106*:6, 1938.
47. Taxin, R. N., Livingston, P. A., and Seaman, W. B.: Multiple gastric ulcers: A radiographic sign of benignity? Radiology, *114*:23, 1975.
48. Bloom, S. M., Paul, R. E., Jr., Matsue, H., et al.: Improved radiologic detection of multiple gastric ulcers. Am. J. Roentgenol., *128*:949, 1977.
49. Keller, R. J., Wolf, B. S., and Khilnani, M. T.: Roentgen features of healing and healed benign gastric ulcers. Radiology, *97*:353, 1970.
50. Bachrach, W. H.: Complete roentgenographic healing of neoplastic ulcers of the stomach. Surg. Gynecol. Obstet., *114*:69, 1962.
51. Sakita, T., Ogura, Y., and Takasu, S.: Observations on the healing of ulcerations in early gastric cancer. Gastroenterology, *60*:835, 1971.
52. Kagan, A. R., and Steckel, R. J.: Diagnostic oncology case studies. Gastric ulcer in a young man with apparent healing. Am. J. Roentgenol., *128*:831, 1977.
53. Kirsh, I. E.: The Veterans' Administration Cooperative Study on Gastric Ulcer. Radiological aspects of cancer after apparent healing. Gastroenterology, *61*:606, 1971.
54. Tedesco, F. J., Best, W. R., Litman, A., et al.: Role of gastroscopy in gastric ulcer patients. Planning a prospective study. Gastroenterology, *73*:170, 1977.
55. Weinstein, W. M.: Gastroscopy for gastric ulcer. Gastroenterology, *73*:1160, 1977.
56. Ming, S-C.: Malignant potential of gastric polyps. Gastrointest. Radiol., *1*:121, 1976.
57. Ming, S-C., and Goldman, H.: Gastric polyps. A histogenetic classification and its relation to carcinoma. Cancer, *18*:721, 1965.
58. Elsborg, L., Andersen, D., Myhre-Jensen, O., et al.: Gastric mucosal polyps in pernicious anemia. Scand. J. Gastroenterol., *12*:49, 1977.
59. Tomasuto, J.: Gastric polyps. Histologic types and their relationship to gastric carcinoma. Cancer, *27*:1346, 1971.
60. Marshak, R. H., and Feldman, F.: Gastric polyps. Am. J. Dig. Dis., *10*:909, 1965.
61. Hoare, A. M., and Elkington, S. G.: Gastric lesions in generalized neurofibromatosis. Br. J. Surg., *63*:449, 1976.
62. Kilman, W. J., and Berk, R. N.: The spectrum of radiographic features of aberrant pancreatic rests involving the stomach. Radiology, *123*:291, 1977.
63. Bonfield, R. E., and Martel, W.: The problem of differentiating benign antral ulcers from intramural tumors. Radiology, *106*:25, 1973.
64. Cooley, R. N.: The diagnostic accuracy of upper gastrointestinal radiologic studies. Am. J. Med. Sci., *242*:628, 1961.
65. Templeton, F. E.: Errors in diagnosis of gastric carcinoma. Gastroenterology, *28*:378, 1955.
66. Fierst, S. M.: Carcinoma of the cardia and fundus of the stomach. Am. J. Gastroenterol., *57*:403, 1972.
67. Winawer, S. J., Posner, G., Lightdale, C. J., et al.: Endoscopic diagnosis of advanced gastric cancer. Gastroenterology, *69*:1183, 1975.

68. Finby, N., and Eisenbud, M.: Carcinoma of the proximal third of the stomach: A critical study of roentgenographic observations in 62 cases. JAMA, *154*:1155, 1954.
69. Kobayashi, S., Yamada, A., Kawai, B., et al.: Study on early cancer of the cardiac region. X-ray findings of the surrounding area of the esophagogastric junction. Australas. Radiol., *16*:258, 1972.
70. Lawson, T. L., and Dodds, W. J.: Infiltrating carcinoma simulating achalasia. Gastrointest. Radiol., *1*:245, 1976.
71. Schulman, A., and Simpkins, K. C.: The definition of radiological signs in gastric ulcer. Assessment of their validity by inter-observer variation study. Clin. Radiol., *26*:311, 1975.
72. Wolf, B. S.: Observations on roentgen features of benign and malignant ulcers. Semin. Roentgenol., *6*:140, 1971.
73. Nelson, S. W.: The discovery of gastric ulcers and the differential diagnosis between benignancy and malignancy. Radiol. Clin. North Am., *7*:5, 1969.
74. Ichikawa, H.: Differential diagnosis between benign and malignant ulcers of the stomach. Clin. Gastroenterol., *2*:329, 1973.
75. Kobayashi, S., Prolla, J. C., Winans, C. S., et al.: Improved endoscopic diagnosis of gastroesophageal malignancy. Combined use of direct vision, brushing, cytology and biopsy. JAMA, *212*:2086, 1970.
76. Segal, A. W., Healy, M. J. R., Cox, A. G., et al.: Diagnosis of gastric cancer. Br. Med. J., *2*:669, 1975.
77. Menuck, L. S.: Gastric lymphoma, a radiologic diagnosis. Gastrointest. Radiol., *1*:157, 1976.
78. Privette, J. T. J., Davies, E. R., and Roylance, J.: The radiological features of gastric lymphoma. Clin. Radiol., *28*:457, 1977.
79. Marshak, R. H., Lindner, A. E., and Maklansky, D.: Lymphosarcoma of the stomach. Am. J. Gastroenterol., *66*:176, 1976.
80. Meyers, M. A., Katzen, B., and Alonso, D. R.: Transpyloric extension to duodenal bulb in gastric lymphoma. Radiology, *115*:575, 1975.
81. Prolla, J. C., Kobayashi, S., and Kirsner, J. B.: Cytology of malignant lymphomas of the stomach. Acta Cytol., *14*:291, 1970.
82. Naqvi, M. S., Burrows, L., and Kark, A. E.: Lymphoma of the gastrointestinal tract: prognostic guides based on 162 cases. Ann. Surg., *170*:221, 1969.
83. Menuck, L. S., and Amberg, J. R.: Metastatic disease involving the stomach. Am. J. Dig. Dis., *20*:903, 1975.
84. Goldstein, H. M., Beydoun, M. T., and Dodd, G. D.: Radiologic spectrum of melanoma metastatic to the gastrointestinal tract. Am. J. Roentgenol., *129*:605, 1977.
85. Dunnick, R., Harell, G. S., and Parker, B. R.: Multiple bull's eye lesions in gastric lymphoma. Am. J. Roentgenol., *126*:965, 1976.
86. Joffe, N.: Metastatic involvement of the stomach secondary to breast cancer. Am. J. Roentgenol., *123*:512, 1975.
87. Laufer, I.: Double contrast radiology in the diagnosis of gastrointestinal cancer. *In:* Glass, G. B. J. (ed.): Progress in Gastroenterology. Vol 3. New York, Grune & Stratton, 1977, pp. 643–669.
88. Laufer, I., Mullens, J. E., and Hamilton, J.: The diagnostic accuracy of barium studies of the stomach and duodenum — correlation with endoscopy. Radiology, *115*:569, 1975.

7

EARLY GASTRIC CANCER

MASAKAZU MARUYAMA, M.D.

INTRODUCTION

The modern technique of double contrast radiography of the stomach was initiated by Shirakabe and his coworkers approximately 20 years ago.[1] They discovered the usefulness of double contrast radiography for delineating superficial gastric erosions while studying this method for visualizing tuberculous lesions of the intestine. In the beginning of their radiologic investigations of gastric lesions attention was focused upon delineation of benign gastric erosions and ulcers. Their earlier experience with these lesions had led to recognition of malignant erosions (type IIc), which had quite different appearances from benign lesions. As a result of enthusiastic efforts to detect gastric cancer, the development of accurate and reliable double contrast radiography was completed in 1965.

Although Shirakabe's *Atlas of X-Ray Diagnosis of Early Gastric Cancer*[2] was published in 1966, the effectiveness of double contrast radiography was not appreciated by Western radiologists for many years.[3] It was not until a few years ago that some re-evaluated its usefulness.[4-6] This method has now been appreciated in South America, where there is a high incidence of gastric carcinoma.[7-9] In the author's view, double contrast radiography of the stomach has not been as readily accepted as the Japanese pioneer radiologists had hoped because too much emphasis has been placed upon its superiority only for the detection of early gastric cancer, which is not common in Western countries. One should, however, be aware that early gastric cancer is only one of the gastric lesions that can be delineated effectively by double contrast radiography. This method is of great value for visualization of the subtle findings of superficial gastric erosions[6] and ulcers, which are the commonest gastric diseases in the West as well as in Japan.

DEFINITION AND CLASSIFICATION OF EARLY GASTRIC CANCER

Definition

The definition and classification of early gastric cancer were first proposed at the annual meeting of the Japan Gastroenterological Endoscopy Society in 1962. Early gastric cancer was defined as carcinoma in which invasion was limited to the mucosa and submucosa, without regard for the presence of lymph node and distant metastases. In 1963, at the annual meeting of the Japanese Research Society for Gastric Cancer, this definition was temporarily modified to "carcinoma limited to the mucosa and submucosa without metastases." However, the original form was later re-adopted by both societies because the presence of metastases could not be detected prior to surgery.

Classification

The macroscopic classification of early gastric cancer was proposed because Borrmann's classification of advanced gastric cancer was not

TABLE 7–1 CLASSIFICATION OF EARLY GASTRIC CANCER

    I. Polypoid (> 0.5 cm in height)
   II. Superficial
          a. Elevated (< 0.5 cm in height)
          b. Flat – minimal or no alteration in height of mucosa
          c. Depressed – superficial ulceration, usually not extending
            beyond the muscularis mucosae
  III. Excavated – prominent depression, usually due to ulceration

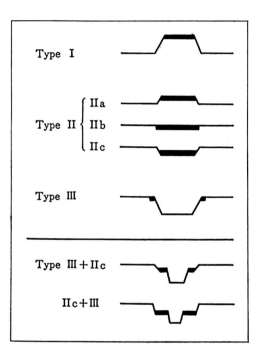

FIGURE 7–1 Classification of early gastric cancer. (*From: Stomach and Intestine, The Research Society for Early Gastric Cancer. Reproduced by permission.*)

considered applicable to cancer that was limited to the mucosa and submucosa. It should be stressed that this classification of early gastric cancer refers to its macroscopic appearance. It can be used for radiologic and endoscopic diagnosis, on the assumption that a one-to-one correspondence is possible between macroscopic, radiologic, and endoscopic findings under ideal conditions.

The macroscopic classification of early gastric cancer includes three basic types, which are summarized in Table 7–1 and illustrated in Figure 7–1. A polypoid early cancer is diagnosed macroscopically as type I if its protrusion into the gastric lumen is over 0.5 cm in height. It is diagnosed as type IIa if its protrusion is less than 0.5 cm. Type IIb is a lesion with almost no recognizable elevation or depression from the surrounding normal mucosa. This type was included in anticipation that an incipient phase of gastric cancer might take such a form, although it had not been identified when the classification was proposed. Recently, however, type IIb has been understood in wider sense, and has been used in radiologic as well as endoscopic diagnosis to indicate a "visible and diagnosable" lesion with the slightest difference in protrusion or depression from the neighboring mucosa. This is called a IIb-simulating or IIb-like lesion. Type IIc is a lesion with a slightly depressed surface, usually not penetrating the muscularis mucosae. Type III refers to a lesion with a prominent excavation that is usually due to ulceration. Occasionally there may be a type III lesion in which the depression is epithelialized and is therefore not an ulcer.

When an early cancer reveals several morphologic patterns, two or more types are described, with the predominant pattern preceding, e.g.,Type IIc + III or Type I + IIa.

Significance

Although the prognosis for early gastric cancer is generally excellent compared with the poor prognosis in advanced disease, there are variations correlating with the macroscopic classification. A report from the Cancer Institute Hospital in Tokyo[10] reveals that the 5-year survival rate of *polypoid* cancer was 95 per cent when the cancer was *intramucosal* without lymph node metastases. It was 78 per cent in polypoid cancers with *submucosal* involvement, mainly due to liver metastases. Patients with *intramucosal* cancer in the *depressed* form had 94 per cent 5-year survival, while in those with *submucosal* involvement it was 89 per cent. Thus in the case of intramucosal cancer, both forms reveal an almost identical prognosis despite the presence of lymph node metastases in the depressed form. But in the case of early cancer with submucosal involvement, the polypoid form has a significantly worse prognosis than the depressed form. It is very important to note the risk of liver metastasis in the polypoid form, which is always a differentiated type* of carcinoma histologically.[11] Thus it might be meaningless to make a simple comparison of the 5-year survival rates by the difference in the histologic type of early gastric cancer. It is obvious that invasion depth plays an important role in the evaluation of prognostic value in any type of classification. Consequently the radiologic investigation of early gastric cancer has recently been directed to estimation of its invasion depth (intramucosal cancer versus submucosal involvement), and further to the distinction of early gastric cancer from advanced cancer with macroscopic findings simulating early cancer.

Western views of early gastric cancer have been described in detail by Johansen[12] and Morson.[13] Johansen, in presenting several cases of early gastric cancer, discussed its macroscopic and microscopic features. Morson stated that carcinoma of the stomach is still a common form of malignant disease in North America and Europe. His statement suggests the possibility that the Japanese experience in the radiologic diagnosis of early gastric cancer may benefit Western radiologists.

---

*In the histologic description of the following cases, "tubular adenocarcinoma" refers to the differentiated type, and "mucinous adenocarcinoma" and "scirrhous adenocarcinoma" refer to the undifferentiated type.

METHOD OF DOUBLE CONTRAST RADIOGRAPHY

Basic Approach

The basic approach to radiologic diagnosis assumes that any lesion that can be seen macroscopically can be diagnosed radiologically. Exact reproduction of macroscopic findings is the foremost requirement for achieving this purpose. It is a process of mapping the macroscopic findings on a radiograph. When the mapping is complete a point on the macroscopic protrusion or depression can be identified as a corresponding point on the radiologic image. The radiologic findings are constructed by a collection of these corresponding points. Thus the main purpose of the detailed examination lies in obtaining radiographs on which a one-to-one correspondence with macroscopic findings is possible. Strictly speaking, there is no definite size to the hollow viscera, such as the stomach and colon. Therefore, the radiologic representation of the macroscopic findings is usually compared with a resected stomach that has been cut open along the greater curvature. In most cases, double contrast radiography is the most suitable procedure for the purpose of demonstrating the macroscopic findings radiologically, because it is easily performed by radiologists and because it is reproducible.

The *routine* examination should be performed so that any kind of abnormality is picked up in any part of the stomach, even if the quality of radiographs is insufficient for a one-to-one correspondence. Once an abnormality has been discovered the *detailed* examination is performed in order to obtain the radiologic findings that reproduce the macroscopic findings with a one-to-one correspondence.

Technical Considerations in the Routine Study

For double contrast radiography of the stomach the principal requirements are an adequate volume of barium and air and frequent positional change of the patient. One must always use more than 200 ml of barium except in some patients with deformity of the stomach. Less than 200 ml of barium does not produce a good quality double contrast image, because such a volume cannot wash the entire mucosal surface. Consequently the influence of mucus and gastric juice cannot be reduced to a minimum. Even as much as 300 ml of barium suspension retained in the fundus flows down mostly along the lesser curvature side when the patient is turned to the right decubitus from the supine position, and it flows up mainly along the greater curvature when the patient is returned to the left decubitus position.

The volume of air required depends on various circumstances. In the routine examination the ideal amount may be that which makes it possible to obtain a double contrast image of the middle portion of the body of the stomach in the supine frontal projection. This volume of air may give the impression that the stomach is overdistended. However, with smaller volumes the entire stomach cannot be visualized in double contrast. At least 300 ml of air is required for this purpose. Frequent positional changes should be made in order to wash the mucosal surface with a rapid flow of barium. By shifting the contrast medium from the fundus to the antrum, adherent mucus is washed away and the gastric juice is mixed together with the barium. It is also very important to vary the speed of the positional change in the detailed examination in order to obtain precise definition of the lesion.

Sequence of Exposures

It is best to administer an antispasmodic agent, such as Buscopan, Coliopan,* or glucagon, intramuscularly 5 to 10 minutes before the examination. This diminishes peristalsis in the stomach and duodenum and results in an easier examination. Table 7–2 summarizes the sequence of exposures in the routine study, and Figure 7–2 is a series of line drawings representing the sequence of exposures obtained at the Cancer Institute Hospital. In most cases the study is performed with a remote-controlled fluoroscopic unit with image intensification and television monitoring. For the routine examination 300 ml of the barium suspension is prepared. At the beginning of the examination a mouthful or about 20 ml of the barium is swallowed, and a mucosal relief picture is taken in the prone position (No. 1). This is necessary for discovering anterior wall lesions. Then the remaining contrast medium is swallowed, and a barium-filled film in the upright frontal position is taken (No. 2). During swallowing the esophagus and cardia are observed carefully by changing the position of the patient from the left posterior to the right posterior** oblique.

Next, effervescent tablets or granules are given to the patient in the upright position to produce gaseous distension of the stomach. These effervescent agents are designed to produce 300 to 400 ml of CO_2. Skill in using a naso- or orogastric tube will lead to better gaseous distension. The table is tilted to the horizontal position, and the patient is turned quickly to the right decubitus position and then to the left decubitus position.

---

*Buscopan and Coliopan are not available in the United States.
**Positions are labeled with respect to the table top.

TABLE 7–2 SEQUENCE OF RADIOLOGIC EXPOSURES IN THE ROUTINE EXAMINATION OF THE STOMACH

1. Mucosal relief image in the prone position
2. Barium-filled image in the upright position
3. Double contrast image in the supine frontal position
4. Double contrast image in the supine left posterior oblique position
5. Double contrast image in the supine right posterior oblique position
6. Double contrast image in the semiupright, right decubitus, or steep right posterior oblique position
7. Barium-filled image in the prone position
8. Double contrast image in the upright frontal position
9. Double contrast image in the upright left posterior oblique position (with barium passing through the cardia)
10. Compression images

After a few seconds the patient is gently returned to the supine position. These are the basic positional changes for obtaining a double contrast radiograph in the supine frontal position (No. 3). The same positional changes are repeated for taking a double contrast radiograph in the left posterior oblique position (No. 4). In this exposure the patient is positioned under fluoroscopic control so that the antrum lies either in the horizontal plane or to the left of the vertebral body. A double contrast radiograph in the right posterior oblique position is taken by turning the patient to the right decubitus from No. 4 and then returning him gently to the oblique position (No. 5). In this exposure the upper part of the gastric body, which is hidden by the contrast medium in the supine frontal position, is visualized.

Film No. 6 is obtained by turning the patient to the right decubitus position with the table horizontal or semiupright. It is important to bring the esophagogastric junction to the central portion of the double contrast image under fluoroscopic control. Following exposure No. 6 a barium-filled film is taken in the prone position (No. 7). The patient is returned to the supine position again, and the table is elevated for a double contrast radiograph in the upright position (No. 8) in order to further scrutinize the upper third of the stomach. Then the patient is given another mouthful of barium so that the passage of barium through the cardia can be observed. Exposures 8 and 9 are best taken by splitting one film.

As the final procedure of the routine examination, several compression pictures are taken, including the duodenal bulb. The antrum and gastric angle are examined with particular attention. In the antrum a search is made for polypoid lesions. Two or three exposures are taken with a degree of compression sufficient to visualize the areae gastricae, even when there is no definite abnormality under fluoroscopy. Compression radiographs around the gastric angle are also necessary, because a small ulcer or a shallow depression of the lesser curvature along the gastric angle is sometimes not visualized by double contrast radiography (Fig. 7–5).

FIGURE 7–2 Line drawings of each exposure in the routine examination of the stomach. (Cancer Institute Hospital, Tokyo.)

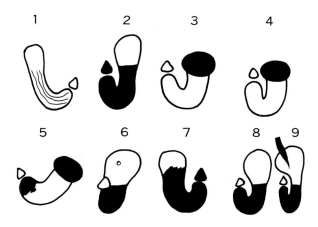

Role of Fluoroscopy

There is little value in prolonged fluoroscopy. The sequence of exposures is designed in such a way as to visualize the entire stomach by a combination of the fixed number of films and the positioning of the patient. For this reason fluoroscopy should be used only for setting the position of the patient for spot filming. The essential emphasis in the routine examination should be placed upon interpretation of the radiographs. The modern radiologic examination of the stomach aims at film diagnosis and reduces radiation dose to a minimum. However, it goes without saying that one is able to convert to a detailed examination and to make use of fluoroscopy if any abnormality is discovered during the routine examination.

Technical Considerations in the Detailed Study

In order to obtain a good double contrast image, colonic gas should be eliminated by preliminary administration of laxatives or by a cleansing enema in the early morning. Administration of antispasmodics usually gives a good result, suppressing peristalsis and avoiding loss of barium and air into the duodenum. Drainage of the gastric juice is indispensable if one wishes to obtain the best double contrast image. If this is not possible the examination should be started as early as possible in the morning.

Plate 44 reveals a resected stomach which is cut open along the greater curvature. There is a IIc lesion measuring 3.0 × 3.0 cm at the posterior wall near the gastric angle. Various appearances of the lesion and the converging folds are demonstrated in the double contrast images in Figure 7–3A to D which were taken by changing the volume of air and barium through the orogastric tube. A double contrast radiograph with approximately 40 ml of air and 100 ml of barium (Fig. 7–3A) reveals some abnormality at the posterior wall near the gastric angle, but this is insufficient for precise diagnosis. A double contrast radiograph with 200 ml of air and 100 ml of barium (Fig. 7–3B) clearly reveals an irregular collection of barium and converging folds. In this radiograph, however, the relationship between the depression and the converging folds is not clear because of insufficient gastric distension. Inflation of another 100 ml of air produces a double contrast radiograph on which the abnormality is well demonstrated (Fig. 7–3C). However, overdistension with 400 ml of air effaces the converging folds almost completely (Fig. 7–3D). This example indicates that the best delineation of the relationship between radiating folds and depressed lesions will be achieved if double contrast radiographs are obtained with at least three degrees of gaseous distension in a range of mild, moderate, and severe.[14]

Polyploid Early Cancer

As was emphasized by Shirakabe,[2] a polypoid lesion is best delineated by the compression method (Fig. 7–4A). Although double contrast radiography is able to suggest the presence of a polypoid lesion in the routine examination, it is not a reliable method for delineation of every feature of the lesion. As the lesion becomes smaller, it is more difficult to detect by double contrast. On the other hand, double contrast radiography gives additional diagnostic detail, including the mucosal pattern surrounding the polypoid lesion (Fig. 7–4B), which is very important in considering the histogenesis of carcinoma with relation to intestinal metaplasia.[15] Therefore, the compression and double contrast methods should always be employed together for the diagnosis of polypoid lesions. At least two double contrast radiographs, taken with different degrees of mucosal coating, are necessary, i.e., one with a thicker layer of barium in which the contrast medium is shed over protrusions (Fig. 7–4C), and the other in which the surrounding mucosal pattern is well delineated by slight mucosal coating with a thin layer of barium (Fig. 7–4B and D). The radiologic and gross pathologic appearances of the lesion are compared in Plate 45.

Depressed Early Cancer

For delineation of a depressed lesion it is necessary to pool the barium within it as much as possible. One must beware of the outflow of the contrast medium from the depression. This is usually caused by an unnecessary postural change (Fig. 7–5A) and is particularly likely to happen with a depression on the posterior wall of the angle and lower body of the stomach when the patient is quickly turned from the right to left decubitus position or from the supine to the left decubitus position. Therefore, a variety of positional changes should be performed when searching for a depressed lesion located in this area. At least one double contrast radiograph should be taken after the patient has been turned from the right decubitus to the supine position. By this procedure the contrast medium is retained in a depression (Fig. 7–5B).

Radiography in the Prone Position

This method was developed by Kumakura in 1968.[17] He succeeded in delineating two cancerous erosions (Type IIc) which were located on the anterior wall of the gastric body. Before this method was developed, mucosal relief and compression methods were the only tools for visualization of anterior wall lesions. However, many anterior wall lesions escaped detection by those methods. Under the best of circumstances, mucosal relief could only suggest the presence of an abnormality without providing precise details. Certainly good compression can delineate anterior wall lesions effectively, but it does not differentiate between posterior and anterior wall lesions. Moreover, the compression method cannot encompass a whole lesion if it is larger than approximately 5 cm in diameter.

The first step in double contrast radiography in the prone position is the passage of an oral tube. After the tip of the tube is positioned in the antrum, the patient is placed in the prone horizontal position. About 30 to 40 ml of barium is injected with a syringe, and the table is tilted to a slightly head-down position.

Gastric secretions mixed with the barium drain spontaneously through the tube by siphonage. Deep abdominal respiration enhances the drainage. This step is very important, because gastric secretions interfere much more with the visualization of a lesion in the prone position than in the supine position. The injected barium produces a changing appearance of the mucosal relief by which the status of drainage can be monitored. If the contrast medium drains out almost completely, about 20 to 30 ml of the contrast medium is injected again. A mucosal relief image is taken as the first step in order to confirm the location of a lesion (Fig. 7–6A). From this point one must adjust the volume of barium and air depending upon the location of the lesion. If the lesion is on the anterior wall of the antrum, not more than 100 ml of barium is desirable. Air should be injected until the antrum is distended such that the anterior wall is separated from the posterior wall. Generally, 400 to 500 ml of air is necessary for this purpose. Good views of the antrum are obtained with the table in a 15 degree head-down position and the patient in an LAO position (the right side slightly elevated).

If the lesion is located around the gastric angle and body, more than 200 ml of barium visualizes it clearly. Air should be injected until both walls are completely separated (Fig. 7–6D). Usually more than 600 ml of air is necessary. A cotton pad placed under the abdomen is very effective for obtaining double contrast detail of the wider area around the lesion. Heaving the patient's abdomen also promotes uniform mucosal coating. If the site of the lesion is higher than the middle part of the body the semi-upright position is always effective. If the lesion is around the gastric angle and in the lower body, the head-down position gives better visualization than the horizontal position.

It must be remembered that there is a completely different quality to the double contrast image in the supine, compared with the prone, position. This is particularly true in the examination of the gastric antrum. In the supine position, even a large barium pool can be accommodated in the capacious gastric fundus. This pool can easily be manipulated into the antrum to improve the coating and then returned to the fundus so that a clear double contrast view of the distal stomach is obtained. However, in the prone position the barium pool tends to collect in the antrum, which has a much smaller capacity than the fundus. Therefore, the antrum becomes very opaque, and in order to get a double contrast effect it is necessary to try to thin out the layer of barium by manipulating the position of the table and the patient and by use of a cotton pad for abdominal compression. In addition, a much greater degree of gastric distension is required.

It should also be remembered that anterior wall lesions may be demonstrated tangentially or by compression in the upright position, although with this technique, precise localization to the anterior or posterior wall is not possible.

Text continued on page 259

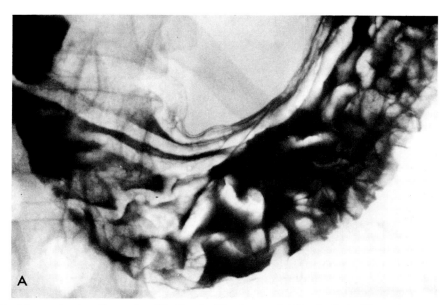

A. Double contrast radiograph with 40 ml of barium and 100 ml of air. There is a suggestion of an abnormality on the posterior wall near the gastric angle, but precise diagnosis is not possible.

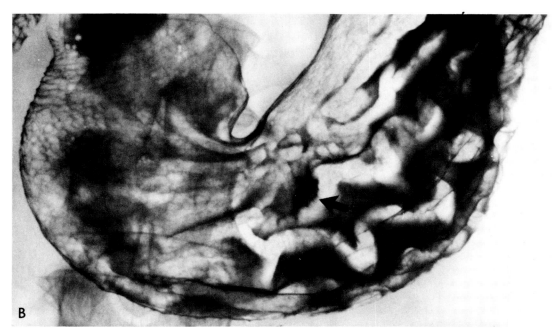

B. Double contrast radiograph with 200 ml of barium and 200 ml of air. This reveals the irregular barium collection in a depressed lesion (*arrow*), but the relationship to the converging folds is not clear.

FIGURE 7–3 Effect of varying degrees of gaseous distension: carcinoma IIc. See Plate 44.

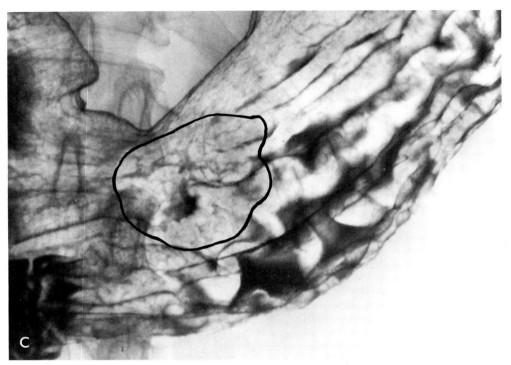

C. Double contrast radiograph with 200 ml of barium and 300 ml of air. This is the optimal distension for demonstration of the lesion (Plate 44).

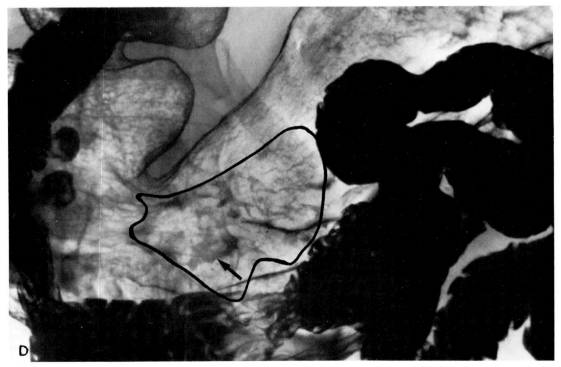

D. Double contrast radiograph with 200 ml of contrast medium and 400 ml of air. Overdistension may efface the converging folds, but the depressed lesion is clearly seen (*arrow*).

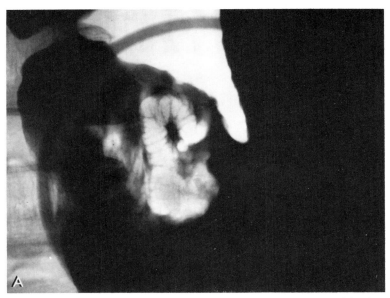

A. Compression radiograph showing an irregular lobulated mass with ulceration.

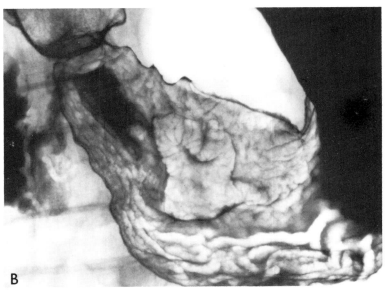

B. Double contrast radiograph. The surface pattern of the polypoid lesion is well seen and can be compared with that of the surrounding normal mucosa of the antrum.

FIGURE 7–4 Value of compression and double contrast in polypoid cancer (47-year-old female). (Plate 45).

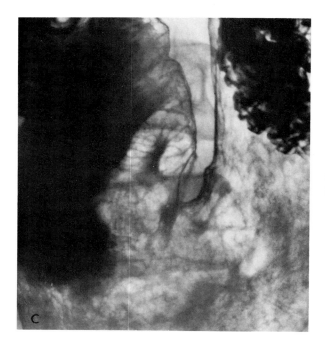

C. Double contrast radiograph with about 300 ml of air and barium surrounding the polypoid lesion.

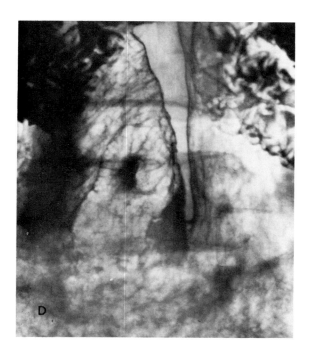

D. With less barium in the antrum, the polypoid lesion is not as apparent, but visualization of surrounding mucosal detail is improved.

FIGURE 7–5 Type IIc + III carcinoma (60-year-old male).

A. Double contrast radiograph in the supine position. Contrast medium is not retained in the deeper depression (part of type III) (*arrow*). Interruption of the converging folds suggests the presence of a IIc lesion, but it is not clearly delineated.

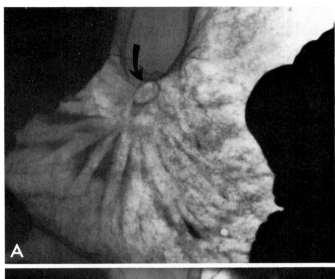

B. Double contrast radiograph in the same position as in *A*. Contrast medium is retained in the deeper portion, but the surrounding IIc lesion is not clearly delineated.

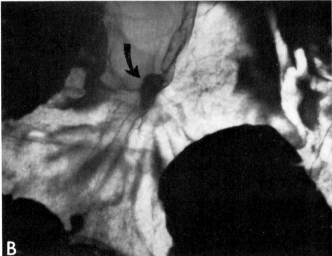

C. Compression radiograph. A part of the IIc lesion is visualized.

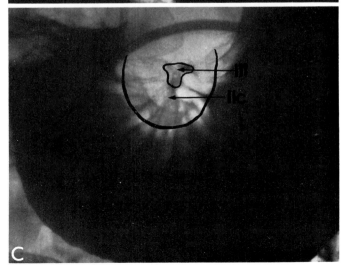

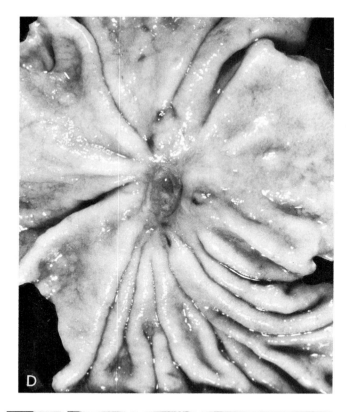

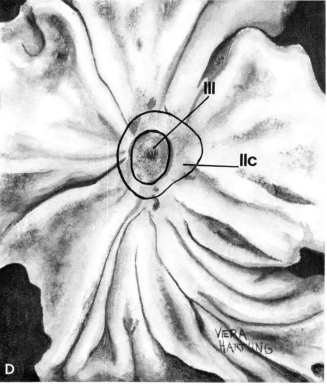

D. Resected specimen and line drawing. A type IIc lesion, measuring 3.8 × 2.5 cm in the largest diameter. The central, more deeply ulcerated, area is a type III lesion. Tubular adenocarcinoma limited to the mucosa without lymph node metastasis (0/21), associated with an ulcer penetrating the muscle layer proper. Severe intestinal metaplasia.

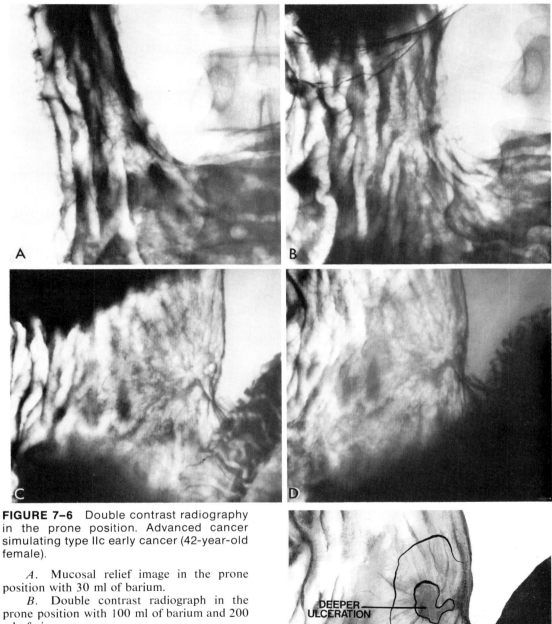

FIGURE 7–6 Double contrast radiography in the prone position. Advanced cancer simulating type IIc early cancer (42-year-old female).

A. Mucosal relief image in the prone position with 30 ml of barium.

B. Double contrast radiograph in the prone position with 100 ml of barium and 200 ml of air.

C. Double contrast radiograph in the prone position with 200 ml of barium and 500 ml of air.

D. Double contrast radiograph in the prone position with 250 ml of barium and 600 ml of air. An irregular ulcerated area is seen surrounded by abnormal mucosa.

E. Line drawing of *D*.

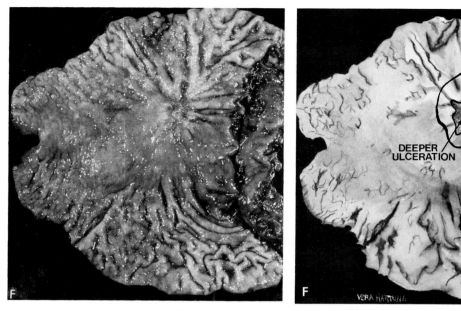

F.   Resected specimen and line drawing. A type IIc-simulating advanced cancer, slightly involving the muscle layer proper, and measuring 3.5 × 3.5 cm in the largest diameter. Tubular adenocarcinoma with lymph node metastases (2/12), and severe intestinal metaplasia.

G.   A cross section of the lesion, showing the involvement of the muscle layer proper.

H.   Line drawing of *G.*

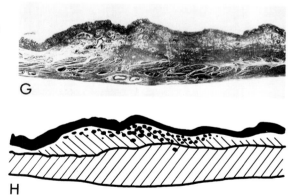

RADIOLOGIC DIAGNOSIS OF EARLY GASTRIC CANCER — CORRELATION WITH ENDOSCOPY

There have been few reports concerning the comparison of radiology, endoscopy, and biopsy examinations for the diagnosis of early gastric cancer. It is difficult to make a comparative study of these examinations, because they are usually performed in different sections of a hospital, and because all patients are not given all examinations from radiology to biopsy. At the present time, a tendency to rely upon biopsy for the final diagnosis has made it impossible to do such a comparative study and has led to the gradual underestimation of the quality of radiologic and endoscopic diagnosis. Shirakabe's report[18] may be the last one to provide a strict evaluation of the radiologic diagnosis of early gastric cancer with correlation with endoscopy and biopsy. Shirakabe stated that the initial *routine* radiologic examination discovered 86 per cent of all the lesions, and the first endoscopy following the routine radiologic examination discovered another 9 per cent. He stated further that the *detailed* radiologic examination following the first endoscopy failed to increase the previous discovery rate. On the other hand, the *routine* radiologic examination diagnosed 32 per cent of all the lesions as malignant, 30 per cent as suggestive of malignancy, and 25 per cent as benign. The first endoscopy reduced the proportion of the "malignancy-suspected" and "benign" lesions to 19 per cent and 17 per cent respectively. The *detailed* radiologic examination diagnosed 68 per cent of all the lesions as malignant, 8 per cent as malignancy-suspected, and 18 per cent as benign. Finally, the collective examination with the detailed radiologic and endoscopic examinations could diagnose 86 per cent of all the lesions as malignant, but there still remained 8 per cent diagnosed as malignancy-suspected, and 6 per cent as benign. Based upon these results, Shirakabe concluded that biopsy was really necessary in 14 per cent of the lesions.

There still remain some problems in the radiologic diagnosis of early gastric cancer. These are the diagnosis of microcarcinoma, Type IIb, and the incipient phase of the linitis plastica type of cancer. Microcarcinoma is incidentally discovered by routine endoscopic examination, and biopsy is the only tool for making the definite diagnosis. Even though it is delineated by double contrast radiography, its radiologic findings are so minute that one cannot always recognize them as indicators of malignancy (Fig. 7–15). A pure IIb lesion cannot be discovered by any examination method at the present time. Nakamura[19] has discussed the theoretical aspects of the early stages of linitis plastica carcinoma from the point of view of pathology, but there have been few clinical examples to support this theory.[20]

RADIOLOGIC DIAGNOSIS OF POLYPOID EARLY CANCER

The radiologic diagnosis of polypoid early cancer starts with recognition of the size, form, and surface pattern. With some exceptions, most lesions are in the range of 1 to 4 cm in the largest diameter.

The height of the polypoid lesion is next estimated either by compression or by a double contrast image. If a polypoid lesion is interpreted as malignant, estimation of the height gives a rough distinction between type I and type IIa. The surface pattern of the lesion is of great importance for the differential diagnosis of malignancy and benignity. Some lesions smaller than 1.0 cm in diameter have a smooth surface pattern, but most lesions larger than 1.0 cm have a granular surface pattern (Fig. 7–4A to C) which is characteristic of early cancer. They also have a lobulated contour (Fig. 7–4A and B). The granularity of the surface, though somewhat irregular and coarse, resembles the surrounding mucosa. As was indicated by Nakamura,[15] a stomach harboring polypoid cancer is lined with moderate to severe intestinal metaplasia. Radiologically this condition appears as uniform granularity of the areae gastricae. In most cases the surface pattern of an early polypoid cancer is comparable to that of the surrounding areae gastricae (Fig. 7–4B and D). In other words, the pattern of areae gastricae is preserved in polypoid cancer when invasion is limited to the submucosa. This observation is the most reliable radiologic sign for the diagnosis of *early* cancer.

In summary, the diagnosis of early polypoid cancer can be established for lesions measuring 2 to 4 cm in the largest diameter. Their surface pattern is comparable to that of the surrounding mucosa. As the cancerous infiltration extends deeper than the submucosa, the similarity of the surface pattern disappears, being replaced by marked erosion or ulceration in most cases. However, a large polypoid cancer preserves the similarity as long as the depth of invasion is limited to the submucosa.

DIFFERENTIAL DIAGNOSIS OF POLYPOID EARLY CANCER

Adenomatous Polyp (Atypical Epithelium)

Polypoid early cancer must be distinguished from two common types of benign polypoid lesions. These are the adenomatous polyp, which has also been termed atypical epithelium by Nakamura[21] and the hyperplastic polyp.

Nakamura[21] reported that malignant transformation in adenomatous polyps was estimated to be not higher than 0.4 per cent. He emphasized the importance of selective follow-up studies when biopsies showed adenomatous polyps. Endoscopic polypectomy was recommended if possible for lesions under 2.0 cm in diameter. Adenomatous polyps arise within an area of intestinal metaplasia of the gastric mucosa. Yamada stated that the surface pattern of adenomatous polyps was more similar to the surrounding areae gastricae than was the case in early polypoid cancer.[22] However, in practice it is usually not possible to distinguish between an adenomatous polyp and an early cancer, type IIa, because there is only a slight difference in the surface pattern between these two lesions (Fig. 7–7). Most adenomatous polyps present as flat or sessile elevations of the mucosa and are less than 2.0 cm in diameter. Polypoid lesions larger than 2 cm in diameter should be considered to be malignant, although a sessile or flat polypoid lesion under 2 cm may be either early cancer or an adenomatous polyp. A pedunculated lesion under 2 cm is almost certainly benign.

Hyperplastic Polyp

Hyperplastic polyps almost always have a smooth surface pattern and contour as opposed to the granular surface and lobulation of adenomatous polyps and early polypoid cancers. The size of hyperplastic polyps is almost always less than 2 cm in diameter. Endoscopic polypectomy is the treatment of choice in order to establish the diagnosis.

Submucosal tumors can be diagnosed rather easily by the presence of a bridging fold or by a gradual sloping of the lesion to the normal mucosal surface (Fig. 2–18).

Gastric Erosions

Various forms of gastric erosions or erosive gastritis may simulate polypoid early cancer. The most common form of gastric erosions is characterized by multiple small flecks of contrast medium surrounded by a radiolucent halo, which Sano[23] named varioliform erosions (see Chapter 6). They often show a "pearl string" arrangement on the crests of the mucosal folds. This type does not present any difficulty in the differential diagnosis of polypoid early cancer. But the other types of gastric erosions with polypoid forms are sometimes difficult to differentiate from malignancy (Fig. 7–8).

Despite early descriptions by Abel,[24] Walk,[25] Frik,[26] and Bücker,[27] the diagnosis of gastric erosions has not attracted the attention of radiologists, but has been exclusively developed by endoscopists.[28] It is just recently that Western radiologists have emphasized the effectiveness of double contrast radiography for delineation of gastric erosions.[6] One must be familiar with the various aspects of the macroscopic pathology of gastric erosions in relation to the differential diagnosis of malignancy. In general the contour of an erosion seems to be indefinite, and its form is changeable in several double contrast or compression radiographs because of its pliability. Usually it has a slight central depression. Sometimes it is on the crest of a mucosal fold. It is also characteristic that there are erosions of varying size, with polypoid forms scattered throughout the stomach.

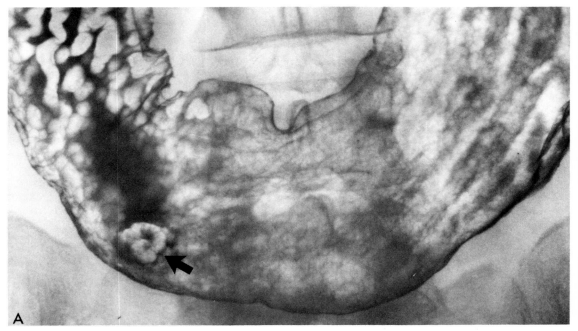

A. Double contrast radiograph in the supine position with 100 ml of contrast medium and 200 ml of air. The antral polyp (*arrow*), with its granular surface, is visible. Note also the coarse nodularity of the antral mucosa (see Plate 46).

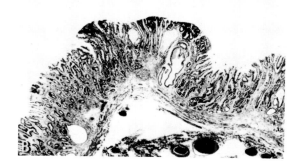

B. A cross section of the lesion.

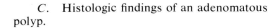

FIGURE 7–7 Adenomatous polyp in the antrum (59-year-old female). (Courtesy of T. Yarita, M. D., Juntendo University, Tokyo.)

C. Histologic findings of an adenomatous polyp.

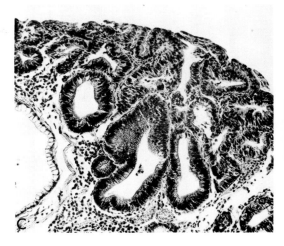

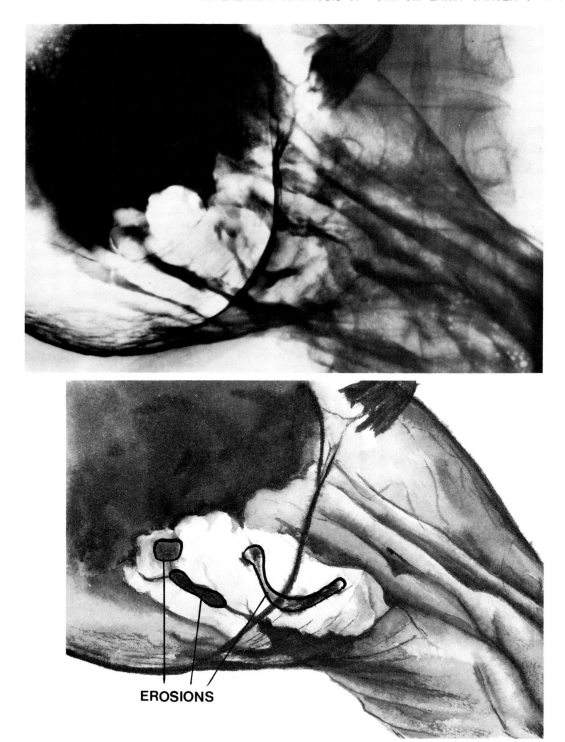

EROSIONS

FIGURE 7–8 Polypoid form of erosive gastritis in a 46-year-old male. Double contrast radiograph in the prone position. There are multiple erosions of varying size and shape, with prominent mucosal mounds that may simulate polypoid carcinoma. This has been termed verrucous gastritis by Sano.[23]

RADIOLOGIC DIAGNOSIS OF DEPRESSED EARLY CANCER

General Considerations

The radiologic diagnosis of depressed early cancer is based upon analysis of a depression and converging folds. The depression is analyzed in terms of its form and surface. Generally the depression is irregular, with a serrated or spiculated margin. The depression is not always clearly demarcated from the normal surrounding mucosa, and it may be difficult to define the precise extent of a lesion.

In most cases of depressed early cancer the surface of the depression is uneven. The converging folds also have characteristic abnormalities, such as tapering, clubbing, interruption, and fusion (Fig. 7–9). The diagnosis of early cancer can be made easily if these converging fold patterns are delineated by double contrast radiography. Moreover, the converging folds are also a very reliable clue, leading to the detection of lesions in many cases. On the other hand, a cancerous erosion not accompanied by converging folds is discovered only with difficulty (Fig. 7–10).

Recent investigation by Baba[29] has revealed the close correlation between radiologic findings and histologic type of early cancer. As Nakamura[15] proposed, it is practical and reasonable to classify gastric cancer into two basic histologic types, namely, undifferentiated carcinoma and differentiated carcinoma. Undifferentiated carcinoma arises from the ordinary gastric mucosa (pyloric and fundic glands), while differentiated carcinoma arises from areas of intestinal metaplasia.

Baba found significant differences in the radiologic appearances of the two histologic types of depressed early cancer. In undifferentiated carcinoma the surface is mostly uneven and coarse, and there is an abrupt transition from normal mucosa to the depression. The converging folds show sudden interruption or tapering, clubbing, and fusion. In differentiated carcinoma the surface is fine and uniform. There is a gradual transi-

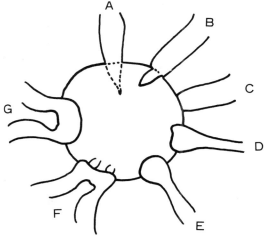

FIGURE 7–9 Various approaches of the converging folds in depressed early cancer.

A : Gradual tapering
B : Abrupt tapering
C : Abrupt interruption

D, E : Clubbing
F, G : Fusion

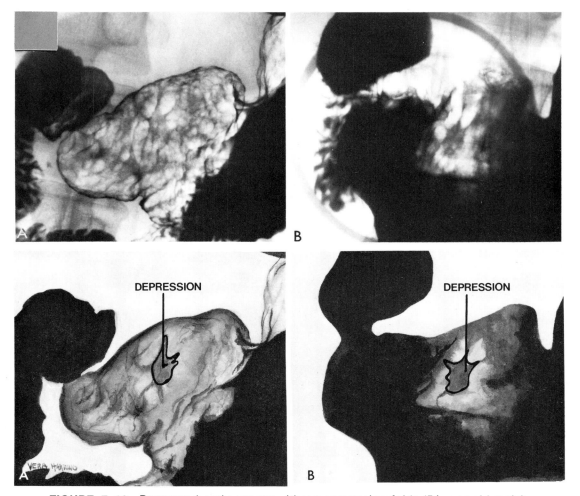

FIGURE 7–10 Depressed early cancer without converging folds (54-year-old male).

A. A small depressed type IIc lesion is surrounded by a somewhat irregular arrangement of areae gastricae in the antrum. The depressed lesion is difficult to detect because of the absence of converging folds.

B. Compression radiograph shows the depression.

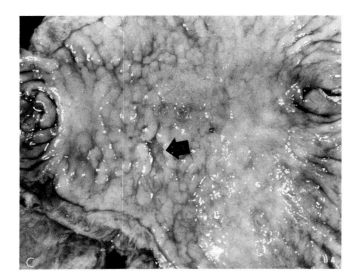

C. Resected specimen. A type IIc lesion (*arrow*) measuring 1.5×0.7 cm in the largest diameter. Tubular adenocarcinoma limited to the mucosa without lymph node metastasis (0/23), with no ulcer but with severe intestinal metaplasia.

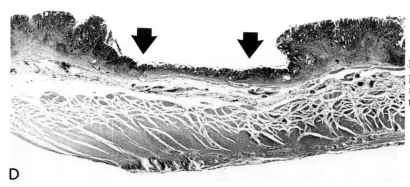

D. A cross section of the lesion. Note that the depressed lesion is covered with malignant epithelium and is therefore not an ulcer.

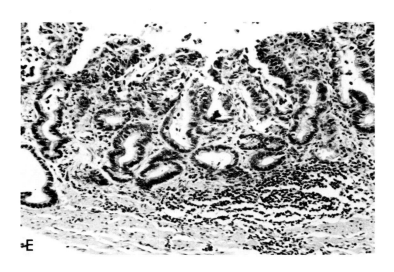

E. Histologic findings.

tion from normal mucosa to the depression, and the borders of the lesion may be difficult to define. The converging folds show gradual tapering. Clinically, recognition of the difference in the histologic type of depressed early cancer is important in determining the extent of gastric resection. Radiologists should consider the histologic type of lesion when reporting on its proximal extension.

Types IIc, IIc + III, and III

The distinction between type IIc and type III is made by the depth of the collection of contrast medium retained in a depression. The depth of the contrast medium in a benign ulcer (Fig. 7–11) can be regarded as typical of type III. A thinner collection of the contrast medium indicates a depression of type IIc. In addition type IIc does not show uniform density of the contrast medium (Fig. 7–3C and D). Irregular proliferation of cancerous tissue or regenerative epithelium usually causes the uneven density. In the superficial spreading type of early cancer (Fig. 7–12) it is difficult to distinguish the boundary between normal mucosa and the depression.

If the depression is variable in its depth it is necessary to decide whether any portion of the depression is comparable to the depth of a benign ulcer. In that case the lesion will be classified as IIc + III (Fig. 7–5) or III + IIc, depending on which appearance predominates.

On the other hand, if an ulcer niche is prominent, one must be alert to the slightest suggestion of a IIc lesion, especially in the profile view, as shown in Figure 7–13. The diagnosis of peptic ulcer is easily made unless attention is paid to the mucosa surrounding the niche. In such a case the IIc lesion becomes clearer during the course of medical treatment (Fig. 7–13C) as the niche decreases in size. This phenomenon is referred to as the malignant cycle of ulceration in early gastric cancer.[30]

In some cases the type III lesion is so predominant that the IIc lesion can scarcely be recognized macroscopically (Fig. 7–14) as the slightest abnormality, either entirely or partially around the III part. Close observation of the niche may lead to recognition of the partial irregularity of its margin (Fig. 7–14A). However, it is expected that the features of the lesion would evolve into III + IIc or IIc + III in a few weeks, especially when treated medically.

Carcinoma Less Than 1.0 cm

Most carcinomas less than 1.0 cm in diameter are not accompanied by ulceration. Consequently it is very difficult to discover the lesion, regardless of its nature. If a lesion is located in an area where double contrast radiography gives good visualization of the mucosal detail, the diagnosis of malignancy can be made by following the general principles of radiologic diagnosis. If a lesion is smaller than 0.5 cm in the largest diameter, the radiologic diagnosis of malignancy is not always possible, because the lesion is too small for the criteria of malignancy to be applied. Sometimes an irregular surrounding translucency, which is unusual in a benign ulcer, gives a strong suggestion of malignancy (Fig. 7–15).

Text continued on page 274

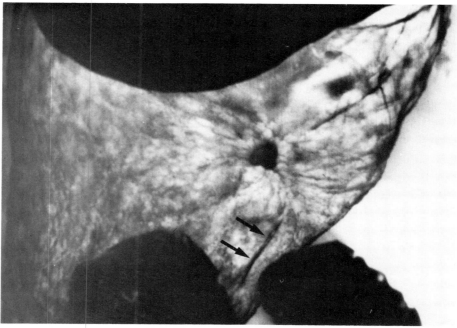

FIGURE 7–11 Typical benign gastric ulcer in a 46-year-old female. A typical double contrast image of a benign ulcer. Note linear extension of the niche toward the greater curvature side (*arrows*).

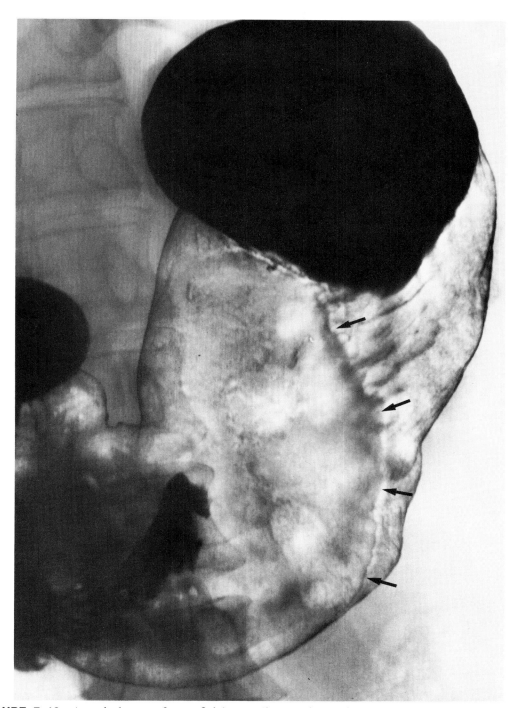

FIGURE 7–12 A typical case of superficial spreading carcinoma in a 47-year-old female. The lateral border is well defined (*arrows*), but the other borders cannot be recognized. See also Plate 47.

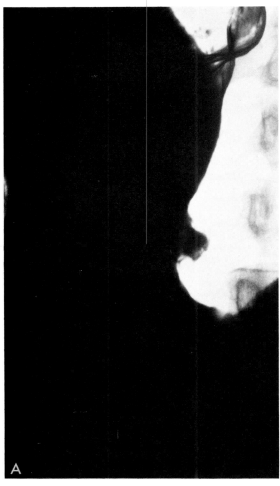

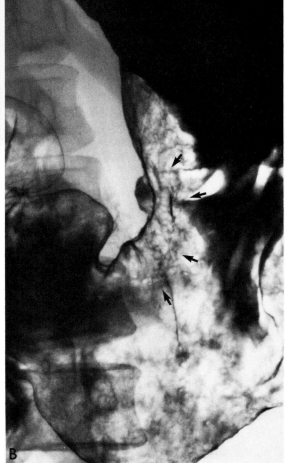

FIGURE 7–13 Type IIc carcinoma with peptic ulcer (31-year-old female).

A. Barium-filled film in the prone position. The lesser curvature ulcer is obvious, but the diagnosis of malignancy cannot be made with this image alone.

B. Double contrast radiograph in the supine position. Note mucusal abnormality of the posterior wall (*arrows*) around the niche.

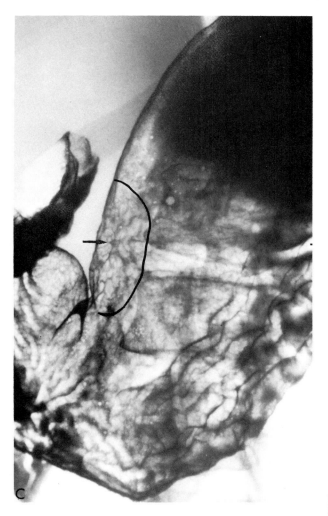

C. Double contrast radiograph in the right posterior oblique position 24 days after the previous examination. The niche (*arrow*) is much smaller, and the surrounding abnormal mucosa of the IIc lesion is more prominent.

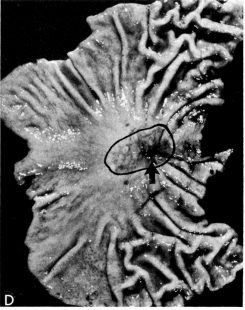

D. Resected specimen. A type IIc + III lesion measuring 4.0 × 2.5 cm in the largest diameter. Mucinous adenocarcinoma limited to the mucosa, without lymph node metastasis (0/16) associated with ulcer scar penetrating the muscle layer proper, and without intestinal metaplasia. There is a small residual ulcer niche (*arrow*) with surrounding nodular mucosa.

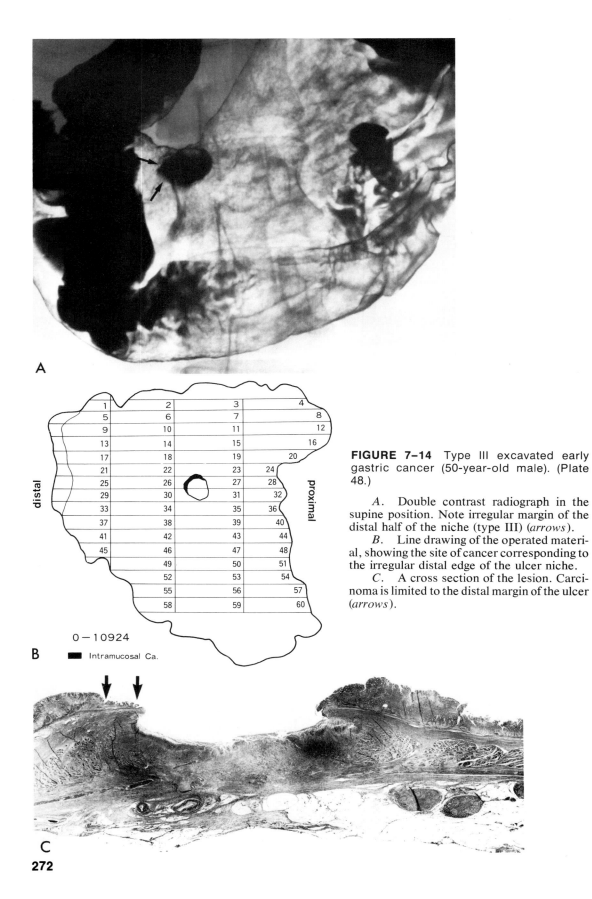

A.

B.

0 − 10924

Intramucosal Ca.

C.

FIGURE 7–14 Type III excavated early gastric cancer (50-year-old male). (Plate 48.)

A. Double contrast radiograph in the supine position. Note irregular margin of the distal half of the niche (type III) (*arrows*).

B. Line drawing of the operated material, showing the site of cancer corresponding to the irregular distal edge of the ulcer niche.

C. A cross section of the lesion. Carcinoma is limited to the distal margin of the ulcer (*arrows*).

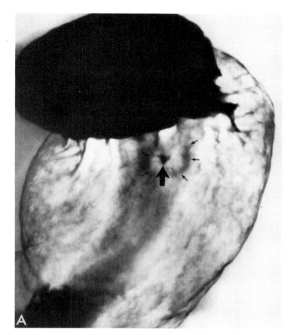

FIGURE 7–15 Very small IIc carcinoma (46-year-old male).

A. Double contrast radiograph in the supine position shows a small irregular depressed lesion (*large arrow*) with asymmetric surrounding radiolucency (*small arrows*).

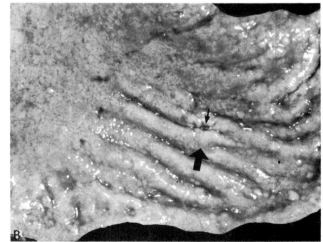

B. Resected specimen shows the swelling (*large arrow*), with a small central depressed area (*small arrow*). A very small type IIc lesion measuring 0.5 cm in the largest diameter.

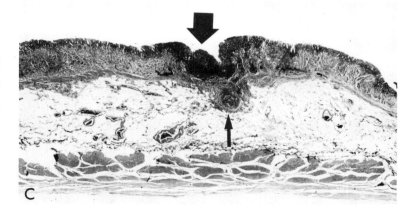

C. A cross section of the lesion showing the depressed area (*large arrow*) with its raised margins and submucosal involvement (*small arrow*).

IIb-like Lesion

Type IIb was initially used to refer to a cancerous lesion in its incipient phase, in which there was no depression or elevation from the normal mucosal surface. This was justified by the fact that pure type IIb lesions, incidentally discovered in the course of operating upon the stomach for some other lesion, have all been smaller than 0.5 cm.[31]

However, many clinical cases have not been classified as pure IIb lesions, but rather as simulating IIb lesions on the basis of a subtle difference in elevation or depression from the normal surrounding mucosa and consequently without clear distinction of their border. These have been called IIb-simulating or IIb-like lesions. This classification can be applied further to describe the border of a depressed lesion with IIb-like peripheral spread (Fig. 7–16). It is important to pay attention to subtle differences in mucosal coating from the surrounding normal mucosa for recognition of IIb-like mucosal spread of cancer.

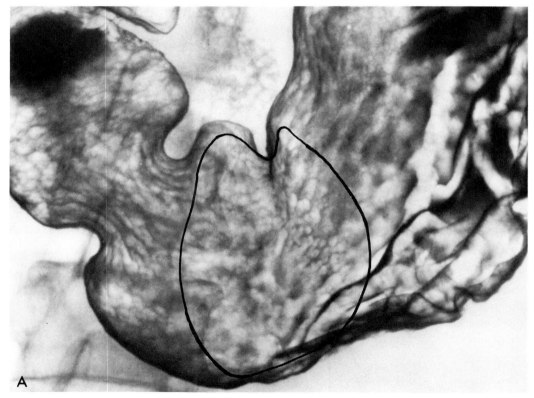

A. Double contrast radiograph in the supine position showing typical findings of a lesion with IIb-like peripheral spread. It is very difficult to define the lesion, but the approximate extent of the lesion is outlined.

FIGURE 7–16 Type IIc lesion with IIb-like peripheral spread (59-year-old female).

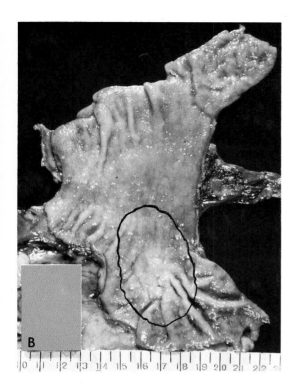

B. Resected specimen. A Type IIc + IIb lesion, with the size estimated to be 6.5 × 4.5 cm in the largest diameter. Tubular adenocarcinoma extensively involving the submucosa without lymph node metastasis. The approximate extent of the lesion is outlined.

C. Schematic representation of the resected specimen showing the extent of cancer.

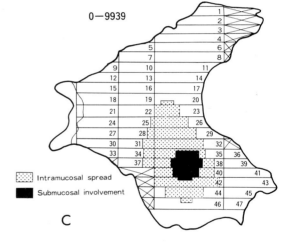

Intramucosal spread

Submucosal involvement

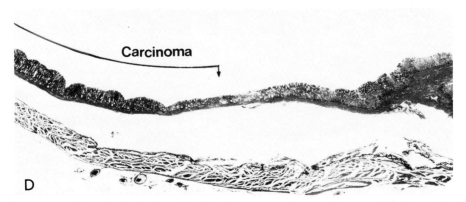

D. A cross section of the lesion showing intramucosal spread extending from the left to the arrow.

DIFFERENTIAL DIAGNOSIS OF DEPRESSED EARLY CANCER

Advanced Cancer Simulating IIc

In the descriptions presented so far, various radiologic aspects of early gastric cancer were discussed without special reference to the differential diagnosis of early gastric cancer and advanced cancer with the same macroscopic appearance. One cannot understand how the radiologic diagnosis of early gastric cancer is made positively unless the essential difference in the radiologic findings between early and advanced cancers is clarified. This raises the question of whether radiologic findings can estimate the depth of invasion in gastric cancer.

The difference is easily understood if early cancer is simply regarded as having a two-dimensional construction in its invasion pattern, and advanced cancer is regarded as having a three-dimensional construction.[32] In other words, the depth of cancerous invasion can be disregarded with early cancer, while the formation of a tumor mass is most prominent in an advanced cancer. The radiologic diagnosis of early gastric cancer can be established by evidence that there is no tumor mass in the radiologic findings. The tumor mass is demonstrated by the compression or double contrast method by changing the volume of air (Fig. 7–17).[32] In the compression image it is visualized as a marked surrounding translucency, which is principally caused by extensive submucosal involvement (Fig. 7–17D).[33]

The submucosal involvement in early cancer is generally slight and is limited to its central part. The presence of marked translucency on the compression study implies extensive submucosal involvement and suggests the possibility of deeper involvement of the gastric wall.[32] On the other hand, minor involvement of the submucosa or muscle layer cannot be detected (Fig. 7–6).

Nishizawa[34] has discussed the radiologic criteria for estimating the depth of invasion. The more sharply demarcated a depression, the deeper the involvement by cancer; the more prominent the converging folds, the deeper the involvement. But these criteria may be somewhat difficult to apply, since the appearance of a depression or of converging folds changes with alterations in the volume of air. It may be useful to estimate the depth of invasion by varying the volume of air. The changing appearance of the depression and the converging folds gives invaluable information regarding the depth of invasion. If there is extensive involvement a tumor shadow is seen on a double contrast image with a small volume of air (Fig. 7–17A). It often disappears with a moderate to excessive volume of air if the invasion does not extend through the entire thickness of the gastric wall (Fig. 7–17C). This is in marked contrast to a so-called advanced cancer which consistently reveals a filling defect and limited distensibility of the affected portion or of the entire stomach. An intramucosal cancer or a cancer with slight submucosal involvement does not reveal a tumor mass on a double contrast image even with a small volume of air.

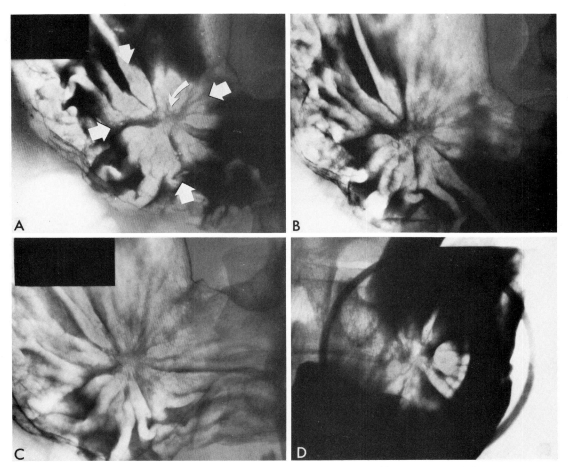

FIGURE 7–17 Advanced cancer simulating type IIc (36-year-old male).

   A.   Double contrast radiograph in the prone position. A tumor shadow (*straight arrows*) is visualized in this radiograph. There is also a central depressed lesion (*curved arrow*).
   B.   Double contrast radiograph in the prone position with additional air. The tumor shadow is faintly visualized.
   C.   Additional air causes overdistension, and the tumor shadow is effaced although the radiating folds are clearly seen.
   D.   Compression radiograph shows a radiolucency owing to the tumor mass.

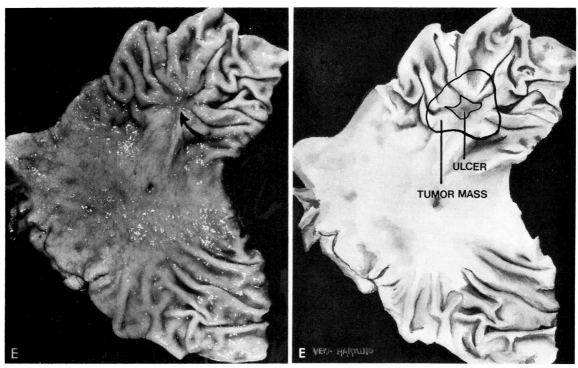

E.   Resected specimen. An advanced carcinoma measuring 3.0 × 4.0 cm in the largest diameter and simulating a type IIc lesion. A tumor mass is visualized. Scirrhous adenocarcinoma extensively involving the muscle layer proper as well as the submucosa, with lymph node metastases (5/10) associated with ulcer (*arrow*) reaching the submucosa.

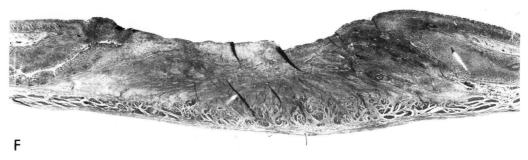

F.   A cross section of the lesion showing tumor invading beyond the submucosa into the serosa.

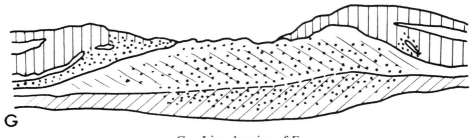

G.   Line drawing of *F.*

Early Malignant Lymphoma

Early malignant lymphoma of the stomach has recently attracted attention in relation to its differential diagnosis from early gastric cancer. Since it has been accepted that malignant lymphoma of the stomach originates from the lymphatic tissue of the lamina propria or the submucosal layer, it may be justified to define its early phase in the same way as early gastric cancer. This definition is supported by the fact that there has been no case reported in the records of the Cancer Institute Hospital or in the world literature in which the proliferation of malignant lymphoma is limited to the muscle layer proper or to the serosa without involvement of the mucosa and submucosa.[35] Thus if the depth of invasion of the malignant lymphoma is limited to the submucosa, it may be considered histologically as an early lesion.

In reviewing the cases at the Cancer Institute Hospital, Sugiyama[35] classified the macroscopic findings of early malignant lymphoma into four forms. Of these, the superficial depressed type is most important in the differential diagnosis of the IIc type of early cancer. Radiologically, the superficial depressed type of malignant lymphoma is characterized by multiple ulcers and slight convergence of the mucosal folds, or sometimes by a depression with a smoothly elevated margin, or by clubbing of the mucosal folds. The polypoid type usually reveals smooth elevation of the mucosa with a bridging fold or sharply demarcated multiple elevations of the mucosa, suggesting a submucosal origin. The polypoid-ulcerated type reveals a combination of multiple elevations of the mucosa, simulating a submucosal tumor and a large ulceration. The giant rugal type reveals a rather smooth, disorganized pattern of the rugal folds without narrowing of the stomach.

It is a particular feature of early malignant lymphoma that marked enlargement or reduction in the size of a tumor may occur during a short period of observation (Fig. 7–18). In other words, a marked change in the macroscopic findings is seen in the follow-up examinations. Takeuchi[36] reported a case of early malignant lymphoma in which the size of the tumor decreased because of ulceration. In Nakano's case[37] a part of the tumor disappeared because of ulceration and reappeared after healing of the ulcer. In this case, invasion of the malignant lymphoma was still limited to the submucosal layer even after the recurrence of the tumor.

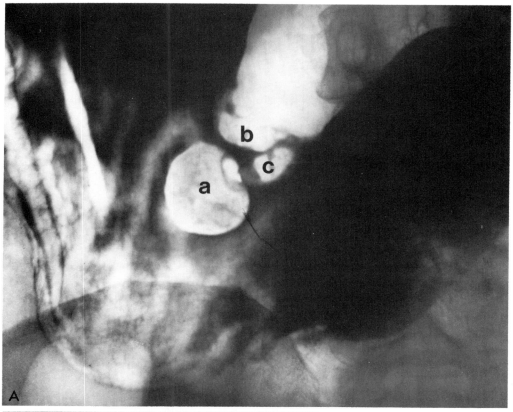

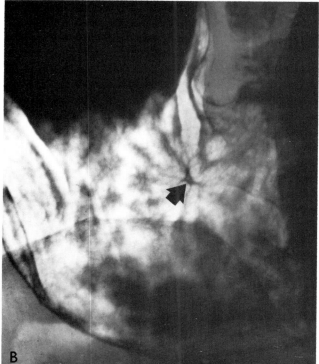

FIGURE 7–18 Early malignant lymphoma (43-year-old male).

A. Double contrast radiograph in the prone position shows three polypoid lesions around the gastric angle.

B. Double contrast radiograph in the prone position taken 20 days later. The largest tumor (*a*) has disappeared and has been replaced by a small ulcer (*arrow*) on the anterior wall with converging folds. The resected specimen showed reticulum cell sarcoma limited to the mucosa and submucosa without lymph node metastasis (0/19), associated with an ulcer reaching the submucosa.

Pseudolymphoma (Reactive Lymphoreticular Hyperplasia)

Localized or diffuse proliferation of lymphoreticular tissue of the stomach is a nonepithelial lesion which may be recognized macroscopically if the proliferation becomes marked. Konjetzny[38] considered this lesion to be a type of chronic gastritis (lymphatisch-hyperplastischer). In 1938 he also reported three cases as "chronisch-lymphatischer gastritis," which was often confused with cancer clinically and radiologically.[39] Schindler[40] described this lesion as "chronic atrophic lymphoblastomatoid gastritis," a type of gastritis that is often misdiagnosed as cancer.

This lesion had not attracted attention until 1958 when Smith and Helwig[41] emphasized its importance in the differential diagnosis of malignant lymphoma. In their statistical investigation of the prognosis of malignant lymphoma they noticed a better prognosis in malignant lymphoma of the stomach compared with other organs. They concluded that the better prognosis could be ascribed to the fact that some benign lesions that were difficult to differentiate histologically from malignancy were included in the cases that had been diagnosed as malignant lymphoma. They called these benign lesions reactive lymphoid hyperplasia. Nakamura[42] called the same lesions reactive lymphoreticular hyperplasia, because lymphocytic as well as reticulum cell hyperplasia is often seen in this lesion. The similarities emphasize the necessity for the differential diagnosis of malignant lymphoma. The term pseudolymphoma has also been applied to this lesion.[43] We prefer the term reactive lymphoreticular hyperplasia, or RLH.

In Japan, RLH has attracted the attention of radiologists and endoscopists as one of the most important lesions in the differential diagnosis of early gastric cancer, and many cases of RLH have been reported in which the diagnosis was made with some difficulty. It has been pointed out by several authors that RLH demonstrates macroscopic findings that may be confused with malignancy. Generally RLH is located in the intermediate zone between pyloric and fundic gland mucosa and has the appearance of gyrus-like hypertrophy of the mucosa or hypertrophy of the mucosal folds (localized hypertrophic form, by Nakamura).[42] In about 70 to 80 per cent of the cases with such macroscopic findings there is ulceration in the center of the lesion. This type of RLH may be difficult to distinguish from IIc + III or sometimes IIa if an ulceration is not present. Another type of RLH is characterized by extensive erosion in the antral portion of the stomach, not extending beyond the intermediate zone (diffuse flat form, by Nakamura).[42] This type is often confused with IIc mucosal carcinoma.

In the radiologic diagnosis, RLH should be distinguished from cancer, malignant lymphoma, peptic ulcer and ulcer scar, erosive gastritis, benign polypoid lesion, and giant rugae. The positive diagnosis of RLH is not difficult if the radiologic examination, including both double contrast radiography and compression method, is performed effectively. The diagnosis of RLH should be considered first if one hesitates to make a diagnosis of early cancer because of the inconsistency of the radiologic findings even after careful review. In IIa-simulating RLH, its outline seems to be obscure compared with that of IIa, or the nodularity is not as densely distributed as in IIa. In IIc + III-simulating RLH the border of the depression has no continuity, i.e., its outline is not circumferential. An ab-

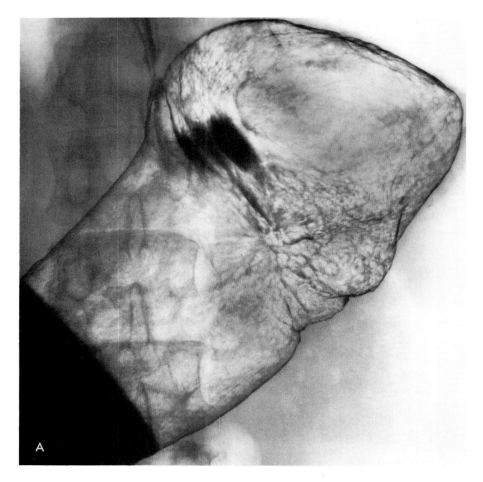

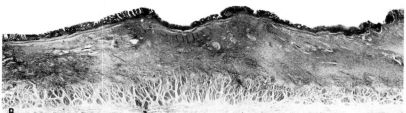

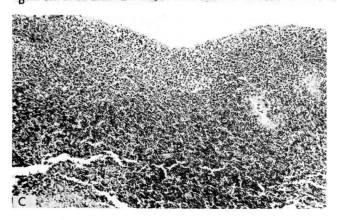

FIGURE 7–19 Reactive lymphoreticular hyperplasia (pseudolymphoma) in a 57-year-old male.

A. Double contrast radiograph in the right posterior oblique position. Typical double contrast findings of reactive lymphoreticular hyperplasia (RLH), with ulcer scar and fine granularity of the mucosa around the converging folds.

B. A cross section of the posterior wall lesion.

C. Histologic findings of RLH.

normality of the converging folds, such as clubbing or interruption, is visualized around part of the depression. Sometimes the surrounding mucosa has fine granularity (Fig. 7–19).

Peptic Ulcer and Erosive Gastritis

There is no problem in the differential diagnosis of depressed early cancer and benign peptic ulcer if only an average double contrast examination is performed. However, multiple peptic ulcers may be difficult to distinguish from IIc or IIc + III. As shown in Figure 7–20, the ulcers and converging folds have a benign appearance, although the intervening mucosa between the ulcers simulates the appearance of a IIc lesion, owing to scar formation. One must be acquainted with another form of multiple ulcers, the so-called symmetrical ulcers, or kissing ulcers which are seen only in the antrum (Fig. 7–21). This refers to ulcers on the opposing anterior and posterior walls. The lesion is characterized by its acute onset and by shallow ulcers with scattered small erosions, different from those in other portions of the stomach. Initially an acute abdomen or pyloric obstruction is suspected. In a few weeks the ulcers show marked reduction in size. Usually anterior wall ulcers heal more rapidly than posterior wall ulcers.

Most lesions of erosive gastritis can be diagnosed radiologically without difficulty, but sometimes they may be difficult to differentiate from polypoid early cancer, i.e., type IIa. Rarely, one encounters an example of erosive gastritis that must be differentiated from type IIc carcinoma, as shown in Figure 7–22. Such a case belongs to a category called hemorrhagic gastritis, or hemorrhagic erosion, which usually shows rapid healing over a short period (Fig. 7–22*B*).

CONCLUSION

Double contrast radiography is an excellent method for the detection of early gastric cancer. However, it should be emphasized that it is also useful in the diagnosis of other gastric diseases. The knowledge gained through efforts to detect early gastric cancer has also facilitated the diagnosis of diseases such as erosive gastritis and peptic ulcers, which are the commonest gastric diseases in most countries. Radiologists must become familiar with the microscopic pathology of early gastric cancer and with the corresponding radiologic appearances utilizing the various components of the double contrast examination. The examination must be tailored to each patient according to the nature, size, and location of the lesion being examined. Constant correlation of the radiologic findings with the appearances at endoscopy and in the resected specimen are of utmost importance for an appreciation of the double contrast method and its application to the diagnosis of early gastric cancer.

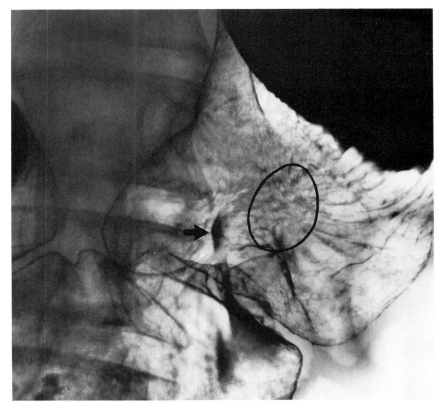

FIGURE 7–20 Multiple benign ulcers (66-year-old male).

Double contrast radiograph in the right posterior oblique position. Typical double contrast findings of multiple ulcers with an active ulcer (*arrow*) and converging folds to an ulcer scar (*circle*). The intervening mucosa has a nodular surface, suggesting malignancy.

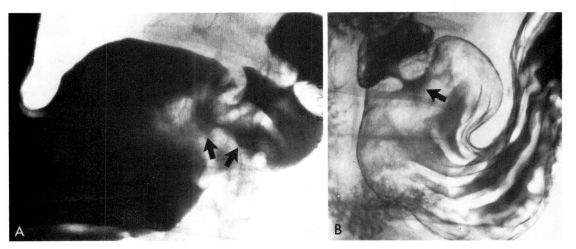

FIGURE 7–21 Kissing ulcers (55-year-old male).

A. Compression radiograph shows two ulcers (*arrows*).

B. Double contrast radiograph with a small volume of air shows only the posterior wall ulcer (*arrow*). The second ulcer is on the anterior wall and is not demonstrated in the supine position.

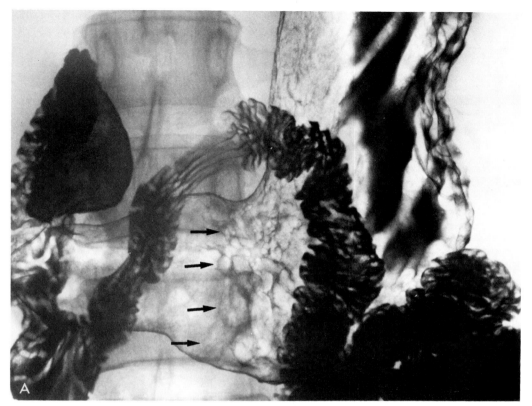

A. Double contrast radiograph in the supine position shows abnormal mucosa due to hemorrhagic gastritis simulating a large IIc lesion. The distal border of the lesion is indicated by the arrows.

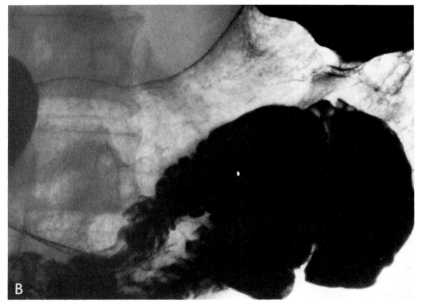

B. Double contrast radiograph 1 month after the previous examination. The lesion has almost disappeared.

FIGURE 7–22 Hemorrhagic gastritis simulating IIc cancer (37-year-old female).

REFERENCES

1. Kumakura, K.: Diagnostic Roentgenology of the Stomach (in Japanese). Kanehara Shuppan Co., Tokyo, 1968.
2. Shirakabe, H., Ichikawa, H., Kumakura, K., et al.: Atlas of X-Ray Diagnosis of Early Gastric Cancer. Philadelphia, J. B. Lippincott, 1966.
3. Gelfand, D. W.: The Japanese-style double-contrast examination of the stomach. Gastrointest. Radiol., 1:7, 1976.
4. Gelfand, D. W.: The double contrast upper gastrointestinal examination in the Japanese style (An experience with 2,000 examinations). Am. J. Gastroenterol., 63:216, 1975.
5. Laufer, I., Mullens, J. E., and Hamilton, J.: The diagnostic accuracy of barium studies of the stomach and duodenum — Correlation with endoscopy. Radiology, 115:569, 1975.
6. Laufer, I., Hamilton, J., and Mullens, J. E.: Demonstration of superficial gastric erosions by double contrast radiography. Gastroenterology, 68:387, 1975.
7. Rubio, H. H., Magnanini, F. L., Pardo, R. F., et al., Cancer Gastrico Temprano. Buenos Aires, Premio Cientifica "F. Antonio Rizzuo," 1971.
8. Strauszer, T., and Csendes, A. (eds.): Cancer Gastrico, Santiago de Chile, Organizacion Mundial de la Salud, 1975.
9. Llorens, P. S.: Diagnóstico Endoscópico del Cáncer Gástrico. Ediciones Sede Santiago Sur, Universidad de Chile, 1975.
10. Takagi, K., and Nakata, K.: Lymph node metastasis and end-result of early gastric cancer (in Japanese). Jap. J. Clin. Surg., 31:19, 1976.
11. Nakamura, K., Sugano, H., Sugiyama, N., et al.: Clinical and histopathological features of scirrhous carcinoma of the stomach (English summary). Stom. Intest., 11:1275, 1976.
12. Johansen, A. A.: Early gastric cancer. In Morson, B. C. (ed.): Current Topics in Pathology No. 63. Pathology of the Gastrointestinal Tract. Berlin, Springer Verlag, 1976.
13. Morson, B. C.: The Japanese classification of early gastric cancer, In: Yardly, J. H., Morson, B. C., and Abell, M. R. (eds.): The Gastrointestinal Tract by 21 Authors. Baltimore, Williams & Wilkins, 1977.
14. Frik, W.: Neoplastic diseases of the stomach. In: Margulis, A. R., and Burhemme, H. J. (eds.): Alimentary Tract Roentgenology. St. Louis, C. V. Mosby, 1973.
15. Nakamura, K., Sugano, H., Takagi, K., et al.: Conception of histogenesis of gastric carcinoma (English summary). Stom. Intest., 6:849, 1971.
16. Kumakura, K.: A guide to double contrast method — X-ray demonstration of type IIc (English summary). Stom. Intest., 4:915, 1969.
17. Kumakura, K., Maruyama, M., and Someya, N.: X-ray demonstration of lesions in the anterior wall of the stomach (English summary). Stom. Intest., 3:873, 1968.
18. Shirakabe, H., Hayakawa, H., Itai, Y., et al.: Comparison of x-ray, endoscopy and biopsy examinations for the diagnosis of early gastric cancer. Jap. J. Clin. Oncol., 12:93, 1972.
19. Nakamura, K., Sugano, H., Maruyama, M., et al.: Histopathological study of primary locus of linitis plastica (English summary). Stom. Intest., 10:79, 1975.
20. Sugiyama, N. and Nakamaura, K.: A clinicopathological study on infiltrating pattern of gastric cancer in relation to its site of origin (English summary). Stom. Intest., 12:1073, 1977.
21. Nakamura, K., and Takagi, K.: Some considerations on lesions of atypical epithelium of the stomach (English summary). Stom. Intest., 10:1455, 1975.
22. Yamada, T., et al.: X-ray diagnosis of borderline lesion between malignancy and benignancy (English summary). Stom. Intest., 10:1479, 1975.
23. Sano, R.: Chronic gastritis observed in various gastric diseases — Analysis of operated materials with special reference to histologic classification of chronic gastritis and its relation to carcinoma. Jap. J. Gastroenterol., 72:1231, 1975.
24. Abel, W.: Die Röntgenbefunde der Gastritis erosiva. Fortschr. Röntgenstr., 80:30, 1954.
25. Walk, L.: Erosive gastritis: Clinical review and analysis of 27 cases. Gastroenterologia, 84:87, 1955.
26. Frik, W., and Hesse, R.: Die Röntgenologische Darstellung von Magenerosionen. Dtsch. Med. Wochenschr., 81:1119, 1956.
27. Bücker, J.: Zur röntgendiagnostik der gastritis erosiva. Radiologe, 4:78, 1964.
28. Rösch, W., and Ottenjann, R.: Gastric erosions. Endoscopy, 2:93, 1970.
29. Baba, Y., Takagi, K., Nakamura, K., et al.: A comparative study between histopathological and radiological findings of depressed early carcinoma of the stomach (English summary). Stom. Intest., 10:37, 1975.
30. Sakita, T., Oguro, Y., Takasu, S., et al.: Observation on the healing of ulcerations in early gastric cancer, the life cycle of the malignant ulcer. Gastroenterology, 60:835, 1971.

31. Nakamura, K., Sugano, H., and Takagi, K.: Carcinoma of the stomach in incipient phase; its histogenesis and histological appearance. Gann, *59*:251, 1968.
32. Maruyama, N., Sugiyama, N., Baba. Y., et al.: Radiodiagnostic possibility of gastric carcinoma involving the proper muscle layer (English summary). Stom. Intest., *11*:855, 1976.
33. Tsukasa, S., et al.: The estimation of invasion depth and extent of the gastric carcinoma by the use of the roentgenogram of resected specimens — special reference of invasion depth (English summary). Stom. Intest., *12*:1017, 1977.
34. Nishizawa, M.: Radologic diagnosis of depressed early cancer — Method of radiologic demonstration (in Japanese). Stom. Intest., 6:221, 1971.
35. Sugiyama, N.: Radiological diagnosis of malignant lymphoma of the stomach based on its macroscopical classification with special reference to early malignant lymphoma (English summary). Jap. J. Gastroenterol., *71*:1118, 1974.
36. Takeuchi, T., Ito, M., Murate, H., et al.: A case of early gastric reticulum cell sarcoma — Follow-up study with x-ray and gastroendoscope during the early stage (English summary). Stom. Intest., 6:211, 1966.
37. Nakano, H., Nakazawa, S., Ito, J., et al.: A case of reticulum cell sarcoma of the stomach (English summary). Stom. Intest., 7:375, 1972.
38. Konjetzyn, G. E.: Die Entzündungen des Magens. *In*: Handbuch spez. Path. Anatomie und Histologie, IV/2, Berlin, Springer Verlag, 1928.
39. Konjetzny, G. E.: Eine besondere Form der chronischen hypertrophischen Gastritis unter dem klinischen und röntgenologischen Bild des Carcinoms. Chirurg., *10*:260, 1938.
40. Schindler, R.: Gastroendoscopy, The Endoscopic Study of Gastric Pathology. 2nd ed. New York, Hofner Publishing Co., 1966.
41. Smith, J. L., and Helwig, E. B.: Malignant lymphoma of stomach, its diagnosis, distinction and biologic behavior (Abstract). Am. J. Pathol., *34*:553, 1958.
42. Nakamura, K., Aoki, M., Sugano, H., et al.: Reactive lymphoreticular hyperplasia of the stomach, Report of 6 surgical cases (English summary). Jap. J. Cancer Clin., *12*:691, 1966.
43. Jacobs, D. S.: Primary gastric malignant lymphoma and pseudolymphoma. Am. J. Clin. Pathol., *40*:379, 1963.

Additional References

Elster, K., Kolaczek, F., Shimamoto, K., et al.: Early cancer-experience in Germany. Endoscopy, 7:5, 1975.

Golden, R., and Stout, A. P.: Superficial spreading carcionoma of the stomach. Am. J. Roentgenol., *59*:157,1948.

Hermanek, P., Rösch, W.: Critical evaluation of the Japanese "early gastric cancer" classification. Endoscopy, 5:220, 1973.

Kawai, L.: Validity rate of concerted diagnosis using various methods. *In*: Murakami, T. (ed.): Early Gastric Cancer. Tokyo, University of Tokyo Press, 1971.

Kumakura, K.: Improvement and advances in double contrast studies. *In*: Murakami, T. (ed.): Early Gastric Cancer. Tokyo, University of Tokyo Press, 1971.

Maruyama, M.: Diagnostic limits for early gastric cancer by radiography. *In*: Murakami, T. (ed.): Early Gastric Cancer. Tokyo, University of Tokyo Press, 1971.

Murakami, K., Misaki, F., Shimamoto, K., et al.: Reevaluation of classification of "Early Gastric Cancer." Endoscopy, 6:209, 1974.

Okabe, H.: Growth of early gastric cancer. *In*: Marakami, T. (ed.): Early Gastric Cancer. Tokyo, University of Tokyo Press, 1971.

Okuda, S.: Differential diagnosis of early gastric cancer from advanced carcinoma. *In*: Murakami, T. (ed.): Early Gastric Cancer. Tokyo, University of Tokyo Press, 1971.

Rösch, W.: Early carcinoma. Endoscopy, 2:64, 1970.

Shirakabe, H.: X-ray diagnosis of early gastric cancer. *In*: Murakami, T. (ed.): Early Gastric Cancer. Tokyo, University of Tokyo Press, 1971.

Shirakabe, H., and Ichikawa, H.: Early gastric cancer. *In:* Stein, N., and Finkelstein. A. K. (eds.): Atlas of Tumor Radiology. Chicago, Year Book Medical Publishers, 1973, pp. 277–357.

Stout, A. P.: Superficial spreading type carcinoma of the stomach. Arch. Surg., *44*:651, 1942.

8

THE POSTOPERATIVE STOMACH

J. ODO OP DEN ORTH, M.D.

INTRODUCTION

A radiologist examining a patient who has had previous gastric surgery should be familiar with the common gastric operations. In order to choose an appropriate examination technique he must know whether or not a surgical anastomosis has been performed. If there has been no anastomosis the examination technique will be essentially the same as that for the intact stomach. However, if an anastomosis has been made the tech-

289

nique must be modified to prevent premature loss of contrast material through the anastomosis. It is therefore of utmost importance that the radiologist collect all available information regarding the surgical procedure. He should also review any preceding radiologic studies if these are available. It these data are not obtainable, the examination must be undertaken on the assumption that an anastomosis has been performed.

OPERATIONS WITHOUT ANASTOMOSIS

The examination technique in these patients is essentially the same as the double contrast examination in patients with an intact stomach. This has been described in detail.[1] We prefer a barium suspension of medium high density, approximately 82% W/V, in order to provide good mucosal coating and to allow for good compression studies.

Simple Closure

Simple closure of a perforated ulcer may result in a localized filling defect.[2, 3] These filling defects disappear with the passage of time.[3, 4] It has been our experience, as well as that of others,[5] that it is often impossible to distinguish between the original ulcer, simple closure, and even a recurrent ulcer in the duodenal bulb.

Vagotomy and Pyloroplasty

The common Heineke-Mikulicz pyloroplasty is performed as a drainage procedure in association with vagotomy. The pyloroplasty consists of a longitudinal incision extending from the antrum across the pylorus. The incision is then closed vertically. This results in a typical deformity, sometimes referred to as the beagle-ear sign (Fig. 8–1).[2, 6-8] In our experience, differentiation between this deformity and recurrent ulcer is extremely difficult, although cineradiography may be of help.[9] Fiberoptic endoscopy may also be very useful for this purpose.

After vagotomy, peristalsis in the stomach is sluggish, and the appearance of the duodenum is similar to that seen during drug-induced hypotonic duodenography. After highly selective vagotomy, peristalsis in the stomach is virtually normal.[5]

Gastropexy and Localized Resections

In an anterior gastropexy, the anterior wall of the stomach is sutured to the anterior abdominal wall. Such an operation produces a characteristic deformity (Fig. 8–2).

Localized resections (wedge resections and segmental resections) result in permanent and often bizarre deformities of the stomach (Fig. 8–3).

Fundoplication

A Nissen fundoplication[10] is often performed to prevent gastroesophageal reflux and to repair a hiatal hernia. A sleeve of the gastric fundus is wrapped around the distal esophagus and is fixed there with plication sutures. On postoperative contrast studies, this produces a typical pseudotumor with variable narrowing of the abdominal esophagus (Figs. 8–4 and 8–5).[11–13] The pseudotumor may diminish or disappear with the passage of time. When neither the pseudotumor nor the narrowing is visualized, one may suspect that the operation has not been successful or that there has been a recurrence.[14]

In the Belsey Mark IV fundoplication the hernia is reduced, and the esophagus is sutured to the stomach and the diaphragm. This can result in a small pseudotumor. In addition, two sharp angles in the intra-abdominal esophagus can be identified.[12, 15]

Text continued on page 295

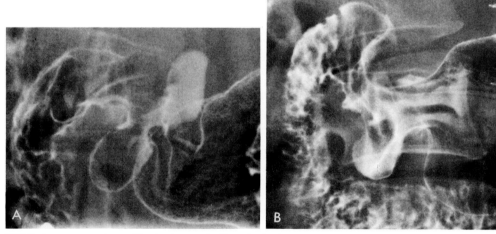

FIGURE 8–1   *A* and *B*   Typical pseudodiverticula in two patients after a Heineke-Mikulicz pyloroplasty. Beagle-ear sign.

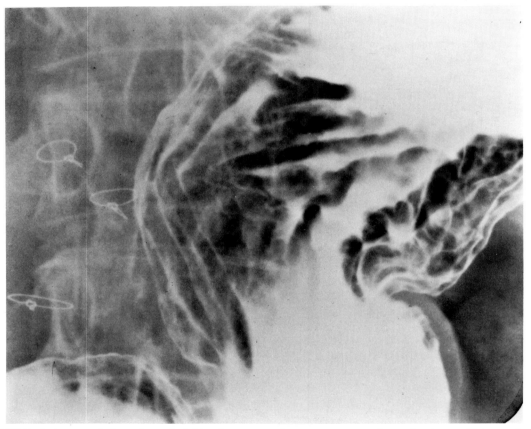

FIGURE 8–2 Angulation of gastric folds after an anterior gastropexy performed to keep a Foley catheter in place after a decompression procedure.

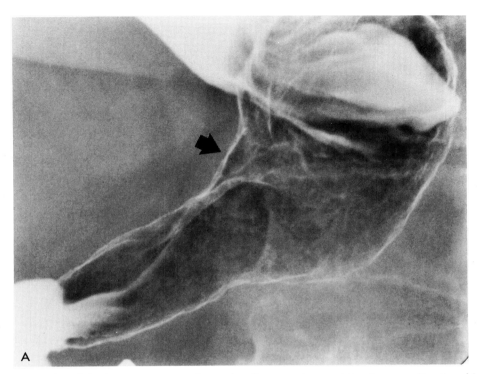

A. Deformity of the lesser curvature 2 months after a wedge excision for a small polypoid carcinoma.

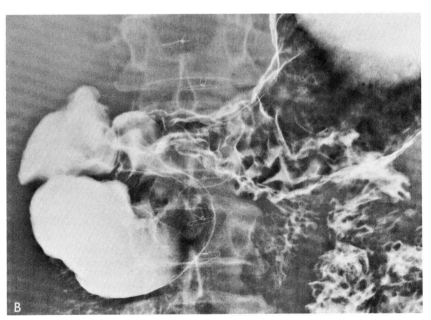

B. Bizarre deformity of the stomach 4 years after wedge resection of the lesser curvature for a benign gastric ulcer.

FIGURE 8–3 Deformity due to local excision.

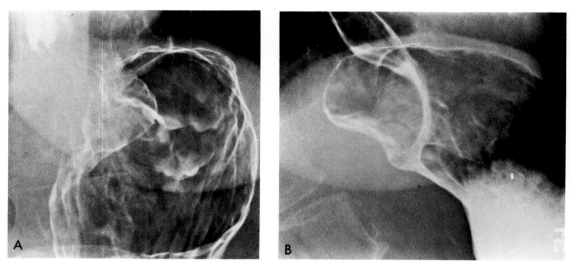

FIGURE 8–4 *A* and *B* Typical pseudotumor and narrowing of the lower esophagus 2 months after a Nissen fundoplication.

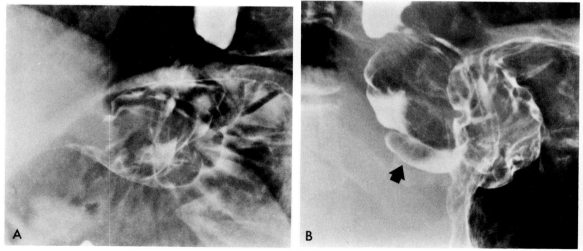

FIGURE 8–5 *A* and *B* Typical pseudotumor and narrowing of the esophagus 10 days after a Nissen fundoplication. On the medial side some barium is in the lumen of the fundal sleeve which has been wrapped around the lower esophagus *(arrow)*.

OPERATIONS WITH ANASTOMOSIS

Examination Technique

In order to prevent rapid loss of contrast material into the small bowel it is necessary to utilize a drug to decrease motility of the upper gastrointestinal tract.[16-18] In our experience an intravenous injection of 1 mg of glucagon is most effective. In addition, tilting the table 20 to 30 degrees anti-Trendelenburg (head-up) helps to prevent loss of gas through the anastomosis.

After gastric surgery the fundus is not accessible to compression, just as in patients without previous surgery. However, the same holds true for the greatest portion of the gastric remnant after distal partial gastrectomy, and for the small bowel segment at the esophagojejunal anastomosis following total gastrectomy. Therefore, double contrast technique is essential for the examination of these segments of the gastrointestinal tract.

Gastroenterostomy

Currently, gastroenterostomy is performed only to provide drainage in cases of distal gastric or duodenal obstruction when no other operation is possible. In most cases the obstruction is caused by a malignant lesion, and a side-to-side anastomosis is fashioned between the stomach and a loop of jejunum (Fig. 8–6). The examination technique is basically the same as that described further on for partial resection with anastomosis. In addition, mucosal relief films are made with the patient in the prone position.

In elderly patients one often encounters a long-standing gastroenterostomy performed for benign disease. In these patients, marked contraction of the antrum, probably due to antral and pyloric hypertrophy, is sometimes seen (Fig. 8–7).[19, 20] Differentiation between such a benign contraction of the antrum and scirrhous carcinoma is often impossible on a purely radiologic basis, so that gastroscopy and biopsy are frequently necessary. It may also be necessary to distinguish this antral contraction from a small partial distal gastrectomy with side-to-side gastrojejunostomy (Fig. 8–8).

Partial Resection with Anastomosis

In common usage the eponym "Billroth I" is used to refer to any partial gastrectomy with gastroduodenostomy, and the eponym "Billroth II" refers to all varieties of partial gastrectomy with gastrojejunostomy.[21]

In a gastroduodenostomy an end-to-end anastomosis is generally used. The cut end of the stomach is usually partially oversewn in order to adapt the size of the gastric opening to the size of the duodenum. The area that is oversewn often produces a persistent deformity or plication defect along the lesser curvature in the preanastomotic area.

In a gastrojejunostomy the end-to-side anastomosis can be made using the entire cut end of the stomach (Fig. 8–10), or the size of the stomach can be reduced by oversewing part of the cut end (Fig. 8–11). The oversewn area produces a plication defect with this type of anastomosis as well.

Text continued on page 302

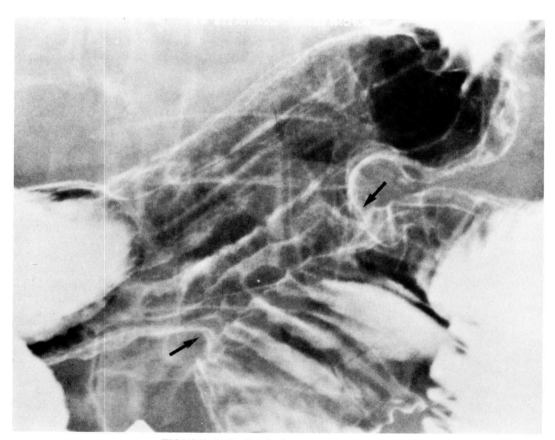

FIGURE 8–6 Typical gastroenterostomy.

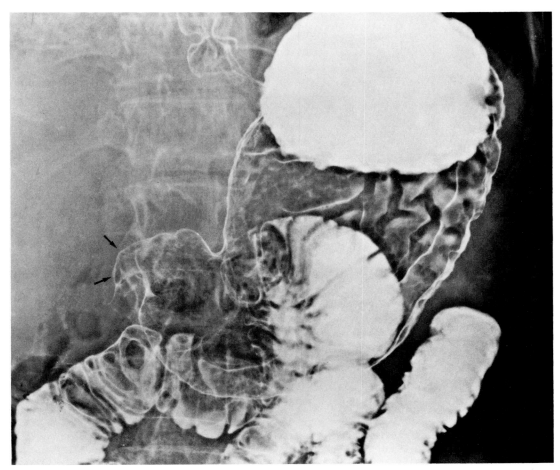

FIGURE 8–7 Gastroenterostomy with antral contraction.

Double contrast examination in the supine position 42 years after a posterior gastroenterostomy. There is contraction of the antrum (*small arrows*). The autopsy performed shortly after the x-ray examination demonstrated a hypertrophic pylorus.

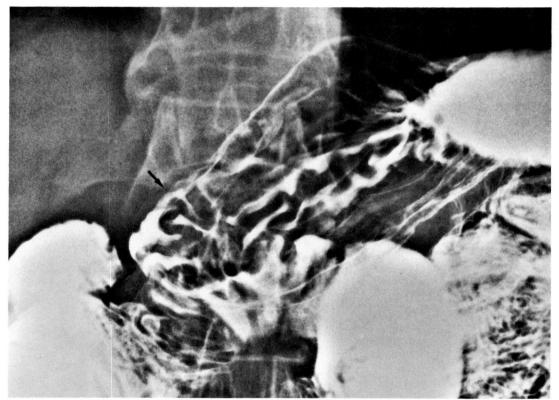

FIGURE 8-8 Billroth II. Small distal partial gastrectomy with a side-to-side gastroenterostomy (patient supine). The configuration of the folds of the distal part of the stomach confirms that a blind pouch (*arrows*) has been formed. This makes it possible to differentiate between this kind of operation and the condition shown in Figure 8–7. This gastrojejunostomy with side-to-side anastomosis represents the original Billroth II operation.

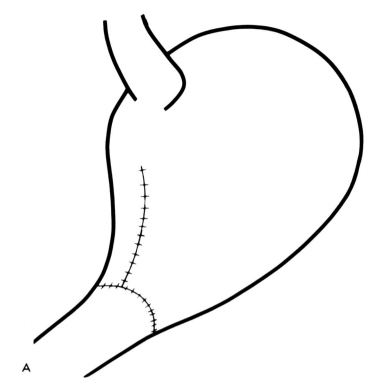

FIGURE 8–9 *A* and *B*   Billroth I. Typical distal partial gastrectomy and gastroduodenostomy and end-to-end anastomosis (patient supine). Despite complete distension there remains a concave defect on the lesser curvature side of the preanastomotic area (*arrow*), probably resulting from the surgical procedure to adapt the size of the distal cut end of the stomach to the duodenum. The surgery had been performed 38 years previously.

A

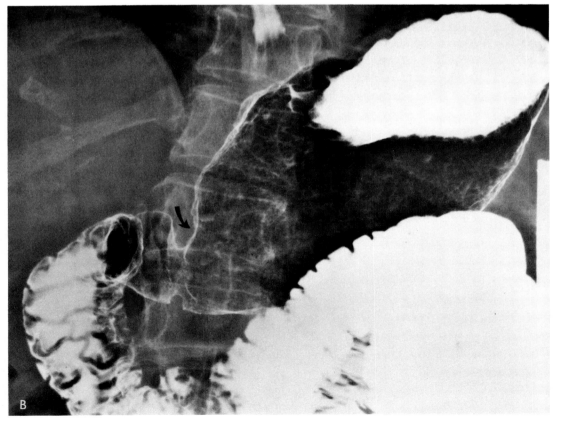

B

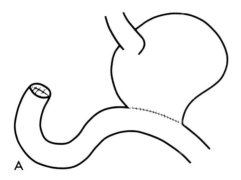

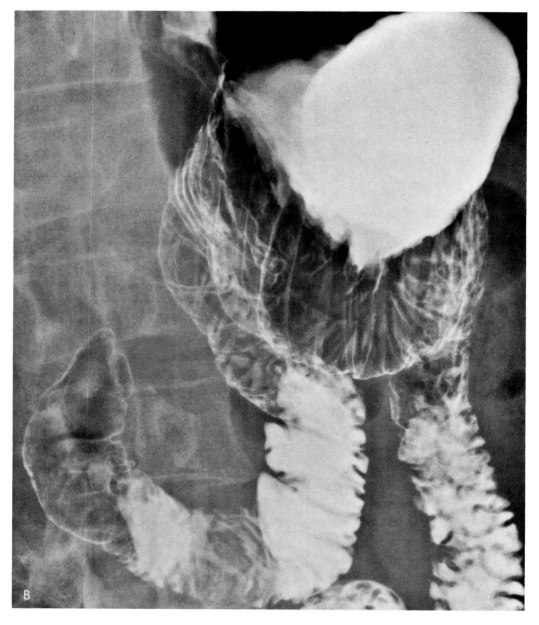

FIGURE 8-10 *A* and *B*   Typical distal partial gastrectomy and gastrojejunostomy with an end-to-side anastomosis (patient supine, right side up). The entire cut end of the stomach has been used for the anastomosis.

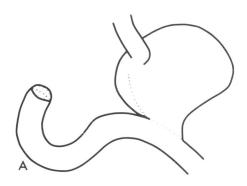

FIGURE 8–11 *A* and *B* Typical distal partial gastrectomy and gastrojejunostomy with an end-to-side anastomosis with a restricted stoma formed 18 years before (patient supine). The concave contour of the gastric remnant just above the anastomosis on the lesser curvature side (*arrow*) results from the operative procedure (plication defect). There is a large diverticulum of the duodenum.

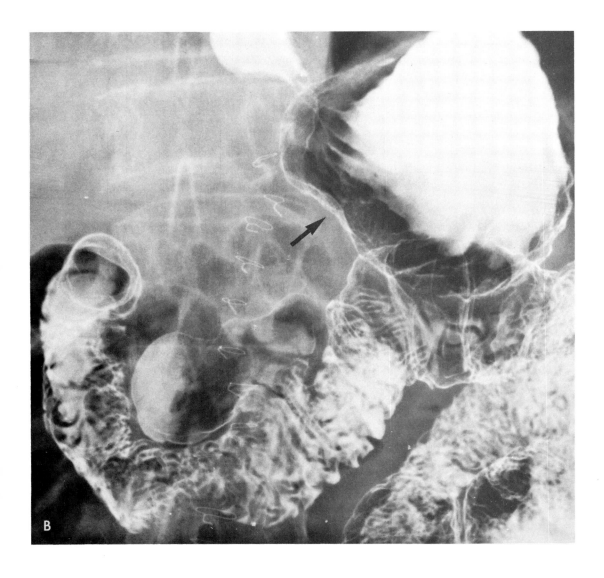

EXAMINATION TECHNIQUE

Immediately before the start of the examination, an intravenous injection of 1 mg of glucagon is given. This renders the gastric remnant and small bowel hypotonic and prevents rapid spilling of contrast material into the small bowel.

Adequate gaseous distension of the gastric remnant and anastomotic loops of small bowel is clearly an important component of this examination. Although satisfactory results can be obtained with the use of effervescent pellets, granules, or powders, we prefer the "bubbly barium" method. This consists of a carbonated barium suspension cocktail which is mixed in a 2-liter soda siphon. It is prepared by slowly adding 2 cartridges of carbon dioxide to 2 liters of refrigerated barium suspension. The "bubbly barium" thus prepared dissociates in 90 seconds to produce 1 part of barium suspension and 2 parts of carbon dioxide.[1, 22, 23]

A barium suspension of moderately high density is preferred in order to allow for good double contrast films (80 to 90 kV with rare earth intensifying screens) as well as for transparency on single contrast compression studies (120 to 150 kV).[1] With such a barium suspension (specific gravity about 1.6), compression studies of the stomal area and the anastomotic loops of small bowel are made. The patient is placed first in the supine and semi-erect positions, and a Holzknecht spoon is used for compression. He is then put in the prone position, and an inflatable paddle is inserted between the patient and the table for compression. The patient then swallows additional barium and an effervescent agent and is placed supine, with the head of the table elevated 20 to 30 degrees.

In order to achieve good mucosal coating the patient rolls to and fro between the right and left decubitus positions, and double contrast films of the gastric pouch and preanastomotic area are made (Figs. 8–12 to 8–14). In order to obtain double contrast views of the stomal area following a Billroth II resection, it is necessary to lower the table to a nearly horizontal position (Fig. 8–15). Careful fluoroscopic control is needed to prevent loss of gas through the anastomosis. The stomal area in a Billroth I resection is easily visualized in a nearly horizontal position with the patient supine and the right side elevated. Double contrast views of the pseudobulb are similar to those of the unoperated duodenal bulb (Fig. 8–16).

The head of the table is again elevated 20 to 30 degrees. The patient lies on the right side and drinks additional barium, and if necessary additional effervescent agent. Frequently the barium will flow spontaneously into the afferent loop to the top of the duodenum. If this does not happen, the Valsalva maneuver or coughing may be of great help. As soon as barium is seen to enter the duodenum the patient is quickly turned to the supine position with the right side up to allow gas to enter the duodenum. To provide good mucosal coating in the duodenum, the patient is rotated approximately 135 degrees between the supine LPO position to the prone position (Fig. 8–17).[22] When good coating has been obtained, films of the duodenum are made with the patient in the supine position, right side elevated and prone (Fig. 8–18). Thereafter large-size survey films are made with the patient in the supine and erect (frontal and lateral) positions (Fig. 8–19).

Text continued on page 308

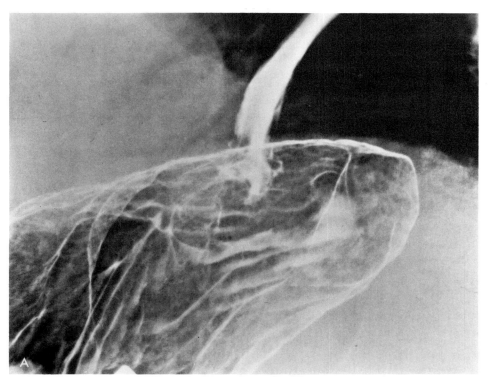

A. Patient supine, left side up. Table 20 to 30 degrees anti-Trendelenburg.

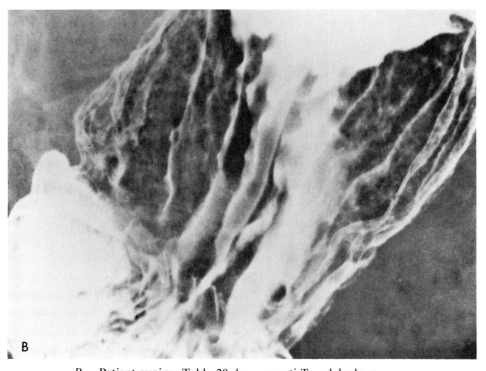

B. Patient supine. Table 20 degrees anti-Trendelenburg.

FIGURE 8–12 Double contrast views of the gastric remnant.

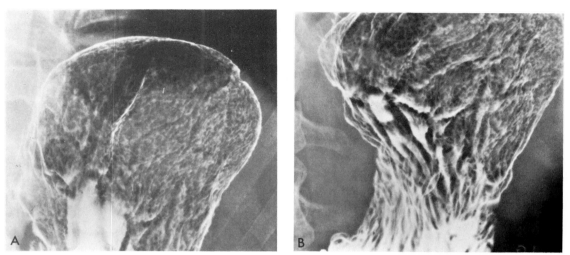

FIGURE 8–13 Double contrast studies of the gastric remnant in another patient. Note the surface pattern or areae gastricae. At endoscopy the appearance of the fundal mucosa was considered to be normal.

A. Patient supine, left side up. Table 20 to 30 degrees anti-Trendelenburg.
B. Patient supine. Table 20 degrees anti-Trendelenburg.

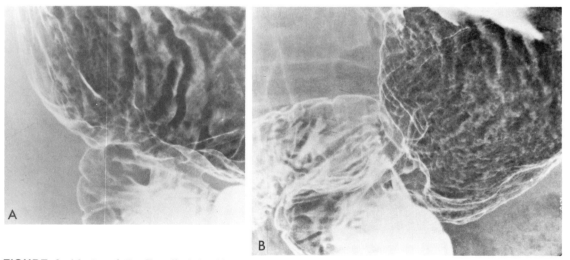

FIGURE 8–14 *A* and *B* Detailed double contrast studies of the preanastomotic area in two different patients with a gastrojejunostomy (patient supine, table only slightly anti-Trendelenburg). Note the areae gastricae.

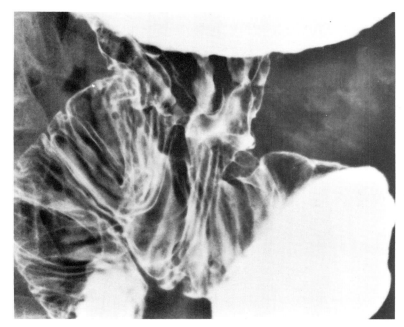

FIGURE 8–15 Detailed double contrast study of an end-to-side gastrojejunostomy (patient supine, table horizontal).

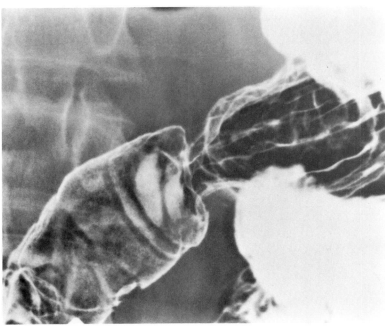

FIGURE 8–16 Detailed double contrast study of an end-to-end gastroduodenostomy (patient supine, right side slightly elevated). A pseudobulb has been formed.

FIGURE 8–17 This schema indicates the movement that must be performed to obtain good mucosal coating of the duodenum. Owing to the dorsal position of the duodenum there is no risk of losing gas when the movements of the patient remain between the indicated limits.

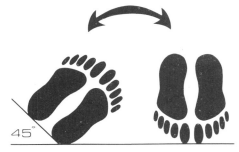

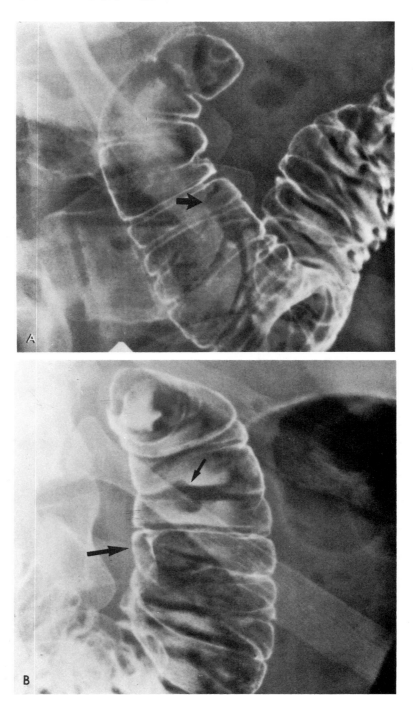

FIGURE 8–18 *A* and *B*   The afferent loop. Note the inverted stump at the top of the duodenum. The major papilla is well visualized in *A* *(arrow)* (patient supine, right side up). The major papilla can also be identified in the prone position in *B* *(large arrow)*. The minor papilla *(small arrow)* can generally only be visualized in the prone position because it is a shallow protrusion which usually has gently sloping edges and is situated on the anterior wall of the descending duodenum.[63] The minor papilla lies cephaloventral of the major papilla, the mean distance 18 to 20 mm.[64, 65]

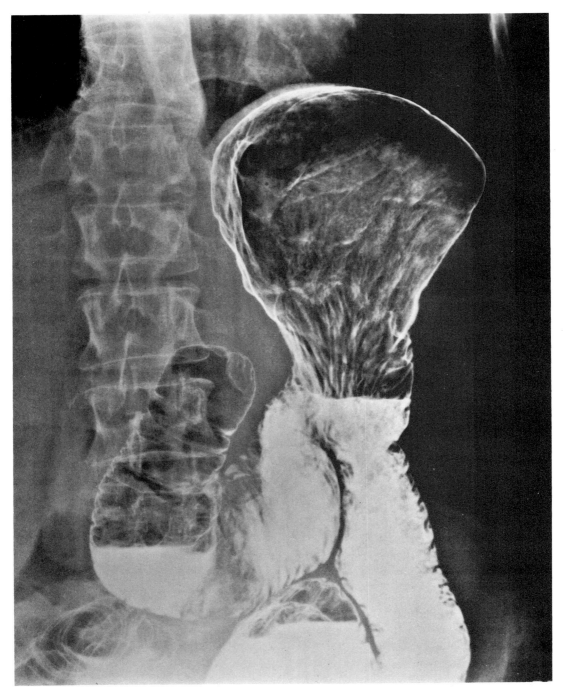

FIGURE 8–19   Survey film after a distal partial gastrectomy and a right-to-left, end-to-side gastrojejunostomy (patient erect). Note the inverted stump at the top of the duodenum.

PLICATION DEFECTS AND OTHER PSEUDOLESIONS

In both the Billroth I and the Billroth II resections, a portion of the cut end of the stomach may be oversewn and inverted to restrict the size of the stoma. These produce typical deformities or plication defects (Fig. 8–20).[24-26] In the differential diagnosis of such defects, foreign body granuloma must also be considered (Fig. 8–28).[27, 28] Typical defects due to an inverted stump with or without a foreign body granuloma also occur in the stump of the duodenum after a Billroth II operation (Fig. 8–21).

At any place where sutures have been placed, distortion of the mucosal relief may occur, causing crater-like patterns (pseudoulcers) which cannot be distinguished from true ulcers on a radiologic basis (Fig. 8–27).

POSTOPERATIVE ULCER

Postoperative ulcers occur more frequently after an operation for duodenal ulcer than for gastric ulcer. In the case of gastrojejunostomy the small bowel just distal to the anastomosis is the site of predilection. The efferent loop is affected more frequently than the afferent loop. Ulceration may also occur in the anastomotic ring. In a gastroduodenostomy the anastomotic ring is affected most commonly, but localization in the pre- and postanastomotic area also occurs. A recurrent ulcer in the rest of the gastric remnant is rare in gastrojejunostomy and in gastroduodenostomy.[3, 29-33]

Just as in the nonoperated stomach, the radiologic diagnosis of such ulcers depends upon the demonstration of an ulcer niche (Figs. 8–22 and 8–23). Both the double contrast and the positive contrast compression

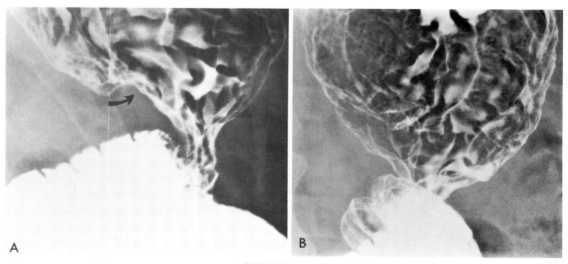

FIGURE 8–20

A. Profile view of the lesser curvature 11 years after a distal partial gastrectomy with an end-to-side gastrojejunostomy: filling defect on the lesser curvature side of the preanastomotic area *(arrow)*.

B. Same patient, face-on view. Gastroscopy and biopsy proved that this was a plication defect.

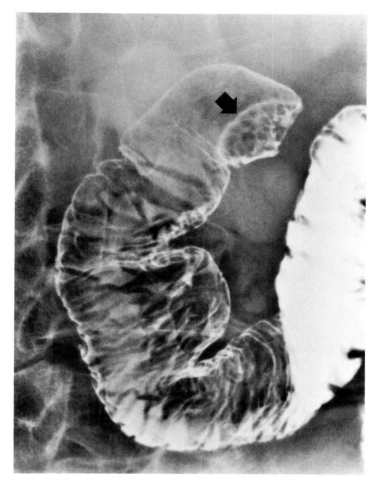

FIGURE 8–21 Afferent loop 6 years after a distal partial gastrectomy with gastrojejunostomy (patient supine, right side up). Large filling defect at the top of the duodenum (*arrow*) caused by a plication defect or a foreign body granuloma.

studies should be used (Figs. 8–24 and 8–25). An ulcer crater in a gastric remnant discovered many years after an operation for a benign condition should be considered potentially malignant (Figs. 8–26 and 8–31).

In the preanastomotic area, pseudolesions resembling an ulcer may be caused by barium trapped between distorted gastric folds. Only the endoscopist can decide whether there is intact mucosa at the base of such a crater-like lesion (Fig. 8–27).

A review of the literature regarding the accuracy of radiologic diagnosis of marginal ulcer shows percentages of correct positive diagnosis ranging from 28 to 60 per cent.[31, 34] Although quantitative studies have not yet appeared, hypotonic double contrast studies are expected to raise the percentage of marginal ulcers demonstrated correctly. However, for demonstrating a *small* marginal ulcer situated in the jejunum, fiber-endoscopy is, until further notice, superior to radiology.[35]

Text continued on page 313

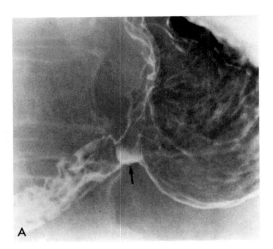
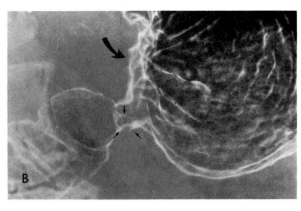

FIGURE 8–22 Stomal ulcer.

    A. Ulcer niche at the stoma (*arrow*), endoscopically confirmed 12 years after distal partial gastrectomy with end-to-end duodenostomy.

    B. The niche is visible only as a ring shadow (*arrows*) after the barium flows out of the niche. Note the large plication defect on the lesser curvature side of the preanastomotic area (*curved arrow*).

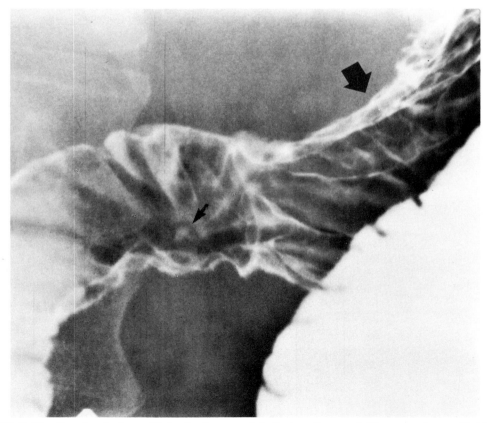

FIGURE 8–23 Duodenal ulcer. Niche in the pseudobulb (*small arrow*) 29 years after a distal partial gastrectomy with end-to-end gastroduodenostomy. Note the large plication defect on the lesser curvature side of the preanastomotic area (*large arrow*). Several weeks after the radiologic examination endoscopy showed inflammation and the remnant of an ulcer niche.

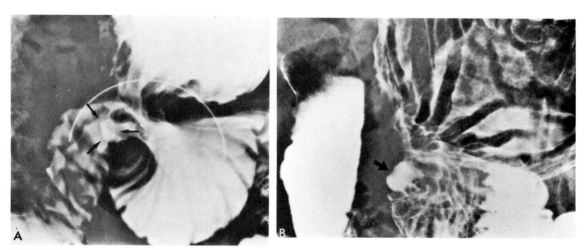

FIGURE 8–24 *A* and *B*   Jejunal ulcer. Endoscopically confirmed jejunal ulcer 9 years after distal partial gastrectomy with end-to-side gastrojejunostomy. The ulcer is demonstrated by both the complete filling/compression technique (*A, arrows*) and the double contrast technique (*B, arrow*).

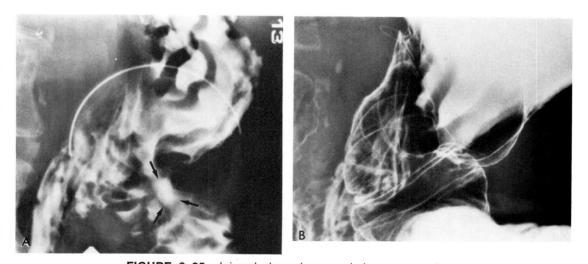

FIGURE 8–25   Jejunal ulcer shown only by compression.

A.   Jejunal ulcer (*arrows*) in the efferent loop 3 years after a distal partial gastrectomy with end-to-side gastrojejunostomy.
B.   The double contrast technique failed to demonstrate the ulcer.

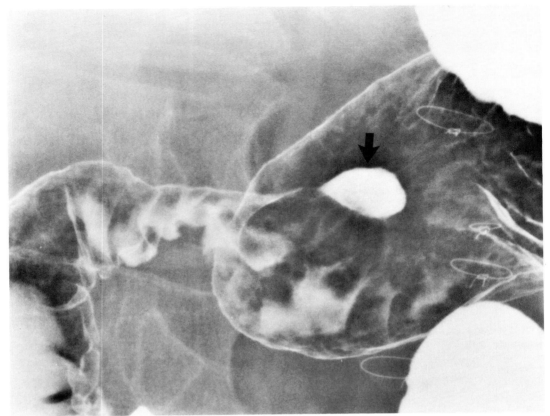

FIGURE 8–26   Gastric ulcer. Large ulcer crater *(arrow)* on the posterior wall (patient supine) of a gastric remnant 28 years after a small distal partial gastrectomy with end-to-end gastroduodenostomy for hypertrophic pyloric stenosis. Because the swollen folds end fairly far from the crater and because of the long postoperative interval, this ulcer was considered to be malignant. However, acid production was demonstrated, and at endoscopy the ulcer looked benign. This was confirmed by multiple biopsies.

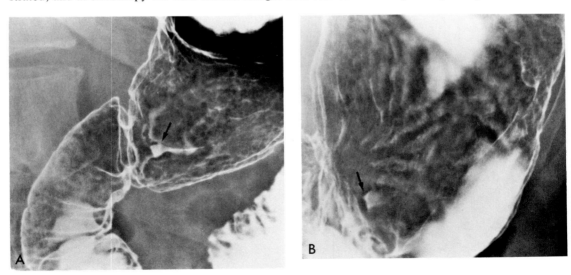

FIGURE 8–27   Pseudoulcers.

A.   A collection of barium in the preanastomotic area of a gastric remnant *(arrow)* 4 years after a distal partial gastrectomy with end-to-end gastroduodenostomy. Gastroscopy showed an intact epithelium. The crater-like pattern is caused by barium trapped between gastric folds.

B.   A crater-like collection *(arrows)* 16 years after a distal partial gastrectomy with end-to-side gastrojejunostomy. Endoscopy demonstrated a configuration of folds which accounted for the radiologic finding. The epithelium at the base of the crater-like lesion was intact.

312

CARCINOMA

The radiologic diagnosis of carcinoma involving the gastric remnant encompasses two distinct conditions. Secondary postgastrectomy carcinoma or recurrent carcinoma refers to those patients who have had gastric surgery for a primary gastric carcinoma. Primary postgastrectomy or gastric stump carcinoma refers to a carcinoma arising in the gastric remnant of a patient in whom the original surgery was for a lesion other than carcinoma. In both cases the detection of carcinoma is difficult, because of the surgical deformity and because the absence of the pylorus makes it difficult to retain contrast in the gastric remnant.

The diagnosis of secondary postgastrectomy carcinoma (recurrent cancer) can be extremely difficult,[36] especially shortly after the operative procedure (Fig. 8–28). An early postoperative baseline study is of great help for comparison with later studies.

Primary postgastrectomy carcinoma or gastric stump carcinoma is often defined as a primary cancer of the gastric remnant arising at least 5 years after a partial gastrectomy in which there was no evidence of malignant disease in the resected portion of the stomach.[37] The incidence seems to be much higher in Europe than in the United States.[37, 38] Stalsberg and Taksdal[39] in Norway studied the frequency of gastric cancer at necropsy after previous gastric surgery (Billroth II resection and gastroenterostomy). Patients who had had their operation less than 15 years prior to death had a lower incidence of gastric carcinoma than matched unoperated controls. However, patients with operations 25 years or more prior to death had a sixfold increase in gastric carcinoma. There was no evidence of a difference in this respect between patients operated on for gastric ulcer and patients operated on for duodenal ulcer, or between partial gastrectomy with gastrojejunostomy and gastrojejunostomy alone. A recent Swiss study by Clémençon and associates[40] reports 21 cases of primary gastric stump carcinoma among 326 patients with a Billroth II resection for benign lesions. The incidence of stump carcinoma after 10 years was 15.1 per cent and after 20 years was 21.43 per cent. These authors advise that gastric resection for benign disease should be avoided whenever possible. An annual endoscopic examination is recommended starting 10 years after the resection. Terjesen and Erichsen[41] in Norway advise that gastric resection be avoided in young patients. They recommend a regular follow-up, thorough x-ray examinations, and gastroscopy starting after a postoperative interval of 15 years.

While performing fiber-endoscopic biopsy examinations in 1005 consecutive patients in the Netherlands, Dekker[42] found 132 cases of adenocarcinoma of the stomach; 11 of them were primary stump carcinomas.

Opinions on the accuracy of the radiologic examination vary greatly,[37, 42-46] although good results were reported by Saegesser and Jämes.[44] Presumably, hypotonic double contrast examinations have improved upon most of these results, but this should be confirmed by a prospective study (Figs. 8–29 to 8–32).

Text continued on page 318

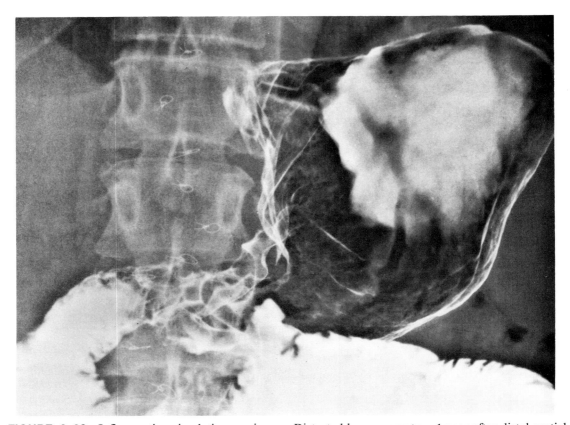

FIGURE 8–28 Inflammation simulating carcinoma. Distorted lesser curvature 1 year after distal partial gastrectomy with end-to-end gastroduodenostomy for carcinoma (early gastric cancer). It is often impossible to exclude secondary postgastrectomy carcinoma (recurrent cancer) on radiologic grounds. The patient refused endoscopy. Shortly after the radiologic examination the patient died. Autopsy showed a large plication defect, swollen folds, gastritis and perigastritis, and persistent sutures with no recurrent carcinoma.

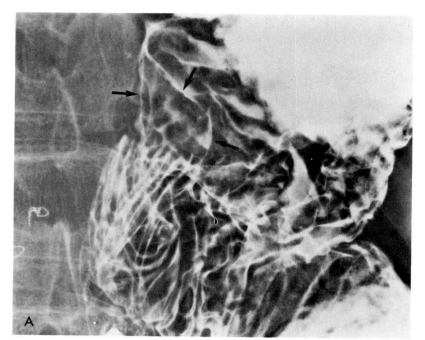

A. Irregular filling defect (*arrows*) on the lesser curvature side just above the anastomosis 20 years after a distal partial gastrectomy with end-to-side gastrojejunostomy. Two years before, the radiologic examination had been completely normal. Gastric biopsy showed adenocarcinoma.

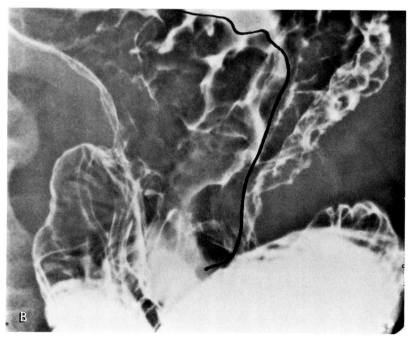

B. Another patient, 30 years after a distal partial gastrectomy with end-to-side gastrojejunostomy. Distortion of folds and nodularity in the preanastomotic area raised the radiologic suspicion of primary postgastrectomy carcinoma which was confirmed by gastrobiopsy.

FIGURE 8–29 Primary gastric carcinoma following Billroth II.

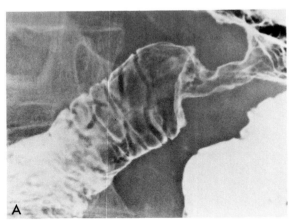
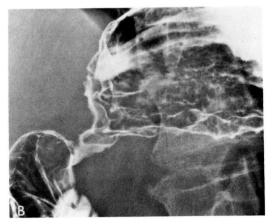

FIGURE 8–30 *A* and *B*   Gastric stump carcinoma following Billroth I. Irregular stricture of the anastomotic area 30 years after a distal partial gastrectomy with end-to-end gastroduodenostomy. The radiologic diagnosis of primary postgastrectomy carcinoma was confirmed by gastroscopy and biopsy.

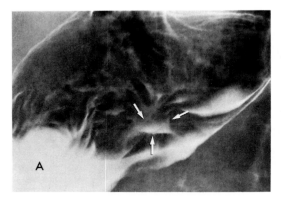
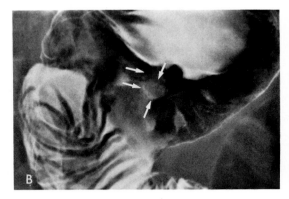

FIGURE 8–31 *A* and *B*   Ulcerated stump carcinoma. Crater *(arrows)* with converging thickened folds on the posterior wall (patient supine) of the gastric remnant 30 years after a distal partial gastrectomy with end-to-side gastrojejunostomy. Gastroscopy and biopsy showed an adenocarcinoma.

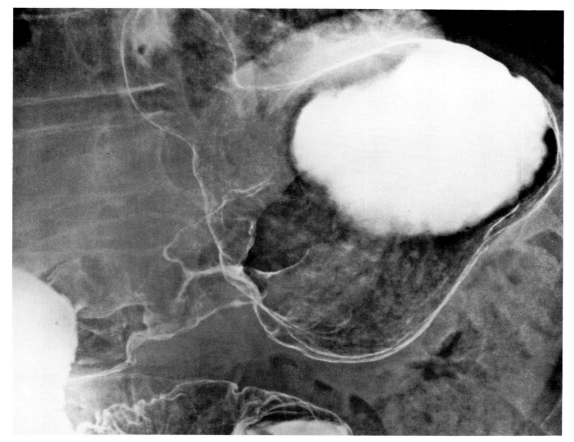

FIGURE 8–32 Irregular stricture of the preanastomotic and anastomotic area 33 years after a distal partial gastrectomy with end-to-end gastroduodenostomy. Gastroscopy and biopsy confirmed the radiologic diagnosis of primary postgastrectomy carcinoma.

MUCOSAL PROLAPSE AND INTUSSUSCEPTION

Gastrojejunal or gastroduodenal mucosal prolapse is a relatively rare condition.[47-50] Its incidence seems to be greater after a restricted stoma has been fashioned. In a series of 24 cases described by Seaman[50] the median time between the initial surgery and the detection of the prolapse was 6 years. It is not an acute condition; bleeding is the commonest clinical manifestation, and partial obstruction may occur. In some cases, awareness of this condition is sufficient for the radiologic diagnosis (Fig. 8–33A and B). When there is an extensive mass, gastric biopsy may be needed to exclude a malignant lesion (Fig. 8–33C and D).

True gastrojejunal intussusceptions are seldom found.[51] Jejunogastric intussusceptions occur more frequently (Fig. 8–34).[52-56] In the acute form this is a potentially lethal condition because of the risk of incarceration. The radiologic diagnosis depends upon the identification of a striated filling defect, representing a part of the small bowel in the gastric remnant.

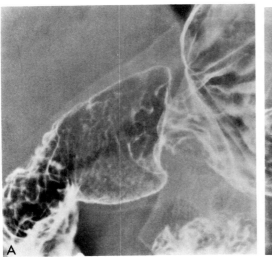 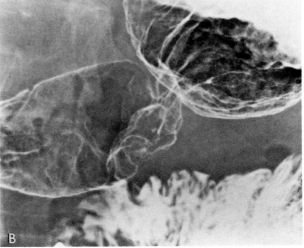

A. Fifteen years after a distal partial gastrectomy with end-to-end gastroduodenostomy. The patient complained of intermittent obstruction. On several occasions gastric retention was found. During the radiologic examination the passage of contrast material through the gastroduodenostomy was unusually slow for such an operation. Gastroduodenal prolapse is obvious.

B. Eighteen years after a distal partial gastrectomy with end-to-end gastroduodenostomy. There is a mass on the greater curvature side of the anastomosis and in the pseudobulb. Gastroscopy and biopsy showed that the mass was caused by prolapsed gastric mucosa.

FIGURE 8–33 Prolapse of gastric mucosa into the duodenum.

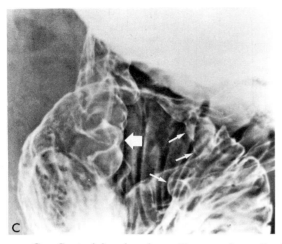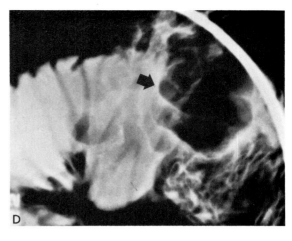

C. Gastrojejunal prolapse 30 years after a distal partial gastrectomy with an end-to-side gastrojejunostomy. Double contrast study, patient supine. There is a mass on the lesser curvature side (*large arrow*) and several smaller masses on the greater curvature side of the anastomosis (*small arrows*).

D. Positive contrast compression study, patient prone. Note the transparency due to the medium high density barium suspension. Gastroscopy and biopsy showed prolapse of gastric mucosa into the jejunum.

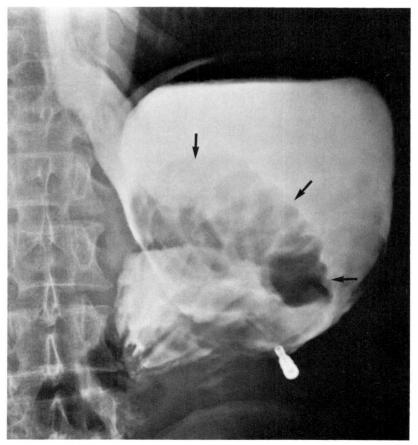

FIGURE 8-34 Retrograde jejunogastric intussusception. Three years following the Billroth II resection, there was sudden onset of abdominal cramps and vomiting. The x-ray study shows obstruction of the gastric remnant owing to retrograde jejunogastric intussusception (*arrows*). The diagnosis was confirmed at laparotomy. (Courtesy of Professor E. Ponette, University Hospital, Leuven, Belgium.)

319

AFFERENT LOOP

With hypotonic technique the afferent loop can be examined much more easily than ever before.[22] Apart from the pathology that is found in hypotonic duodenography (Figs. 8–35 and 8–36), the relationship between the gastric remnant and the anastomosed loop can be studied very easily. According to Burhenne,[57] an iatrogenic afferent loop syndrome can occur if the afferent loop has been attached to the greater curvature instead of to the lesser curvature. Such a left-to-right anastomosis can, particularly when an oblique plane of anastomosis exists, result in preferential filling of the afferent loop, which might cause symptoms (Fig. 8–37). There is however, sometimes a striking discrepancy between the radiologic findings and the absence of complaints (Fig. 8–38).

Text continued on page 324

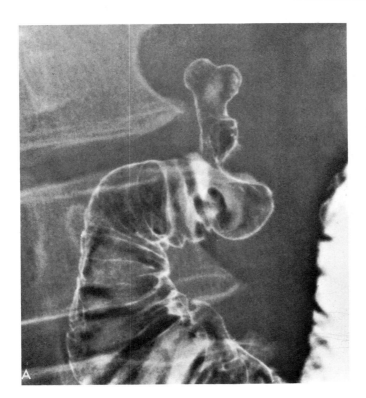

A. Hypotonic duodenogram of the afferent loop after a distal partial gastrectomy with gastrojejunostomy (patient supine, right side up) showing an irregular configuration of the proximal part of the duodenum. Probably the remnants of the deformed duodenal bulb; confirmation by duodenoscopy.

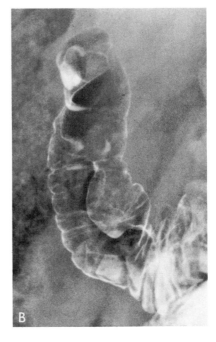

FIGURE 8–35 Scarred duodenal bulb.

B. Extramucosal mass. Hypotonic duodenogram of the afferent loop, 35 years after a distal partial gastrectomy with gastrojejunostomy (patient supine, right side up). Smooth-surfaced indentation along the inner aspect of the descending duodenum. Duodenoscopy showed an extramucosal indentation.

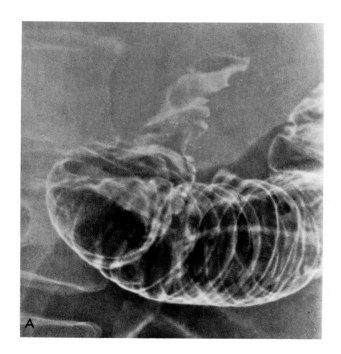

A. Supine, right side up.

FIGURE 8–36 Duodenal involvement by cholecystitis. Hypotonic duodenogram in a patient with a distal partial gastrectomy and gastrojejunostomy with clinical features of cholecystitis.

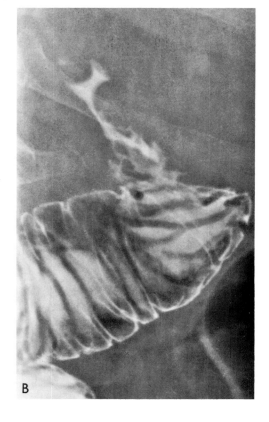

B. Prone. Compression of the duodenum by pericholecystitis caused by a perforation of the gallbladder.

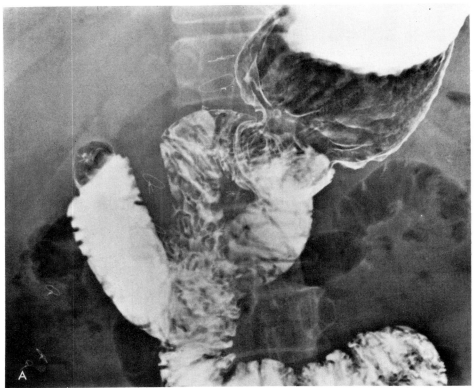

A. Distal partial gastrectomy with end-to-side gastrojejunostomy. There is a left-to-right anastomosis resulting in preferential filling of the afferent loop. Following the operation the patient complained of nausea and vomiting after meals.

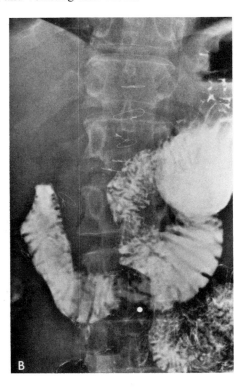

FIGURE 8–37 Afferent loop syndrome.

B. Follow-up film after 90 minutes showed hyperperistalsis of the afferent loop, which was still filled with barium. An example of an iatrogenic afferent loop syndrome.

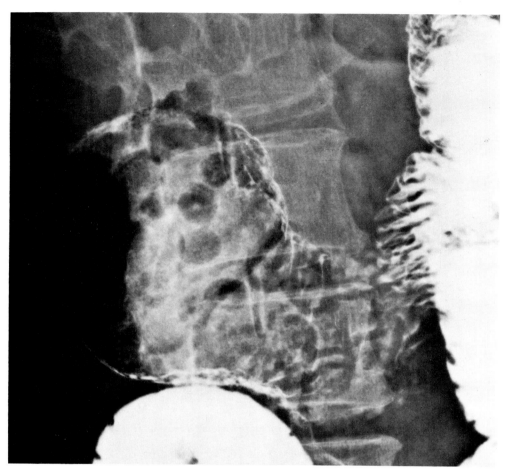

FIGURE 8–38 Afferent loop obstruction 19 years after a distal partial gastrectomy with gastrojejunostomy. Patient supine, right side up. There is huge dilatation of the afferent loop with dilution of the barium suspension and residual food (green peas). The patient denied any complaints.

FIGURE 8–39 Forty years after a distal partial gastrectomy with end-to-side gastrojejunostomy. Small polypoid lesions (*arrows*) on the greater curvature side of the preanastomotic area. Gastroscopy and biopsy showed that they were benign.

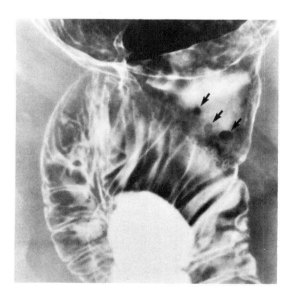

LIMITATIONS OF RADIOLOGIC EXAMINATION

Owing to the many surgical procedures and their variations it is not possible to describe the *normal* stomach after partial distal gastrectomy. Examples of plication defects and other pseudolesions have been given in this chapter (Figs. 8–20, 8–21, and 8–27). Furthermore, acute and chronic inflammatory changes of the mucosa of the gastric remnant due to bile reflux frequently complicate the picture.[58, 59] Benign polypoid lesions, the significance of which is uncertain, are often found in the stomal area after gastrojejunostomy (Fig. 8–39).[60-62] Figures 8–40 to 8–42 illustrate the limitations of the radiologic examination, the need for baseline studies, and in many instances the need for endoscopy with multiple biopsies.

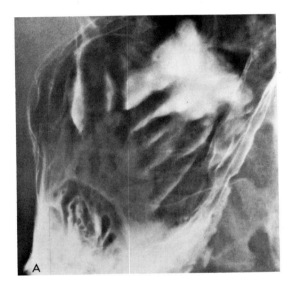 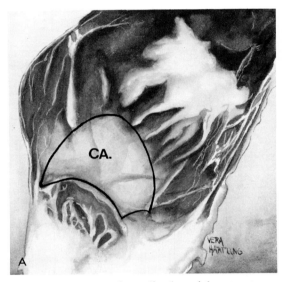

A. Face-on view of the lesser curvature of the gastric remnant 9 years after a distal partial gastrectomy with gastrojejunostomy. The mucosal folds are interrupted by an area of flattened mucosa.

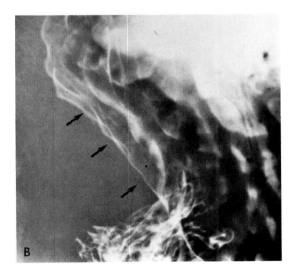

FIGURE 8–40 Early cancer of the gastric remnant.

B. Same patient, profile view. Unusual appearance on the lesser curvature side of the preanastomotic area (*arrows*). Radiologic diagnosis indeterminate; no baseline studies. Gastroscopy and biopsy: adenocarcinoma. Resected specimen: carcinoma restricted to the mucosa, i.e., early cancer of the gastric remnant.

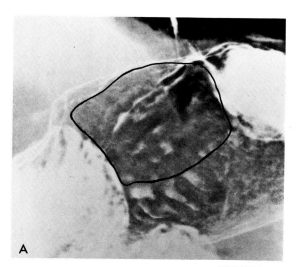 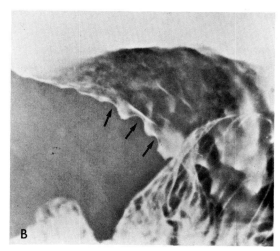

FIGURE 8–41 Gastritis.

A. Face-on view of the lesser curvature of a gastric remnant 25 years after a distal partial gastrectomy with gastrojejunostomy.

B. Same patient, profile view. Swollen irregular folds on the lesser curvature side. No radiologic diagnosis. Gastroscopy: swollen folds. Gastroscopy and biopsy: inflammatory changes.

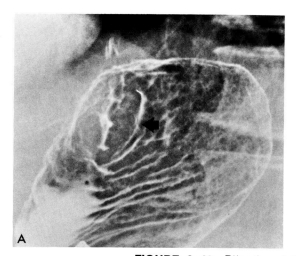 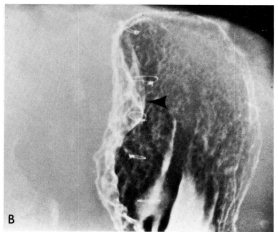

FIGURE 8–42 Plication defect simulating carcinoma.

A. Face-on view of the gastric remnant 17 years after a distal partial gastrectomy.

B. Same patient, profile view. Large filling defect on the lesser curvature side, suggestive of carcinoma. In this case, however, postoperative baseline and follow-up studies were available and demonstrated that the lesion had not changed over many years. A malignant lesion was therefore excluded.

Total Gastrectomy

A detailed description of the large number of operative techniques used to restore continuity in the digestive tract after total gastrectomy is beyond the scope of this chapter. We feel, however, that the hypotonic double contrast technique is of help in the visualization of the postoperative result, as shown in Figure 8–43.

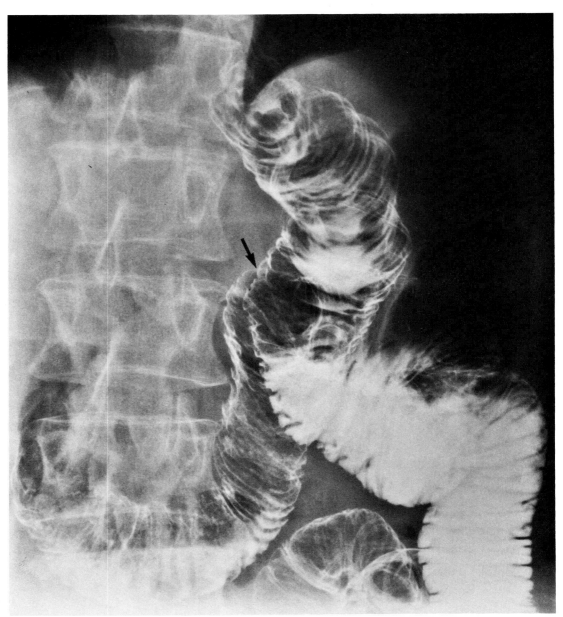

FIGURE 8–43 Esophagojejunostomy 12 days after a total gastrectomy. The hypotonic examination clearly demonstrates the end-to-side jejunojejunal (Roux-en-y) anastomosis (*arrow*).

CONCLUSION

An optimal hypotonic double contrast study proves in many instances that there is no macroscopic abnormality in the stomach. After suturing, however, particularly when a restricted stoma has been made, artifacts may occur. In some cases they cannot be differentiated from malignant tumors or ulcer craters on a purely radiologic basis, although postoperative baseline studies may be helpful. For this purpose, endoscopy and biopsy are often necessary.

The possibility of *recurrent* carcinoma must be considered even after a short interval following surgery for gastric carcinoma. However, if the surgery was undertaken for a benign lesion, a higher rate of malignancy (primary gastric stump carcinoma) is not to be expected before a postoperative interval of at least 5 years. In our experience, gastroscopy has proved to be superior to radiology for detecting a small jejunal ulcer following a Billroth II resection.

The hypotonic technique allows for excellent visualization of the afferent loop, the normal anatomic landmarks, the sequelae, and the complications of surgery as well as unrelated diseases affecting the duodenum.

ACKNOWLEDGMENTS

I wish to express my gratitude to Willem Dekker, M.D., Ph.D., who performed the endoscopies and confirmed or refuted my initial diagnoses. With the cooperation of such an excellent endoscopist, the radiologist can improve his techniques. He also gave valuable advice after reading the manuscript. My thanks also go to M. Pertaap Chandie Shaw, M.D., who gave such constructive criticism on a second reading. I gratefully acknowledge the assistance of my colleagues, Henry E. Schutte, M.D., Ph.D.; J. Dick Wackwitz, M.D.; and Carel A. van Hees, M.D., who made this work possible. The same holds true for Rein J. Meelker, Chief Technician, and his staff. Meindert G. Popkes, a superb medical photographer, made the prints. Last but not least, I want to thank Sonia Dorst for her help in the preparation of this chapter.

REFERENCES

1. Op den Orth, J. O., and Ploem, S.: The standard biphasic-contrast gastric series. Radiology, *122*:530, 1977.
2. Burhenne, H. J.: Postoperative defects of the stomach. Semin. Roentgenol. *6*:182, 1971.
3. Prévôt, R.: Die Röntgendiagnostik des operierten Magens. Dtsch. Med. Wochenschr., *88*:942, 1963.
4. Norberg, P. B.: Results of the surgical treatment of perforated peptic ulcer; a clinical and roentgenological study. Acta Chir. Scand., Suppl. *249*, 1959.
5. Nahum, H., and Fékété. F.: Radiologie de l'appareil digestif opéré. Paris. Masson et Cie., 1976. pp. 54–58.
6. Gleecon, J., and Ellis, H.: Vagotomy and pyloroplasty, a cineradiographic study. Am. J. Dig. Dis., *14*:84, 1969.
7. Toye, D. K. M., Hutton, J. F. K., and Williams, J. A.: Radiological anatomy after pyloroplasty. Gut, *11*:358, 1970.
8. Wilson, W. J., and Weintraub, H. D.: The postpyloroplasty antrum. Am. J. Roentgenol. Radium Ther. Nucl. Med., *96*:408, 1966.

9. Bloch, C., and Wolf, B. S.: The gastroduodenal channel after pyloroplasty and vagotomy: a cineradiographic study. Radiology, *84*:1965.

10. Nissen, R., and Rossetti, M.: Surgery of hiatal and other diaphragmatic hernias. J. Int. Coll. Surg., *43*:663, 1965.

11. Cohen, W. N.: The fundoplication repair of sliding esophageal hiatus hernia: its roentgenographic appearance. Am. J. Roentgenol. Radium Ther. Nucl. Med., *104*:625, 1968.

12. Feigin, D. S., James, A. E., Stitik, F. P., et al.: The radiological appearance of hiatal hernia repairs. Radiology, *110*:71, 1974.

13. Kuyk, P. J., van: Diagnostic radiology in fundoplication according to Nissen. Radiol. Clin., *45*:115, 1976.

14. Kuyk, P. J., van: Fundoplication according to Nissen. Personal communication, 1978.

15. Skucas, J., Mangla, J. C., Adams, J. T., et al.: An evaluation of the Nissen fundoplication. Radiology, *118*:539, 1976.

16. Régent, D., Bigard, M. A., Hodez, Cl., et al.: Exploration radiologique en double contraste de l' estomac opéré. J. Radiol. Electrol., *57*:683, 1976.

17. Gold, R. P., and Seaman, W. B.: The primary double-contrast examination of the postoperative stomach. Radiology, *124*:297, 1977.

18. Op den Orth, J. O.: Experiences with a standard biphasic-contrast examination after partial gastrectomy. RSNA Educational Materials Center: audiovisual program RS 88, 1977.

19. Carter, T. L., and Martel, W.: Contraction of the gastric antrum following a long-term gastroenterostomy. Radiology, *91*:514, 1968.

20. Hajdu, N., Hyde, D. M. R. I., and Riddell, V.: Antro-pyloric hypertrophy in patients with longstanding gastroenterostomies; a study of thirteen cases. Br. J. Radiol., *41*:49, 1968.

21. Burhenne, H. J.: Roentgen anatomy and terminology of gastric surgery. Am. J. Roentgenol. Radium Ther. Nucl. Med., *91*:731, 1964.

22. Op den Orth, J. O.: Tubeless hypotonic examination of the afferent loop of the Billroth II stomach. Gastrointest. Radiol., *2*:1, 1977.

23. Pochaczevsky, R.: "Bubbly barium," a carbonated cocktail for double-contrast examination of the stomach. Radiology, *107*:465, 1973.

24. Kim, S. Y., and Evans, J. A.: The roentgen appearance of the stomach and duodenum following the Billroth I gastric resection. Am. J. Roentgenol. Radium Ther. Nucl. Med., *81*:576, 1959.

25. Fisher, M. S.: The Hofmeister defect: a normal change in the postoperative stomach. Am. J. Roentgenol. Radium Ther. Nucl. Med., *84*:1082, 1960.

26. Sasson, L.: Tumor-simulating deformities after subtotal gastrectomy. JAMA, *174*:142 (280–283), 1960.

27. Eklöf, O., and Ohlsson, S.: Postoperative plication deformity with foreign-body granuloma simulating tumour of the stomach; report of three cases. Acta Chir. Scand., *123*:125, 1962.

28. Gueller, R., Shapiro, H. A., Nelson, J. A., et al. Suture granulomas simulating tumors. Am. J. Dig. Dis., *21*:223, 1976.

29. Frik, W.: Digestive Tract. *In*: Schinz, H. R., Baensch, W. E., Frommhold, W., et al. (eds.): Lehrbuch der Rëntgendiagnosik. Band V. Stuttgart, Georg Thieme Verlag, 1965, p. 223.

30. Wychulis, A. R., Priestley, J. T., and Foulk, W. T.: A study of 360 patients with gastrojejunal ulceration. Surg. Gynecol. Obstet., *122*:89, 1966.

31. Schulman, A.: Anastomotic gastrojejunal ulcer: accuracy of radiological diagnosis in surgically proven cases. Br. J. Radiol., *44*:422, 1971.

32. Demling, L., Ottenjann, R., and Elster, K.: Endoskopie und Biopsie der Speiseröhre und des Magens. Stuttgart, F. K. Schattauer Verlag, 1972, p. 121.

33. Burhenne, H. J.: The postoperative stomach. *In*: Margulis, A. R., and Burhenne, H. J. (eds.): Alimentary Tract Roentgenology. Vol I. St. Louis, C. V. Mosby, 1973, p. 766.

34. Moulinier, B., Lambert, R., Russo, A., et al.: Diagnostic endoscopique de l'ulcère anastomotique après chirurgie gastrique; à propos de 150 cas. Ann. Gastroentérol. Hépatol., *11*:209, 1975.

35. Dekker, W., and Op den Orth, J. O.: Correlations and discorrelations between endoscopy and radiology of the upper GI tract. Scientific exhibit shown at the Scientific Assembly and Annual Meeting of the Radiological Society of North America, Chicago, 1977.

36. Bachman, A. L., and Parmer, E. P.: Radiographic diagnosis of recurrence following resection for gastric cancer, Radiology, *84*:913, 1965.

37. Feldman, F., and Seaman, W. B.: Primary gastric stump cancer. Am. J. Roentgenol. Radium Ther. Nucl. Med., *115*:257, 1972.

38. Dahm, K., and Werner, B.: Das Karzinom im operierten Magen. Dtsch. Med. Wochenschr., *100*:1073, 1975.

39. Stalsberg, H., and Taksdal, S.: Stomach cancer following gastric surgery for benign conditions. Lancet, 2, 1175, 1971.

40. Clémençon, G., Baumgartner, R., Leuthold, E., et al.: Das Karzinom des operierten Magens. Dtsch. Med. Wochenschr., 101:1015, 1976.

41. Terjesen, T., and Erichsen, H. G.: Carcinoma of the gastric stump after operation for benign gastroduodenal ulcer. Acta Chir. Scand., 142:256, 1976.

42. Dekker, W.: Fiberendoscopisch-bioptisch onderzoek van maagmaligniteiten. Amsterdam, Academische Pers, 1976, p. 148.

43. Pygott, F., and Shah, V. L.: Gastric cancer associated with gastroenterostomy and partial gastrectomy. Gut, 9:117, 1968.

44. Saegesser, F., and Jämes, D.: Cancer of the gastric stump after partial gastrectomy (Billroth II principle) for ulcer. Cancer, 29:1150, 1972.

45. Kriedeman, E., Rotte, K. -H., Mateev, B., et al.: Probleme der Diagnostik des magenstumpfkarzinoms und des Tumorrezidivs; ein Vergleich zwischen Röntgen diagnostik und Endoskopie. Arch. Geschwulstforsch., 45:552, 1975.

46. Dobroschke, J., Feustel, H., and Filler, D.: Das Karzinom am resezierten Magen; secondary carcinoma after gastric resection. Akt. Gastrologie, 5:369, 1976.

47. LeVine, M., Boley, S. J., Mellins, H. Z., et al.: Gastrojejunal mucosal prolapse. Radiology, 80:30, 1963.

48. Grimoud, M., Moreau, G., and Lemozy, J.: Le prolapse post-opératoire transanastomotique de la muqueuse gastrique. Arch. Mal. Appar. Dig., 53:649, 1964.

49. Shane, M. D., Amberg, J. R., and Szemes, G.: Gastrojejunal mucosal prolapse after subtotal gastrectomy. California Medicine, 111:177, 1969.

50. Seaman, W. B.: Prolapsed gastric mucosa through a gastrojejunostomy. Am. J. Roentgenol. Radium Ther. Nucl. Med., 110:403, 1970.

51. Poppel, M. H.: Gastric intussusceptions. Radiology, 78:602, 1962.

52. Aleman, S.: Jejuno-gastric intussusception—a rare complication of the operated stomach. Acta Radiol., 29:384, 1948.

53. Bradford, B., and Boggs, J. A.: Jejunogastric intussusception — an unusual complication of gastric surgery. Arch. Surg., 77:201, 1958.

54. Bret, P., Amiel, M., and Lescos, L.: Les images lacunaires des moignons de gastrectomie. Ann. Radiol., 7:519, 1964.

55. Reyelt, W. P., Jr., and Anderson, A. A.: Retrograde jejunogastric intussusception. Surg. Gyn. Obstet., 119:1305, 1964.

56. Devor, D., and Passaro, E.: Jejunogastric intussusception: review of 4 cases—diagnosis and management. Ann. Surg., 173:93, 1966.

57. Burhenne, H. J.: The iatrogenic afferent loop syndrome. Radiology, 91:942, 1968.

58. Bushkin, F. L., Wickbom, G., DeFord, J. W., et al.: Postoperative alkaline reflux gastritis. Surg. Gyn. Obstet., 138:933, 1974.

59. Drapanas, T., and Bethea, M.: Reflux gastritis following gastric surgery. Ann. Surg. 179:618, 1974.

60. Kobayashi, S., Prolla, J. C., and Kirsner, J. B.: Late gastric carcinoma developing after surgery for benign conditions: endoscopic and histologic studies of the anastomosis and diagnostic problems. Am. J. Dig. Dis., 15:905, 1970.

61. Domellöf, L., Eriksson, S., and Janunger, K.-G.: Late occurrence of precancerous changes and carcinoma of the gastric stump after Billroth II resection. Acta Chir. Scand., 141:292, 1975.

62. Domellöf, L., Eriksson, S., and Janunger, K.-G.: Carcinoma and possible precancerous changes of the gastric stump after Billroth II resection. Gastroenterology, 73:462, 1977.

63. Op den Orth, J. O.: Radiologic visualization of the normal duodenal minor papilla. Fortschr. Roentgenstr., 128:572, 1978.

64. Baldwin, M.: The pancreatic duct in man, together with a study of the microscopical structure of the minor duodenal papilla. Anat. Rec. 5:197, 1911.

65. Poppel, M. H., Jacobson, H. R., and Smith, R. W.: The Roentgen Aspects of the Papilla and Ampulla of Vater. Springfield, Charles C Thomas, 1953, pp. 4–8, 12–20, 110.

9

DUODENUM

GILES W. STEVENSON, M.D., AND IGOR LAUFER, M.D.

INTRODUCTION

Fiberoptic endoscopy has exposed the limitations of radiology of the duodenum, in that 20 to 35 per cent of lesions may be missed[1-2] and false positive diagnoses occur frequently.[3] It has been shown that double contrast examinations of the upper GI tract may reduce the overall error rate to 5 or 6 per cent, as judged by endoscopy.[4-6] The majority of remaining false negatives occur with examinations that the radiologist can recognize and report as less than ideal. Burhenne has written that it is of much greater importance not to miss a lesion than it is to accurately diagnose its nature,[7] and this is increasingly true as duodenal endoscopy becomes more readily available. The first part of this chapter therefore is devoted to some aspects of technique that may help radiologists to declare with confidence that the duodenum is normal. This will depend upon the clear

331

demonstration of normal anatomic landmarks. The second part of the chapter deals with some of the common abnormalities found in and around the duodenum.

TECHNIQUE

Double contrast duodenography has been performed as a selective examination, utilizing a duodenal tube and hypotonia for evaluation of suspected pancreaticoduodenal disorders.[8-10] Subsequently "tubeless" hypotonic duodenography was described, whereby air was introduced into the stomach either by drinking through a perforated straw or by an effervescent agent.[11-14] With appropriate positioning of the patient, double contrast views were obtained. The modified technique of double contrast hypotonic duodenography described in this chapter is a part of our routine upper gastrointestinal study.

Routine Study

Ideally, examination of the duodenum would include all the standard radiologic techniques. These include fluoroscopic diagnosis, mucosal relief films, high kV dilute barium-filled films, compression spots, double contrast films with high density, low viscosity barium, and multiple projections, including prone, supine, and erect views. A compromise is forced by the facts that only one type of barium can be used; that examination of the duodenum follows examination of the stomach; and that parts of the duodenum are inaccessible to compression. The technique to be described relies heavily on double contrast, but overreliance on double contrast, particularly when coating is poor, will result in errors. Compression remain an integral part of the examination, and films in the prone position are necessary, especially for anterior wall lesions. Erect views in double contrast films in particular may miss superficial lesions (Fig. 9–17C).

The materials utilized are those described in Chapter 3 for the double contrast examination of the upper gastrointestinal tract. Hypotonic agents are particularly important for consistent demonstration of the normal anatomic landmarks in the duodenum. Either intravenous glucagon in a dose of from 0.05 to 1.0 mg or Buscopan in a dose of 20 mg is satisfactory[15-17] (see Chapter 3, page 63). The hypotonic agent is given at the beginning of the study to provide hypotonia for the examination of the stomach. If glucagon is being used, a very small dose should be administered in order not to delay filling of the duodenum.

DUODENAL LOOP

Most of the examination of the stomach may have been completed without barium being permitted to flow into the duodenum. However, when the patient is turned onto the right side to obtain films of the lesser curve of the upper body, cardia, and fundus, barium will flood through the pylorus and fill the duodenal bulb and loop. If barium passes well around the duodenum, followed by some air when the patient is turned into the supine right-side-up position, then the two duodenal loop films may conveniently be taken before the duodenal bulb is examined. In this case the patient is turned further to the left, a pad is placed against the upper abdomen, and the patient turns still further to lie semiprone with the right side raised. In this position the pad compresses the lower body of the stomach against the patient's spine, trapping a large volume of air in the antrum. The patient's respiration then massages this air through the pylorus and around the duodenal loop. In this oblique position the air-filled second part of the duodenum can be seen projected through the air-filled antrum (Fig. 9–35). If the patient is now turned further fully prone, the second part of the duodenum and the proximal third part come clear of the stomach and a double contrast film can be taken (Fig. 9–1A). The patient is then immediately rotated back onto the left side into the supine right-side-up position for the second duodenal loop film (Fig. 9–1B).

DUODENAL BULB

Spot films of the duodenal bulb are then taken (Fig. 9–2A). Although good double contrast views are frequently obtained, sometimes the volume of gas in the stomach creates difficulties by rotating the duodenum more posteriorly. This problem can be overcome by a variety of maneuvers. These include turning the patient slightly to the right (Fig. 9–2B), or employing a series of projections turning the patient to the left to show the duodenum between the stomach and jejunum (Fig. 9–2C), through the air-filled antrum (Fig. 9–2D), or anterior to the stomach in the semiprone position (Fig. 9–2E). A good double contrast view of the duodenum can also be obtained in the upright position (Fig. 9–2F). In some patients these maneuvers may all fail, and a conventional examination of the duodenal bulb can be carried out at the end of this study when there is less air in the stomach.[18] Erect compression films of the duodenal bulb frequently do show lesions, including ulcers, and both oblique views may be taken. The right posterior oblique projection in particular occasionally shows ulcers not visible on other views.[19]

SELECTIVE HYPOTONIC DUODENOGRAPHY

The technique just described is suitable for use during routine double contrast examinations of the upper GI tract. Occasionally one is interested only in examining the duodenum. In such patients a modified technique for hypotonic duodenography can be utilized. The patient is given the effervescent agent and is allowed to drink the barium suspension while lying on the right side. In this position the barium passes freely into the duodenum. As soon as the duodenum is seen to fill with barium, the hypotonic agent, usually glucagon 0.5 mg, is injected intravenously. The patient is then turned to the left to allow air to enter the duodenum, and the examination proceeds as described earlier. If the examination is directed toward the duodenal loop, an additional dose of effervescent agent may be administered. As a last resort one may perform hypotonic duodenography with a duodenal tube.[8-10]

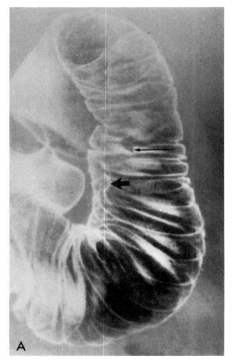

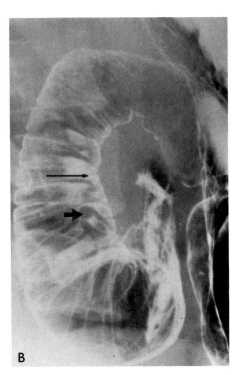

FIGURE 9–1 Duodenal loop with the major papilla (*thick arrow*) and minor papilla (*thin arrow*).

    A. Prone position.

    B. Supine, LPO. The minor papilla is found on the anterior wall, 1 to 2 cm proximal to the major papilla.

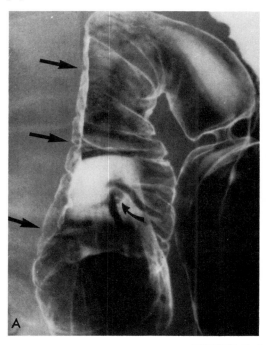

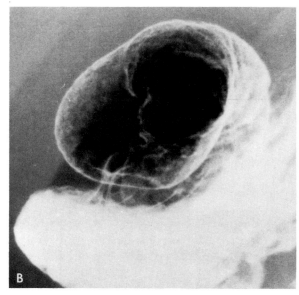

FIGURE 9–2 The duodenal bulb.

    A. Ideal visualization of the duodenal bulb and loop. Note the right renal impression along the lateral aspect of the descending duodenum (*straight arrows*) and the ampulla of Vater (*curved arrow*).

    B. Duodenal bulb in right posterior oblique projection.

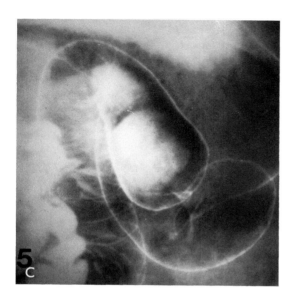

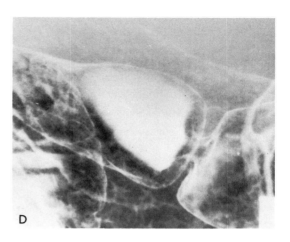

C. Steep left posterior oblique projecting the duodenum between the stomach and jejunum.
D. Left lateral or slightly prone view, projecting the duodenal bulb through the air-filled stomach.

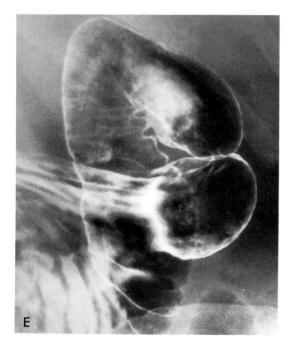

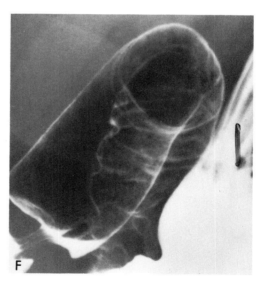

E. Semiprone, left anterior oblique view, with a pad between the abdomen and the table to show the bulb clear of the stomach.
F. Upright, right posterior oblique view.

NORMAL APPEARANCES

Duodenal Bulb

When Buscopan or glucagon is used the pylorus is frequently shown as an opened ring, with a diameter varying from a few millimeters to more than a centimeter (Fig. 9–3*A*). It is normally centrally placed in the base of the duodenal bulb and is circular. A triangular shape or an eccentricity on either the duodenal or gastric side may indicate previous ulceration (Fig. 9–3*B*). The surface pattern of the duodenum is finer than that of the areae gastricae (Fig. 9–4), though the latter is variable. The duodenal pattern is composed of innumerable tiny interlacing circles of barium enclosing 1 to 2 mm lucencies representing the villous pattern of the duodenal mucosa. Not infrequently small surface elevations are present, and occasionally these may appear large and numerous (Fig. 9–4*C* and *D*). Endoscopic biopsy results in these patients have been normal, although when surface nodularity is prominent Brunner's gland hyperplasia, duodenitis, or lymphoid nodular hyperplasia (Fig. 9–30) may be suspected. The superior duodenal fold at the junction of the first and second parts appears as a crescent-shaped fold. However, not uncommonly there is redundant mucosa at this point. Buckling of the mucosa may trap barium in some crevices and produce the flexural pseudopolyp which may be mistaken either for a polyp, apical ulcer, or ectopic pancreatic tissue (Fig. 9–5).[20, 21]

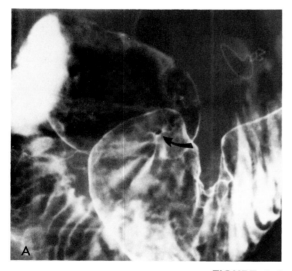
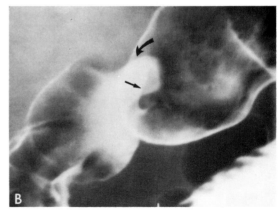

FIGURE 9–3 The pylorus.

A. Normal pylorus seen as a circular lucency (*arrow*) with small radiating folds.

B. Eccentric pylorus (*straight arrow*) due to a pyloric channel ulcer (*curved arrow*). See also Plate 52.

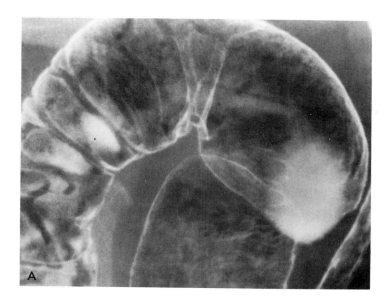

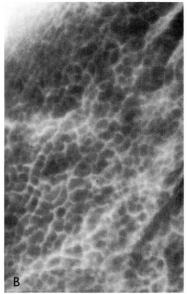

A. The normal fine, villous surface pattern.
B. This is compared with the much coarser pattern seen in the stomach.

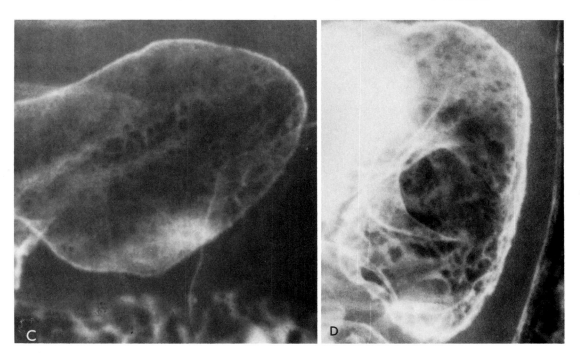

C and *D.* Surface elevations may be seen in the duodenum. Biopsy results in both cases showed normal duodenal mucosa.

FIGURE 9–4 Surface pattern of the duodenum.

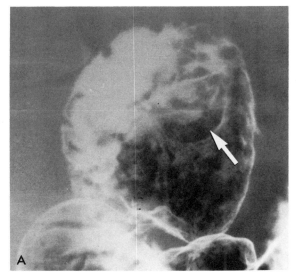

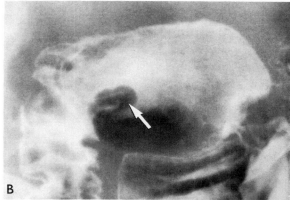

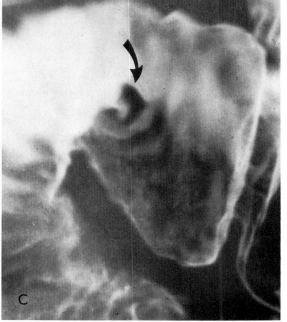

FIGURE 9–5 *A* to *C*   Three examples of a duodenal pseudopolyp due to redundant mucosa at the superior duodenal flexure. This may be mistaken for a polyp, ulcer, or pancreatic rest.[20, 21]

Duodenal Loop

The major landmarks are the circular valvulae conniventes and the papillae.[22-24] Ferrucci[22] and Eaton[23] have described in detail the internal anatomy of the duodenal loop, including the major papilla, promontory, straight segment, and longitudinal fold. They found that the minor papilla was almost never visible on hypotonic duodenography. This was probably due to the fact that they did not selectively examine the anterior wall of the descending duodenum by double contrast.

The ampulla of Vater usually lies on the medial aspect of the second part of the duodenum and is about 5 mm in diameter. Its position may vary from approximately the midpoint of the second part of the duodenum to as distal as the third part. Endoscopically three common types of ampulla are found — hemispheric, flat, and papillary (Fig. 9–6). Radiologically the ampulla is usually identified by its associated mucosal folds (Figs. 9–7 and 9–8). The distal longitudinal fold is present in approximately 90 per cent of patients, as is a hooding fold. Oblique folds are often seen, and less often there may be a proximal longitudinal fold.

The accessory papilla marking the orifice of Santorini's duct is usually not patent. It seldom has a distal longitudinal fold, and even the hooding fold is rarely very prominent. The accessory papilla lies about 1 cm proximal to the major papilla and 30 to 45 degrees anterior to it. Thus if in the supine oblique position the ampulla of Vater can be seen lying posteriorly a little nearer the medial than the lateral wall of the second part of the duodenum, the accessory papilla, when identifiable, will be seen tangentially on the medial aspect (Fig. 9–1B). Conversely, if in the prone position the ampulla of Vater can be identified lying on the medial aspect of the second part of the duodenum, Santorini's accessory papilla will be seen anteriorly en face, a short distance proximal to the major papilla (Fig. 9–1A). The relationship between the major and minor papillae is astonishingly constant. The minor papilla varies greatly in size, and it is sometimes as large as the major papilla. In two such patients the minor papilla has been patent and draining a portion of the pancreas (Figs. 9–9 and 9–10).

The demonstration of the villous surface pattern of the duodenal bulb and of the papillae may seldom be of importance in itself (but see Fig. 9–31). However, clear demonstration of these anatomic landmarks may serve as an indication that the examination has been technically satisfactory and will allow increased confidence that a radiologic report of a normal duodenum is reliable.

Text continued on page 345

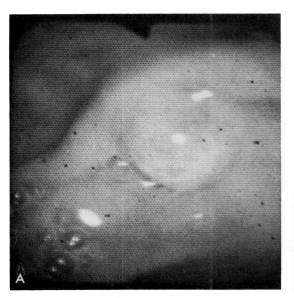
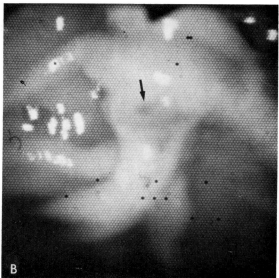

A. Hemispheric papilla with a hooding fold, but no distal longitudinal fold.

B. Flat papilla with the dark central spot (*arrow*) representing the orifice. The hooding fold, distal longitudinal fold, and oblique folds are all clearly visible.

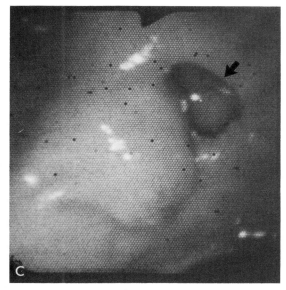

C. Papillary papilla with no prominent folds. The neck of a duodenal diverticulum (*arrow*) is seen beside the papilla.

FIGURE 9–6 Endoscopic appearance of the major types of papilla.

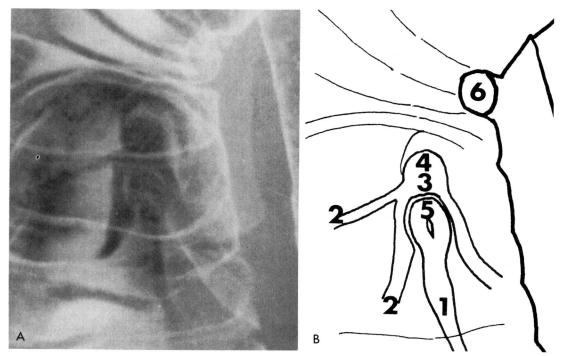

A and *B* Anatomic landmarks in the descending duodenum. *1.* Distal longitudinal fold. This is present in the vast majority of patients. *2.* Oblique folds — variable. *3.* Hooding fold. This also is present in the majority of patients. *4.* Proximal longitudinal fold — variable. *5.* Ampulla of Vater. *6.* Accessory papilla.

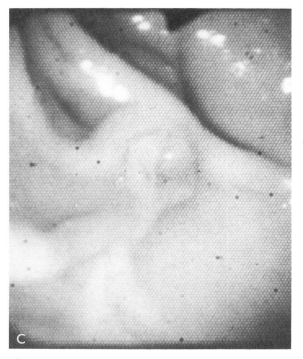

C. This endoscopic photograph was taken from a patient with a similar arrangement of folds.

FIGURE 9–7 The ampulla of Vater and its associated folds.

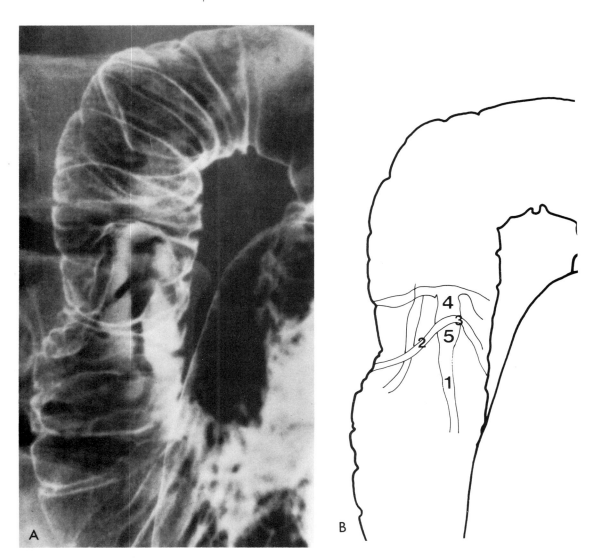

FIGURE 9–8 *A* and *B*   Another example of the ampulla of Vater and its associated folds. See Legend for Figure 9–7.

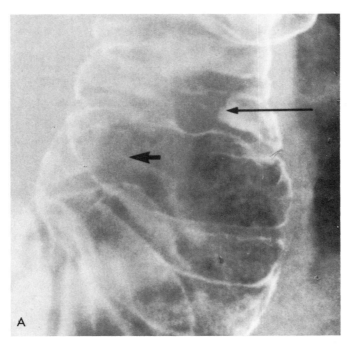

A. The major papilla is indicated by the short arrow, and the accessory papilla, which is unusually large, is indicated by the long arrow.

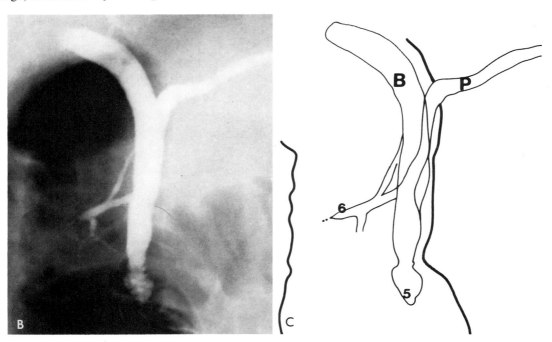

B. and *C.* At ERCP injection into the major papilla filled both the biliary and pancreatic ducts. When the cannula was removed, clear fluid was seen coming from the orifice in the accessory papilla[6] as well as from the ampulla of Vater. This is documented by two small droplets of contrast emerging from the accessory papilla which drains the duct of Santorini. In this patient there is persistent fetal communication between the dorsal and ventral pancreas.

FIGURE 9–9 Unusually large accessory papilla.

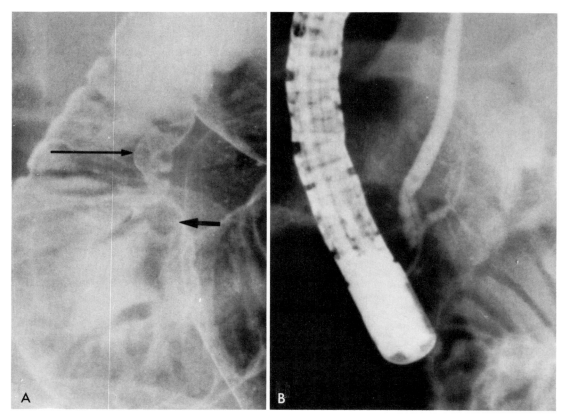

FIGURE 9–10 Another patient with an unusually large accessory papilla.

A. The ampulla of Vater (*short arrow*) and the unusually large accessory papilla (*long arrow*) are seen.

B. At ERCP there was filling of the common bile duct and a small dorsal pancreatic duct system. There was no communication with the rest of the pancreatic duct system which must be draining through the enlarged accessory papilla. The accessory papilla could not be cannulated.

DUODENAL ULCER

The technical considerations described earlier become important in the detection of duodenal ulcers. In the presence of poor mucosal coating an ulcer crater can easily be missed (Fig. 9–11). Duodenal deformity and spasm can also mask an ulcer crater. This can be relieved to a large extent by hypotonic agents (Fig. 9–12).

Duodenal ulcers may occur on the superior, inferior, anterior, and posterior walls of the duodenal bulb (Fig. 9–13). The ulcer craters are frequently very small, but are still clearly demonstrated (Fig. 9–14A). In many cases there is no recognizable duodenal deformity (Fig. 9–14B). However, even in the presence of deformity an ulcer crater is frequently clearly demonstrated (Fig. 9–14C and D).

Anterior wall ulcers are common, and unfortunately are easily missed radiographically (Figs. 9–13C and 9–15 to 9–17). The supine double contrast study may show only a ring shadow in the duodenal bulb owing to coating of the ulcer base with barium. The crater can be filled with barium either by turning the patient into the prone position or by compression in either the prone or upright positions (Figs. 9–13C, 9–16, and 9–17). Although most ulcer craters are more or less rounded in configuration, linear ulcers are seen in approximately 15 per cent of cases (Figs. 9–18 and 9–19).[2]

Duodenal ulcer scars are also clearly demonstrated with good coating and relaxation of the duodenal bulb (Fig. 9–20). Postbulbar ulcers are relatively infrequent (Fig. 9–21). They are often associated with narrowing of the postbulbar duodenum, and in many cases only the postbulbar stricture is seen.[25-26] The presence of multiple postbulbar ulcers should raise the possibility of Zollinger-Ellison syndrome (Fig. 9–22).[27]

Overreliance on double contrast views, particularly erect double contrast films, must be avoided (Fig. 9–17). Prone oblique views with compression, erect compression of the duodenal bulb, both oblique views when possible, and even supine compression will all increase the diagnostic yield.[19, 28, 29] While double contrast extends the scope of examination of the bulb and increases accuracy in the diagnosis of duodenal ulcers, it complements but in no way replaces conventional techniques.

Endoscopy has increased our understanding of the morphologic pattern of duodenal ulcer. For example, 16 per cent of duodenal ulcers are linear (Figs. 9–18 and 9–19); they are multiple in 10 to 15 per cent of cases. They occur on the anterior, posterior, superior, and inferior walls of the bulb in 50, 23, 5, and 22 per cent of cases, respectively.[2] Indeed, endoscopic papers comparing the results of endoscopy and radiology of the duodenum may lead one to wonder if radiology is worthwhile. But it must be remembered that endoscopy has a false negative rate in the duodenum (12 per cent in one series)[2] partly because of overreliance by endoscopists on forward-viewing instruments. In attempting diagnosis of duodenal ulcer disease, the barium meal examination has twin aims. The first is that the confident diagnosis of either a normal duodenal bulb or an active duodenal ulcer should be accurate. The corollary of this is accepting the necessity to report on a substantial group of patients that good demonstration has not been achieved, and that endoscopy would be necessary to determine whether an active ulcer is present or not. Denial of the existence of this last group simply decreases the reliablility of the normal or active ulcer crater reports. Attention to detail and double contrast techniques may decrease the size of the last group of patients, in whom a report of uncertainty or deformity must be given, and should increase the number of confident normal or active ulcer crater reports.[28]

Text continued on page 354

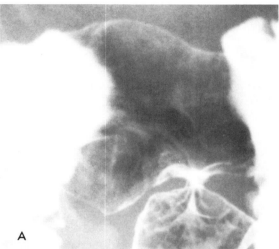

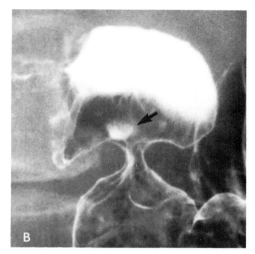

FIGURE 9–11 Importance of mucosal coating for demonstrating an ulcer.

A. Well-distended but poorly coated duodenal bulb. No ulcer crater is seen.
B. With improved coating the ulcer crater at the base of the duodenal bulb is clearly seen.

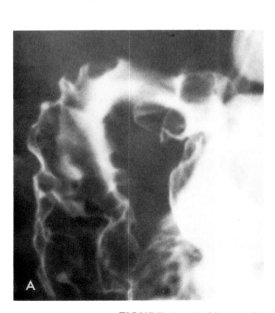

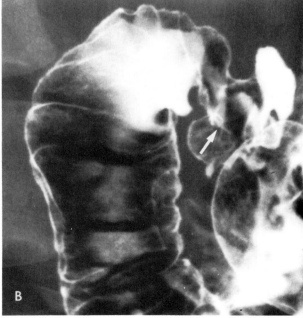

FIGURE 9–12 Value of hypotonia for demonstrating an ulcer.

A. Without a relaxant drug the duodenum is poorly distended, and no definite diagnosis is possible.

B. With intravenous glucagon there is much better distension of the duodenum. The duodenal deformity and ulcer crater (*arrow*) are more easily appreciated.

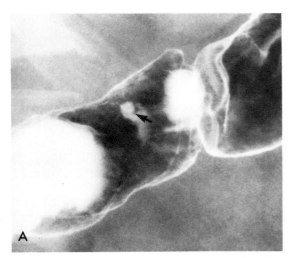
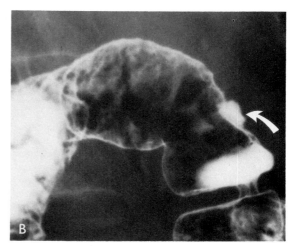

A. Posterior wall.
B. Superior surface.

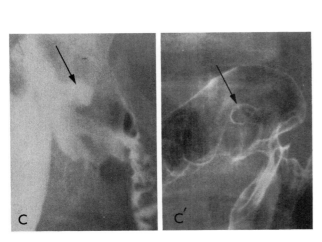
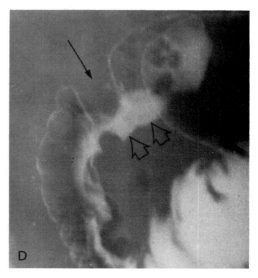

C. Anterior wall, prone projection. *C'.* Same ulcer, supine position, showing the typical ring shadow of an ulcer crater on the nondependent surface.

D. Large penetrating ulcer on the inferior surface (*broad arrows*) with an incisure (*long arrow*). There is a reverse 3 sign, indicating swelling of the head of the pancreas owing to pancreatic penetration by the ulcer.

FIGURE 9–13 Duodenal ulcers in various locations.

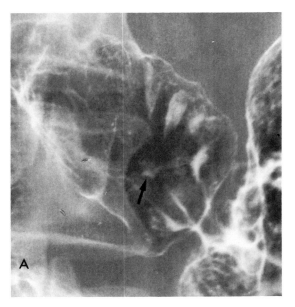

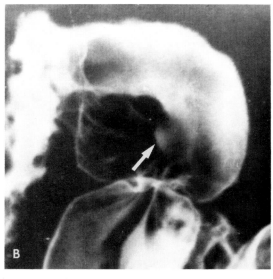

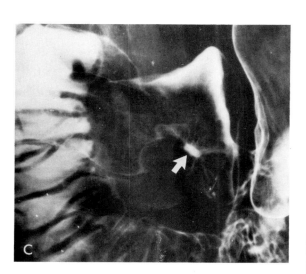

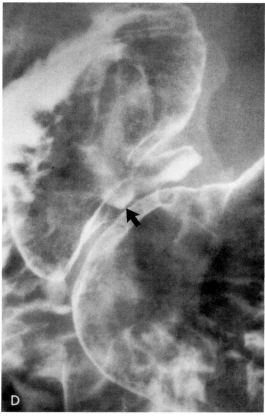

FIGURE 9–14 Variety of small duodenal
ulcers.

A and B.   With little or no deformity.
C and D.   With duodenal deformity.

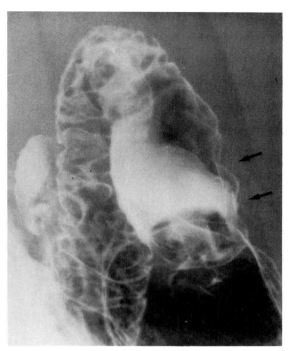

FIGURE 9-15 Anterior wall duodenal ulcer (unrecognized). The significance of the irregularity of the anterior wall of this duodenal bulb (*arrows*) was not appreciated (prone, left anterior oblique projection). Supine and erect views were normal. Prone double contrast and compression views were not obtained. This anterior wall duodenal ulcer perforated 3 weeks later.

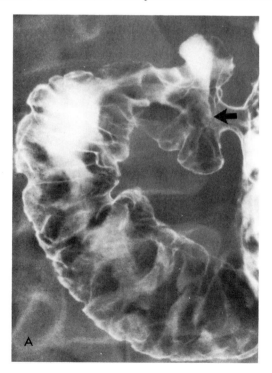
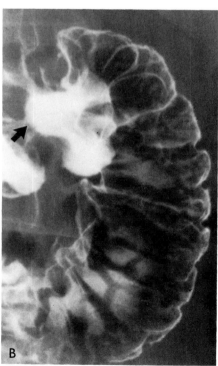

FIGURE 9-16 Anterior wall duodenal ulcer.

A. The supine view shows a deformed duodenal cap with a faint ring shadow at the base of the duodenum (*arrow*).

B. The film in the prone position shows barium filling the ulcer crater (*arrow*).

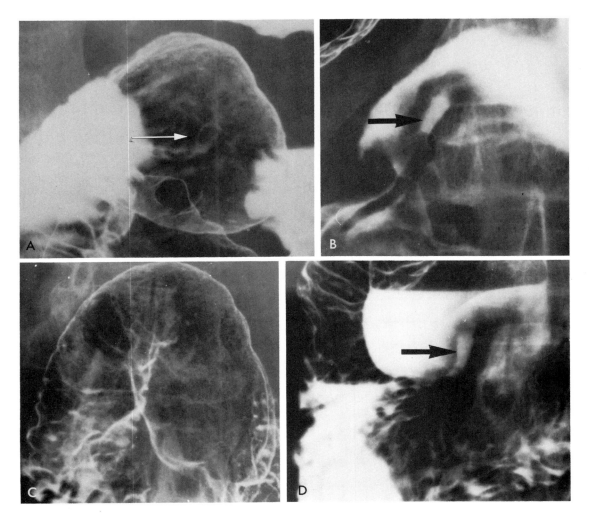

FIGURE 9–17 *A* to *D*   Anterior wall ulcer in multiple projections. A 34-year-old female with a history of four major gastrointestinal bleeding episodes over 5 years. She had had four negative conventional barium meals, three negative endoscopies, two negative colonoscopies and negative abdominal arteriography. The anterior wall ulcer was seen with difficulty with the small bowel enteroscope at this presentation. Early supine double contrast films were normal. Only when excellent coating was achieved could the ulcer be seen as a ring shadow (*A*). Prone compression (*B*) and erect compression (*D*) show the ulcer and surrounding rim of edema clearly. The ulcer was not detectable on the erect double contrast films despite good coating (*C*).

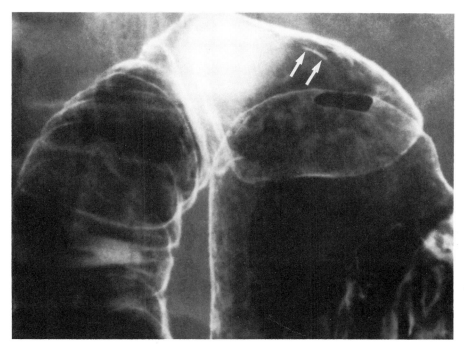

FIGURE 9–18 Linear duodenal ulcer without deformity of the duodenal bulb or pylorus.

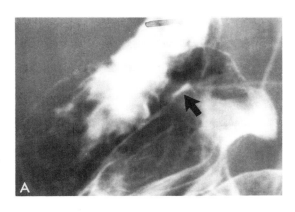

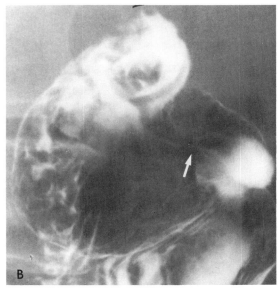

FIGURE 9–19 *A* and *B*　Linear ulcer with scarring and radiating folds.

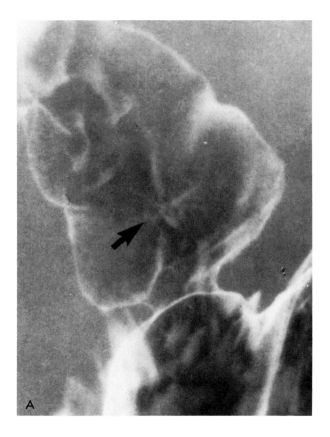

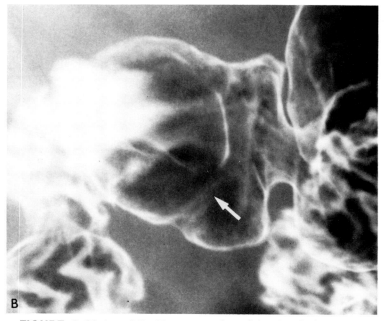

FIGURE 9–20 *A* and *B*   Two examples of duodenal ulcer scar.

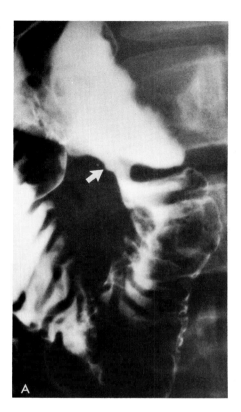

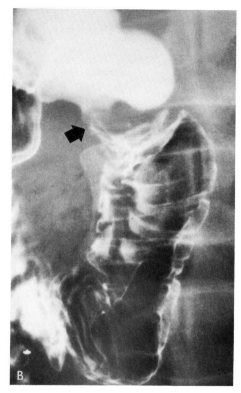

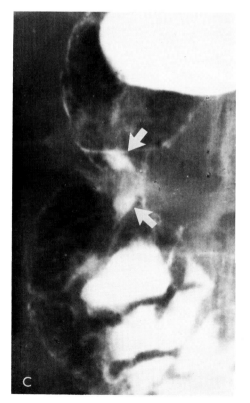

FIGURE 9–21 Three examples of postbulbar ulcer.

A. Postbulbar ulcer (*arrow*) with ring stricture.

B. Postbulbar ring stricture with no active ulcer. Note in both *A* and *B* the prominent longitudinal and oblique folds.

C. Postbulbar narrowing with two ulcer craters (*arrows*).

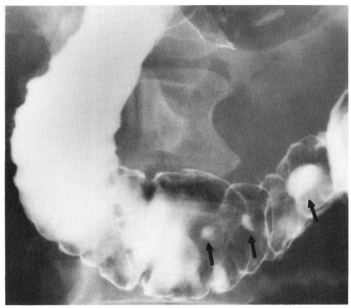

FIGURE 9–22 Multiple postbulbar ulcers in a patient with Zollinger-Ellison syndrome. (Courtesy of Wylie J. Dodds, M.D., Milwaukee.)

DUODENITIS

Erosive Duodenitis

The clinical significance of duodenitis has been a subject of great controversy.[30-32] It is generally considered that this condition cannot be accurately diagnosed radiologically.[33-34] The endoscopic spectrum of duodenitis ranges from erythema, to thickened and nodular folds, to duodenal erosions. Erosive duodenitis has been found to be the cause of gastrointestinal hemorrhage in 8 per cent of patients presenting with gastrointestinal bleeding.[30] These erosions are demonstrable by double contrast techniques, and their appearance is very similar to the appearance of erosions in the stomach. There is a central collection of barium surrounded by a radiolucent halo. Erosions are seen most frequently in the duodenal bulb (Fig. 9–23*A* and *B*),and they may be associated with a duodenal ulcer (Fig. 9–23*C*).

Hemorrhagic duodenitis may be a complication in patients with myocardial infarction or congestive heart failure.[35] These patients frequently present with gastrointestinal hemorrhage, and although the site of bleeding has been demonstrated by angiography,[36-37] the erosions may also be demonstrated by double contrast technique (Fig. 9–24).

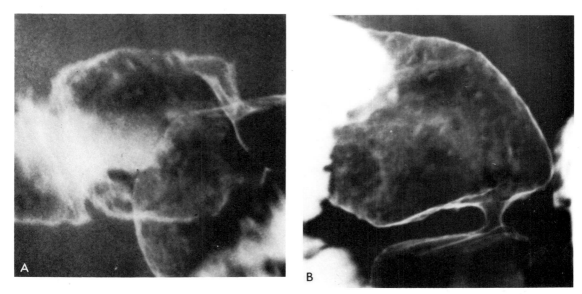

FIGURE 9–23

A and *B*.   Multiple small barium collections surrounded by radiolucent halo representing duodenal erosions. Confirmed by endoscopy.

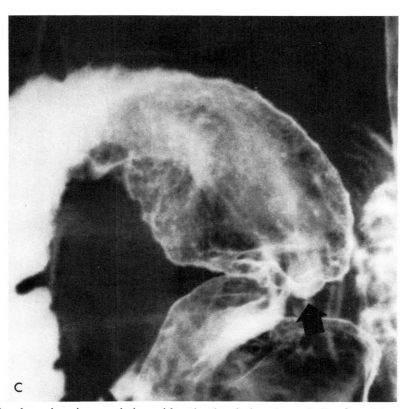

C.   Duodenal erosions in association with a duodenal ulcer (*arrow*). Confirmed by endoscopy.

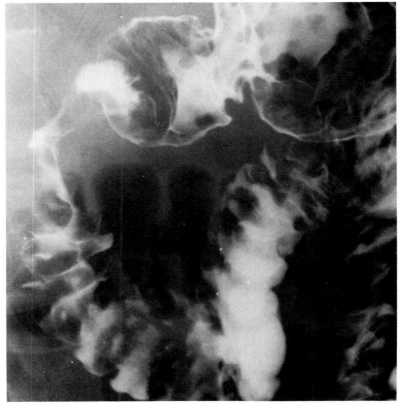

FIGURE 9–24 Erosions in the descending duodenum in a patient with congestive heart failure.

Crohn's Disease

Involvement of the upper gastrointestinal tract has been reported in only 1 to 2.8 per cent of patients with Crohn's disease.[38-40] However, in these patients the duodenal disease is usually advanced, with thickened folds, narrowing, and scarring (Fig. 9–25). It seems likely that many cases of early duodenal involvement remain undetected. The early lesions of Crohn's disease in the duodenum consist of superficial erosion and "aphthoid ulcers" similar to those seen elsewhere in the gastrointestinal tract in Crohn's disease (Figs. 9–26 to 9–28) (see Chapter 16).[41] The duodenal lesions usually affect the bulb and proximal half of the second part of the duodenum. The antrum is frequently affected as well (Figs. 9–26*D*, 9–27, and 9–28*A*).

Early lesions are easily overlooked (Figs. 9–26*A* and 9–28). Although gastroduodenal lesions usually become apparent after Crohn's disease has been diagnosed in the small intestine or colon, patients occasionally present with proximal disease (Fig. 9–28). Biopsy findings are often positive in the duodenum or antrum in these patients,[42] and the presence of these characteristic lesions may help in the diagnosis of individuals with nonspecific ileal abnormalities (Fig. 9–27). Severe duodenal disease (Fig. 9–28*A*) is usually associated with severe disease elsewhere in the GI tract.

Review of patients with Crohn's disease seen at McMaster University Medical Center showed that routine double contrast upper GI examination detected gastroduodenal abnormalities in 40 per cent of patients. In half of these the changes were histologically documented to be caused by Crohn's disease.[42] In the remaining patients with gastroduodenal abnormalities, endoscopic biopsies failed to yield granulomata, but it seems likely that at least some of these patients had gastroduodenal Crohn's disease. Therefore, in this series there was gastroduodenal involvement in 20 to 40 per cent of patients with Crohn's disease. The radiologic finding of thickened antral or duodenal folds was often associated with erosions at endoscopy and has become one of the relative indications for endoscopy in Crohn's disease.

Text continued on page 361

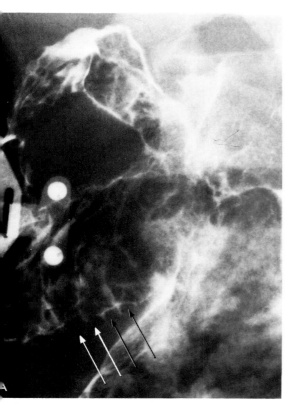
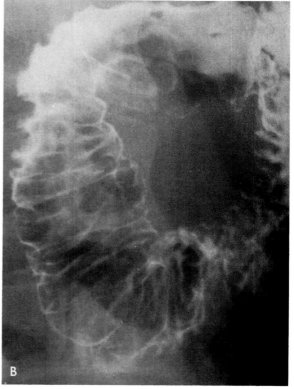

FIGURE 9–25 Advanced duodenal Crohn's disease.

A. Narrowing of the second part of the duodenum with cobblestoning and fissuring in the third part (*arrows*) in a patient with Crohn's disease involving the small bowel. He later required gastroenterostomy because of gastric outlet obstruction.

B. Characteristic signs of earlier or milder disease, with thickening of the folds, marginal irregularities, and slight limitation of distensibility. Hypotonia relieves spasm and improves the demonstration of these features.

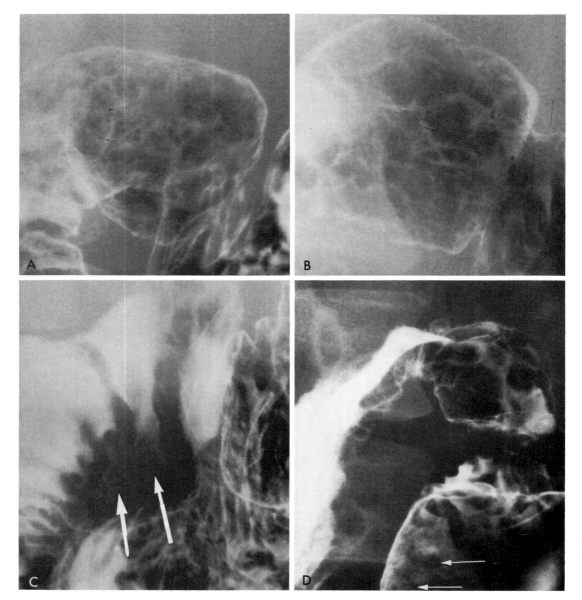

FIGURE 9–26 Crohn's disease in the duodenal bulb.

A. Minimal change, initially reported as normal. There were numerous tiny superficial erosions at endoscopy and biopsy findings showed a histiocytic granuloma.

B. More obvious flecks and irregular crisscross lines of barium. At endoscopy there were erosions in the duodenal bulb and antrum, with a positive antral biopsy result for Crohn's disease.

C. Two discrete erosions in the duodenal bulb (*arrows*).

D. This 43-year-old female was referred for epigastric pain. There were antral erosions (*arrows*), with deformity of the duodenal mucosa, crisscross barium lines, poor distension, and thickened folds in the second part of the duodenum. Because of these findings a small bowel follow-through study was performed, and extensive distal ileal disease was discovered.

All four of these patients had ileal or colonic Crohn's disease or both.

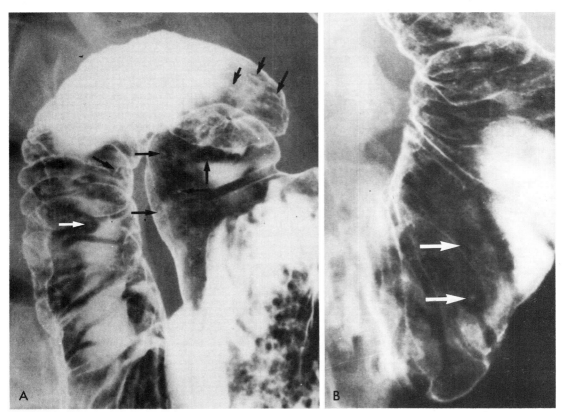

FIGURE 9–27 *A* and *B*   Aphthoid ulcers in the stomach and duodenum in an 18-year-old female with nonspecific changes in the terminal ileum. Aphthoid ulcers were also present in the colon. These aphthoid ulcers represent the early lesions of Crohn's disease (see also Plate 55).[41]

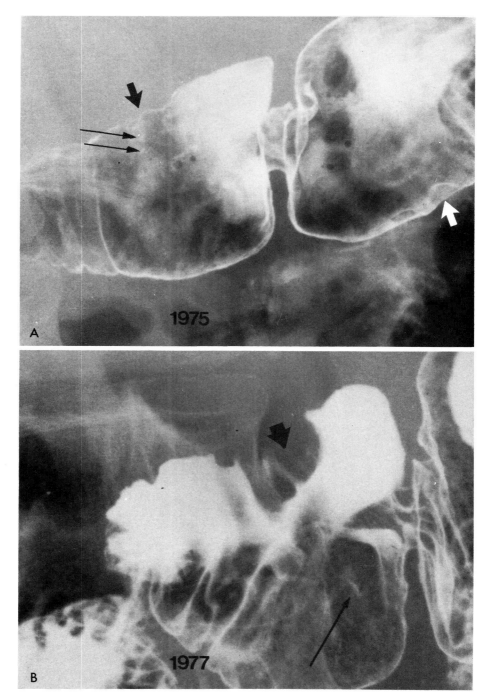

FIGURE 9–28 In 1975 Crohn's disease was diagnosed by rectal biopsy in this 19-year-old male.

 A. There was an irregularity of the superior aspect of the duodenal bulb with erosions, and there was also a polypoid swelling in the antrum. The terminal ileum was normal.

 B. By 1977 there was extensive distal ileal disease. The superior deformity of the bulb had increased (*short arrow*) and discrete erosions (*long arrow*) in the bulb were confirmed at endoscopy.

MASS LESIONS

Duodenal Tumors

Neoplastic lesions in the duodenum are quite uncommon. In fact most polypoid lesions in the duodenal bulb are actually gastric polyps that have prolapsed into the duodenum (Fig. 9–29). Multiple small filling defects in the duodenal bulb can be due either to hyperplasia of Brunner's glands or to lymphoid hyperplasia (Fig. 9–30).

Malignant tumors become more common around the ampulla of Vater and in the distal duodenum.[43-44] In some cases the polypoid tumor may be quite small when the patient presents with obstructive jaundice (Fig. 9–31). The tumor itself may not be seen, but there is a broad impression on the duodenum owing to the markedly dilated common bile duct (Fig. 9–32). Other tumors, such as villous adenomas[45] and lymphoma (Fig. 9–33),[46] also involve the duodenum.

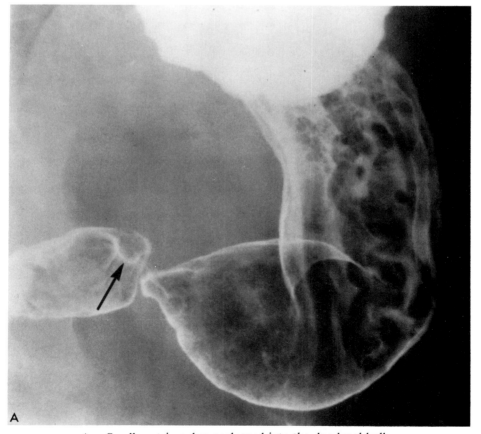

A. Small gastric polyp prolapsed into the duodenal bulb.

FIGURE 9–29 Prolapsed gastric polyps.

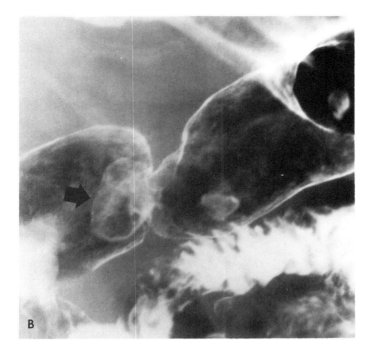

B. Polypoid mass in the duodenum, representing a polypoid gastric carcinoma that had prolapsed into the duodenum.[47]

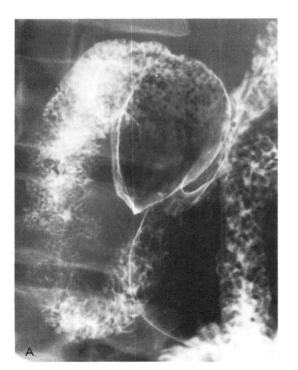

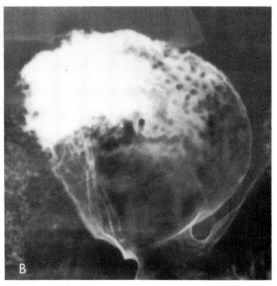

FIGURE 9–30 *A* and *B*   Lymphoid hyperplasia of the duodenum in a patient with hypogammaglobulinemia.

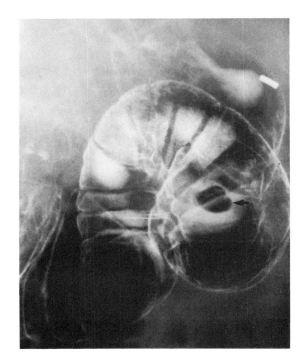

FIGURE 9–31 Polypoid ampullary carcinoma in a 75-year-old man presenting with obstructive jaundice (see also Plate 56).

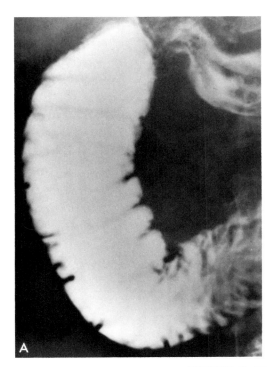

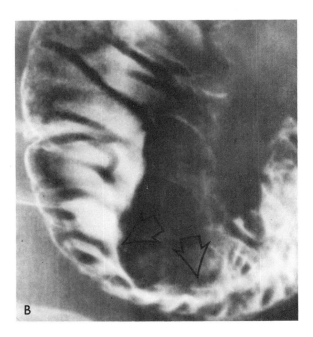

FIGURE 9–32 Ampullary carcinoma.

A.   Barium-filled view of the duodenal loop shows no abnormality.

B.   Hypotonic duodenography with double contrast shows a broad impression in the distal descending duodenum. This impression was due to a dilated common bile duct secondary to a small ampullary carcinoma. (Courtesy of Harald Stolberg, M.D., Hamilton, Ontario. Reproduced by permission of Progress in Gastroenterology[48].)

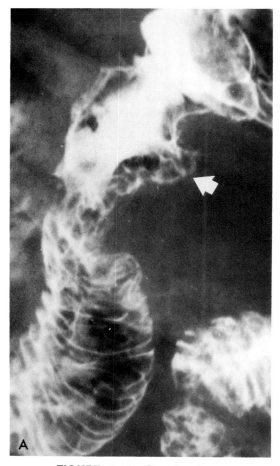

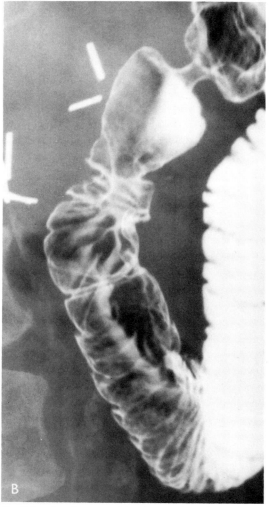

FIGURE 9–33 Duodenal lymphoma.

A. There is a mass lesion involving the medial wall of the duodenum with a large ulcer (*arrow*). At operation, this was found to be lymphoma involving the wall of the duodenum.

B. Follow-up study after radiation therapy shows resolution of the mass lesion, with scarring in the region of the previous ulcer. Note the prominent longitudinal and oblique folds.

Masslike Lesions

A number of innocuous findings may simulate duodenal tumors. These include prolapsed gastric mucosa (Fig. 9–34*A*), see-through artifacts (Fig. 9–34*B*), and surgical defects (Fig. 9–34*C*).

The ampulla of Vater may become quite large and may simulate a tumor in patients with an impacted common duct stone or pancreatitis. A prominent longitudinal fold seen tangentially may also suggest an intrinsic or extrinsic mass lesion. This situation is usually easily clarified by hypotonic duodenography (Fig. 9–35).

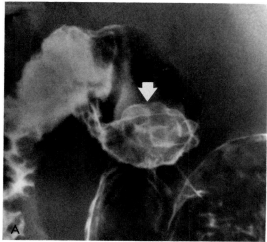

A. Prolapsed gastric mucosa.

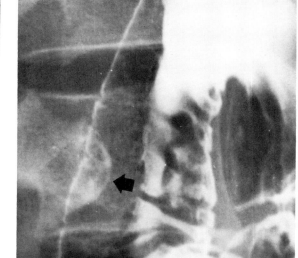

B. Vertebral pedicle seen through the descending duodenum.

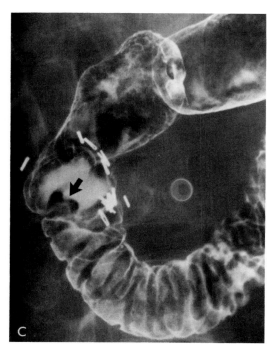

FIGURE 9–34 Masslike lesions.

C. Surgical defect.

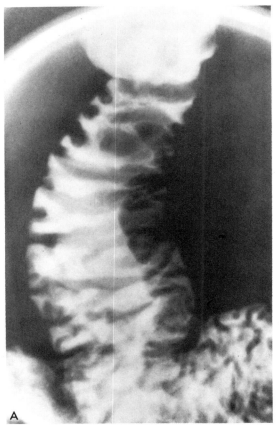
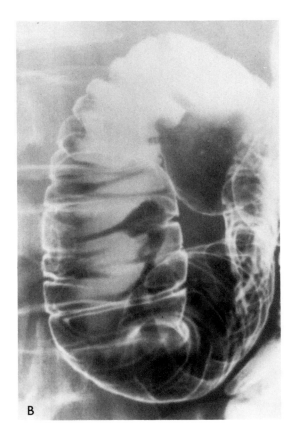

FIGURE 9–35

A. Prominent longitudinal fold, suggesting a lesion in the medial duodenum or head of the pancreas.

B. Hypotonic double contrast duodenography shows a prominent longitudinal fold with no evidence of a mass lesion (Courtesy of Harvey M. Goldstein, M.D., Houston.)

PANCREATIC DISEASES

The duodenal manifestations of pancreatic disease have been covered in detail by Eaton and Ferrucci.[23] In patients with pancreatitis the duodenal changes consist of a combination of compression due to enlargement of the head of the pancreas (Fig. 9–36) and mucosal inflammatory changes (Fig. 9–37). In pancreatic carcinoma, the predominant finding is compression and nodularity on the medial aspect of the duodenum (Fig. 9–38*A*). As the tumor erodes into the duodenum, ulceration may occur (Fig. 9–38*B*).

The "reverse 3" sign of pancreatic carcinoma may be simulated by underfilling of the duodenum, particularly in the presence of a duodenal diverticulum (Fig. 9–39).

Text continued on page 370

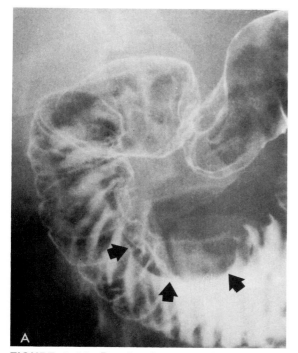 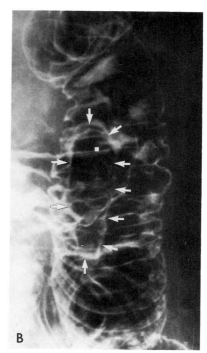

FIGURE 9–36 Duodenal compression from chronic pancreatitis in a 46-year-old man with abdominal pain and weight loss.

A. Hypotonic duodenography shows a mass projecting into the duodenum (*arrows*).

B. The prone oblique view shows the outline of the periampullary mass en face. This configuration was confirmed at endoscopy. Mucosal biopsy results were normal. The ampulla was not identifiable, but the orifice was found on the mass at the point marked by a dot. ERCP showed chronic pancreatitis which was confirmed by the subsequent clinical course.

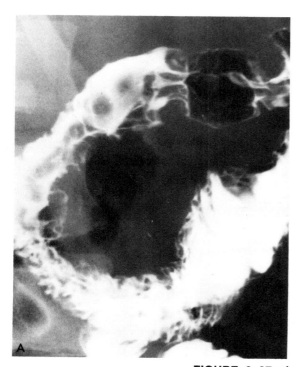 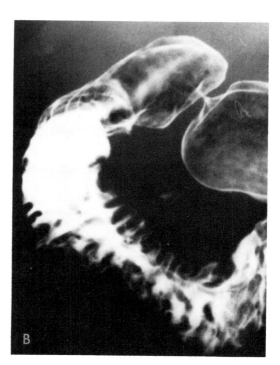

FIGURE 9–37 Acute pancreatitis.

A. Compression and widening of the duodenal loop, with thickening of the folds.

B. Thickening of the folds and spiculation in the descending duodenum.

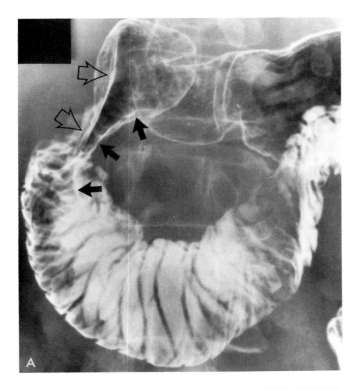

A. Compression of the medial aspect of the duodenum by the pancreatic tumor. There is also compression on the lateral aspect owing to an enlarged gallbladder (Courtesy of Harvey M. Goldstein, M.D., Houston. Reproduced by permission of Clinics in Gastroenterology.[49])

FIGURE 9–38 Pancreatic carcinoma.

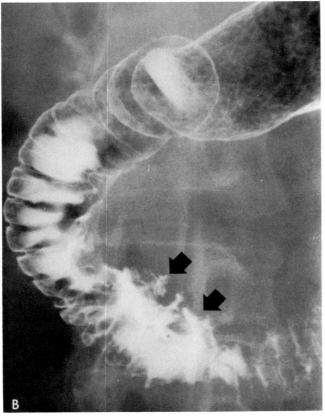

B. Pancreatic carcinoma with irregular ulceration of the descending duodenum.

A. There is a suggestion of medial compression of the duodenum with a reverse 3 sign.

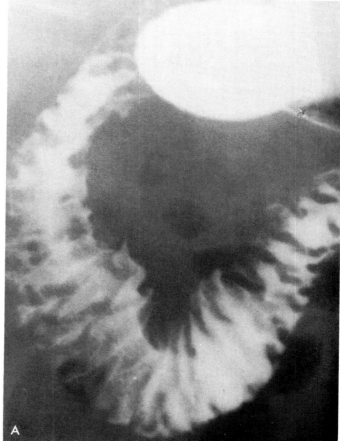

FIGURE 9–39 Spurious reverse 3 sign due to a duodenal diverticulum.

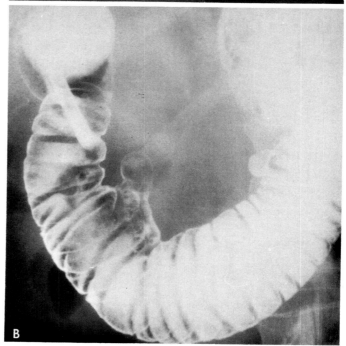

B. Hypotonic duodenography with a tube shows the duodenal diverticulum, with no other evidence of pancreatic or duodenal disease.

REFERENCES

1. Salmon, P. R., Brown, P., Htut, T., et al.: Endoscopic examination of the duodenal bulb: Clinical evaluation of forward- and side-viewing fibreoptic systems in 200 cases. Gut, *13*(1):170, 1972.
2. Classen, M: Endoscopy in benign peptic ulcer. Clin. Gastroenterol., *2*(2):315, 1973.
3. Belber, J. P.: Endoscopic examination of the duodenal bulb: a comparison with x-ray. Gastroenterology, *61*:55, 1971.
4. Herlinger, H., Glanville, J. N., and Kreel, L.: An evaluation of the double contrast barium meal (DCBM) against endoscopy. Clin. Radiol., *28*:307, 1977.
5. Laufer, I., Mullens, J. E., and Hamilton, J.: The diagnostic accuracy of barium studies of the stomach and duodenum: correlation with endoscopy. Radiology, *115*:569, 1975.
6. Laufer, I.: Assessment of the accuracy of double contrast gastro-duodenal radiology. Gastroenterology, *71*:874, 1976.
7. Burhenne, H. J.: Technique of examination of stomach and duodenum. *In*: Alimentary Tract Roentgenology, Vol. 1. 2nd ed. St. Louis, C. V. Mosby, 1973., p. 593.
8. Bilbao, M. K., Frische, L. H., and Dotter, C. T.: Hypotonic duodenography. Radiology, *89*:438, 1967.
9. Raia, S., and Kreel, L.: Gas-distension double-contrast duodenography using the Scott-Harden gastroduodenal tube. Gut, *7*:420, 1966.
10. Eaton, S. B., Benedict, K. T., Jr., Ferrucci, J. T., Jr., et al.: Hypotonic duodenography. Radiol. Clin. North Am., *8*:125, 1970.
11. Martel, W., Scholtens, P. A., and Lim, L. W.: "Tubeless" hypotonic duodenography: Technique, value and limitations. Am. J. Roentgenol., *107*:119, 1969.
12. Goldstein, H. M., and Zboralske, F. F.: Tubeless hypotonic duodenography. JAMA, *210*:2086, 1969.
13. Sear, H. S., and Friedenberg, M. J.: Simplified technique for tubeless hypotonic duodenography. Radiology, *103*:210, 1972.
14. Op den Orth, J. O.: Hypotonic duodenography without the use of a stomach tube. Radiol. Clin. Biol., *42*:173, 1973.
15. Kreel, L.: Pharmacoradiology in barium examinations with special reference to glucagon. Br. J. Radiol., *48*:691, 1975.
16. Miller, R. E., Chernish, S. M., Skucas, J., et al.: Hypotonic roentgenography with glucagon. Am. J. Roentgenol., *121*:264, 1976.
17. Miller, R. E., Chernish, S., Brunelle, R., et al.: Double blind radiographic study of dose response to intravenous glucagon for hypotonic duodenography. Radiology, *127*:55, 1978.
18. Saxton, H. M.: Starting the double contrast barium meal. Br. J. Radiol., *50*:610, 1977.
19. Sim, G. P. G.: The diagnosis of craters in the duodenal cap. Br. J. Radiol., *41*:792, 1968.
20. Nelson, J. A., Sheft, D., Minagi, H., et al.: Duodenal pseudopolyp — the flexure fallacy. Am. J. Roentgenol., *123*:262, 1975.
21. Burrell, M., and Toffler, R.: Flexural pseudo-lesions of the duodenum. Radiology, *120*:313, 1976.
22. Ferrucci, J. T., Jr., Benedict, K. T., Page, D. L., et al.: The radiographic features of the normal hypotonic duodenogram. Radiology, *96*:401, 1970.
23. Eaton, S. B., and Ferrucci, J. T., Jr.: Radiology of the Pancreas and Duodenum. Philadelphia. W. B. Saunders, 1973.
24. Kirby, J. R.: Observations on the duodenal mucosa with reference to problems associated with its three-dimensional structure. Clin. Radiol., *24*:139, 1973.
25. Bilbao, M. K., Frische, L. H., Rösch, J., et al.: Postbulbar duodenal ulcer and ring-stricture. Radiology, *100*:27, 1971.
26. Rodriguez, H. P., Aston, J. K., and Richardson, C. T.: Ulcers in the descending duodenum. Am. J. Roentgenol., *119*:316, 1973.
27. Nelson, S. W., and Christoforidis, A. J.: Roentgenologic features of the Zollinger-Ellison syndrome: ulcerogenic tumor of the pancreas. Semin. Roentgenol., *3*:254, 1968.
28. Sim, G. P. G.: A personal assessment of the gas contrast barium meal. Australas. Radiol., *18*:175, 1974.
29. Stein, G. N., Martin, R. D., Roy, R. H., et al.: Evaluation of conventional roentgenographic techniques for demonstration of duodenal ulcer craters. Am. J. Roentgenol., *91*:801, 1964.
30. Wechsler, R. L., and Jaffer, S. S.: Duodenitis. *In*: Bockus, H. L. (ed.): Gastroenterology. Philadelphia, W. B. Saunders, 1976.
31. Palmer, E. D.: Common duodenitis — of any clinical importance? JAMA, *230*:599, 1974.
32. Thomas, W. O., Robertson, A. G., Jinrie, C. W., et al.: Is duodenitis a dyspeptic myth? Lancet, *1*:1197, 1977.
33. Cotton, P. B., Price, A. B., Tighe, J. R., et al.: Preliminary evaluation of "duodenitis" by endoscopy and biopsy. Br. Med. J., *3*:430, 1973.
34. Gregg, J. A., and Garabedian, M.: Duodenitis. Am. J. Gastroenterol., *61*:177, 1974.

35. Katz, A. M.: Hemorrhagic duodenitis in myocardial infarction. Ann. Intern. Med., *51*:212, 1959.
36. Baum, S., Ward, S., and Nusbaum, M.: Stress bleeding from the mid-duodenum. An often unrecognized source of gastrointestinal hemorrhage. Radiology, *95*:595, 1970.
37. Blakemore, W. S., Baum, S., and Nusbaum, M.: Diagnosis and management of massive hemorrhage from postoperative stress ulcers of the descending duodenum. Surg. Clin. North Am., *50*:979, 1970.
38. Legge, D. A., Carlson, H. C., and Judd, E. S.: Roentgenologic features of regional enteritis of the upper gastrointestinal tract. Am. J. Roentgenol., *110*:355, 1970.
39. Wise, L.: Crohn's disease of duodenum. Am. J. Surg., *121*:184, 1971.
40. Thompson, W. H., Cockrill, H., Jr., and Rice, R. P.: Regional enteritis of the duodenum. Am. J. Roentgenol., *123*:252, 1975.
41. Laufer, I., and Costopoulos, L.: Early lesions of Crohn's disease. Am. J. Roentgenol., *130*:307, 1978.
42. Stevenson, G. W., Hyland, J., Laufer, I., et al.: Gastroduodenal lesions in Crohn's disease. Submitted for publication.
43. Blumgart, L. H., and Kennedy, A.: Carcinoma of the ampulla of Vater and duodenum. Br. J. Surg., *60*:33, 1973.
44. Bosse, G., and Neeley, J. A.: Roentgenologic findings in primary malignant tumors of the duodenum. Am. J. Roentgenol., *170*:111, 1969.
45. Ring, E. J., Ferrucci, J. T., Jr., Eaton, S. B., et al.: Villous adenomas of the duodenum. Radiology, *104*:45, 1972.
46. Balikian, J. P., Nassar, N. T., Shamma'a, M. H., et al.: Primary lymphomas of the small intestine including the duodenum. Am. J. Roentgenol., *107*:131, 1969.
47. Joffe, N., Goldman, H., and Antonioli, D. A.: Transpyloric prolapse of polypoid gastric carcinoma. Gastroenterology, *72*:1326, 1977.
48. Laufer, I.: Double contrast radiology in the diagnosis of gastrointestinal cancer. *In*: Glass, G. B. J. (ed.): Progress in Gastroenterology. Vol. 3. New York, Grune & Stratton, 1977, pp. 643–669.
49. Dodd, G. D., and Goldstein, H. M.: Newer radiologic techniques in the diagnosis of gastrointestinal cancer. Clin. Gastroenterol., *5*:597, 1976.

10 RADIOLOGIC-ENDOSCOPIC CORRELATION

The purpose of this chapter is to facilitate the development of skill in the interpretation of double contrast studies by correlating the radiologic appearances in a variety of normal and abnormal states with the corresponding gross pathologic appearances. In most cases the gross pathology is illustrated by endoscopic photographs, since these are taken under conditions that closely resemble the conditions of the radiologic examination. However, in a few cases we have had to use the surgical specimen to demonstrate the gross pathology. For the most part we have tried to present radiologic and endoscopic findings on the same patient. In some cases both studies were not available, and we have substituted studies from other patients with similar findings.

We hope that this chapter will emphasize the importance of constant endoscopic and pathologic correlation as an unexcelled tool for the development of expertise in gastrointestinal radiology.

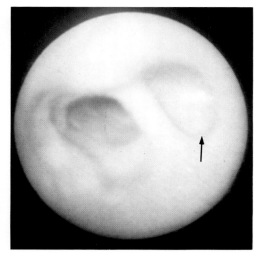
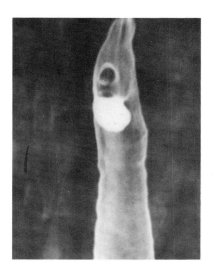

PLATE 1

Two esophageal diverticula shown on esophagram. The endoscopic photograph shows one of the diverticula (*arrow*).

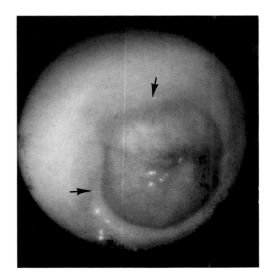

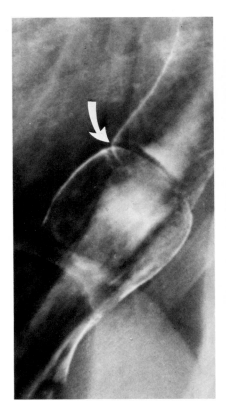

PLATE 2

Hiatal hernia with a widely patent lower esophageal ring *(arrows)*.

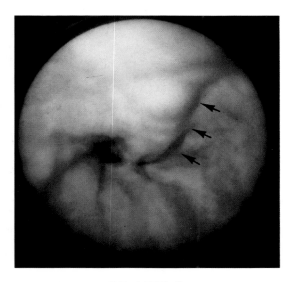

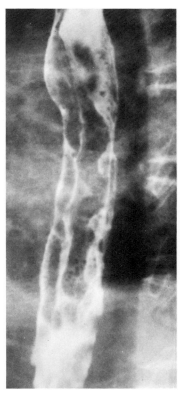

PLATE 3
Esophageal varices.

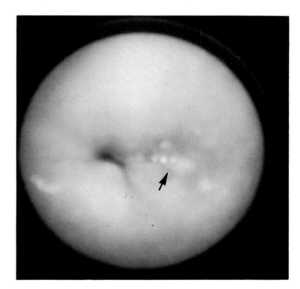

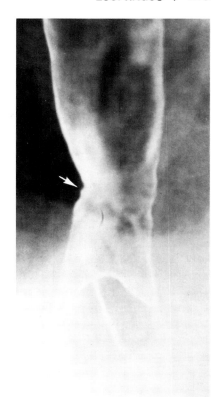

PLATE 4
Superficial linear ulcer due to reflux esophagitis.

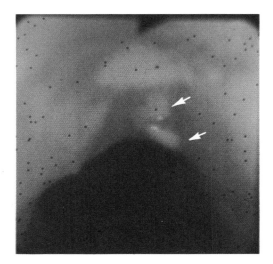

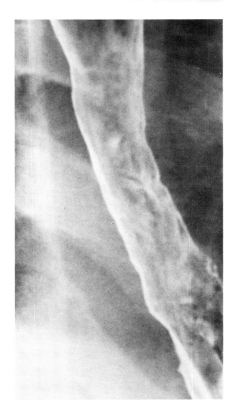

PLATE 5
Multiple superficial ulcers due to reflux esophagitis. (See Fig. 4–18)

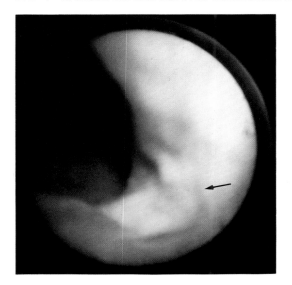

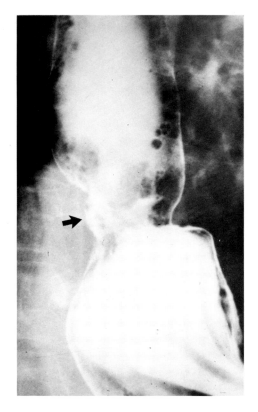

PLATE 6

Large ulcer at the gastroesophageal junction secondary to reflux esophagitis.

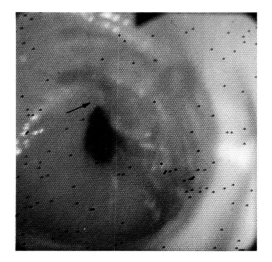

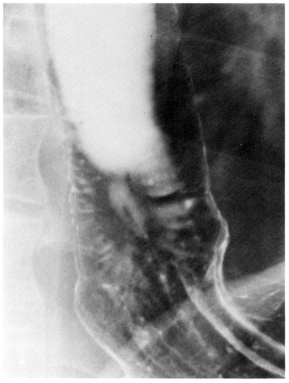

PLATE 7

Linear ulcer due to reflux esophagitis. (See Fig. 4–28)

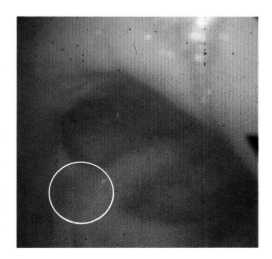

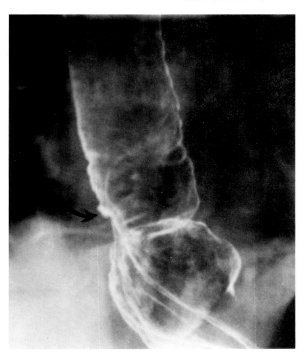

PLATE 8

Esophageal ulcer secondary to reflux esopha-gitis. Endoscopic photograph was taken several weeks after the radiograph when there was partial healing of the ulcer *(arrow)*.

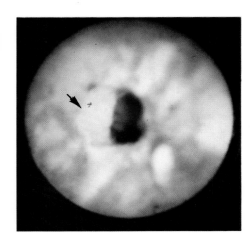

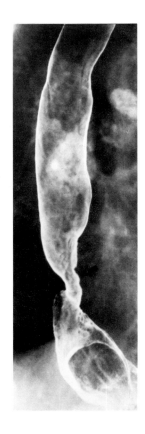

PLATE 9

Severe esophagitis with stricture and ulcer *(arrow)*.

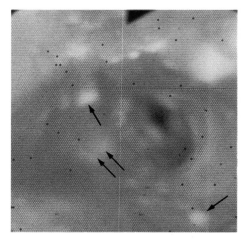

PLATE 10
Monilial esophagitis with linear, plaque-like filling defects *(arrows)*. (See Fig. 4–37.)

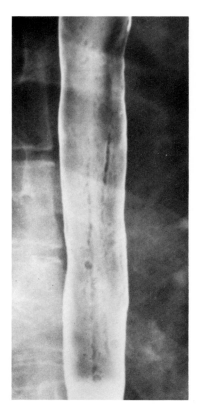

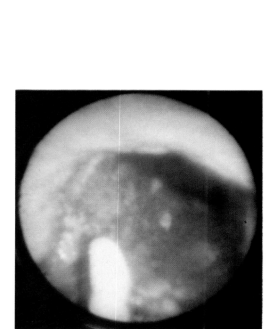

PLATE 11
Chronic monilial esophagitis with polypoid cheesy exudates.

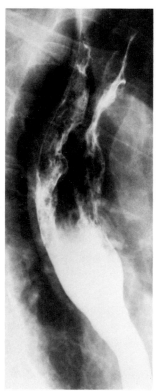

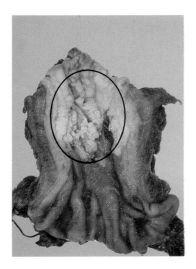

PLATE 12
Esophageal papillomatosis.

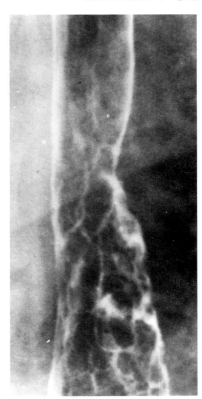

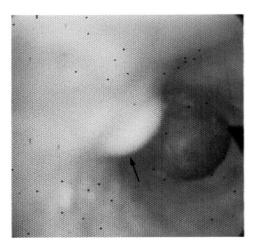

PLATE 13
Flat submucosal tumor in the midesophagus, probably a lipoma.

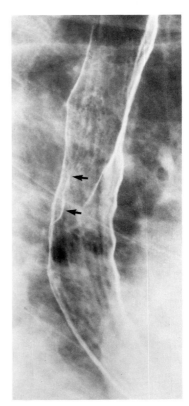

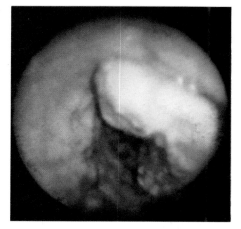

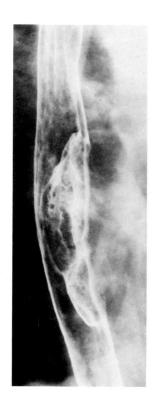

PLATE 14

Polypoid tumor in a patient with malabsorption due to nontropical sprue. (*From:* Laufer, I. *In:* Glass, G. B. J. (ed.): Progress in Gastroenterology. New York, Grune & Stratton, 1977.[7] Reproduced by permission.)

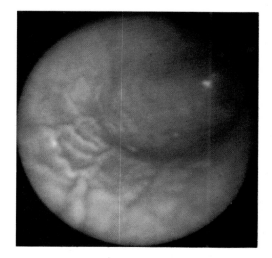

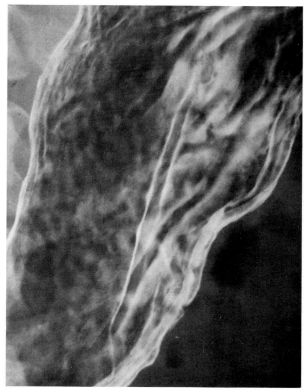

PLATE 15

The rugal pattern of the stomach, most prominent along the greater curvature.

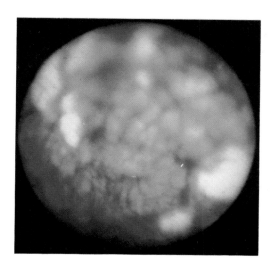
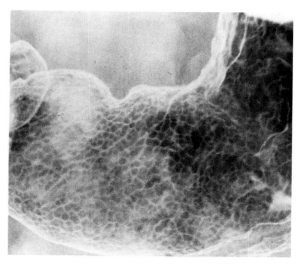

PLATE 16

Methylene blue dye scattered over the surface of the stomach shows the reticular appearance of the areae gastricae.

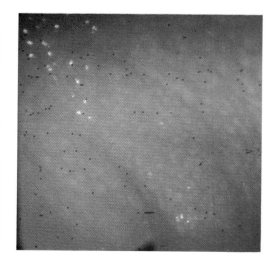
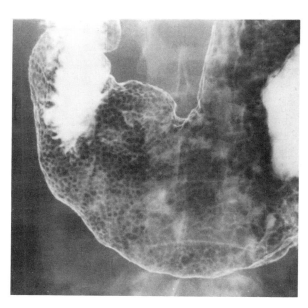

PLATES 17 AND 18

Coarsening of the areae gastricae resulting in a finely nodular appearance due to intestinal metaplasia in a young female.

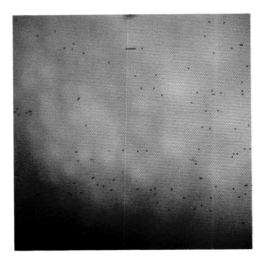

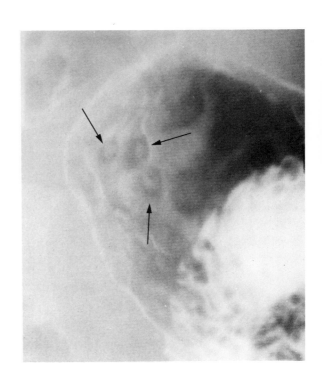

PLATE 18
See legend with Plate 17.

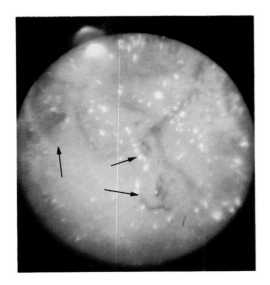

PLATE 19
Superficial gastric erosions with an edematous mound surrounding each erosion. (*From*: Laufer, I., Hamilton, J., and Mullens, J. E.: Gastroenterology, *63*:387, 1975.[1] Reproduced by permission.)

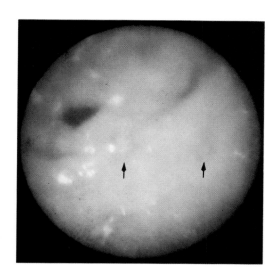 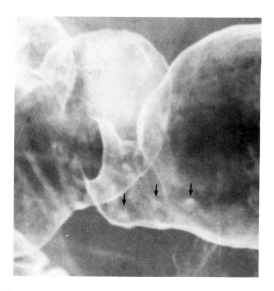

PLATE 20

Incomplete erosions. There are multiple superficial erosions with very little surrounding inflammatory reaction.

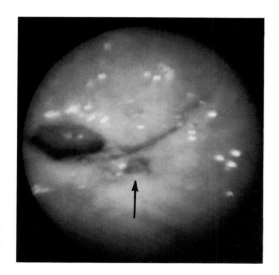 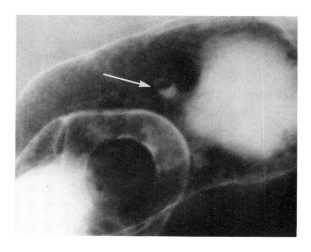

PLATE 21

Superficial erosion with a blood clot. (*From* Laufer, I., Hamilton, J., and Mullens, J. E.: Gastroenterology, *63*:387, 1975.[1] Reproduced by permission.)

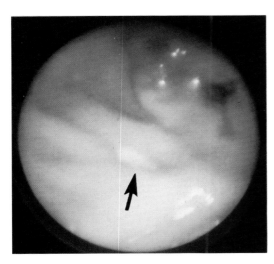

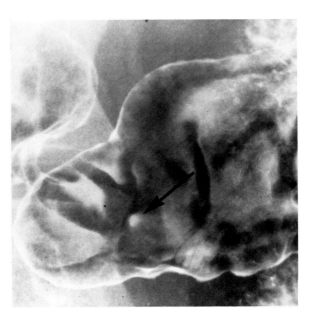

PLATE 22

Shallow posterior wall ulcer with radiating folds.
(Radiograph from: Laufer, I., Mullens, J. E.,
and Hamilton, J.: Radiology, *115*:569, 1975.[2]
Reproduced by permission.)

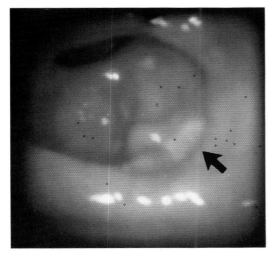

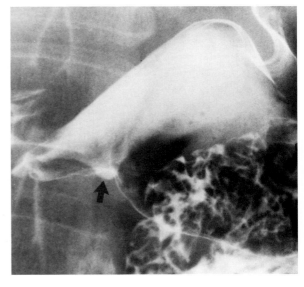

PLATE 23

Greater curvature ulcer (aspirin-induced).

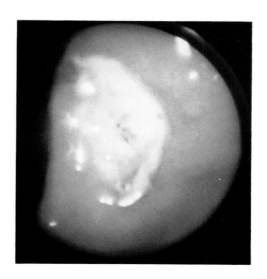
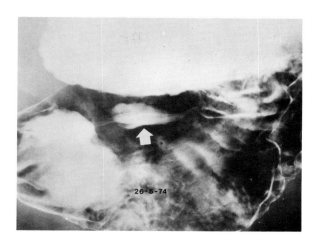

PLATE 24
Large benign ulcer near the lesser curvature. (Radiograph from: Laufer, I.: Radiology, *117*:513, 1975.[3] Reproduced by permission.)

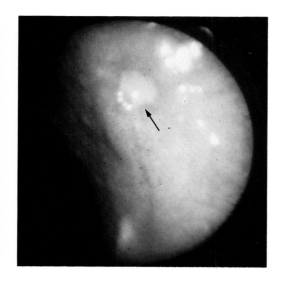
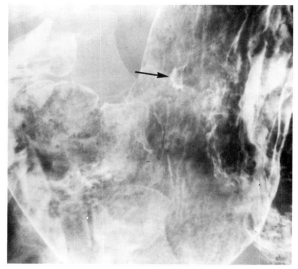

PLATE 25
Shallow posterior wall ulcer near the lesser curvature.

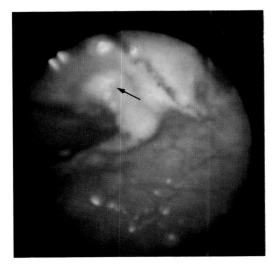

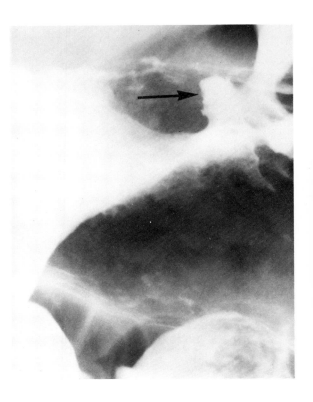

PLATE 26

Small benign ulcer adjacent to the cardia. The endoscope is seen passing through the esophageal hiatus and is retroflexed to demonstrate the ulcer (arrow).

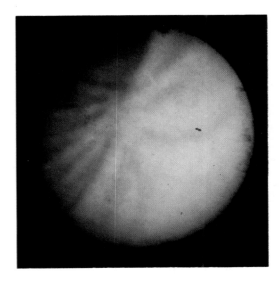

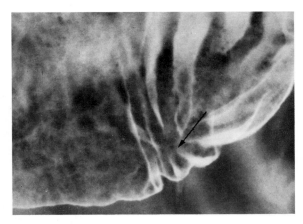

PLATE 27

Radiating folds to an ulcer scar near the greater curvature. (Radiograph from: Laufer, I., Gastroenterology, 71:874, 1976.[5] Reproduced by permission.)

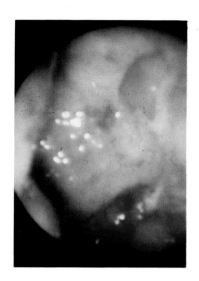

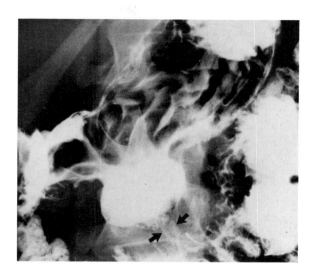

PLATES 28 AND 29

Gastrocolic fistula due to a benign gastric ulcer. The gastric side of the fistula is demonstrated in Plate 27. The endoscope then passed through the fistula into the colon (Plate 28), showing nodularity of the wall of the colon secondary to serosal inflammation. (*From*: Laufer, I., Thornley, G. D., and Stolberg, H.: Radiology, *119*:7, 1976.[4] Reproduced by permission.)

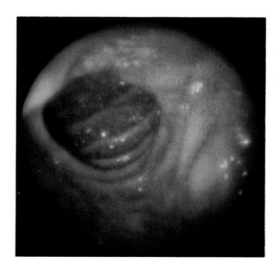

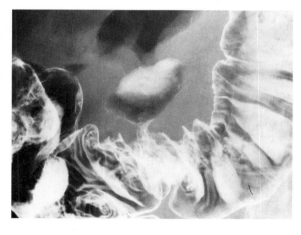

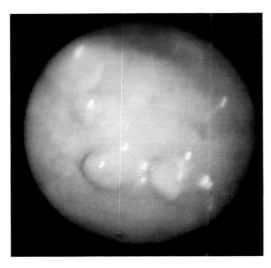

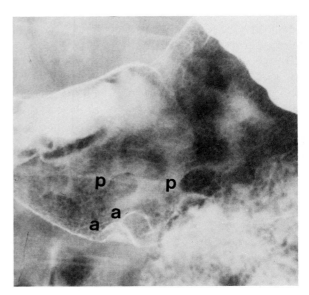

PLATE 30

Multiple hyperplastic polyps on the posterior (p) and anterior (a) walls.

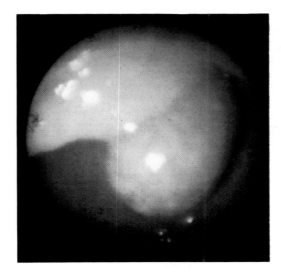

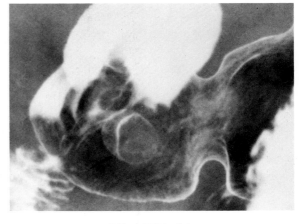

PLATE 31

Gastric antral polyp.

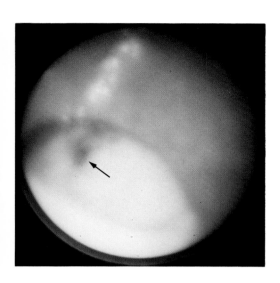

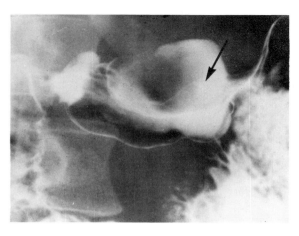

PLATE 32
Antral leiomyoma with a central ulcer *(arrow)*.

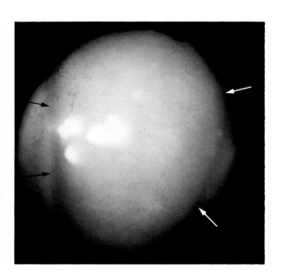

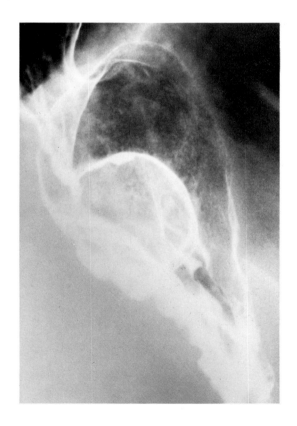

PLATE 33
Leiomyoma in a gastric remnant.

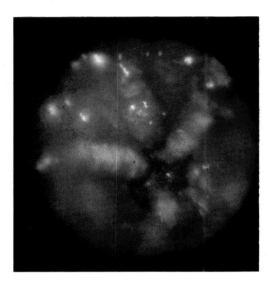
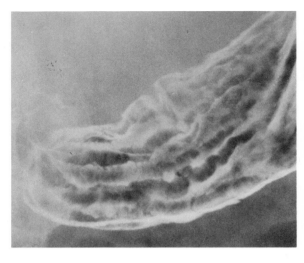

PLATE 34

Thickened tortuous folds due to an arteriovenous malformation of the antrum. Confirmed by angiography and surgery. (*From*: Lewis, T. D., Laufer, I., and Goodacre, R. L.: Am. J. Dig. Dis., *23*:467, 1978.[6] Reproduced by permission.)

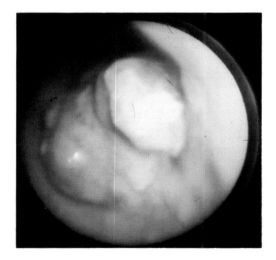
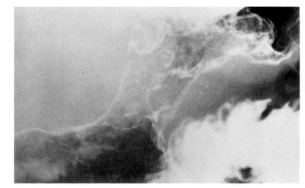

PLATE 35

Polypoid gastric carcinoma.

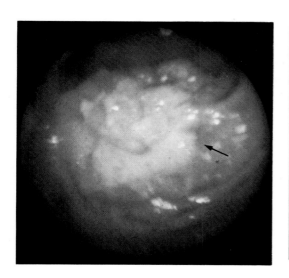
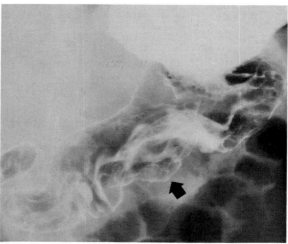

PLATE 36

Ulcerated gastric carcinoma along the greater curvature. There is a rim of tumor tissue with a large central ulcer having a necrotic base (*arrow*).

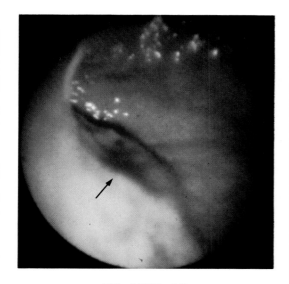
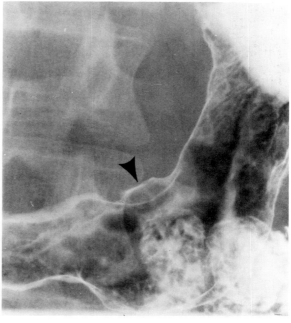

PLATE 37

Linitis plastica carcinoma with a lesser curvature ulcer (*arrow*).

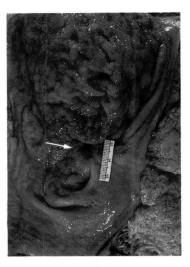

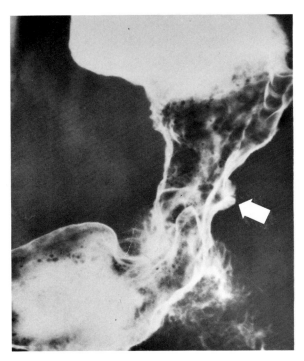

PLATE 38

Linitis plastica carcinoma with a greater curvature ulcer *(arrow)*, large folds, and diffuse infiltration.

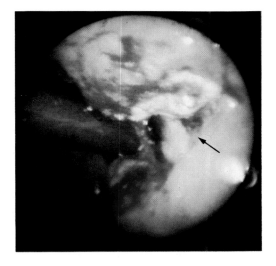

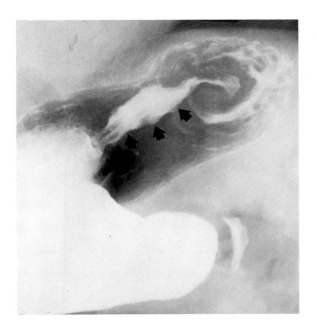

PLATE 39

Large malignant ulcer adjacent to the cardia. (Radiograph from: Laufer, I.: *In*: Glass, G. B. J. (ed.): Progress in Gastroenterology. New York, Grune & Stratton, 1977.[7] Reproduced by permission.)

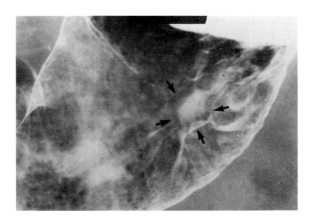

PLATE 40

Malignant ulcer with radiating folds. There is nodularity in the wall of the ulcer with nodularity, clubbing, and fusion of the radiating folds. (Courtesy of Fredrick M. Kelvin, M.D., Duke University. From: Laufer, I.: *In*: Glass, G. B. J. (ed.): Progress in Gastroenterology. New York, Grune & Stratton, 1977.[7] Reproduced by permission.)

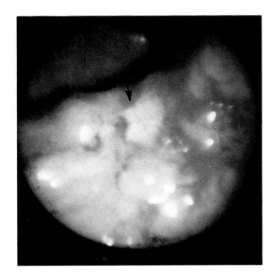

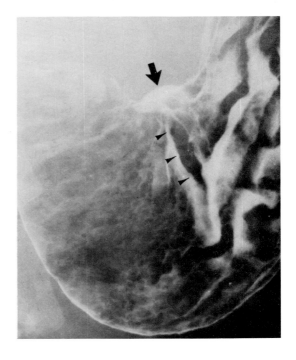

PLATE 41

Superficial spreading carcinoma with ulceration. There is a lesser curvature ulcer *(arrow)* with nodular folds and nodularity to the margin of the ulcer.

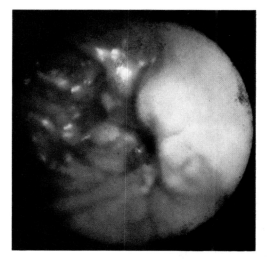

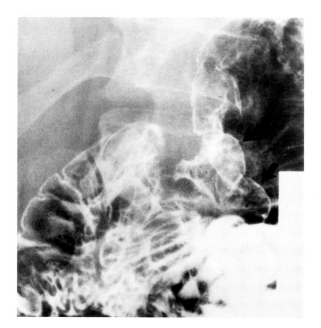

PLATE 42

Gastric stump carcinoma 20 years following surgery for benign ulcer. There is a polypoid mass in the gastric remnant *(arrows)*, extending to involve the anastomosis. (Radiograph from Gold, R. D., and Seaman, W. B.: Radiology, *124*:297, 1977.[8] Reproduced by permission.)

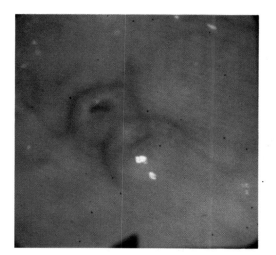

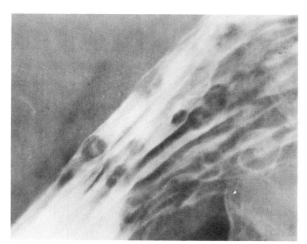

PLATE 43

Multiple bull's-eye lesions representing ulcerated metastases.

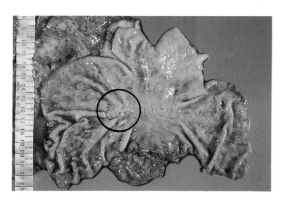 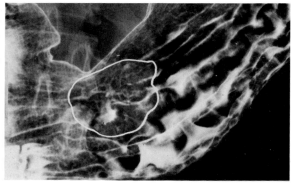

PLATE 44

A type IIc lesion measuring 3.0 × 3.0 cm in the largest diameter with depressed lesion and radiating folds. Histologic diagnosis: mucinous adenocarcinoma limited to the mucosa, without lymph node metastasis (0/12), associated with ulcer scar reaching the submucosa and slight intestinal metaplasia (see Figure 7–3).

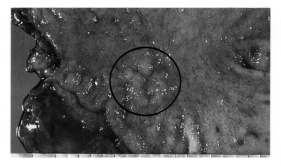 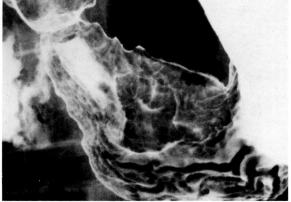

PLATE 45

A type IIa + IIç lesion measuring 2.0 × 2.0 cm in the largest diameter. Polypoid lesion with central ulceration. Tubular adenocarcinoma extensively involving the submucosa with lymph node metastases (3/14) and severe intestinal metaplasia (see also Figure 7–4).

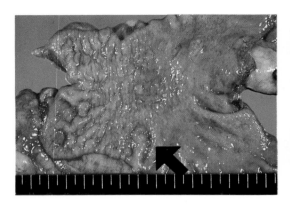
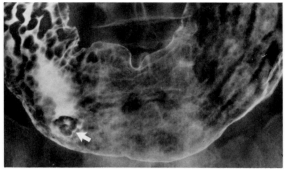

PLATE 46

Adenomatous polyp measuring 1.3 × 0.8 cm in the largest diameter, with severe intestinal metaplasia (see also Figure 7–7).

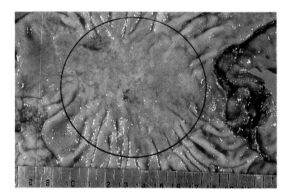

PLATE 47

Superficial spreading carcinoma. A large type IIc lesion measuring 13 × 12 cm in the largest diameter (superficial spreading type). Mucinous and scirrhous adenocarcinoma slightly involving the submucosa without lymph node metastasis (0/16), with moderate intestinal metaplasia (see also Figure 7–12).

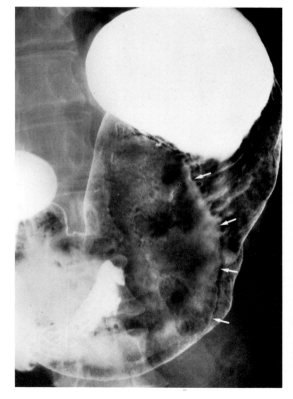

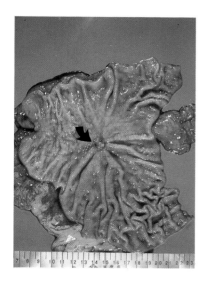

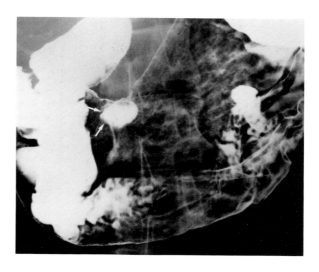

PLATE 48

Type III carcinoma. Tumor was restricted to the distal margin of the ulcer *(arrows)*. (see Figure 7–14).

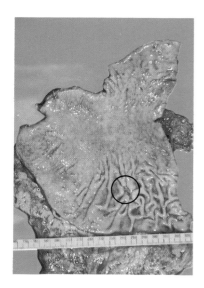

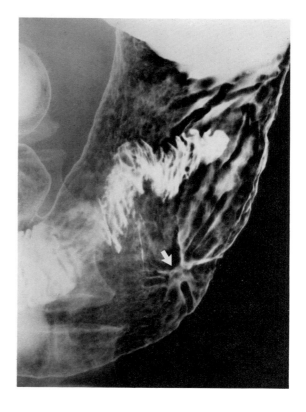

PLATE 49

Type IIc lesion in the fundic gland mucosa in a 57-year-old female. Double contrast radiograph in the supine position.

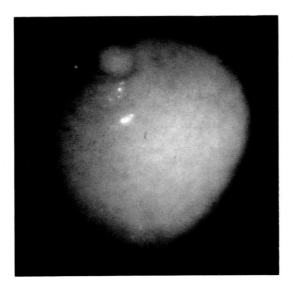

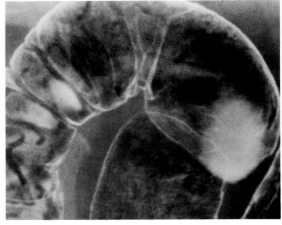

PLATE 50
Normal mucosal relief in the duodenal cap.

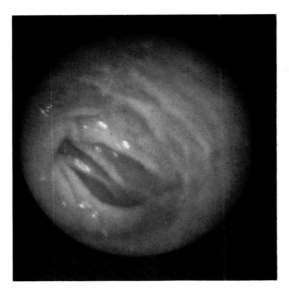

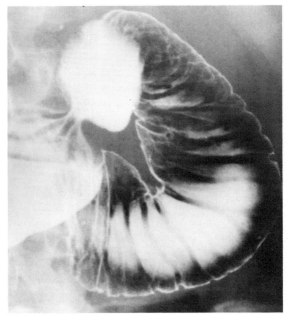

PLATE 51
Normal circular folds in the descending duodenum.

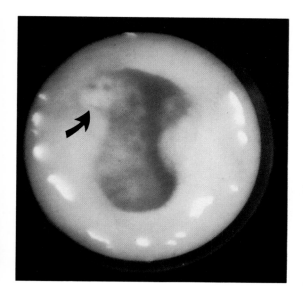

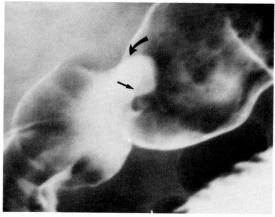

PLATE 52

Distortion of the pyloric canal *(straight arrow)* by an ulcer in the duodenal cap *(curved arrow)*.

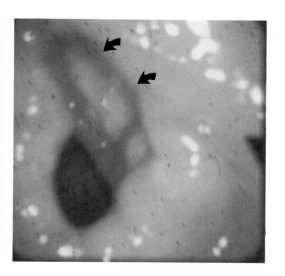

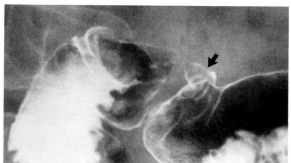

PLATE 53

Duodenal ulcer presenting in the pyloric channel.

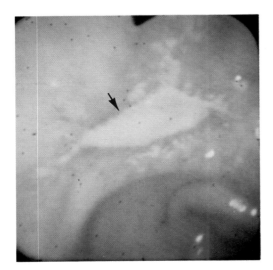
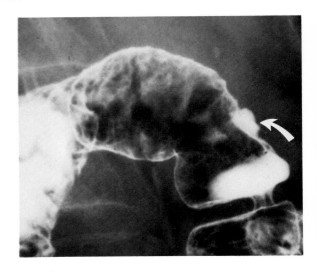

PLATE 54
Ulcer along the superior aspect of the duodenum.

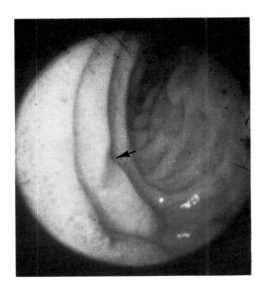

PLATE 55
Aphthous ulceration in the descending duodenum in a patient with Crohn's disease.

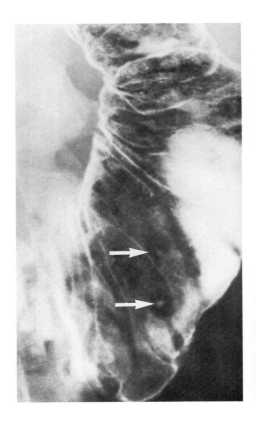

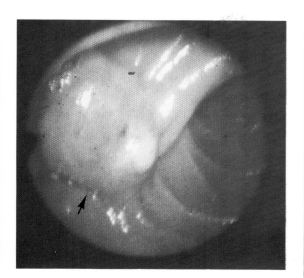

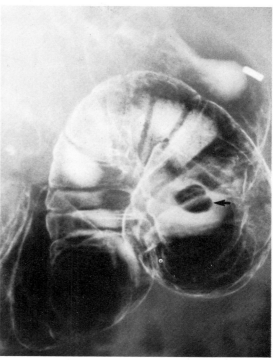

PLATE 56
Polypoid carcinoma of the ampulla of Vater.

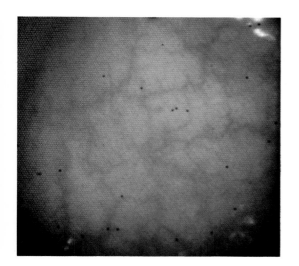

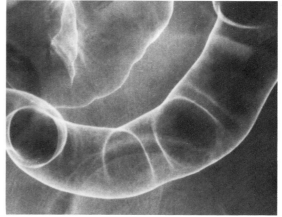

PLATE 57
Normal colonic mucosa with clear visualization of
the submucosal vascular plexus.

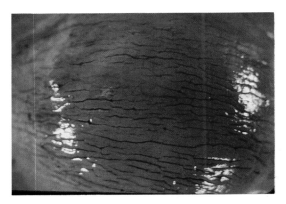

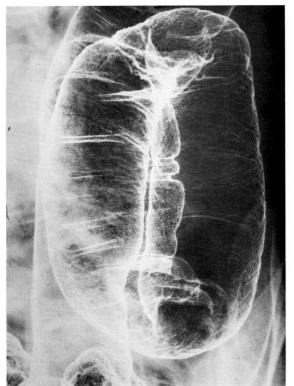

PLATE 58

The surface pattern (innominate lines) of the colon. (Specimen photograph courtesy of Drs. H. Shirakabe, M. Nishizawa, A. Kariya, Juntendo, Univ. Tokyo).

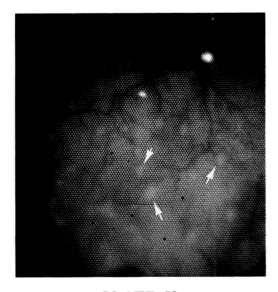

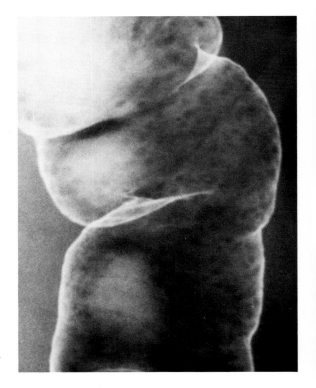

PLATE 59

The lymphoid follicular pattern of the colon in an adult. The lymphoid follicles are represented by small filling defects on the x-ray study. At endoscopy, these appear as tiny white plaques (different patient). (Endoscopic photograph courtesy of E. Burbige, M.D., Martinez, California. *From*: Burbige, E., and Sobyk, R. Z. F.: Gastroenterology, *72*:524, 1977.[9] Reproduced by permission.)

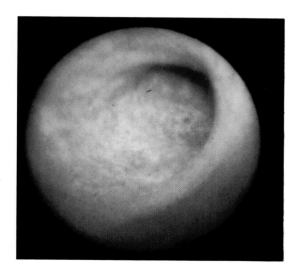

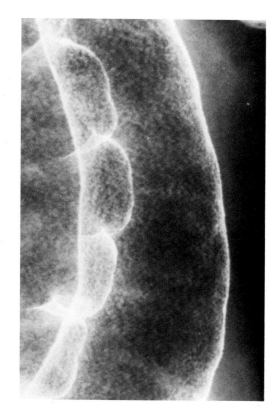

PLATE 60

Ulcerative colitis with fine granularity of the mucosa due to mucosal edema and hyperemia. The normal vascular plexus is obscured. (*From*: Laufer, I., Mullens, J. E., and Hamilton, J.: Radiology, *118*:1, 1976.[10] Reproduced by permission.)

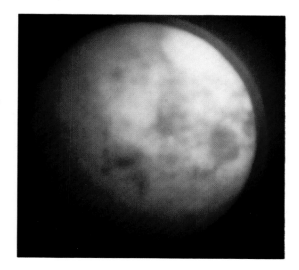

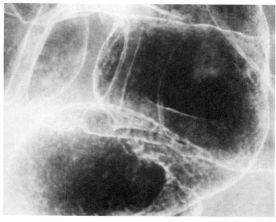

PLATE 61

Stippling of the mucosa due to superficial erosions in ulcerative colitis. (Plates 61 and 62 from Laufer, I., Mullens, J. E., and Hamilton, J.: Radiology, *118*:1, 1976.[10] Reproduced by permission.)

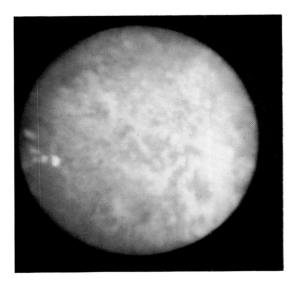

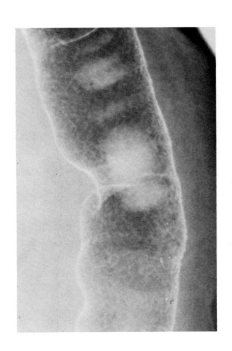

PLATE 62

Coarse granularity, typical of chronic ulcerative colitis.

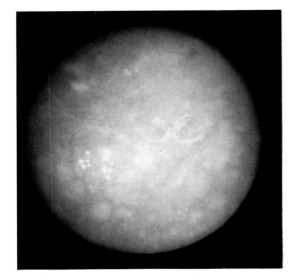

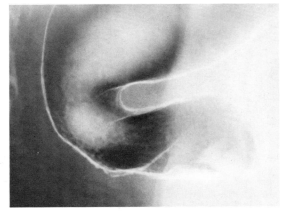

PLATE 63

Edema of the rectal mucosa in ulcerative proctitis confined to the distal portion of the rectum. (Radiograph from Laufer, I.: J. Can. Assoc. Radiol., 26:116, 1975.[11] Reproduced by permission.)

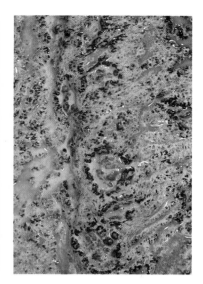

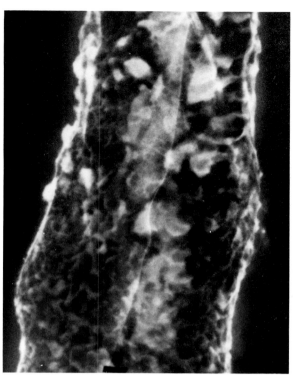

PLATE 64

Ulceration on a background of diffusely granular mucosa in ulcerative colitis. The ulcers are seen in profile and en face as amorphous collections of barium. The specimen has been lightly coated with barium to highlight the ulcers and the granularity of the mucosa. (*From*: Laufer, I.: CRC Crit. Rev. Diagnost. Imaging, *9*:421, 1977.[2] Reproduced by permission.)

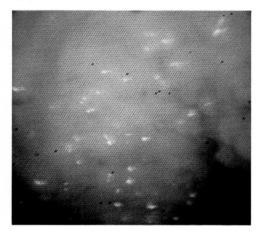

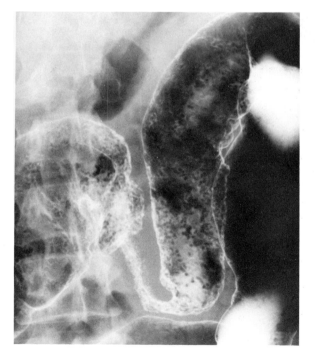

PLATE 65

Postinflammatory polyposis in a patient with a previous episode of severe ulcerative colitis. (Radiograph from Zegel, H., and Laufer, I.: Radiology, *127*:615, 1978.[13] Reproduced by permission.)

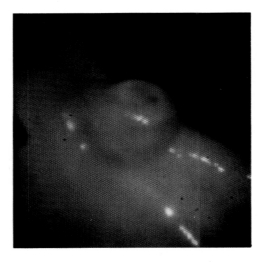

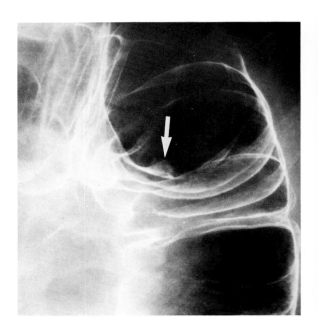

PLATE 66

Postinflammatory polyp in a patient with quiescent ulcerative colitis.

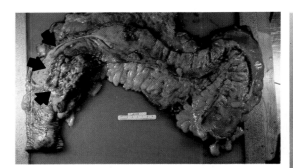

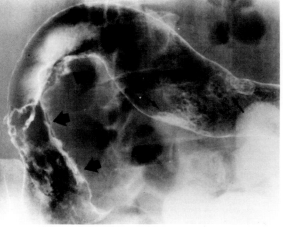

PLATE 67

Carcinoma of the ascending colon in a patient with a 10-year history of ulcerative colitis (*large arrows*). There are other smaller polypoid lesions which are adenomatous polyps (*small arrows*). There is minimal granularity of the mucosa, suggesting a background of chronic ulcerative colitis.

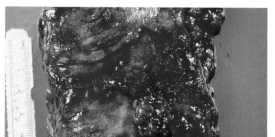

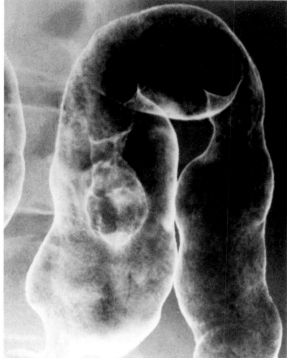

PLATES 68 AND 69

Two inflammatory polyps in a patient with minimally active ulcerative colitis, as evidenced by the granular appearance of the mucosa.

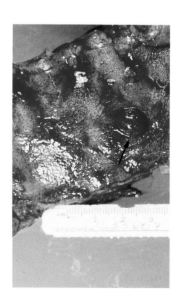

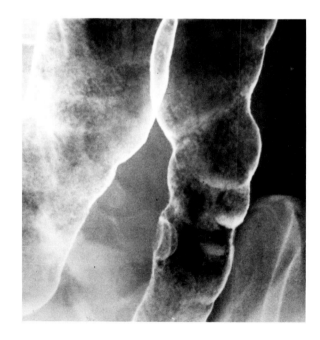

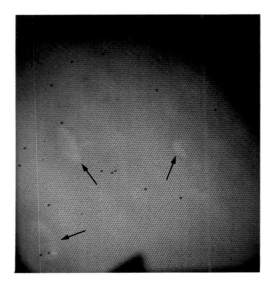

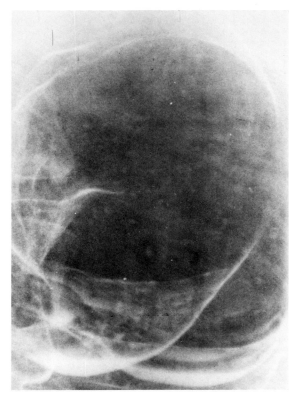

PLATE 70

Multiple small target lesions representing aphthous ulcers in Crohn's disease. The ulcers have a white base and a red, elevated margin on a background of normal mucosa. (*From*: Laufer, I.: CRC Crit. Rev. Diagnost. Imaging, 9:421, 1977.[12] Reproduced by permission.)

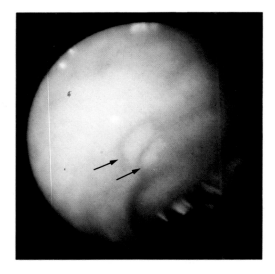

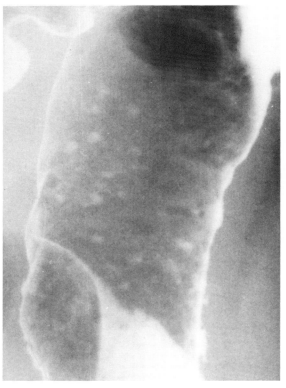

PLATE 71

Slightly larger aphthous ulcers. Note the background of normal mucosa. (Radiograph from Laufer, I.: J. Can. Assoc. Radiol., 26:116, 1975.[11] Reproduced by permission.)

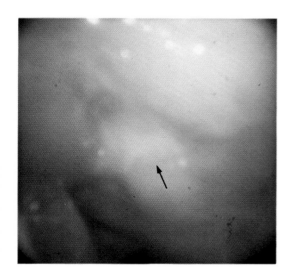

PLATE 72

Larger ulcers throughout the splenic flexure on a background of normal mucosa in Crohn's disease. One of these ulcers is demonstrated in the endoscopic photograph.

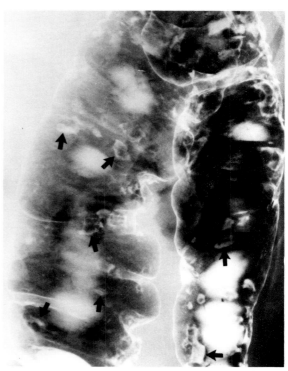

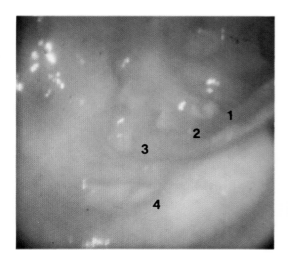

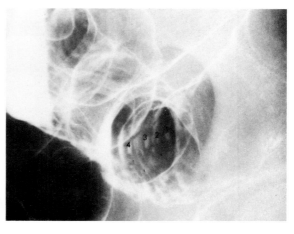

PLATE 73

Crohn's disease with four ulcers in a linear arrangement. (*From:* Laufer, I., Mullens, J. E., and Hamilton, J.: Radiology, *118*:1, 1976. Reproduced by permission.)

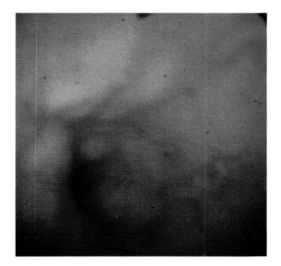

PLATE 74

Chronic granulomatous colitis with mucosal thickening.

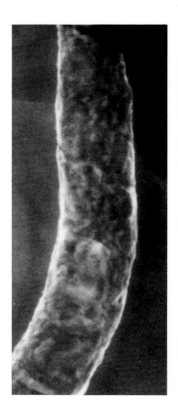

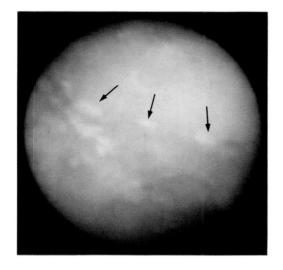

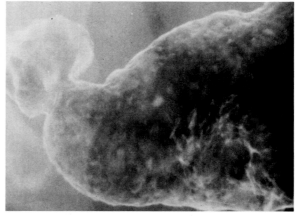

PLATE 75

Erosive gastritis due to Crohn's disease of the stomach.

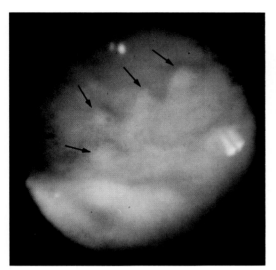 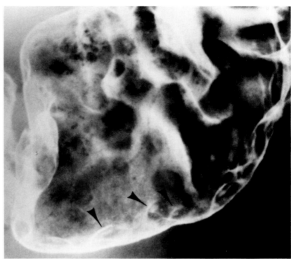

PLATE 76

Another example of gastric erosions due to Crohn's disease. The endoscopic photograph shows primarily the edematous mounds of mucosa surrounding the erosions.

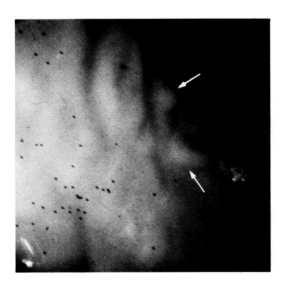 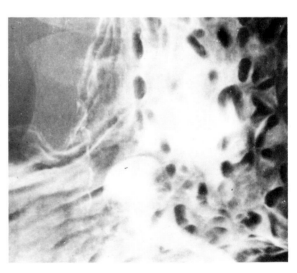

PLATE 77

Filiform polyps in the stomach in a patient with Crohn's disease. (Radiograph from Zegel, H., and Laufer, I.: Radiology, *127*:615, 1978.[13] Reproduced by permission.)

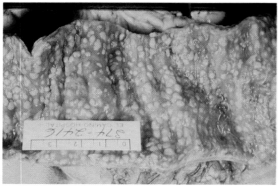

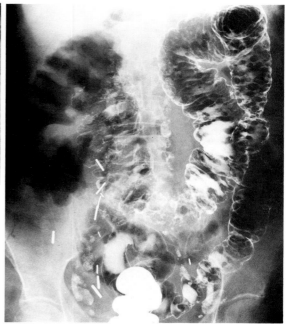

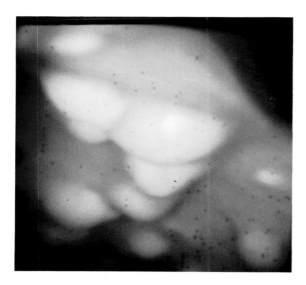

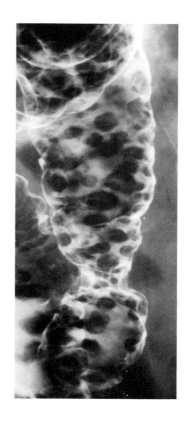

PLATES 78 AND 79

Pseudomembranous colitis with multiple small filling defects representing the plaques of pseudomembrane. (Endoscopic photograph courtesy of The Upjohn Company. Surgical specimen courtesy of Saul Eisenstadt, M.D., Los Altos, California. *From*: Hyson, E. A., Burrell, M., and Toffler, R.: Gastrointest. Radiol., 2:183, 1977. Reproduced by permission.)

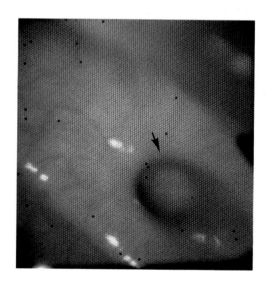

PLATE 80
Colonic diverticulum.

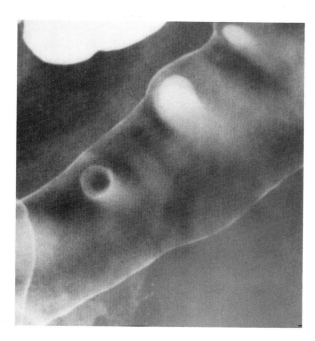

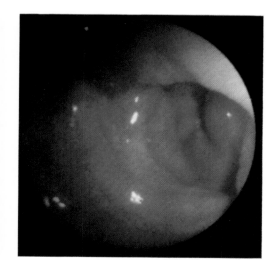

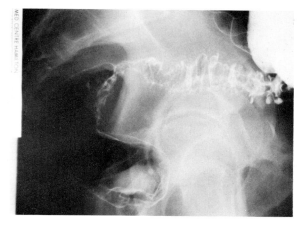

PLATE 81
Acute diverticulitis with intact but inflamed mucosal folds.

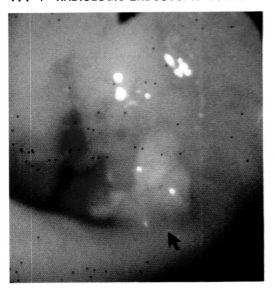 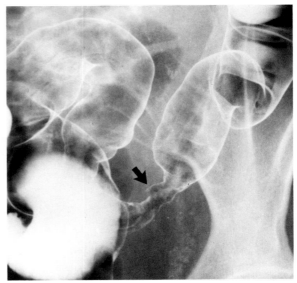

PLATE 82
Radiation colitis with mucosal edema, hyperemia, and ulceration *(arrow)*.

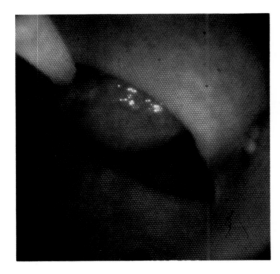 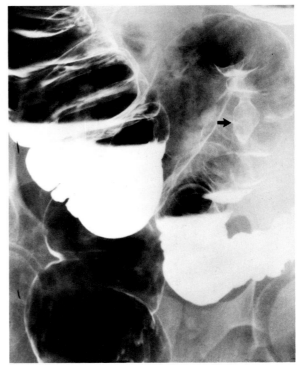

PLATE 83
Pedunculated sigmoid polyp. The sheath containing the snare is seen advancing towards the polyp.

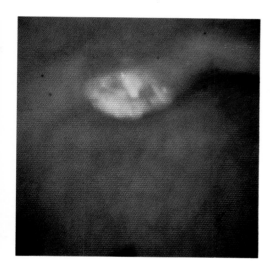

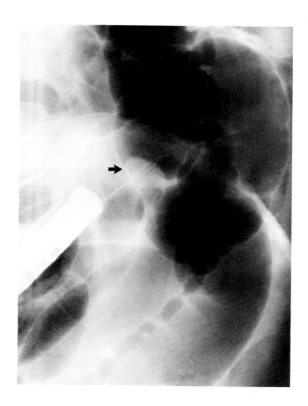

PLATE 84
The snare is looped around the stalk of the polyp. The appearance of the transected stalk is shown.

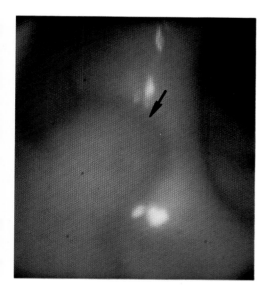

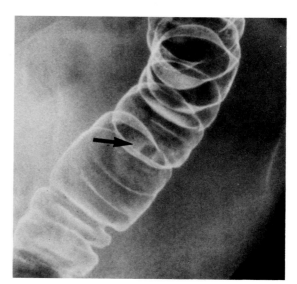

PLATE 85
Small hyperplastic polyp in the descending colon.

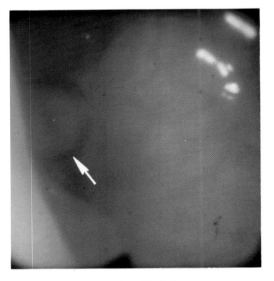

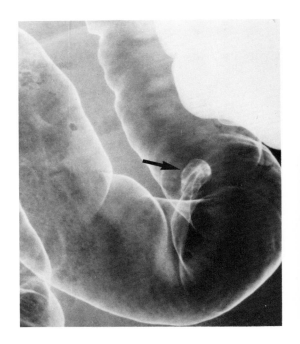

PLATE 86

Polyp at the junction of the sigmoid and descending colon, missed at colonoscopy. Note that the polyp is just behind an area of sharp angulation, and as it lies against the mucosal surface it can easily be missed. (Radiograph from Laufer, I., Smith, N. C. W., and Mullens, J. E.: Gastroenterology, *70*:167, 1976. Reproduced by permission.)

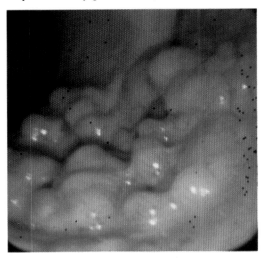

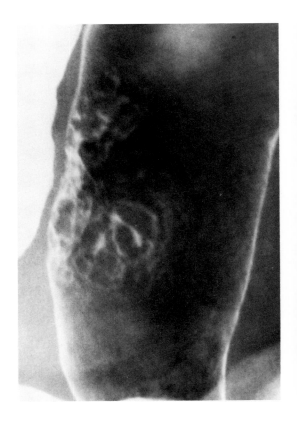

PLATE 87

Flat, lobulated, villoglandular polyp in the descending colon.

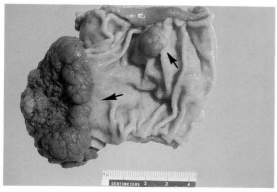

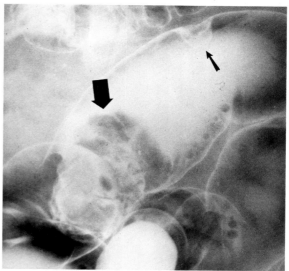

PLATE 88

Two polypoid tumors in the sigmoid colon. The radiologic findings suggest that the distal lesion is malignant because of its size, while the proximal lesion might be malignant because of its irregular base. Both lesions turned out to be benign adenomatous polyps.

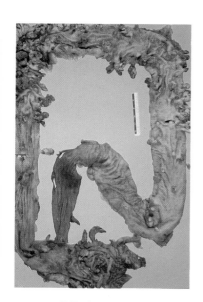

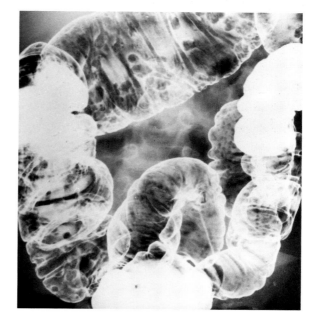

PLATE 89

Juvenile colonic polyposis in an 8-year-old girl.

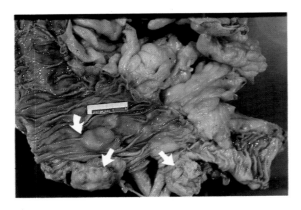

PLATE 90

Bilobed lipoma of the ascending colon *(curved arrow)* and a polypoid carcinoma arising from the superior lip of the ileocecal valve *(straight arrow)*.

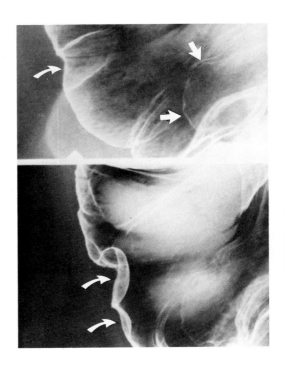

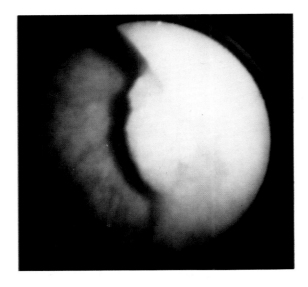

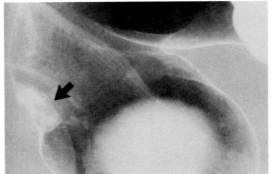

PLATE 91

Flat polypoid carcinoma of the rectum.

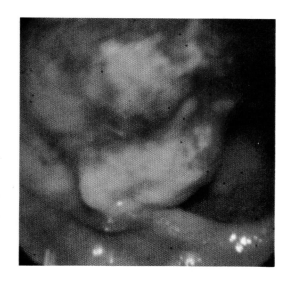
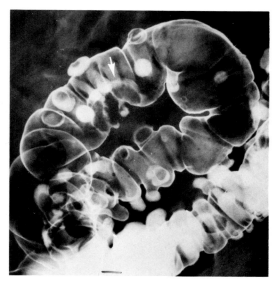

PLATE 92
Polypoid carcinoma with surface ulceration in the sigmoid colon.

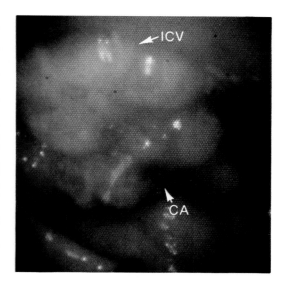

PLATE 93
Polypoid carcinoma of the cecum. In the endoscopic photograph, the ileocecal valve (ICV) is seen just proximal to the tumor (CA).

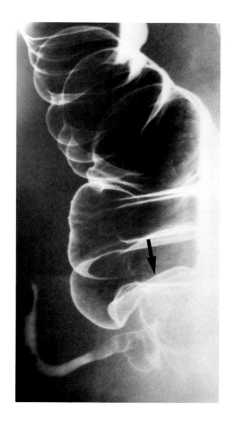

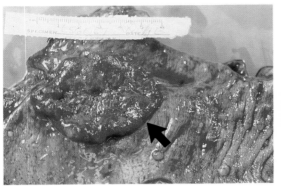

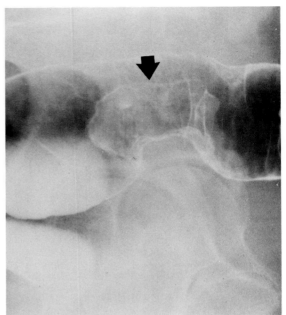

PLATE 94

Flat plaque-like carcinoma representing a recurrence at a colorectal anastomosis.

REFERENCES

1. Laufer, I., Hamilton, J., and Mullens, J. E.: Demonstrations of superficial erosions by double contrast radiography. Gastroenterology, 63:387, 1975.
2. Laufer, I., Mullens, J. E., and Hamilton, J.: The diagnostic accuracy of barium studies of the stomach and duodenum — correlation with endoscopy. Radiology, 115:569, 1975.
3. Laufer, I.: A simple method for routine double contrast study of the upper gastrointestinal tract. Radiology, 117:513, 1975.
4. Laufer, I., Thornley, G. D., and Stolberg, H.: Gastro-colic fistula as a complication of benign gastric ulcer. Radiology, 119:7, 1976.
5. Laufer, I.: Assessment of the accuracy of double contrast gastroduodenal radiology. Gastroenterology, 71:874, 1976.
6. Lewis, T. D., Laufer, I., and Goodacre, R. L.: Arteriovenous malformation of the stomach: radiologic and endoscopic features. Am. J. Dig. Dis., 23:467, 1978.
7. Laufer, I.: Double contrast radiology in the diagnosis of gastrointestinal cancer. In: Glass, G. B. J. (ed.): Progress in Gastroenterology. Vol. 3. New York, Grune & Stratton, 1977, pp. 643–669.
8. Gold, R. P., and Seaman, W. B.: The primary double-contrast examination of the postoperative stomach. Radiology, 124:297, 1977.
9. Burbige, E. J., and Sobyk, R. Z. F.: Endoscopic appearance of colonic lymphoid nodules: a normal variant. Gastroenterology, 72:524, 1977.
10. Laufer, I., Mullens, J. E., and Hamilton, J.: Correlation of endoscopy and double contrast radiography in the early stages of ulcerative and granulomatous colitis. Radiology, 118:1, 1976.
11. Laufer, I.: The radiologic demonstration of early changes in ulcerative colitis by double contrast technique. J. Can. Assoc. Radiol., 26:116, 1975.
12. Laufer, I.: Air-contrast studies of the colon in inflammatory bowel disease. CRC Crit. Rev. Diagnost. Imaging, 9:421, 1977.
13. Zegel, H., and Laufer, I.: Filiform polyposis. Radiology, 127:615, 1978.
14. Hyson, A. E., Burrell, M., and Toffler, R.: Drug-induced gastrointestinal disease. Gastrointest. Radiol., 2:83, 1977.
15. Laufer, I., Smith, N. C. W., and Mullens, J. E.: The radiologic demonstration of colorectal polyps undetected by endoscopy. Gastroenterology, 70:167, 1976.

11

SMALL BOWEL

HANS HERLINGER, M.D.

INTRODUCTION

The small intestine, a winding tube of uncertain length and variable position within the abdomen, is an environment potentially hostile to ingested barium suspensions. A torrent of fluid that contains most substances present in plasma and about 250 g of shed epithelial cells pours into its lumen every day, most of it being continuously reabsorbed together with ingested materials.[1] Added to this are pancreatic secretions containing protein and electrolytes, gastric juice, and bile with pigments, salts, and mucus. In the fasting state this outpouring diminishes considerably, although there is still an estimated daily outflow that includes 10 to

423

25 g of fat,[2] most of it reabsorbed. Little is known about the mucus that covers the whole of the mucosa.[3] In this environment even flocculation-resistant barium may occasionally flocculate in patients whose fecal fats are normal.[4]

Normal variations of bowel wall tonus[5] and transit time[6] can affect the radiologic appearance of the mucosal surface, showing the valvulae conniventes as either circular bands surrounding a wider lumen or a feathery pattern in the collapsed small bowel.

The variable appearance of the normal surface of small bowel, coating difficulties due to gut contents, unpredictable transit time, and problems caused by overlap of loops have made it difficult to be confident either of normality or of the early changes in disease. Moreover, even the most carefully done small bowel studies produce a very low yield of organic disease.[7] It is not surprising that many radiologists show little interest in the small bowel and that clinicians have been induced to accept, as sufficient radiodiagnostic effort, overview radiographs of barium-filled loops with the assurance that major pathology had not been revealed.

The purpose of this chapter is to describe an intubation method that produces a double contrast form of lumen delineation and aims to bring the small bowel examination into line with the now widely practiced double contrast radiology of the upper and lower gastrointestinal tracts. As the investigation of the duodenum forms part of the barium meal routine, the term small intestine in the context of this chapter will refer to the jejunum and ileum only. The examination has not been employed in children, and only adolescent and adult patient material is included.

HISTORICAL REVIEW

Duodenal intubation for radiodiagnostic purposes goes back a long way. Cole in 1911,[8] dissatisfied with the way the duodenum was outlined during the intermittent passage of a bismuth-buttermilk mixture through the pylorus, used a modified Einhorn tube to obstruct the distal duodenum by balloon inflation. In this way the contrast material was held up until the duodenum had filled to an acceptable degree. A modification of the tube, Cole suggested, would make it possible to introduce contrast material directly into an unobstructed duodenum. However, no further report of this method could be traced.

Max Einhorn,[9] in the second edition of his monograph, discussed the then widespread use of duodenal intubation in the diagnosis of duodenal, pancreatic, and biliary disease. Among an assortment of specialized duodenal tubes, he described a "duodenal obturator" for balloon obstruction of the distal duodenum and the injection of a bismuth-acacia mixture above the obstruction. The illustrated example of this procedure shows the balloon only partly distended and the contrast medium flowing into the jejunum — an unintended, but first ever, small bowel enema. Dr. Cole was not mentioned in Einhorn's bibliography.

The first attempt at double contrast study was reported by Pribram and Kleiber in 1927. Their "pneumoduodenography" required intubation and the introduction of barium followed by air in patients given atropine "for the better adherence of barium."[10] Pesquera[11] in 1929 referred to the difficulty of follow-through x-ray diagnosis in the small bowel because of the "irregularity of its action, its motility and the flaky distribution that the menstrum assumes in this position of the gastrointestinal tract''; he therefore introduced a barium-acacia-water mixture by gravity through a duodenal tube, observed its progress, and exposed x-ray plates at intervals. Ghelew and Mengis (1938) intubated through the mouth and instilled 1200 to 1400 ml of thorium and water. They were the first to stress the importance of a clean colon.[12]

A blood transfusion type of syringe was used by Gershon-Cohen and Shay[13] to inject barium through a tube in the duodenum; after small bowel filling and imaging they introduced air to obtain double contrast views. Schatzki (1943) also intubated by the oral route. He reported 75 examinations using 500 to 1000 ml of dilute barium;[14] the average time to reach the cecum was 15 minutes, but problems of reflux into the stomach were encountered. In the discussion that followed that paper, Ross Golden suggested that injecting barium through a Miller-Abbott (MA) tube advanced into the jejunum would avoid gastric reflux. Lura in 1951 reported 300 intubation studies, all without complications.[15]

Earlier intubations had been made by means of an Einhorn or a Rehfuss tube; more easily manageable types of tube now became available. In 1960 Scott-Harden[16] described a coaxial tube system with an outer catheter to be taken to the vicinity of the pylorus, and a more pliable inner tube to advance into the duodenum. The long, 1.5 mm lumen inner tube allowed the introduction of only dilute barium, given in surprisingly small amounts and then flushed along with injected water.[17, 18] Intubation was further facilitated by Gianturco's[19] application of a modified Volkswagen speedometer cable to serve as a guide in a duodenal tube described by Bilbao and coworkers.[20]

The small bowel enema (SBE) came of age with the publications of Sellink.[21-23] His method essentially consists of the infusion of barium by gravity via a nasoduodenal tube. The density of the suspension is adjusted to the patient's body thickness, the whole small bowel is filled with an uninterrupted column, and the examination is completed with the injection of water.

Most publications concerning the intubation examination of the small bowel have come from innovators and enthusiasts who have not critically questioned the clinical value of this more complex procedure. Fleckenstein and Pedersen (1975) were the first to report a series of small bowel enemas and follow-through examinations carried out in the same patients.[24] In 52 evaluation pairs they considered the enema to be superior in the jejunum and upper ileum, but found no significant difference in the terminal ileum. Sanders and Ho[25] were able to compare the conventional small bowel examination with the enema in 26 patients; the latter gave relevant additional information in half their patients. In a comparison of the oral technique with the double contrast small bowel enema in 43 patients with Crohn's disease,[26] intubation was found to demonstrate pathology more clearly and to delineate the proximal extension of disease more accurately. Fistulae were shown equally well by both modalities.

TECHNICAL CONSIDERATIONS

Distension

Is distension desirable? The undistended jejunum, as usually presented in a small bowel follow-through (SBFT), shows a feathery mucosal pattern of crisscrossing radiolucent channels which are replaced by a circular arrangement of folds as the lumen distends. According to Haworth and colleagues,[27] its diameter should not exceed 25 mm in the normal adult. Others[28] regard 30 mm as the normal diameter limit.

The SBE method increases the upper limit of diameter normality to a degree that will depend on injection speed and quantity. Dilatation as a sign of disease is not as obvious as in the SBFT, in which fold pattern change as well as diameter increase attracts attention.

A number of valuable advantages compensate for this flaw of the SBE.

A. The uniformly spaced circular arrangement of folds which replaces the crisscross pattern in small bowel distension makes accurate measurement possible (see further on).

B. In the SBFT, owing to the superimposition of contracted loops, fold intersection frequently gives a false impression of fine nodulation (Fig. 11–1). This is avoided in the SBE.

C. Small mucosal nodules are easily missed unless the lumen is distended (Fig. 11–2).

D. Short narrowed segments can be overlooked in a SBFT until they have progressed to cause proximal dilatation. They are recognized in an earlier stage against the distended background of the SBE (Fig. 11–3).

Transradiation of Loops

In the stomach or colon filled with barium of approximately 100% W/V only lesions demonstrated in profile are visible unless compression is employed. If barium density is reduced, filling defects in the lumen may be shown without compression, although there may be some loss of detail. This difficulty has been resolved by the double contrast method of examination, now commonly used in the stomach and colon.

The situation is more complex in the small bowel, where lumen visibility is influenced by overlap of loops and by the degree of loop filling as well as by the density of the barium suspension used. With greater distension, crowding of loops must increase within the limited space of the peritoneal cavity. In the case of the SBE two or even three loops may become superimposed and compression may no longer be able to isolate segments, although the combined volume to be transradiated can be reduced.

In the well-filled loops of the SBE the density level of instilled barium is crucial, a fact stressed by Sellink.[22] Yet even an optimal combination of x-ray exposure and barium density adjusted to the body thickness of the patient may fail to outline with sufficient clarity an intraluminal lesion where superimposition of filled loops exists (Fig. 11–4). Given the unavoidable overlap characteristic of the SBE, the combined small bowel diameter can amount to 5 to 7 cm, comparable to the transradiation requirements found in the stomach or colon. Thus a double contrast form of examination seems equally necessary in the small bowel. Compression of double contrast–filled overlapping loops will reduce patient thickness and combined lumen diameter, and therefore will improve detail (Fig. 11–5).

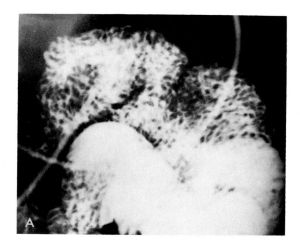

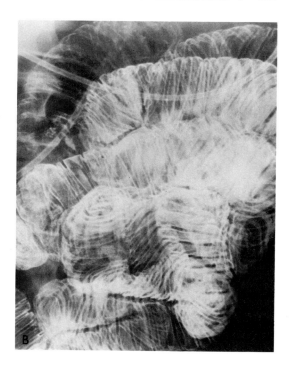

FIGURE 11–1

A. Intersection of superimposed folds in contracted loops produces a false impression of nodularity.

B. Distension and double contrast demonstrate normal appearance and absence of nodules.

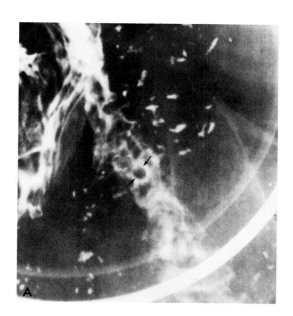

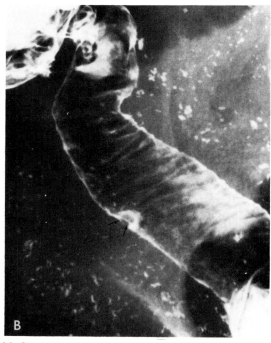

FIGURE 11–2

A. Collapsed terminal ileum. Arrows indicate a small polyp.

B. Distension and air double contrast (by pneumocolon) clearly demonstrate the small adenomatous polyp. (Courtesy of Herbert Y. Kressel, M.D., Philadelphia.)

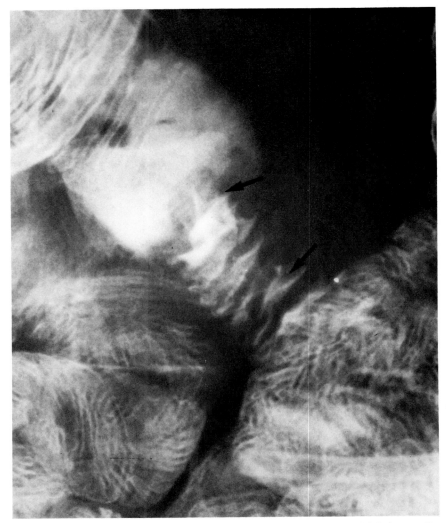

FIGURE 11–3 Short segment of early Crohn's disease in lower jejunum which is nondistensible with swollen folds. Such a lesion would not be recognized in the nondistended small intestine.

Double Contrast Agents

The term double contrast implies the delineation of the barium-coated mucosal surface against a radiolucent contrast agent distending the lumen, making possible the recognition and study of structures en face (Fig. 11–6) as well as in profile.

Water and air have been the most frequently used radiolucent materials for distension.

A. *Water.* Sellink[22] often introduces 600 ml or more of water after barium has reached the distal ileum. This will produce more adequate distension of ileal loops at a desired level of contrast medium dilution, but a true state of double contrast is confined to the jejunum where it may last less than 1 minute. Not only does water wash the barium rapidly from

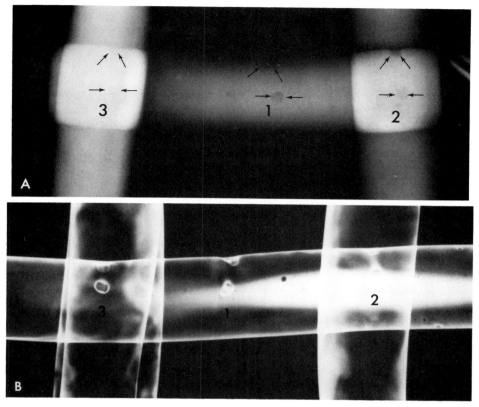

FIGURE 11–4

   A. A rubber tube (2 cm in diameter) was fitted with pairs of 3 mm nodules at three sites, placed to project them en face and in profile; it was filled with barium of varying concentration. It was crossed by three additional tubes filled with the same barium suspension, arranged so that x-ray imaging of one pair of nodules required the transradiation of only one tube; of the other pair, of two tubes; and of the third, of three tubes. The barium concentation and the x-ray kilovoltage were repeatedly changed. No satisfactory image of all three nodule pairs could be obtained on one film (see best example).

   B. Same experimental situation, but using double contrast with MC. All three nodule pairs are clearly shown.

FIGURE 11–5 Effect of compression on double contrast distended loops. Area 1 shows a single noncompressed segment; area 2 shows two superimposed segments with compression (segments outlined by dots).

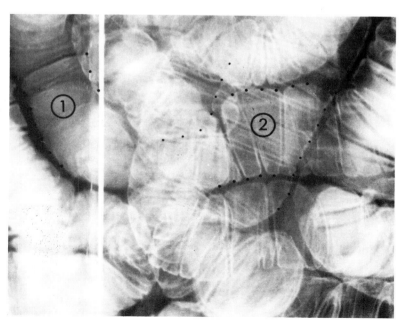

the mucosa, but excessive dilution with water leads to disintegration of the barium suspension.[22]

B.   *Air.*   Air is an ideal double contrast medium in the stomach or colon, but its use in the small bowel presents problems.

   1.   Air bubbles can cause confusion, and excessive density differences may be difficult to interpret.[22]

   2.   Air does not propel barium through the small bowel. Although it excites strong peristaltic activity, this serves only its own rapid advance without appreciably moving the barium suspension,[29] which remains in dependent pools separated from the anterior bowel wall.

Nevertheless, the double contrast study of the terminal ileum can in many cases be achieved by no means other than air. It may be introduced from above by duodenal tube after barium has reached the cecum; via the rectum (Fig. 11–2) by the method of Kellet and associates[30] (see Chapter 12, Figures 12–3 and 12–4), or as an extension of the double contrast barium enema (Fig. 12–10). As far as the greater part of the small bowel is concerned, the introduction of air will not produce a double contrast examination in the full sense. As in the colon, a vertical x-ray beam through air- and barium-filled loops may fail to demonstrate small lesions submerged in a barium pool or may show them inadequately against the background of pooled barium. In the colon this is overcome by taking opposing lateral decubitus views with a horizontal beam. This cannot be usefully applied to the small bowel where the lateral decubitus position increases loop crowding, and the alteration of loop distribution within the abdomen in response to the change of position would render orientation between decubitus film pairs an impossible task (Fig. 11–7).

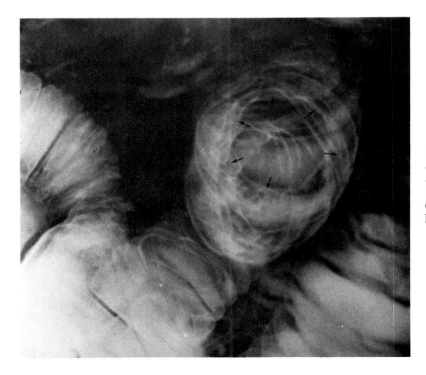

FIGURE 11–6   A segment of jejunum in double contrast distension is seen end-on. Barium coats the mucosa (*arrows*); the lumen is translucent.

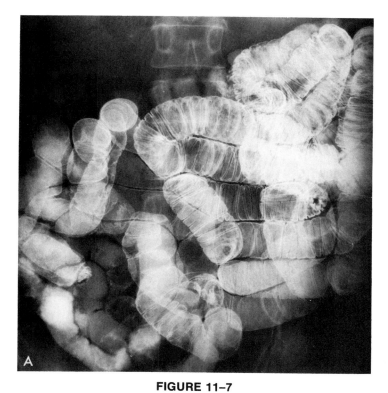

FIGURE 11–7

A. Double contrast overview of entire small intestine.

B. Patient turned on side; horizontal ray film. Very few fluid levels. Loops have become crowded together, and their relative position has changed.

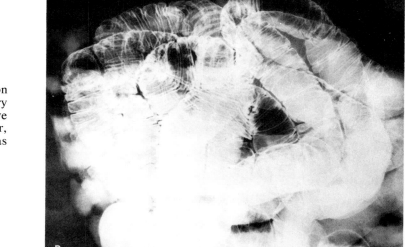

Flocculation

Manufacturers' additives hold barium in suspension by giving a protective coating to individual particles. Coating prevents particle-to-particle contact.[31] Nevertheless, in the presence of mucin even protected particles can show mucoprotein absorption, and such altered particles will agglomerate into "flocs." Flocculated barium is no longer capable of adherence to mucosal surfaces. The degree of degradation of a barium suspension in the presence of flocculation depends on the amount of coatable, unaltered barium left over. Radiologically, a mild degree of flocculation would show a granular pattern, still capable of imaging, although of suboptimal quality. (Fig. 11–8). A severe degree of flocculation will lead to the gradual accumulation of larger amounts of altered barium (Fig. 11–9), no longer depicting surfaces, but presenting patterns that reflect its own physical-chemical change ("segmentation," "moulage").

A direct relationship could be demonstrated in vitro[32] between the degree of flocculation, the relative quantity of interacting fluid, and the time of exposure to it. In our experience the comparatively small quantities of barium intermittently leaving the stomach in a SBFT examination, and passing rather slowly through the small intestine, are readily overwhelmed by flocculation-inducing small bowel contents in even mild forms of steatorrhea. In the SBE the larger quantity of barium introduced almost as a bolus and pushed along rapidly will be able to coat the mucosa and produce images before flocculation develops.[33]

When reviewing Sellink's *Atlas,*[23] Wittenberg expressed surprise at the author's lack of interest in flocculation as a radiologic sign. Laws and coworkers[4] have been able to show lack of correlation between the degree of flocculation and the degree of steatorrhea or villous atrophy. In fact, patients passing as much as 20 g of fat per day did not have flocculation, while others with normal fat contents did. Miller and Skucas[35] also consider flocculation an unreliable sign.

Though flocculation will eventually occur even with the SBE in the presence of abnormal fluid material, its deferment allows imaging of the whole small bowel mucosa to be completed first. Information on morphologic normality or disease can thus be obtained.

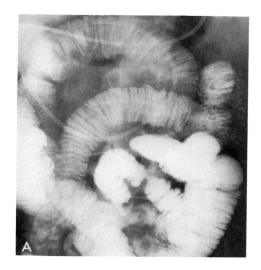

A. Jejunum, start of MC injection. Granular pattern of the barium suspension.

FIGURE 11-8 Mild celiac disease.

B. Later development of slight flocculation in the jejunum. Granularity of barium suspension in ileum.

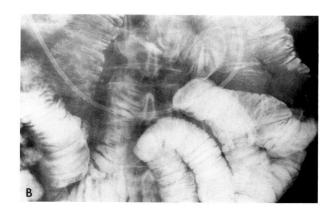

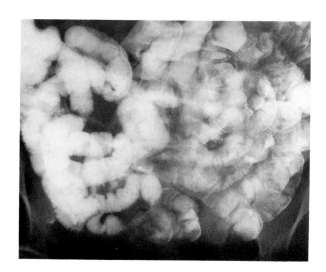

FIGURE 11-9 Severe celiac disease showing more pronounced barium flocculation, approaching the maximum found in this form of SBE.

Methyl Cellulose (MC)

Historical Review. Having found the "water flush" method[17, 18] to produce too much dilution of barium in the ileum, Trickey and coworkers (1963) searched for a "flush" that would not readily mix with barium, that would be able to propel the barium toward the colon, and that would distend the lumen while rendering it radiolucent.[36]

They introduced a 0.7 per cent solution of water containing hydroxyethylcellulose with a wetting agent, a proprietary preparation no longer available. A 1 per cent suspension of methyl cellulose MC in water had been employed as a contrast agent for barium enemas,[37] and it was claimed that removal of barium coating from the bowel wall was minimized in this way. For their method of double contrast SBE Gmünder and Wirth[38] used a "flush" of MC, 2 teaspoonfuls in 900 ml of water, following the injection of only 50 ml of Micropaque.*

MC in the SBE. During the last 12 years the author has employed a 0.5 per cent solution of MC in water for the SBE examination. MC has the following advantages:

1. Employed with a compatible barium suspension, e.g., Micropaque liquid* or reconstituted powder,† it shows a very low degree of diffusivity compared with that of water (Fig. 11–10).

2. It efficiently propels an unbroken and gradually diluting barium column toward the cecum and will overtake it only if a very inadequate quantity of barium has been injected (Fig. 11–11).

3. Small bowel loops distended with MC remain in a state of relaxation and low activity and retain their double contrast pattern for 15 to 20 minutes (Fig. 11–12).

4. The combination of Micropaque and 0.5 per cent MC appears to resist flocculation long enough for the examination to be completed.

5. On entry into the colon the desiccation-resistant MC and barium mixture provokes rapid evacuation.

PREPARATION. It is essential to use MC powder of correct viscosity, correctly prepared. We employ methyl cellulose (USP or BP) giving a viscosity of 350 to 550 centistokes in a 2 per cent solution at 20°C. We prepare our solution by adding 10 g of MC to about 400 ml of water at 85 to 90°C, stirring well until the powder is fully wetted and dispersed and no aggregates are seen.[39] Cold water with ice cubes is then added, with continued stirring until a total quantity of 1.6 liters is reached and all dispersed powder is in solution. It is advisable to store this mixture at 4°C for 24 to 36 hours, by which time viscosity will have stabilized. It is taken out of refrigeration just before use, when 400 ml of warm water is stirred in to render the solution comfortably cool. Refrigeration until use is important, as MC solutions lack fungistatic activity; in the refrigerated state the solution can be safely stored for several days. No toxic effects have been reported.

---

*Nicholas Laboratories, Slough, England
†Picker Co., Cleveland, Ohio, U.S.A.

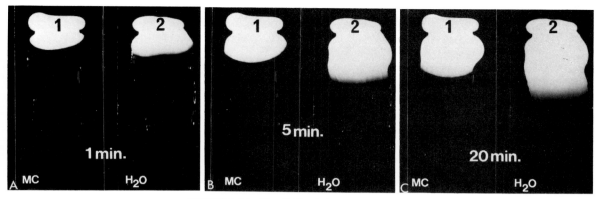

FIGURE 11-10   Diffusivity experiment.

Undiluted Micropaque (MP) placed at ends of slides 1 and 2. Slide 1 was covered with 1/2% MC, and slide 2 with water in amounts sufficient to make contact with the barium. Both slides were left undisturbed and were photographed at intervals.

A.   At 1 minute the interface between the barium and MC and water is maintained, with no diffusion of barium into the liquid.

B.   At 5 minutes there is lack of sharpness of the interface in slide 2 owing to diffusion of barium into the water.

C.   At 20 minutes there is further lack of sharpness in slide 2, while the interface between the barium and MC in side 1 remains sharp, indicating that the barium has not diffused into the MC.

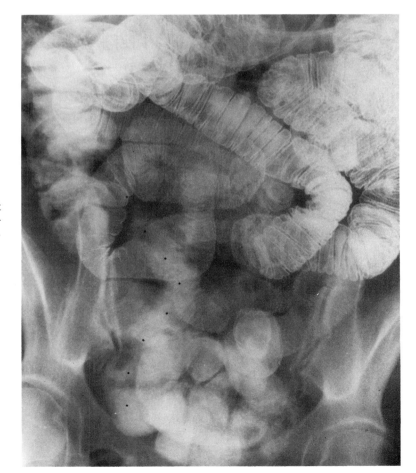

FIGURE 11-11   Insufficient barium left to outline the terminal ileum adequately (*dots*).

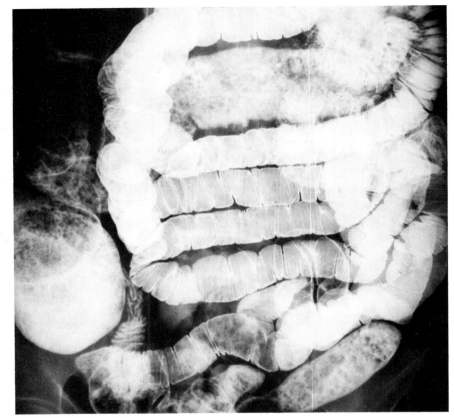

FIGURE 11–12 Late film of a normal examination, showing persistence of double contrast effect throughout the small bowel.

THE DOUBLE CONTRAST SMALL BOWEL ENEMA (SBE)

In the last 10 years we have performed approximately 1000 examinations by this method.

Patient Preparation

We agree that a clean right colon is important.[12, 22] The presence of feces in the cecum is often associated with reflux of fecal material into the terminal ileum, and it tends to retard the ileal passage of barium. Food material in the ileum increases the barium requirement to wash the food through before the double contrast effect can be obtained (Fig. 11–13).

Four teaspoons of a saline laxative in cold ginger ale are taken on the two nights before the examination. A nonresidue liquid diet is given on the day before the study — synthetic juices, carbonated drinks, Sanka, or tea (no milk), clear broth, gelatin dessert, not too much sugar. Nothing is permitted by mouth on the day of the examination. The reduction of normal fluid and cell outpouring into the small bowel lumen as a result of diet restriction[1] will improve the quality of the examination. Drugs that de-

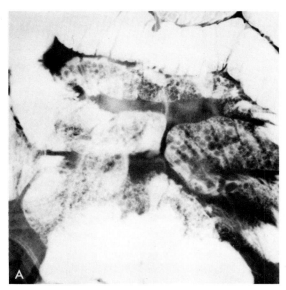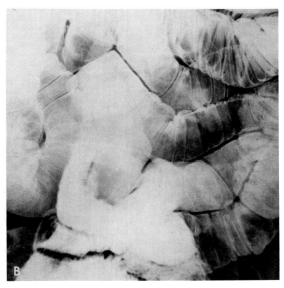

FIGURE 11–13 Unprepared patient.

A. Large amount of food material in the ileum.
B. Double contrast effect after wash-through (cecum lying deep in the pelvis).

crease bowel activity, e.g., tranquilizers or anticholinergics, should be discontinued.

Intubation

We advise the oral administration of 20 mg of metoclopramide in tablet or syrup form 15 minutes before the examination to shorten intubation time.[41] We believe that it also promotes the onward passage of injected barium and prevents excessive distension of the small bowel during injection. Partial anesthesia of the throat with a brief spraying of Cetacaine* is recommended.

We have used a modified Bilbao-Dotter tube.† It is 135 cm long and has only an end-hole. The flexible, rotationally rigid guide is slightly shorter, has a curved end, and is Teflon-coated. The catheter system is thoroughly lubricated inside and out with a silicone spray. We prefer intubation through the mouth, with the patient sitting and encouraged to make swallowing movements. Occasionally it is necessary to pass the tube while the patient sips water. If several small bowel examinations are to be grouped into one session, we leave it to a nurse to introduce the tube in an anteroom; this is done without the guide, with the patient lying

---

*Cetylite, Long Island City, N.Y.
†SBD-2 Herlinger Modification. Cook, Inc., Bloomington, Ind.

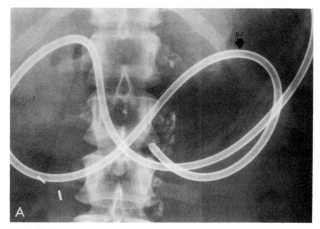

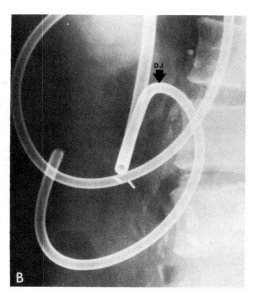

FIGURE 11-14 Tube introduced beyond the duodenojejunal junction (DJ).

A.   Frontal view.
B.   Lateral view.

on the right side and encouraged to advance the tube slowly beyond the expected level of the gastric fundus.

We aim to position the end of the tube beyond the duodenojejunal junction (Fig. 11-14) in order to reduce the likelihood of reflux into the stomach.

INTUBATION PROBLEMS

Tube Coiled in the Fundus (Fig. 11-15).   The tube is withdrawn until its tip lies at the cardia. The guide is then introduced fully, and the patient is turned toward the right. The knob at the end of the guide is turned to bend

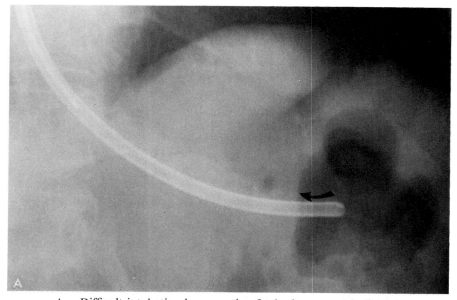

A.   Difficult intubation because tip of tube is arrested in fundus.

FIGURE 11-15

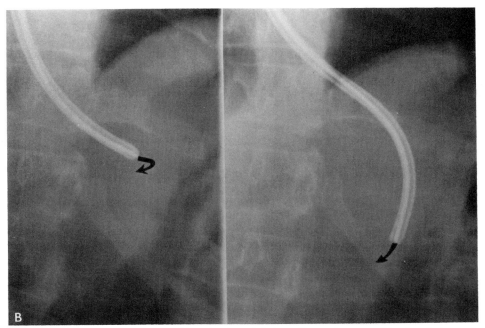

B. Tube is withdrawn, and guide wire is twirled to direct tip toward body of stomach.

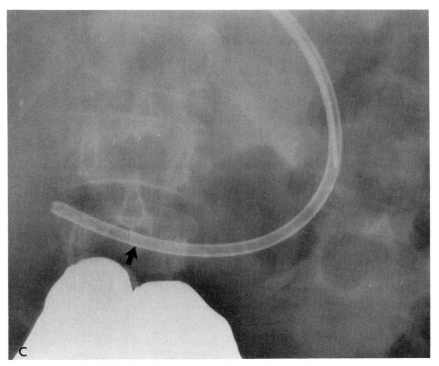

C. Tube is advanced over the guide into the antrum.

the tube toward the body of the stomach. It is essential to advance the tube at the right moment, and as soon as it passes in the direction of the body of the stomach to advance the tube itself over the wire guide.

Tube Doubled Back in the Antrum (Fig. 11–16 *A* to *C*). The tube is withdrawn slowly while the guide is advanced until the tube end flicks forward again. The guide is then pulled back and held at the level of the angulus. The gloved hand applies craniad pressure to the greater curvature of the antrum to establish a caudad tube concavity during the advance of the tube through the pylorus and the first part of the duodenum. Should it still be difficult to find the way out of the stomach the guide wire is pulled out, and 50 to 100 ml of air are injected as a bolus, with the patient turned well to the left. Air excites gastric peristalsis and will outline the pyloric area.

Tube Arrested at the Superior Duodenal Flexure. The patient should turn sharply to the left in order to open up the hairpin bend. The guide is held in midstomach, the gloved right hand firmly pressing against the left rib cage to try to prevent bulging of the tube toward the fundus during further introduction.

Tube Arrested at the Inferior Duodenal Flexure. If possible the guide is advanced beyond the superior flexure. The left hand helps the tube end round the flexure while the right hand presses against the left rib cage.

In the absence of real difficulty (patient's noncooperation, organic disease, hernias) intubation should succeed every time and should take 5 to 10 minutes. Occasionally in uncooperative patients, nasal intubation may be necessary. Intubation after gastric surgery presents few problems as long as the type of operation is known.

When intubation is arrested at unexpected levels it is important to investigate the cause by injecting a small amount of barium. In one patient, a duodenal leiomyoma was discovered in this way (Fig. 11–16*D*)

Barium Injection

Barium injection is done with 20 ml syringes at the rate of 80 to 100 ml/min. The barium used is Micropaque, either as powder suspended in an equal volume of water (85% W/V) or (in Great Britain and continental Europe) as undiluted suspension. A total of 150 to 200 ml is normally injected, somewhat less if the patient is very thin or has had small bowel resections; more if the patient is stout or if the diagnostic problem is specifically related to the distal ileum. Considerably more may have to be given (up to 400 ml) if there is small bowel dilatation with fluid excess.

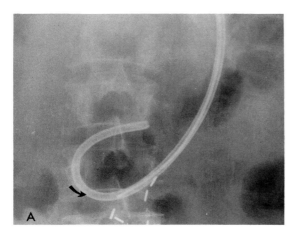

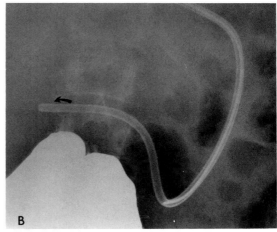

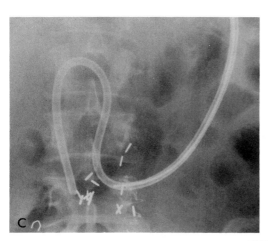

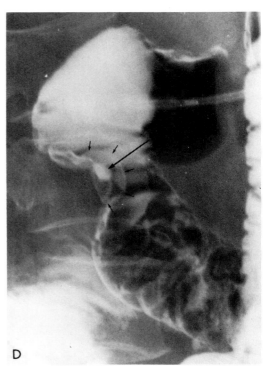

FIGURE 11–16

   A. The tip of the tube is coiled in the antrum. This is remedied by withdrawing the tube while advancing the guide wire until the tip of the tube flicks forward.

   B. The gloved hand applies craniad pressure along the greater curvature of the antrum in order to prevent the tube from coiling.

   C. The tube will then pass through the pylorus into the duodenum.

   D. Duodenal leiomyoma discovered as it gave rise to intubation difficulty. Small arrows outline its mucosal surface, the larger arrow its central ulcer.

Barium must not be injected at a rate that will cause jejunal distension. The aim is to achieve forward movement of an uninterrupted column of barium through the nondistended small bowel, and the speed of the injection must be adjusted to this purpose. Introduction of barium is discontinued when ileum overlying the left iliac bone starts to become opacified. If there is any indication of increased fluid contents (Fig. 11–17) the injection of barium is continued well into the midileum.

MC Injection

The comfortably cool solution of 0.5 per cent MC is introduced by 50 ml syringes, the usual injection rate being 100 to 150 ml/min. This is continued until a sufficient degree of transradiancy and filling have been achieved in the distal and terminal ileum (Fig. 11–18). Should barium reach the sigmoid colon before this (transit in the colon is rapid!) it may be necessary to interrupt the examination briefly and place the patient on a bedpan.

Normally 1 to 2 liters of MC solution are injected. The tube is withdrawn as soon as sufficient MC has been given.

Filming

While we observe the progress of the barium column by intermittent fluoroscopy, we do not normally expose films until the MC solution is injected. Most films are taken with compression, positioned and adjusted by fluoroscopy. The jejunum and upper ileum are usually best shown with the patient turned slightly to the right, the more distal ileum with the patient turned to the left. The terminal ileum can cause difficulty. Because barium in the cecum may interfere with visualization, it may be important to film the cecum during passage of the first bolus.

A not-to-be-neglected part of the examination is the observation of peristaltic activity, best seen before distension with MC. Most important is the careful palpation of all accessible loops. We particularly evaluate the *mobility* of small bowel loops to identify any adhesions or adherence due to disease and their *pliability*, i.e., the ability to change shape in response to palpation and compression. Mural infiltration will stiffen loops and reduce or abolish pliability. An examination without undue complexity will last 15 to 25 minutes, including intubation, and will require about 14 spot films. A prone overhead view on a 14/17 film is taken after fluoroscopy. In the case of obstruction or in adynamic states it will often be necessary to follow up with later spot and overhead films, and such an examination may not be completed for 24 hours or more.

A successful SBE will present the whole of the small bowel in double contrast (Fig. 11–18), although the distal ileum may be seen in a just sufficiently transulucent and distended state. It will give measurable evidence of normality or of disease.

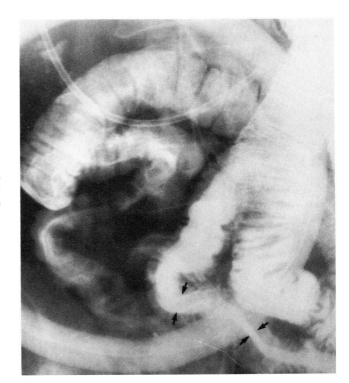

FIGURE 11–17 Fluid accumulation within small bowel, as shown by streaming of barium within the lumen (*arrows*) and by increasing dilution.

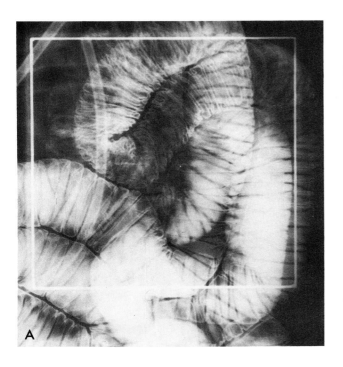

FIGURE 11–18 A successful normal double contrast examination by SBE.

A. Jejunum.

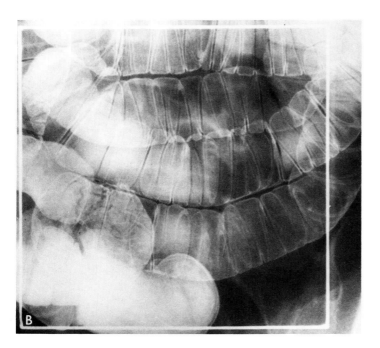

B. Upper ileum.

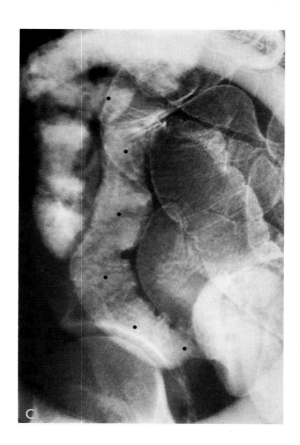

C. Terminal ileum.

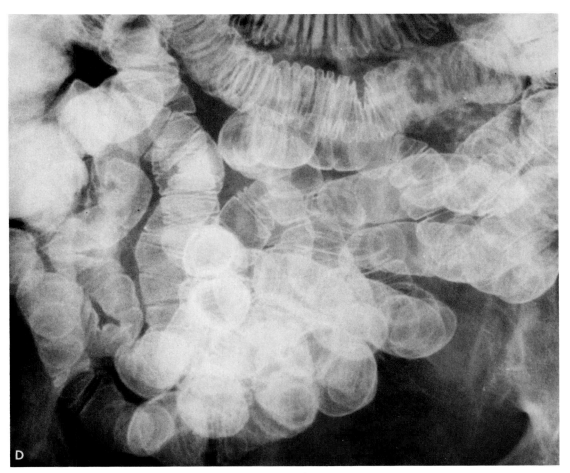

D. Overview.

Problems

Misjudged Quantities. To the experienced examiner it is advantageous to be able to adapt to each patient's problem and anatomy the quantities and injection speeds of barium and MC. By the same token, this facility can lead to examination failure.

If too little barium has been introduced, visualization of the distal ileum will suffer and MC may actually overtake the barium column. Once this has occurred it is impossible to salvage the examination (Fig. 11–11). If too much barium has been given, filling of the colon may occur before the double contrast effect has reached the more distal ileum (Fig. 11–19). Evacuating the colon before continuing with the injection of MC may salvage such an examination. If one is to err in matters of barium quantity, it is clearly preferable to give too much rather than too little.

Reflux into the Stomach. This can be a real problem (Fig. 11–20). Intubation beyond the ligament of Treitz reduces, but does not abolish, its incidence. An overrapid or uneven rate of injection seems to provoke reflux, and once begun it tends to continue.[23] It is important to prevent it, since sudden projectile vomiting without any warning is the likely outcome. If it is not possible to intubate the jejunum we keep the injection rate at a much lower level and tilt the x-ray table slightly head-up. At the first sign of any reflux we inject more slowly still, turn the patient well to the left, and tilt the table up further.

Slowing the injection rate means less complete filling of the loops and will compromise the quality of the examination (Fig. 11–20). A balloon catheter for duodenal intubation which has recently been described[42] may well overcome the reflux problem, but it has not yet become available.

Ileal Loops in the Pelvis. We advise patients not to empty their bladders immediately before the examination (the introduction of the desiccation-resistant MC solution will not add to their discomfort). It is only too frequent, however, to find ileal loops lying low in the pelvis, inaccessible to compression or palpation. For a successful examination we must achieve a double contrast appearance throughout these loops while attempting, through compression, head-down tilt of the table, and prone-positioning of the patient, to displace the loops out of the pelvis.

Food Material in Distal Ileum. Adequate patient preparation will reduce its incidence. If food matter is found, the situation can be remedied provided there is sufficient barium available to wash the material into the colon (Fig. 11–13) and still leave enough for double contrast coating.

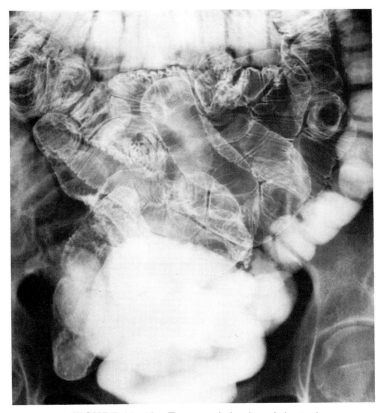

FIGURE 11–19 Too much barium injected.

Double contrast is seen in jejunum and upper ileum, but ileal loops in pelvis are obscured by barium that has reached the sigmoid.

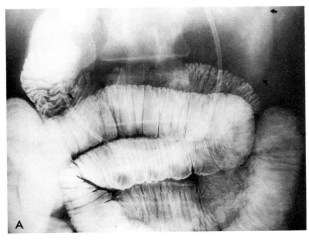

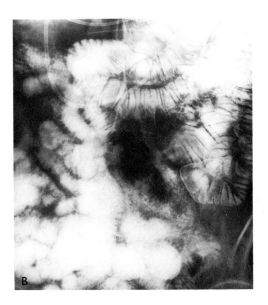

FIGURE 11–20 Reflux into stomach.

A.   Reflux, mostly of MC (*arrows*).
B.   Slowing of MC injection to avoid further reflux produces suboptimal demonstration of the ileum.

SBE Through a Miller-Abbott (MA) Tube

Patients in whom an MA tube has been inserted in the clinical management of small bowel obstruction may require a barium study to demonstrate the level, degree, and nature of the obstructing lesion. The MA tube can be successfully used for the introduction of contrast material provided attention is given to the following points:

A.   The MA tube should lie as close as possible to the site of obstruction. At the very least it must reach 6 inches into the jejunum to insure that all side holes are beyond the ligament of Treitz.

B.   The balloon must be deflated.

C.   Since the lumen of the long tube is narrow, it will be necessary to inject a barium suspension of reduced viscosity. Micropaque powder should be suspended 4 parts in 5 parts of water, giving a W/V concentration of only 75 per cent.

D.   Enough barium must be introduced to reach the site of obstruction, overinjection being preferable to an insufficient amount.

E.   MC injection is begun only after barium has reached the obstructing lesion to delineate the features of the lesion more clearly. In the presence of pre-existing distension and considerable fluid retention the addition of MC would serve no purpose.

NORMAL APPEARANCES

Characteristics

The combination of distension, double contrast, and abdominal compression makes it possible to study fold shapes and to measure a number of parameters (Fig. 11–21).

Fold Shapes.   Valvulae conniventes are found throughout the small bowel, but can be less pronounced and occasionally absent in the ileum. We do not consider their accentuated presence in the ileum ("jejunization") to be of significance. With the bowel distended, these folds run fairly straight across the long axis, their sides parallel, joining the bowel wall in the form of "rounded corners" (Fig. 11–21A).[23] At times, more often in the ileum than in the jejunum, a few of the folds crowd together on the concave aspect of a bend in a bowel loop. Such triangular fold patterns can be found in the ileum, even where segments are straight, when their direction of convergence is seen to alternate (Fig. 11–21B).

Fold Thickness.   Jejunal folds are normally 1.7 to 2.0 mm thick, ileal folds 1.4 to 1.7 mm thick (Fig. 11–21A to C). Thickness does not vary with lumen diameter. Fold thickness is considered pathologic if it exceeds 2.5 cm in the jejunum and 2 mm in the ileum. Abnormal narrowness of folds is not considered of pathologic significance.

Number of Folds.   In the more distended, possibly somewhat elongated, small bowel in this form of SBE, the number of circular folds per inch of length was less than that reported by Sellink.[23] We found four to six folds per inch in the jejunum, and three to five folds in the ileum (Fig. 11–21D to E). In the occasional patient in whom small bowel tonus appeared increased, particularly in young persons, a greater number of folds was seen in what was probably shortened bowel (Fig. 11–21F).

Fold Height. In this respect, jejunum and ileum differ significantly. The usual fold height varies between 3.5 and 7 mm in the jejunum and between 2.0 and 3.5 mm in the ileum, the height decrease being a gradual process. However, fold height has been found to vary considerably within the same segment of bowel, and height measurement has not been of diagnostic value (Fig. 11–21 A, C, and D).

Lumen Diameter. In this form of SBE, diameters for the upper jejunum are between 3.0 and 4.0 cm., 2.5 to 3.5 cm in the lower jejunum, and 2.0 to 2.8 cm in the ileum. Diameters are considered abnormal if they exceed 4.5 cm in the upper jejunum, 4.0 cm in the mid- small bowel, and 3.0 cm in the ileum. Care must be taken not to measure diameters in front of a peristaltic wave.

Wall Thickness. Wall thickness is considered measurable if two luminal surfaces are seen to be strictly parallel over at least 4 cm during abdominal compression. We then consider the loops to lie in the same plane and think it justified to regard the distance between the two mucosal surfaces as representing the combined thickness of the two bowel walls. Of normal patients, 75 per cent showed a wall thickness of 1.0 to 1.5 mm, 12.5 per cent of 1.6 to 2.0 mm, and 12.5 per cent below 1.0 mm. This measurement was found to be the same throughout the small bowel (Fig. 11–21 E and G). A wall thickness greater than 2 mm is considered abnormal.

Length of the Small Bowel. No remotely accurate estimate can be made of this three-dimensional reality on the basis of two-dimensional x-ray films. There is no doubt that individuals vary enormously in this respect and that racial differences exist. Muscle tone is likely to be an important factor. Withdrawing an MA tube under x-ray control will show that approximately two thirds of it can be pulled back through an increasingly telescoping gut before the tip of the tube even begins to move back.

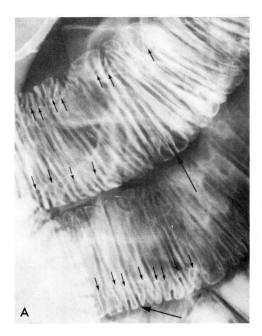

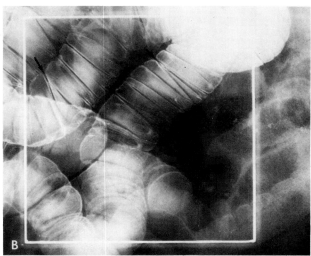

FIGURE 11–21 Normal appearances.

A. Jejunal folds of normal thickness and height (*small arrows*). Large arrows show "rounded corners."

B. Triangular arrangement of the fold pattern in parts of the ileum.

C. Ileal folds of normal thickness and height (*small arrows*). Large arrows show "rounded corners."

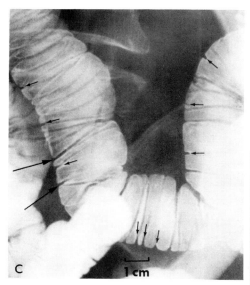

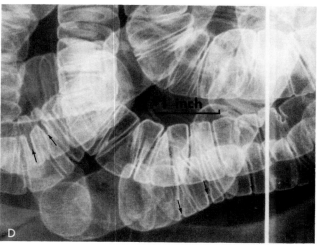

D. Mid-small bowel fold height and number per inch of length.

E. Number of jejunal folds per inch of length. Wall thickness measurement.

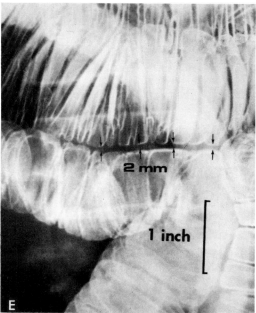

F. Small bowel shortened with normal folds close together. Young person, with no evidence of disease in the shortened gut; Crohn's disease, terminal ileum.

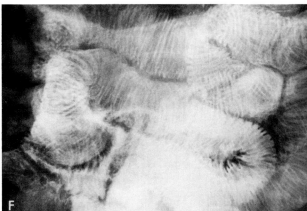

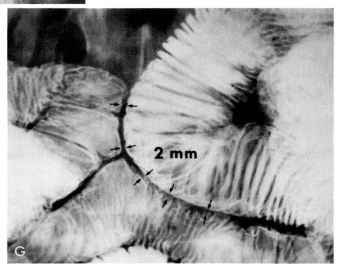

G. Measurement of bowel wall thickness with a normal value of 2 mm.

Variations

Positional Variant. While rotational anomalies of development are rarely seen, we have not infrequently encountered patients with a normally placed jejunum in whom the ileum was in the right upper abdomen. In such a case the terminal ileum had to descend vertically to reach the cecum. This positional variant makes it more difficult to gage the correct amount of barium to be injected.

Fixation. Developmentally premature fixation of the cecum is rare. More frequently found is a freely mobile cecum, either folded upward, in which case the terminal ileum will enter from the right and below, or a cecum prolapsed into the pelvic cavity. In the latter case it may be difficult to demonstrate the terminal ileum fully once the cecum has filled with barium. With this in mind we always attempt to record terminal ileum opacification by the initial barium bolus, using later films taken during the MC wash-through to show mucosal detail (Fig. 11–22).

Lymph Follicles. Numerous 2 to 3 mm rounded elevations may normally be present in the terminal ileum of children and adolescents (Fig. 12–10*B*).

Hypertonicity. The entire small bowel may present a shortened appearance with folds of normal thickness close together. This may occur in the absence of disease, particularly in young people. We have also found it in the normal small bowel proximal to a segment of Crohn's disease (Fig. 11–21*F*).

Meckel's Diverticulum. This is found in 1 to 4 per cent of autopsies, but its roentgen demonstration with barium is uncommon.[43] Meckel's di-

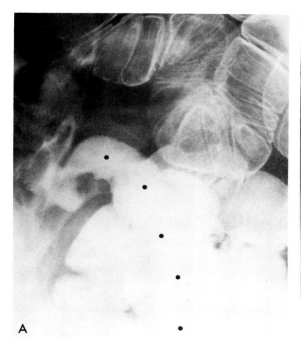
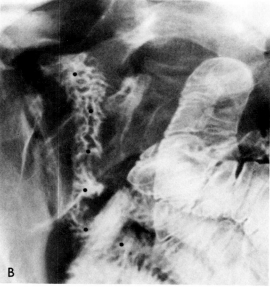

FIGURE 11–22

A. Terminal ileum recorded during passage of initial bolus.
B. Lateral view of terminal ileum after wash-through of barium.

verticulum is situated on the antimesenteric surface within 90 cm of the ileocecal valve. We have diagnosed only one case by the SBE. It made itself unmistakable by retaining its barium-filled density during the development of double contrast in the ileum (Fig. 11–23).

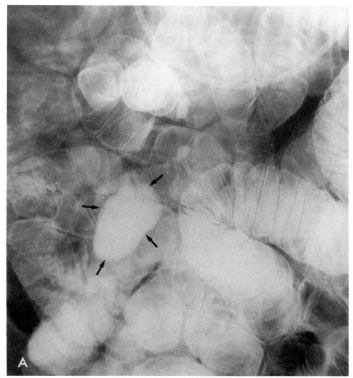

FIGURE 11–23 A Meckel's diverticulum retains barium.

A. During early wash-through with MC.

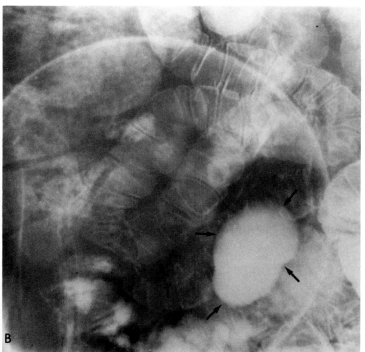

B. Late in the wash-through phase.

THE SMALL BOWEL ENEMA IN DISEASE

Examples rather than complete descriptions of disease processes will be presented. The aim is to show the versatility and increased accuracy of the double contrast method and its relevance to clinical management. Its application to pediatric diagnosis is not included.

Malabsorption State

The term malabsorption refers to the failure of transport of digested or maldigested particles as well as vitamins and minerals from the gut lumen into body fluids. Most generalized small bowel diseases will be accompanied by a degree of malabsorption which may be accentuated by actual loss of nutrients due to increased secretions. The disturbance of absorption is usually multifactorial, although in mild forms of even generalized small bowel disease it may be limited to selected materials. More localized intestinal disease will on the whole affect only substances that are normally absorbed at those levels. In most conditions, steatorrhea, the disturbance of fat absorption, is the distinctive clinical marker of malabsorption.

STEATORRHEA

The amount of fat excreted is expressed as grams per day. Reported upper limits of normality vary between 5 g[44] and 12 g.[45] The fact that the fecal fat content will vary with the amount of dietary fat taken may explain this considerable difference. According to Losowsky and coworkers,[1] a fat excretion of no more than 7 per cent of intake would more accurately express the upper limit of normality. It has also been shown that fecal fat excretion relates to intake in patients who have steatorrhea. In this way steatorrhea may be masked by a low-fat diet and accentuated by an increased intake. Clearly a single measurement of fecal fat content or a radiologist's attention to possible flocculation of barium in a single examination cannot provide useful information on which to exclude or to base a diagnosis of steatorrhea.

The clinical diagnosis of steatorrhea requires the chemical examination of feces after diet stabilization. Flocculation of barium, as has already been discussed, relates to fecal fat in an unreliable way.[4, 35] Moreover, it may be caused by other abnormal fluid contents of the small bowel, e.g., mucus, inflammatory exudate, or increased digestive juices.

Not only is flocculation an unreliable indicator of steatorrhea, but it will make it impossible — owing to the associated reduction of the imaging ability of the barium — to discharge the real purpose of diagnostic radiology in this situation. In malabsorption states the clinician should look to the radiologist for the demonstration of small bowel morphology to the highest possible degree of accuracy, and thereby to exclude gross morphologic abnormalities as the cause of the malabsorption.

In order to simplify radiologic diagnosis, several authors have presented useful lists of x-ray findings in steatorrhea.[46-48] A further list is presented here which relates to the increased imaging accuracy of this method of SBE (Table 11-1).

TABLE 11–1   SMALL BOWEL ENEMA IN STEATORRHEA

Radiologic Feature	No Fluid Increase	Fluid Increase
Normal	Maldigestion — bile salt or pancreatic enzyme deficiency Gastric surgery Alactasia	Celiac disease Tropical sprue Dermatitis herpetiformis
Dilatation	Scleroderma Dermatomyositis Pseudo-obstruction	Celiac disease Obstruction Blind loops
Folds Thickened, Straight	Amyloidosis Radiation Ischemia Lymphoma (rarely) Macroglobulinemia	Zollinger-Ellison syndrome Abetalipo-proteinemia
Folds Unevenly Thickened; nodulation	Lymphoid hyperplasia Lymphoma Crohn's disease Whipple's disease Mastocytosis	Lymphangiectasia Giardiasis Whipple's disease (rarely)
Other Structural Lesions	Stricture, blind loop, fistula, resection, diverticulosis	

Celiac Disease

The clinical diagnosis can be difficult. Not every patient will have steatorrhea; some may present with anemia (iron or folate malabsorption) or even osteomalacia. Essential to the diagnosis is the demonstration of subtotal villous atrophy in the jejunum (best confirmed by multiple biopsy), with a clinical and histologic return to normality after a period of total gluten withdrawal. Another important element in the diagnosis is a normal small bowel mucosal pattern, as shown by a double contrast SBE. This is valuable because subtotal villous atrophy may accompany other small bowel disorders associated with malabsorption,[1] in which the SBE will be able to demonstrate an abnormal small bowel surface.

The particular value of the SBE in celiac disease is its ability to complete the imaging of the entire small intestine before significant flocculation can occur, even in severe disease (Fig. 11–24). It will, however, be necessary to inject a larger amount of barium suspension, as in any patient with increased fluid within the bowel.

It has been said that jejunal folds are thickened in celiac disease.[49] Marshak and Lindner[50] have recently explained that folds may appear thickened because of the amount of secretion present. We agree with this observation (Fig. 11–25) and have found circular folds of normal diameter in uncomplicated celiac disease. We have never found evidence of fold *thinning*.

Dilatation can be a feature of celiac disease, and its degree has been shown[4] to correlate well with the severity of steatorrhea (Fig. 11–26). It is, however, by no means a frequent finding.[3]

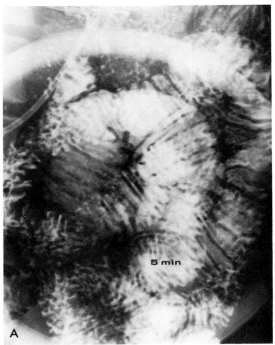

A

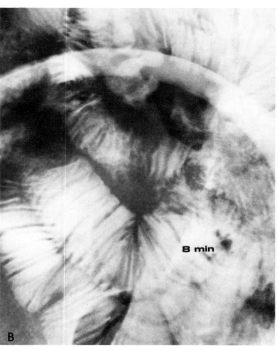

B

FIGURE 11-24 Severe celiac disease.

A. At 5 minutes, adequate imaging of the jejunum.

B. At 8 minutes, ileal detail shown to acceptable standard.

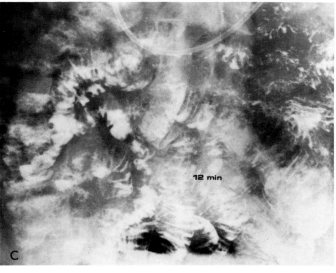

C

C. At 12 minutes, extreme degree of flocculation (as shown by this method); imaging now impossible.

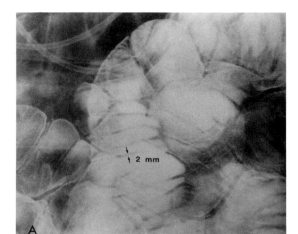

FIGURE 11-25 False impression of fold-thickening in active celiac disease.

A: Initial double contrast film shows straight and normal jejunal folds that measure 2 mm in thickness.

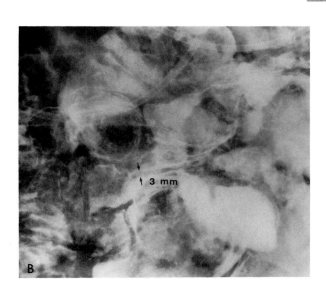

B. A few minutes later, same folds give a thickness measurement of 3 mm.

C. Later, fold outline has become unsharp and uneven; the thickness measurement is now 4 mm.

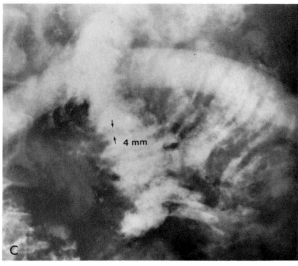

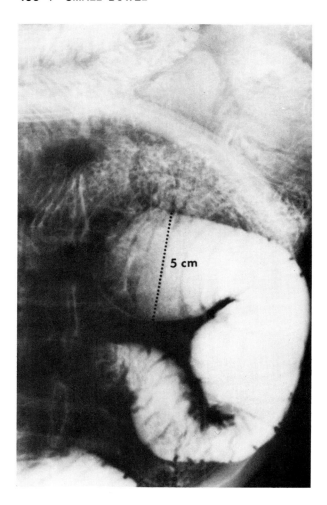

FIGURE 11–26 Severe celiac disease. Jejunum dilated to 5 cm

COMPLICATIONS

Patients with chronic celiac disease may occasionally develop strictures, probably at sites of earlier ulcerations. The relationship of celiac disease to gastrointestinal malignancy has been well documented.[51] A significantly increased incidence of small bowel and esophageal carcinoma occurs in patients with long-established disease who have not adhered strictly to a gluten-free diet. Males are particularly at risk. Lymphoma has long been known to complicate celiac disease, and its prevalence does not seem to relate to the avoidance of gluten-containing foods. It has been suggested[52] that depression of cell-mediated immunity in celiac disease may relate to the high risk of malignancy. Collins and coworkers[53] have presented examples of the radiologic changes that accompany malignancy complicating celiac disease. They stress the premalignant nature of the disease and the opportunity it may provide for the early radiologic detection of tumor, both in the small bowel and esophagus.

Lymphoma (see further on) tends to be diffuse and nodular (Fig. 11–27). Our example of adenocarcinoma (Fig. 11–28) occurred in a male patient with long-established celiac disease and a history of dietary lapses. Numerous strictures and intervening dilatations were found. One of the strictures showed an irregularly nodular mucosal pattern, and carcinoma was found at this site; liver metastases had already occurred.

Tropical Sprue. Jejunal biopsy appearances and SBE findings are the same as in nontropical sprue or celiac disease. Improvement follows folic acid administration, not gluten withdrawal.

Dermatitis Herpetiformis. This shows a distinct association with celiac disease, including its typical histologic changes; there is also a favorable response to gluten withdrawal.[1] X-ray appearances are indistinguishable from those of celiac disease.

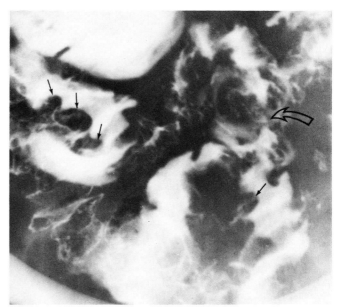

FIGURE 11–27 Lymphoma complicating celiac disease. Arrows indicate nodules in the jejunum. Open arrow to a jejunojejunal fistula.

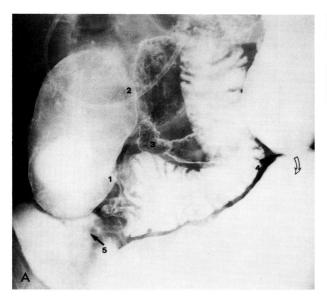
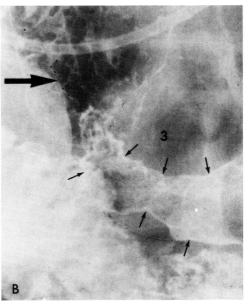

FIGURE 11–28 Long-standing celiac disease.

A. Multiple strictures, probably secondary to ulceration.

B. Stricture 3 presents a nodular surface pattern. Adenocarcinoma found at laparotomy.

Systemic Sclerosis (Scleroderma). The esophagus is commonly affected with changes caused by replacement of the muscular layers with collagen tissue. The small bowel may be involved in the same way. Dilatation, atony, and delayed emptying are more likely to be found in the duodenum and upper jejunum. Although malabsorption may exist, there is no fluid increase or barium flocculation.

Dilated loops may show sacculation (Fig. 11–29*A*) or the "hidebound" small bowel sign,[54] which presents as tightly packed folds of normal thickness within a dilated segment (Fig. 11–29*B*). It occurs in 60 per cent of cases and is most helpful in the differential diagnosis of other conditions that present with an atonic small bowel.

Dermatomyositis. This disorder resembles scleroderma in its involvement of the gastrointestinal tract. Dilatation may be pronounced.

Pseudo-obstruction. This has been defined[1] as a condition with clinical manifestations of small bowel obstruction in the absence of mechanical obstruction. Barium passes through extremely slowly and without visible peristaltic activity. The examination of such patients may commence as a SBE, but this will soon be abandoned and replaced by follow-through filming, which may have to be continued for well over 24 hours.

Amyloidosis. Gastrointestinal involvement is frequent, malabsorption unusual. Uniform fold thickening throughout the small intestine is typical of primary amyloidosis. Scattered, nonuniform amyloid deposits, some of them large, may occur in the secondary form of the disease.

Ischemia. Small bowel ischemia may lead to a range of changes between necrosis and a transient disturbance. If involvement is extensive, long-lasting, and mild, absorption disturbances may appear. More usually it presents as segmental ischemic disease, mostly of the nonocclusive variety. The barium appearances have been described as mild dilatation with fold thickening, often of the "picket fence" type, with spasm, irritability, and scalloping of the contour.[55] A stricture may be the result of incomplete recovery. A recent editorial[56] draws attention to the relationship of

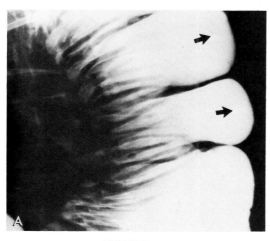
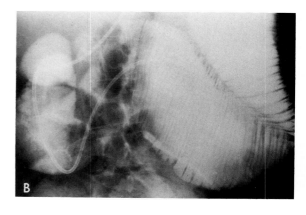

FIGURE 11–29 Two cases of systemic sclerosis (scleroderma).

A. Pseudodiverticula in dilated jejunum (sacculation).

B. The "hidebound" small bowel sign, a combination of dilatation and crowded circular folds.

ischemia and the contraceptive pill and the often serious prognosis of the condition.

A psychotic patient who presented with partial obstruction and slight melena showed typical SBE features of segmental ischemia in the distal ileum (Fig. 11–30).

Macroglobulinemia. The primary form (Waldenström's syndrome) is rare, and associated steatorrhea is rarer still. Khilnani and coworkers[57] have described the barium appearances and the clinicopathologic findings in three cases.

Abetalipoproteinemia. This is a rare inherited disease that combines steatorrhea with acanthocytosis, retinal abnormalities, and central nervous system damage. Betalipoproteins are absent from the plasma.[1] The SBE has shown dilatation, fold thickening throughout, and a fluid increase which soon caused barium flocculation.

Lymphoid Hyperplasia and Dysgammaglobulinemia. Marshak and associates[58] have described the small bowel x-ray appearance in a number of conditions that could be grouped together owing to recent better understanding of immunologic processes. Steatorrhea is not often the presenting clinical feature.

Nodular lymphoid hyperplasia has been found associated with dysgammaglobulinemia by Hermans and coworkers.[59] IgA and IgM are mostly diminished, and a high incidence of *Giardia lamblia* infection is found. Nodular changes of the mucosa predominate in the jejunum, but the whole small bowel may be involved. There is neither dilatation nor fold thickening (Fig. 11–31). With giardiasis, changes of an inflammatory type (irritability, fold thickening, increased secretions) are superimposed mostly in the duodenum and jejunum. Giardiasis may also occur without immunoglobulin deficiency.

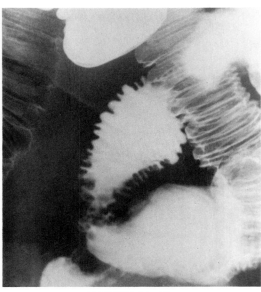

FIGURE 11–30

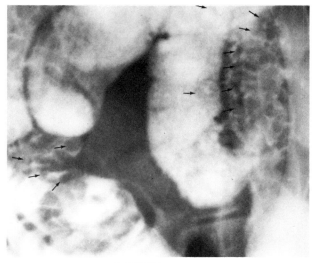

FIGURE 11–31

FIGURE 11–30 Ischemic enteritis. Thick parallel folds, increased peristaltic activity, and diminished pliability.

FIGURE 11–31 Lymphoid hyperplasia and dysgammaglobulinemia. Mucosal surface nodularity throughout jejunum.

Whipple's Disease. Valvulae conniventes are thickened and may show a finely nodular surface pattern, most pronounced in the duodenum.[60] This is due to extensive infiltration of mucosa and submucosa by macrophages containing PAS-positive material; this allows for definitive diagnosis by jejunal biopsy. The SBE (Fig. 11–32) demonstrates the undulating shape of the thickened jejunal folds, as emphasized in other reports.[61] Secretions may be increased, but this is variable.

Mastocytosis. This is a rare disorder not necessarily associated with urticaria pigmentosa. Segments of the small intestine show fold thickening with nodules. Wall thickening may also be found.[62] There is an interesting relationship to celiac disease with the finding of subtotal villous atrophy and improvement on gluten withdrawal. Jejunal biopsy establishes the diagnosis by demonstrating an excess of mast cells.[63]

Lymphangiectasia. This is a rare but important condition, with protein loss into the gut resulting in hypoalbuminemia and hypogammaglobulinemia. It is usually due to a congenital malformation of intestinal lymphatics.[64]

Valvulae conniventes are extensively enlarged and nodular. There is considerable fluid increase in the lumen. Surface detail is seen only in the early stages of the SBE before dilution and degradation of barium has gone too far (Fig. 11–33). Diagnosis needs to be confirmed by jejunal biopsy and by documentation of protein loss. Occasionally lymphatic blockage due to extensive malignancy produces a similar clinical picture of secondary lymphangiectasia.[65]

Structural Lesions. These are mostly the result of surgery and easily recognized, or the result of inflammation (to be discussed later).

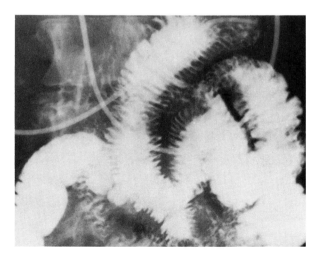

FIGURE 11–32 Whipple's disease. Markedly thickened, somewhat undulating jejunal folds. Slight fluid increase. Diagnosis confirmed by biopsy.

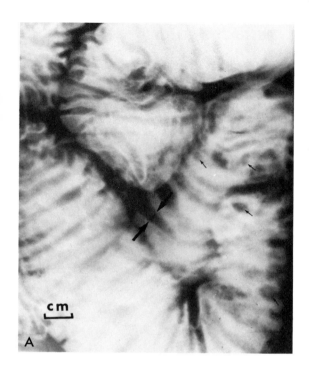

FIGURE 11–33 Lymphangiectasia.

A. Upper jejunum. Folds thick and uneven; nodules.

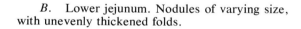

B. Lower jejunum. Nodules of varying size, with unevenly thickened folds.

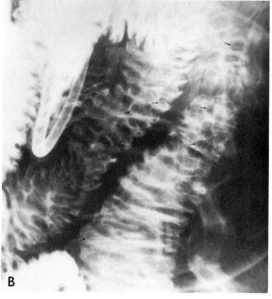

Jejunal Diverticulosis. The diverticula are herniations of mucosa through the muscularis on the mesenteric side of the bowel. These atonic sacs can produce significant metabolic abnormalities, even if they are few or solitary.[66] The reported incidence varies widely; we have found 5 cases in about 1000 examinations. Erect views taken in the course of the SBE readily show characteristic fluid levels in the usually numerous atonic sacs (Fig 11–34).

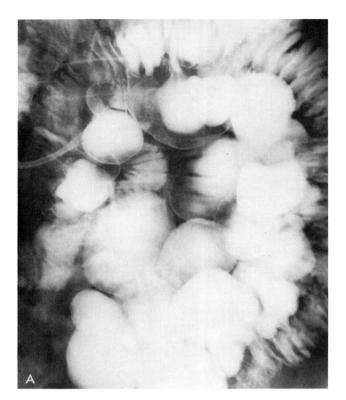

FIGURE 11–34 Jejunal diverticulosis.

A. Supine.

B. Erect.

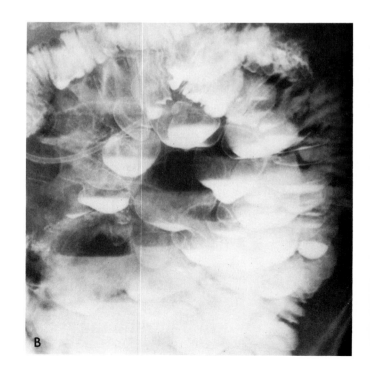

Inflammatory Conditions

CROHN'S DISEASE

A chronic nonspecific granulomatous process, Crohn's disease when fully developed involves and thickens the entire wall of a small bowel segment together with its mesentery and lymph nodes. Segments with established disease can be readily identified by simple follow-through examination, as they stand away from other closely folded, noninvolved loops of bowel.

However, the SBE has a distinctly useful application in Crohn's disease.

A. It is more accurate in showing the proximal limit of the disease process in patients in whom surgery is contemplated (Fig. 11–35).

B. In addition to readily shown, established distal disease at least 1 in 10 patients presents additional, more proximal skip lesions with the disease at an earlier stage. The SBE is capable of demonstrating this appearance (Fig. 11–3); this would be significant should surgery be contemplated.

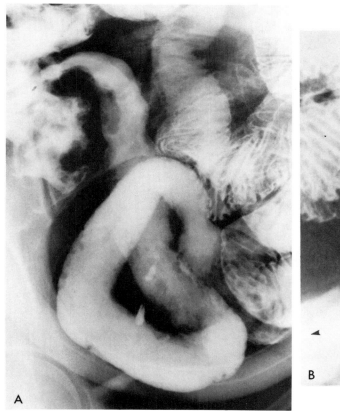
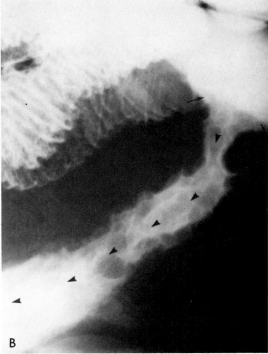

FIGURE 11–35 Crohn's disease of terminal ileum.

A. Any kind of small bowel examination could establish this diagnosis.

B. The SBE is best suited to demonstrate the proximal extent of the disease process (*arrow*).

C. At lease one third of patients with Crohn's disease have steatorrhea and malabsorption.[1] Its causation is multifactorial: loss of absorptive surface by disease, resection, or bypass; stagnant loops with abnormal bacterial flora; and increased gastrointestinal loss of nutrients.[67] As explained earlier, the SBE is the method of choice for imaging in malabsorption.

D. Postresection problems seem to be shown more accurately by the SBE (Figs. 11–36 to 11–38).

E. In the presence of strictures, distension, and stagnation the SBE is capable of providing information relevant to surgical management (Figs. 11–38 and 11–39).

F. Crohn's disease of unusual proximal distribution is by no means rare; the SBE may be able to demonstrate normality of the distal segments (Fig. 11–40).

G. Enterocolic fistulae due to Crohn's disease can be missed by the follow-through examination.

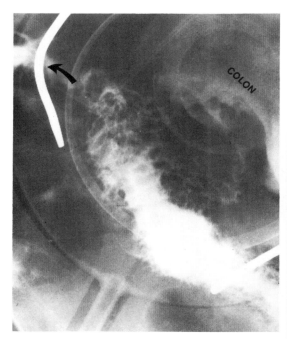

FIGURE 11–36 Crohn's disease. Recurrence in neoterminal ileum after resection. Cobblestone pattern of diseased ileum proximal to and at anastomosis. Arrow indicates cutaneous fistula.

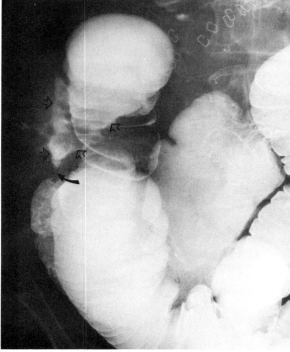

FIGURE 11–37 Recurrence of Crohn's disease in ileum at anastomosis with transverse colon. Dilated normal ileum, narrowing at anastomosis (*arrows*), with multiple tracking into the soft tissues proximal to the anastomosis.

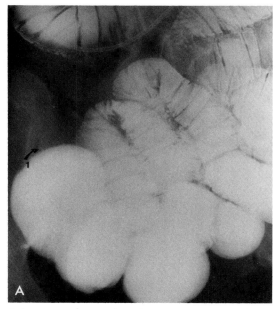

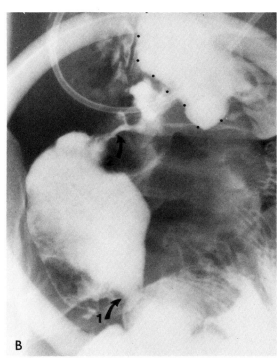

FIGURE 11–38 Two strictures with recurrence of Crohn's disease in neoterminal ileum after right hemicolectomy.

    A. Dilated normal ileum proximal to first stricture.

    B. Both strictures shown *(arrows)*, with active Crohn's disease extending to end-to-end anastomosis with transverse colon *(dots)*.

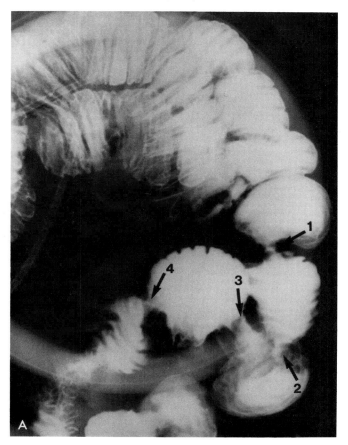

    A. At least four strictures *(arrows)* in jejunum.

FIGURE 11–39 Crohn's disease of proximal small bowel with strictures.

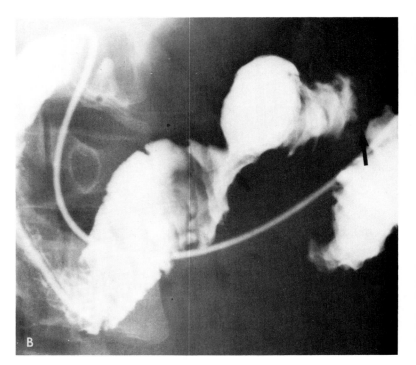

B. Two years later. Involvement of duodenum and upper jejunum.

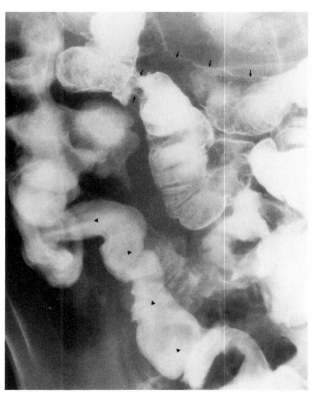

FIGURE 11–40 Crohn's disease, upper small intestine. Normal terminal ileum (*arrowheads*) with two areas of disease shown more proximally (*arrows*).

The early radiologic features of Crohn's disease are discussed in detail in Chapter 16. These include (a) mucosal swelling and nodularity with limited distensibility (Figs. 11–3 and 11–41*A*); (b) shallow, aphthous ulceration, as described histopathologically by Morson (Fig. 16–48);[69] and (c) shallow ulceration on the mesenteric side, with decrease in length and redundancy on the antimesenteric side (Fig. 11–41*B*).

The appearances of the well-established disease are readily recognized — linear ulceration, cobblestoning, strictures, fistulae, and sinus tracks (Fig. 11–42).

Yersinia Ileitis. This is a short-term benign disease in which a bacteriologic or serologic diagnosis of infection with *Yersinia enterocolitica* must be made.[70] The terminal ileum is involved predominantly and presents a pattern of nodules and edema (Figs. 11–43 and 16–52). Resolution within 10 weeks provides the definitive differential diagnosis from Crohn's disease.

Ileocecal Tuberculosis. A rare condition in Western countries, it now almost exclusively relates to autoinfection with tuberculosis-positive sputum. In some tropical countries the bovine strain is still the major source of infection of the gastrointestinal tract.

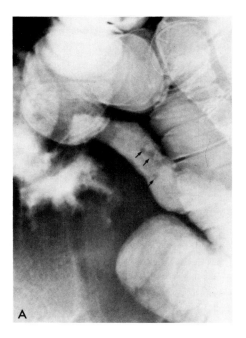

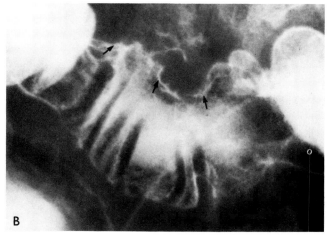

FIGURE 11–41 Early Crohn's disease of the terminal ileum.

A. Rigidity, angular outline. Numerous mucosal nodules (*arrows*).

B. Short segment of jejunum with unmistakable Crohn's disease. Mesenteric border shortened, ulcerated (*arrows*). Redundant antimesenteric side is thrown into thickened folds.

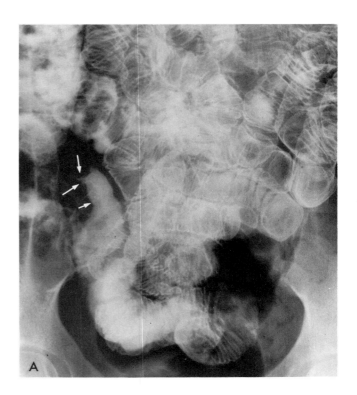

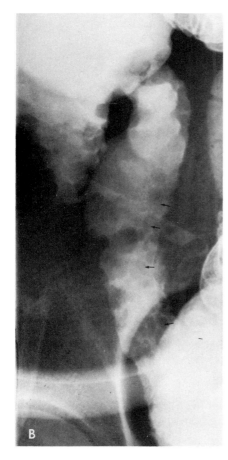

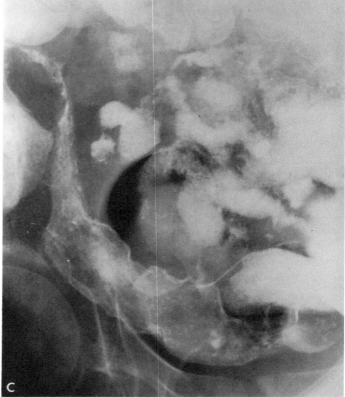

FIGURE 11–42

A. Normal small bowel study, but with terminal ileum slightly dilated owing to narrowing and ulceration (*arrows*) of its final 2 to 3 centimeters. Established Crohn's disease.

B. Many shallow ulcers, mostly on mesenteric border (*arrows*).

C. Double contrast view. Linear ulcers, irregular contours.

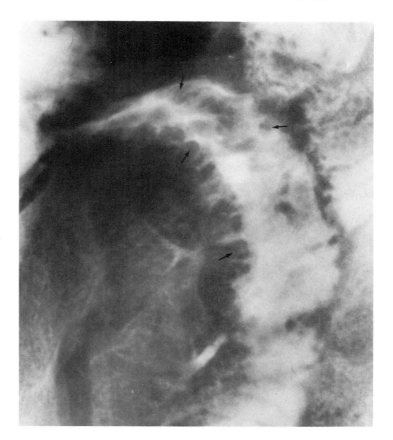

FIGURE 11–43 Yersinia ileitis. Nodules (*arrows*), wall thickening, fold still visible. Return to normal appearance within 6 weeks.

A firm diagnosis based on the findings of barium studies is not possible. Features that suggest tuberculosis rather than Crohn's disease are:

A. cecal involvement in excess of disease in the terminal ileum or even without it (Fig. 11–44A).

B. a cephalad retraction of the cecum, with straightening of the ileocecal junction (Fig. 11–44A).[71]

C. an abrupt change from normality to disease,[72] with much inflammatory exudate in the terminal ileum (Fig. 11–44B).

Appendix Abscess. The obvious point of differentiation from Crohn's disease is that in the latter the inflammatory mass surrounds the terminal ileum, which exhibits a deranged mucosal pattern (Fig. 11–45). The appendix abscess must arise and lie extrinsic to the terminal ileum which may be deformed and displaced by it, but will merely show swollen, compressed mucosal folds (Fig. 11–46).

In the case of a 24-year-old patient with abdominal pain, distension, and pyrexia, a follow-through examination of the small bowel was believed to show Crohn's disease of the terminal ileum. Steroid treatment seemed to produce clinical improvement. An SBE was done and showed clearly that terminal ileum changes could only represent extrinsic disease, probably an appendiceal abscess. Steroid administration was stopped, and surgery soon followed (Fig. 11–47).

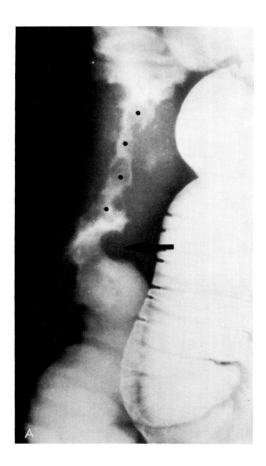

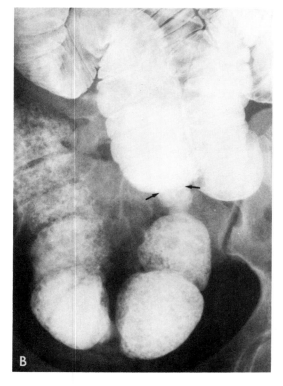

FIGURE 11–44   Two examples of ileocecal tuberculosis.

   A.   Terminal ileum slightly dilated, but normal to
the thickened ileocecal valve area (*arrow*). The cecum
is totally contracted; the extensively ulcerated ascending colon (*dots*) seems to be the direct continuation of
the terminal ileum.

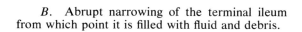

   B.   Abrupt narrowing of the terminal ileum
from which point it is filled with fluid and debris.

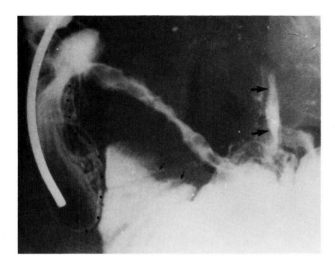

FIGURE 11–45 Inflammatory mass in Crohn's disease around narrow terminal ileum which shows nodules and ulcers. Cecum is deformed (*dots*), and displaced segments of adjacent distal ileum adhere to the mass (*arrows*).

FIGURE 11–46 Appendix abscess. Terminal ileum is deformed, and mucosal folds along its lateral border are swollen and compressed (*arrows*).

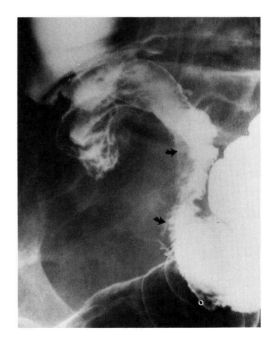

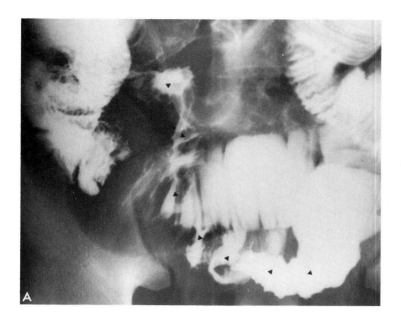

A. Follow-through examination. Terminal ileum (*arrowheads*) seems abnormal. Crohn's disease diagnosed. Patient given steroids; initial improvement.

FIGURE 11–47 Male patient with abdominal pain, distension, pyrexia.

B. SBE shows terminal ileum to be relatively normal (*arrowheads*). Deformity of segment proximal to it (*arrows*) with intact mucosa, although folds are swollen and compressed. Appendix abscess confirmed at laparotomy.

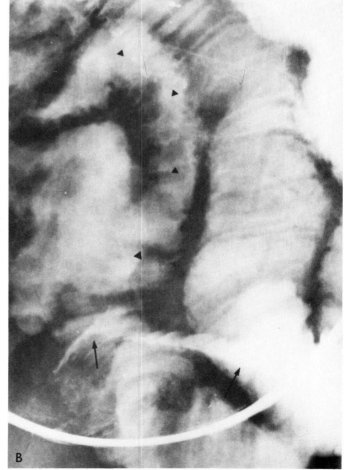

Tumors

Small bowel tumors are rare. Benign tumors occur with slightly greater relative frequency than malignant neoplasms. The overall incidence is 1.5 to 6 per cent of all tumors of the gastrointestinal tract.[73] In the conventional barium examination, small bowel tumors are more often missed than diagnosed.[74]

BENIGN TUMORS

Leiomyomas, adenomas, lipomas, hemangiomas, and fibromas, occurring in this order of relative frequency, account for 95 per cent of benign tumors in the small bowel. Bleeding, obstruction, a palpable mass, and weight loss are the presenting features. Angiography being the primary radiologic method of investigation in gastrointestinal bleeding in our hospital, most leiomyomas and hemangiomas have been demonstrated in this way and not by the SBE.

A typical duodenal leiomyoma, discovered accidentally during the intubation for an SBE, is seen in Figure 11–16D. Adenomas occur slightly more often in the ileum than in the jejunum; a small adenomatous polyp of the terminal ileum is illustrated in Figure 11–2. Duodenal polyposis has recently been shown to frequently accompany polyposis coli;[75] duodenojejunal adenomatous polyps could be demonstrated in one patient with familial polyposis (Fig. 11–48). A lipoma of the terminal ileum presented with intermittent intussusception and an intermittently palpable mass (Fig. 11–49).

The antegrade barium demonstration of an intussusception differs from the appearance usually met in the colon on retrograde studies. The somewhat dilated lumen narrows abruptly to a beaklike shape. If barium is able to pass through the obstruction, the distal lumen will be outlined, possibly demonstrating the leading tumor at the apex of the intussusceptum. The "coil-spring" appearance of stretched folds will be faintly visible only after retrograde entry of barium into the space between intussusceptum and intussuscipiens (Fig. 11–49).

MALIGNANT TUMORS

About two thirds of all malignant neoplasms of the small intestine produce clinical manifestations as compared with only one fifth of benign tumors.[73] Most carcinomas are symptomatic, but carcinoid tumors cause symptoms in only one third of patients. Pain and weight loss are the most frequent manifestations; bleeding and a palpable mass occur somewhat less often.

Carcinoid. The commonest small bowel neoplasm, this occurs most frequently in the distal ileum and is twice as common in males as in females. Most lesions neither invade nor metastasize. If they invade the bowel wall, a desmoplastic reaction ensues and produces a characteristic deformity. The carcinoid syndrome,[76] an expression of its systemic effect, occurs only in the presence of liver metastases, usually after the primary tumor has reached a diameter approaching 2 cm. Carcinoid tumors may be multiple and may ulcerate and bleed.

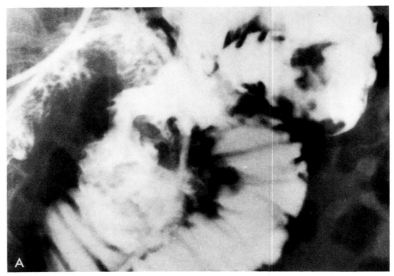

A.   Before MC.

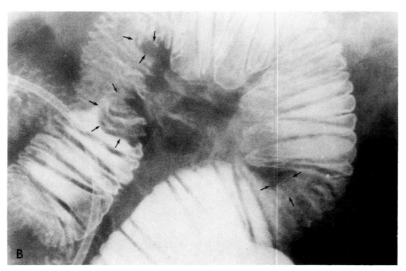

B.   With MC.

FIGURE 11–48   Familial polyposis coli with multiple duodenojejunal polyps shown.

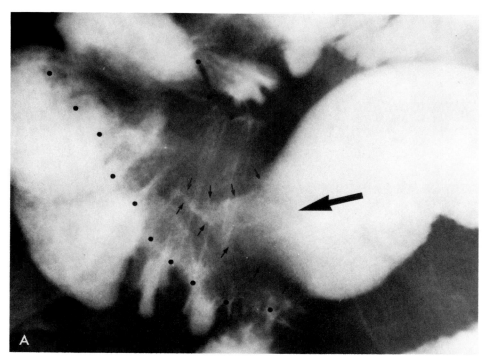

A. Beak-shaped narrowing at entry of intussusceptum (*arrows*). Barium flowing back from beyond the intussusception outlines its soft tissue mass from outside (*dots*), and by entry between intussuscipiens and intussusceptum, faintly shows the stretched "coil-spring" pattern of folds.

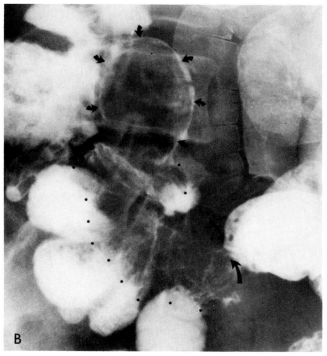

B. Lipoma at apex of intussusception (*smaller arrows*).

FIGURE 11–49 Lipoma of terminal ileum causing intussusception.

In a patient with right iliac fossa pain and weight loss, but without the carcinoid syndrome, a carcinoid of the ileocecal valve was outlined by a combination of SBE and pneumocolon (Fig. 11–50).

Carcinoma. Most are infiltrative adenocarcinomas and are found in the upper small intestine. They soon encircle the gut and cause obstruction. Other presentations are pain, weight loss, and melena.

An increased incidence of small intestinal carcinoma is found in celiac disease (Fig. 11–28). Crohn's disease also carries a higher risk of carcinoma,[77] particularly in bypassed loops; these tumors are more difficult to diagnose, are more frequent in the ileum, and have a worse prognosis.

Of two carcinomas found by the SBE, one presented with pain and weight loss (Fig. 11–51A), the other with subtotal obstruction (Fig. 11–51B). Both were located in the ileum.

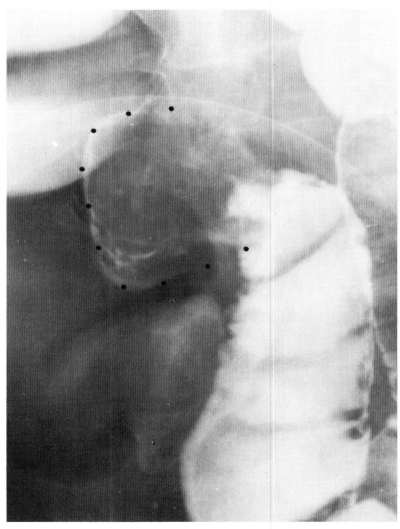

FIGURE 11–50 Carcinoid tumor at ileocecal valve *(dots)* shown by combination of SBE and pneumocolon.

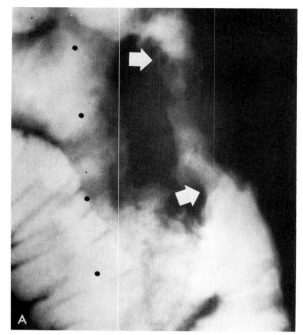
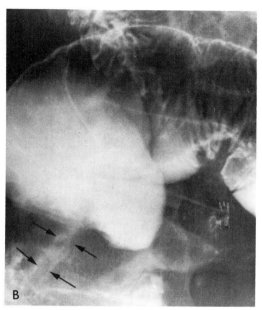

FIGURE 11–51 Two examples of carcinoma of the ileum.

A. Annular carcinoma of the ileum *(arrows)*. Dots outline terminal ileum.
B. SBE through MA tube demonstrates an annular carcinoma causing subtotal obstruction of the ileum. Irregular strictured lumen within the carcinoma *(arrows)*.

Lymphoma. Lymphoma should be considered in three groupings:[1]

A. Lymphoma arising elsewhere, involving the small intestine secondarily.
B. Primary small bowel lymphoma.
C. Lymphoma complicating celiac disease.

The SBE appearances are the same for primary and secondary lymphoma. The recognition of the rarer primary lymphoma has important prognostic implications, and its diagnostic criteria have been clearly defined.[78] Primary lymphoma may present with malabsorption and villous atrophy, and may even show an initial response to a gluten-free diet.[1] Jejunal biopsy can give diagnostic evidence of lymphoma, provided the upper jejunum is involved. This is more likely to occur in celiac-related lymphoma and in the Mediterranean type. Barium studies are essential to the diagnosis of lymphoma in most cases.

The disease arises in lymphoid patches,[79] which become bulky and produce nodular imprints into the barium column (Fig. 11–27). Some areas show larger polypoid lesions which may even intussuscept. The bowel wall may be invaded, with destruction of muscle and flaccid dilatation. Extension into the mesentery and mesenteric nodes may produce exoenteric masses. Ulceration of mural lymphoma into an exoenteric mass may result in considerable excavation (Fig. 11–52).

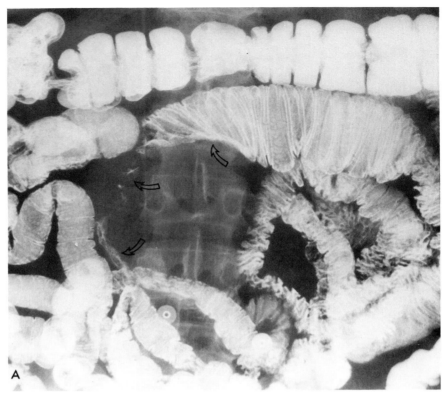

A. Exoenteric mass involving a segment of jejunum, causing partial obstruction *(arrows).*

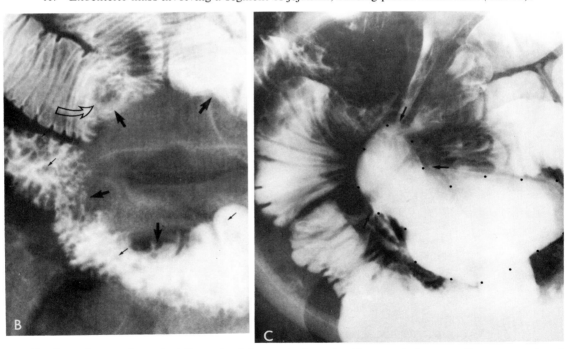

B. Lymphoma of terminal ileum (nodules up to 6 mm) with exoenteric mass *(large arrows)* and secondary involvement of an adjacent loop *(open arrow).*

C. Excavated mass of mainly exoenteric lymphoma *(dots)* surrounded by a loop of mid-small bowel with thickened mucosal folds drawn into it *(arrows).*

FIGURE 11–52 Lymphoma with exoenteric mass.

Hodgkin's Disease. Small bowel localization is rare. Unlike lymphoma, it does not present with excavation, fistulae, or dilatation, but shows fibrosis with narrowing of the lumen.[80] It may give rise to secondary spruelike malabsorption.

Metastatic Tumors. The primary sites, in decreasing order of frequency, are usually the colon, stomach, breast, ovary, uterus, melanin cells (melanoma), and bronchus. Our experience in the diagnosis of metastatic carcinoma relates largely to referrals of patients with advanced malignancy of the cervix or ovary. The SBE was done as part of the staging of such carcinomas or in the assessment of patients with known spread before further surgery was carried out.

According to Smith and coworkers[81] the radiographic findings in secondary neoplastic disease of the small intestine include:

A. Fixation and stretching of folds across the long axis, the "transverse stretch," in patients with mesenteric or peritoneal involvement.

B. Thickening or flattening of folds with intramural deposits.

C. Obstruction due to kinking, annular constriction, or a larger polypoid mass.

D. Compression by direct extension of a primary tumor or involved nodes.

Secondary neoplasms involve the bowel by direct invasion, intraperitoneal seeding, or hematogenous spread.[82] Seeded deposits are most likely to be found within the lower recesses of the small bowel mesentery, in relation to the terminal ileum. Ascitic fluid flow from the pelvis, and with it seeding of pelvic cancers, occurs preferentially upward toward the right paracolic gutter. The appearance and clinical effect of deposits also relate to the degree of local fibrous reaction they provoke. In almost all cases of small bowel involvement by metastases there are multiple lesions. Of the hematogenous metastases, those arising from melanoma may provide characteristic appearances on barium studies.[83, 84]

The SBE has shown metastases clearly. Seeded deposits from ovarian or cervical carcinoma seem to involve the right iliac fossa area preferentially. Serosal deposits show sharp demarcation with folds flattened, stretched, curved, or obliterated (Fig. 11–53). A mural deposit may protrude and narrow the lumen (Fig. 11–54), or incite a desmoplastic response with kinking and obstruction. The cecum may also show the effects of mural or serosal deposits (Fig. 11–55). Rarely are metastases clearly of peritoneal origin (Fig. 11–56). Direct extension of the primary tumor or involved nodes may invade and constrict a segment of ileum. In grossly advanced disease, combinations of direct extension and implants or tumor encasement with fistula formation can be demonstrated very clearly by the SBE.

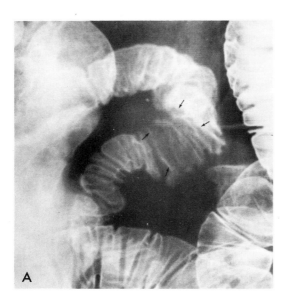

A. Carcinoma of cervix with metastasis to terminal ileum. Folds flattened; fairly sharp demarcation *(fine arrows)*.

FIGURE 11–53 Serosal metastatic deposits from gynecologic carcinoma.

B. Ileal metastasis from carcinoma of cervix *(arrows)*. Lumen narrowed, folds curved *(dots)*.

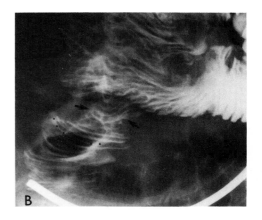

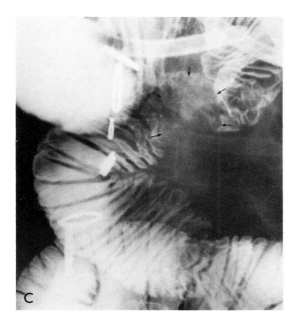

C. Metastasis to jejunum from an ovarian carcinoma. Folds virtually obliterated, outline sharp *(arrows)*.

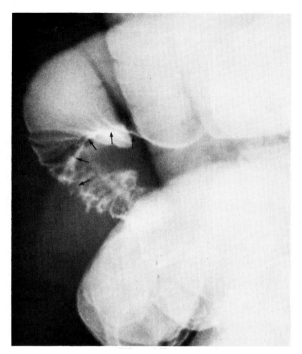

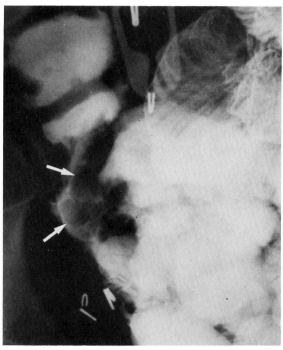

FIGURE 11-54 Mural deposit in ileum from a cervical carcinoma. Protrusion into lumen, fold obliteration, and displacement. Presented as small bowel obstruction.

FIGURE 11-55 Cecum involved by metastases from gynecologic carcinoma.

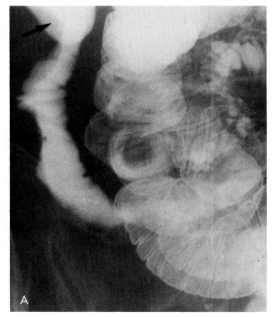

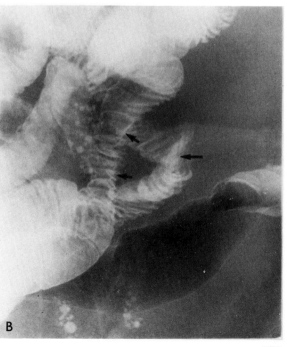

FIGURE 11-56 Mostly peritoneal metastases from ovarian carcinoma. Ascites.

A. Metastases indenting lateral border of terminal ileum (*arrows*).

B. Metastases displacing ileal loops in the left abdomen (*arrows*).

Radiation Damage

The small intestine is very radiosensitive.[85] With higher radiation doses to the pelvis, it will escape injury only if free to move out of the beam. Bowel tethered by past surgery is likely to suffer damage from a dose of about 5000 rads.

Chronic radiation damage makes its appearance 1 to 12 years later and demonstrates recognizable changes on barium examination. The injury is essentially an endarteritis with vascular occlusion. Superficial patchy mucosal denudation occurs, with infiltration of mucosa and submucosa leading to thickening of the bowel wall by edema and fibrosis.[86] This produces the characteristic radiologic appearances of thickened folds with compressed interfold spaces. Added to this there are often irregular nodular defects, bowel wall thickening, rigidity, and fixation. Strictures are seen with severe radiation damage. Adhesions may be revealed by the finding of mucosal folds drawn out and "tacked down." Such appearances cannot always be distinguished from metastases. Loops may be extensively matted and encased, showing neither peristalsis nor distensibility. In such circumstances it may be necessary to abandon the SBE, as

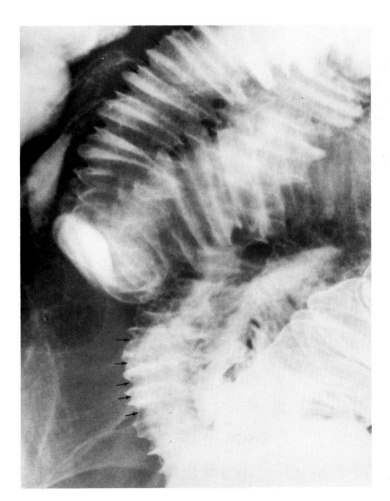

FIGURE 11–57 Radiation damage to ileum. Folds thick, straight, and parallel *(arrows)*. Compressed interfold spaces appear as sharp projections of barium between arrows.

further injections of barium or MC cannot be accommodated and reflux into the stomach will occur. Follow-through over many hours may have to take its place.

All of our cases of radiation enteritis shown by the SBE have followed irradiation of the pelvis for malignancy of the cervix or ovary. Thick, straight folds with compressed and spiky interfold spaces are unmistakable (Fig. 11–57). Fold thickening may be more uneven, with variable lumen diameter and longitudinal shortening (Fig. 11–58). Thick folds may be fewer with nodules and wall thickening (Fig. 11–59). Mucosal tacking is well demonstrated by the SBE (Fig. 11–60). We found only one example of radiation stricture (Fig. 11–61).

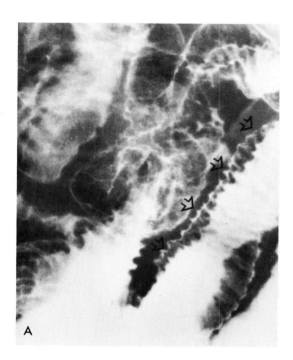

A. Evenly thickened folds with sharp projections of barium representing the compressed interfold spaces (*arrows*). Irregular fold thickening proximally.

FIGURE 11–58 Extensive radiation damage to ileum.

B. Less thickened folds are crowded by longitudinal shortening (*arrows*). Nodules seen above (*fine arrows*).

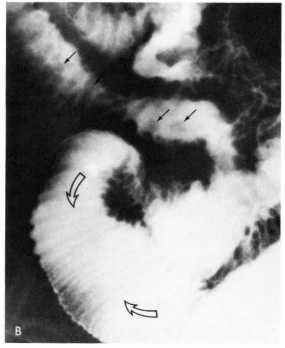

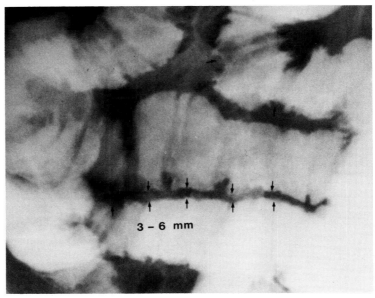

FIGURE 11–59 Radiation damage, midileum. Irregular nodulation produces uneven lumen outline. Wall thickening *(arrows)*.

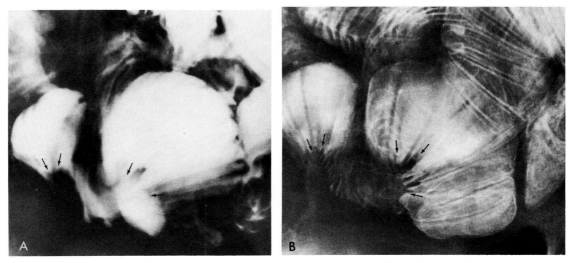

FIGURE 11–60 Radiation damage or malignancy? Carcinoma of cervix; previous surgery with extensive resection; radiotherapy. Presented with malabsorption and intermittent bleeding.

A. Fixed loop of ileum at pelvic inlet. Could be encased by tumor, (?) malignant stricture.

B. Development of double contrast. Tacked-down normal mucosal folds demonstrated *(arrows)*. No mucosal destruction; narrowed segment widens. Loop is incorporated in fibrous tissue, a sequela of radiation.

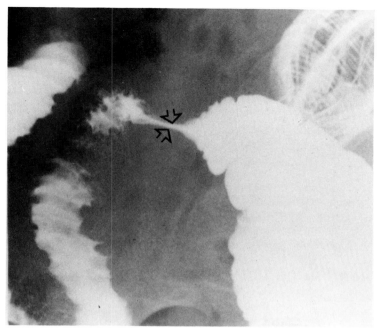

FIGURE 11–61 Radiation stricture. History of carcinoma of ovary treated with high radiation dosage. Presented with small bowel obstruction; SBE via MA tube.

Miscellaneous

Edema. Edema is probably the most frequent abnormality of the small intestine. It is usually submerged in the primary symptomatology of a patient and is not investigated radiologically. Hypoalbuminemia is the commonest cause,[87] related to protein loss from the gastrointestinal tract, cirrhosis, or nephrosis. Protein-losing enteropathy may also occur in conditions such as congestive heart failure, constrictive pericarditis, and allergy. Cell-free fluid accumulates in the bowel wall and causes uniform fold thickening, thickening and stiffening of the bowel wall, and often an increase in intraluminal fluid. Figure 11–62 shows an SBE with edema and hypoalbuminemia due to cirrhosis.

Bleeding. Intramural bleeding may occur with trauma, in patients on anticoagulant treatment, or with coagulopathies, such as hemophilia and thrombocytopenia.[88] The roentgen changes are readily demonstrated by any form of barium study of the small bowel. These changes are usually segmental, producing a rigid, separated loop with uniformly swollen, straight, parallel folds — the "stacked coin" appearance. Spasm or peristalsis is absent; early resolution is usual. Figure 11–63 illustrates a segment of jejunum with intramural bleeding in a patient with thrombocytopenia.

Obstruction. Obstruction by bands or adhesions is shown with great accuracy by the SBE, either through routine intubation or through a Miller-Abbott tube already in position. The barium suspension should be brought to the site of abrupt change in caliber from a dilated lumen proximal to the obstruction to a collapsed lumen beyond. With the aid of MC

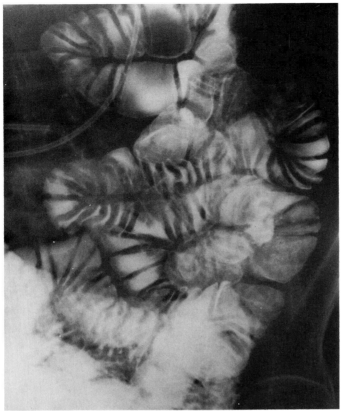

FIGURE 11–62 Cirrhosis and hypoalbuminemia. Small bowel edema. Folds thickened; slight wall thickening.

FIGURE 11–63 Patient with thrombocytopenia. "Stacked-coin" appearance of jejunum due to intramural bleeding.

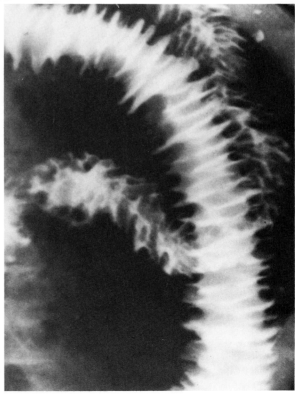

it is then usually possible to identify the imprint of the causative lesion as either a band or as more extensive adhesions (Fig. 11–64). Adhesions show fixation and fold distortion which are best seen during compression (Fig. 11–65).

Hernia. Internal hernias are rare and are responsible for less than 1 per cent of mechanical bowel obstruction. They are usually the result of abnormalities of small bowel fixation and are most common in the paraduodenal area. Pericecal hernias are the rarest forms of internal herniation and include the ileocolic, ileocecal, retrocecal, and retroappendiceal types.[89] A hernia through a defect in the mesoappendix has been described at surgery.[90] In a patient with a history of intermittent partial small bowel obstruction and without previous laparotomy, the SBE was able to demonstrate prolapse of a loop of distal ileum through a narrowed neck into a space lateral to the terminal ileum and below the cecum (Fig. 11–66). Surgery confirmed an internal herniation through an opening in the mesentery of the appendix.

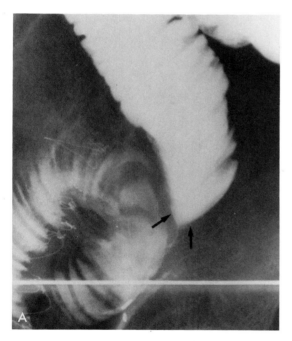

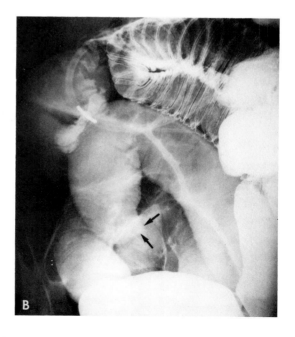

FIGURE 11–64 Obstruction by bands.

A. Partial obstruction of the lower jejunum by a band (*arrows*).

B. A band related to previous surgery causing complete obstruction of the ileum. SBE through MA tube.

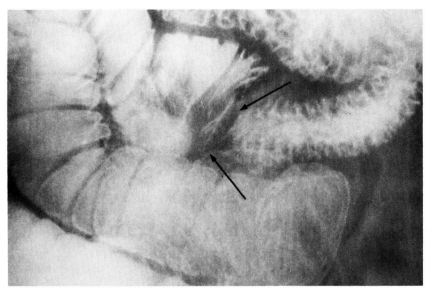

FIGURE 11–65 Adhesions to the anterior abdominal wall produce abrupt caliber change, fixation, and fold distortion during compression (*arrows*).

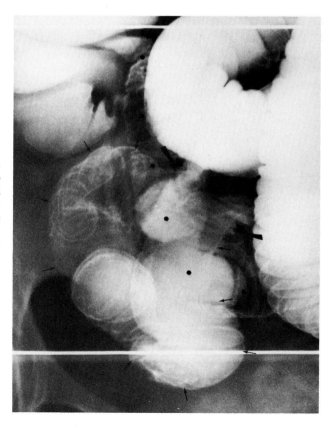

FIGURE 11–66 Internal hernia. Intermittent partial small bowel obstruction. A loop of distal ileum (*small arrows*) in constant position, its afferent and efferent limbs confined to a narrow space (*larger arrows*). Dots mark the terminal ileum. Laparotomy confirmed the diagnosis of internal hernia and showed it to have passed through an opening in the mesentery of the appendix.

CONCLUSION

It is the author's belief[40] that whenever a small bowel investigation is indicated for management purposes in a given patient, the SBE should be the routine and primary form of examination. There are no contraindications to its use. Abnormally apprehensive patients can be sedated with diazepam, and the throat can be fully anesthetized. The SBE is a radiologist's timesaver and lends itself to grouping into special small bowel study sessions, with intubation started in a side room. We have had no difficulty in carrying out six consecutive, well-documented examinations in a 2-hour session.

Many departments, however, will prefer to undertake screening small bowel examinations on demand. It would in those circumstances make sense to have two levels of small bowel investigation by barium.

A. The follow-through examination with overhead films and, whenever indicated, spot filming. This can be in addition to a barium meal or could be used wth only token gastroduodenal effort in patients in whom only small bowel investigation is requested in the absence of good indication of small bowel pathology.

B. The SBE when small bowel disease seems likely to exist and in circumstances in which this form of examination can be expected to make a useful contribution. Such indications are:

1. All forms of *malabsorption*. The vast majority will present normal appearances which will rule out an underlying morphologic abnormality. In a few patients, surface abnormalities shown by the SBE may be the only or the major feature to lead to full diagnosis.

2. *Crohn's disease*. In its well-established form a diagnosis is readily made by any barium study. The SBE is essential when early disease is looked for, or whenever surgery is contemplated to demarcate the true extent of involvement and to show possible discontinuous disease at other levels.

3. *Tumors*. They will always be more accurately delineated, and mainly because of the distensibility and distension of normal gut on either side will be diagnosed at an earlier stage.

4. *Secondary malignancy* to the small bowel which the SBE will demonstrate with considerable accuracy. This will help in the staging of carcinoma and in the planning of major resective surgery.

5. *Radiation damage* involving the small bowel which can be difficult to assess by other means. Distinction from metastatic malignancy can be a problem — clearly a differential diagnosis of important consequence for management. The SBE seems the most precise method available for this differential diagnostic purpose.

6. *Small bowel obstruction* of any cause. The SBE by means of routine intubation or through a Miller-Abbott tube has been found accurate in disclosing the site of an obstruction and in indicating the nature of the lesion responsible for it.

REFERENCES

1. Losowsky, M. S., Walker, B. E., and Kelleher, J.: Malabsorption in Clinical Practice. Edinburgh, Churchill Livingstone, 1974.
2. Creamer, B.: Loss from the small intestine. J. R. Coll. Physicians Lond., 5:323, 1971.
3. Creamer, B.: The Small Intestine. London, William Heinemann, Ltd., 1974.
4. Laws, J. W., Booth, C. C., Shawdon, H., et al.: Correlation of radiological and histological findings in idiopathic steatorrhoea. Br. Med. J., 1:1311, 1963.
5. Frik, W.: Small bowel. In: Schinz, H. R. (ed.): Roentgen Diagnosis. Vol. 5. 6th ed. London, William Heinemann, Ltd., 1965.
6. Kreel, L.: Pharmacoradiology in barium examinations with special reference to glucagon. Br. J. Radiol., 48:691, 1975.
7. Friedman, J., and Rigler, L. G.: A method of double contrast roentgen examination of the small intestine. Radiology, 54:365, 1950.
8. Cole, L. G.: Artificial dilatation of the duodenum for radiographic examination. Am. J. Roentgenol., 3:204, 1911.
9. Einhorn, M.: The Duodenal Tube and its Possibilities. 2nd ed. Philadelphia, F. A. Davis, 1926.
10. Pribram, B. O., and Kleiber, N.: Ein neuer Weg zur röntgenologischen Darstellung des Duodenums (Pneumo-duodenum). Fortschr. Geb. Roentgenstr. Nuklearmed., 36:739, 1927.
11. Pesquera, G. S.: A method for the direct visualization of lesions in the small intestine. Am. J. Roentgenol., 22:254, 1929.
12. Ghelew, B., and Mengis, O.: Mise en évidence de l'intestin grêle par une nouvelle technique radiologique. Presse Med., 46:444, 1938.
13. Gershon-Cohen, J., and Shay, H.: Barium enteroclysis. Am. J. Roentgenol., 42:456, 1939.
14. Schatzki R. Small intestinal enema. Am. J. Roentgenol., 50:743, 1943.
15. Lura, A.: Enema of the small intestine with special emphasis on the diagnosis of tumours. Br. J. Radiol., 24:264, 1951.
16. Scott-Harden, W. G.: In: McLaren, J. W. (ed.): Modern Trends in Diagnostic Radiology. 3rd series. London, Butterworth, 1960.
17. Pygott, F., Street, D. F., Shellshear, M. F., et al.: Radiological investigation of the small intestine by small bowel enema technique. Gut, 1:366, 1960.
18. Scott-Harden, W. G., Hamilton, H. A. R., and McCall-Smith, S.: Radiological investigation of the small intestine. Gut, 2:316, 1961.
19. Gianturco, C.: Rapid fluoroscopic duodenal intubation. Radiology, 88:1165, 1967.
20. Bilbao, M. K., Frische, L. H., Dotter C. T., et al.: Hypotonic duodenography. Radiology, 89:438, 1967.
21. Sellink, J. L.: Examination of the Small Intestine by Means of Duodenal Intubation. Leiden, H. E. Stenfert Kroese B. V., 1971.
22. Sellink, J. L.: Radiologic examination of the small intestine by duodenal intubation. Acta Radiol., 15:318, 1974.
23. Sellink, J. L.: Radiological Atlas of Common Diseases of the Small Bowel. Leiden, H. E. Stenfert Kroese B. V., 1976.
24. Fleckenstein, P., and Pedersen, G.: The value of the duodenal intubation method (Sellink modification) for the radiological visualization of the small bowel. Scand. J. Gastroenterol., 10:423, 1975.
25. Sanders, D. E., Ho, C. S.: The small bowel enema. Experience with 150 examinations. Am. J. Roentgenol., 127:743, 1976.
26. Ekberg, O.: Crohn's disease of the small bowel examined by double contrast technique: A comparison with oral technique. Gastrointest. Radiol., 1:355, 1977.
27. Haworth, E. M., Hodson, C. J., Joyce, C. R. B., et al.: Radiological measurement of small bowel calibre in normal subjects according to age. Clin. Radiol., 18:417, 1967.
28. Bluestone, R., MacMahon, M., and Davison J. M.: Systemic sclerosis and small bowel invovlement. Gut, 10:185, 1969.
29. Ekberg, O.: Double contrast examination of the small bowel. Gastrointest. Radiol., 1:349, 1977.
30. Kellett, M. J., Zboralske, F. F., and Margulis, A. R.: Per oral pneumocolon examination of the ileocecal region. Gastrointest.-Radiol., 1:361, 1977.
31. Miller, R. E.: Barium sulphate in small bowel examinations. Radiol. Clin. North Am., 7:185, 1969.
32. Knoefel, P. K., Davis, L. A., and Pilla, L. A.: Agglomeration of barium sulfate and roentgen visualization of the gastric mucosa. Radiology, 67:87, 1956.
33. Dyet, J. F., Pratt, A. E., and Flouty, G.: The small bowel enema: description and experience of a technique. Br. J. Radiol., 49:1039, 1976.
34. Wittenberg, J.: Book review. Radiology, 125:612, 1977.

35. Miller, R. E., and Skucas, J.: Radiographic Contrast Agents. Baltimore, University Park Press, 1977.
36. Trickey, S. E., Halls, J., and Hodson, C. J.: A further development of the small bowel enema. Proc. R. Soc. Med., *56*:1070, 1963.
37. Sinclair, D. J., and Buist, T. A. S.: Water contrast barium enema technique using methyl cellulose. Br. J. Radiol., *39*:228, 1966.
38. Gmünder, U., and Wirth, W.: Dündarmdoppelkontrastdarstellung. Schweiz. Med. Wochenschr., *100*:1236, 1970.
39. Marriott, P. H., and John, E. G.: Influence of electrolytes on the hydration of methyl-cellulose in solution. J. Pharm. Pharmacol., *25*:633, 1973.
40. Herlinger, H.: A modified technique for the double contrast small bowel enema. Gastrointest. Radiol., *3*:201, 1978.
41. Christie, D. L., and Ament, M. E.: A double blind crossover study of metoclopramide versus placebo for facilitating passage of multipurpose biopsy tube. Gastroenterology, *71*:726, 1976.
42. Loubière, M., Grimaud, A., Coussemet, A., et al.: L'étude radiologique en double contraste de l'intestin grêle sous intubation doudéno-jéjunale. J. Radiol. Electrol., *58*:75, 1977.
43. Dalinka, M. K., and Wunder, J. F.: Meckel's diverticulum and its complications with emphasis on roentgenologic demonstration. Radiology, *106*:295, 1973.
44. Stewart, J. S., Pollock, D. J., Hoffbrand, A. V., et al.: A study of proximal and distal intestinal structure and absorptive function in idiopathic steatorrhea. Q. J. Med., *36*:425, 1967.
45. Thaysen, T. E. H.: Absorption of Fat and Protein. Non-tropical Sprue. Copenhagen, Levin and Munksgaard, 1932.
46. Nelson, S. W.: Abnormal small bowel fold patterns. In categorical course on gastrointestinal radiology. Am Roentgen Ray Soc., 1977.
47. Tully, T. E., and Feinberg, S. B.: Roentgenographic classification of diffuse diseases of the small intestine presenting with malabsorption. Am. J. Roentgenol., *121*:283, 1974.
48. Osborn, A. G., and Friedland, G. W.: A radiological approach to the diagnosis of small bowel disease. Clin. Radiol., *24*:281, 1973.
49. Kalser, M. H.: Celiac sprue. *In:* Bockus, H. L. (ed.): Gastroenterology. 3rd ed. Philadelphia, W. B. Saunders, 1976.
50. Marshak, R. H., and Lindner A. E.: Malabsorption syndrome: Sprue. *In:* Radiology of the Small Intestine. 2nd ed. Philadelphia, W. B. Saunders, 1976.
51. Stokes, P. L., and Holmes, G. K. T.: Malignancy in celiac disease. Clin. Gastroenterol., *3*:159, 1974.
52. Scott, B. B., and Losowsky, M. S.: Depressed cell-mediated immunity in celiac disease. Gut, *17*:900, 1976.
53. Collins, S. M., Hamilton, J. D., Lewis, T. D., et al.: Small-bowel malabsorption and gastrointestinal malignancy. Radiology, *126*:603, 1978.
54. Horowitz, A. L., and Meyers, M. A.: The "hide-bound" small bowel of scleroderma: characteristic mucosal fold pattern. Am. J. Roentgenol., *119*:332, 1973.
55. Joffe, N., Goldman, H., and Antonioli, D. A.: Barium studies in small bowel infarction: radiological-pathological correlation. Radiology, *123*:303, 1977.
56. Editorial: Small-bowel ischaemia and the contraceptive pill. Br. Med. J., *1*:4, 1978.
57. Khilnani, M. T., Keller, R. J., and Cuttner, J.: Macroglobulinemia and steatorrhoea: Roentgen and pathological findings in the intestinal tract. Radiol. Clin. North Am., *7*:43, 1969.
58. Marshak, R. H., Hazzi, C., Lindner, A. E., et al.: Small bowel in immunoglobulin deficiency syndromes. Am. J. Roentgenol., *122*:227, 1974.
59. Hermans, P. E., Huizenga, K. A., Hoffman, H. N., et al.: Dysgammaglobulinemia associated with nodular lymphoid hyperplasia of small intestine. Am. J. Med., *40*:78, 1966.
60. Clemett, A. R., and Marshak, R. H.: Whipple's disease. Roentgen features and differential diagnosis. Radiol. Clin. North Amer., *7*:105, 1969.
61. Benozio, M., Legendre, H., Rymer, R., et al.: Diagnostic radiologique de la maladie de Whipple. A propos de huit observations. Ann. Radiol., *20*:461, 1977.
62. Clemett, A. R., Fishbone, G., Levine, R. J., et al.: Gastrointestinal lesions in mastocytosis. Am. J. Roentgenol., *103*:405, 1968.
63. Scott, B. B., Hardy, G. J., and Losowsky M. S.: Involvement of the small intestine in systemic mast cell disease. Gut. *16*:918, 1975.
64. Shimkin, P. M., Waldmann, T. A., and Krugman, R. L.: Intestinal lymphangiectasia. Am. J. Roentgenol., *110*:827, 1970.
65. Vigne, J., Marambat, G., Lechat, S., et al.: Stéatorrhée par blocage du retour lymphatique au cours d'une affection maligne des ganglions lymphatiques profonds. Presse Med., *76*:1601, 1968.

66. Cooke, W. T., Cox, E. U., Fone, D. J., et al.: The clinical and metabolic significance of jejunal diverticula. Gut., 4:115, 1963.
67. Smith, A. N., and Balfour T. W.: Malabsorption in Crohn's disease. Clin. Gastroenterol., 1:433, 1972.
68. Laufer, I., Mullens, J. E., and Hamilton, J.: Correlation of endoscopy and double contrast radiography in the early stages of ulcerative and granulomatous colitis. Radiology, 118:1, 1976.
69. Morson, B. C.: Histopathology of regional enteritis (Crohn's disease). In: Engel, A., and Larsson, T. (eds.): Skandia International Symposia on Regional Enteritis (Crohn's disease). Stockholm, Nordiska Bokhandelns Forlag, 1971, pp. 15–33.
70. Ekberg, O., Sjostrom, B., and Brahme, F. J.: Radiological findings in Yersinia ileitis. Radiology., 123:15, 1977.
71. Brombart, M., and Massion, J.: Radiologic differential diagnosis between ileocecal tuberculosis and Crohn's disease. Am. J. Dig. Dis., 6:589, 1961.
72. Herlinger, H.: Angiography in the diagnosis of ileocecal tuberculosis. Gastrointest. Radiol., 2:371, 1978.
73. Carlson, H. C., and Good, C. A.: Neoplasms of the small bowel. In: Margulis, A. R., and Burhenne, H. J. (eds.): Alimentary Tract Radiology. 2nd ed. St. Lousis, C. V. Mosby, 1973.
74. Martel, W., Whitehouse, W. M., and Hodges, F. J.: Small bowel tumors. Radiology, 75:368, 1960.
75. Ushio, K., Sasagawa, M., Doi, H., et al.: Lesions associated with familial polyposis coli: Studies of lesions of the stomach, duodenum, bones and teeth. Gastrointest. Radiol., 1:67, 1976.
76. Marshak, R. H., and Lindner, A. E.: Carcinoid tumors and the carcinoid syndrome. In: Radiology of the Small Intestine, 2nd ed. Philadelphia, W. B. Saunders, 1976.
77. Hoffman, J. P., Taft, D. A., Wheelis, R. F., et al.: Adenocarcinoma in regional enteritis of the small intestine. Arch. Surg., 112:606, 1977.
78. Dawson, I. M. P., Cornes, J. S., and Morson, B. C.: Primary malignant lymphoid tumours of the intestinal tract. Br. J. Surg., 49:80, 1961.
79. Theros, E. G.: RPC of the month from the AFIP. Radiology, 92:1363, 1969.
80. Ornstein, D. H., and Ruoff, M.: Hodgkin's disease of the small intestine. Am. J. Gastroenterol., 68:182, 1977.
81. Smith, S. J., Carlson, H. C., and Gisvold, J. J.: Secondary neoplasms of the small bowel. Radiology., 125:29, 1977.
82. Meyers, M. A.: Dynamic Radiology of the Abdomen. Normal and Pathologic Anatomy. New York, Springer Verlag, 1976.
83. Goldstein, H. M., Beydoun, M. T., and Dodd, G. D.: Radiologic spectrum of melanoma metastatic to the gastrointestinal tract. Am. J. Roentgenol., 129:605, 1977.
84. Zornoza, J., and Goldstein, H. M.: Cavitating metastases of the small intestine. Am. J. Roentgenol., 129:613, 1977.
85. Roswit, B.: Complications of radiation therapy: The alimentary tract. Semin. Roentgenol., 9:51, 1974.
86. Mason, G. R., Dietrich, P., Friedland, G. W., et al.: The radiological findings in radiation-induced enteritis and coilitis. A review of 30 cases. Clin. Radiol., 21:232, 1970.
87. Marshak, R. H., Khilnani, M. T., Eliasoph, J., et al.: Intestinal edema. Am. J. Roentgenol., 101:379, 1967.
88. Marshak, R. H., and Lindner, A. E.: Intramural intestinal bleeding. In: Radiology of the Small Intestine. 2nd ed. Philadelphia, W. B. Saunders, 1976.
89. Lawler, R. E., and Duncan, T. R.: Retrocecal hernia. A case report. Radiology, 87:1051, 1966.
90. Rooney, J. A., Carroll, J. P., and Keeley, J. L.: Internal hernias due to defects in the meso-appendix and mesentery of small bowel and probable Ivemark syndrome. Report of two cases. Ann. Surg., 157:254, 1963.

12

DOUBLE CONTRAST ENEMA: TECHNICAL ASPECTS

PATIENT PREPARATION

MATERIALS

PROCEDEDURE

PERORAL PNEUMOCOLON (PNC)

NORMAL APPEARANCES
   Transverse Folds
   Lymph Follicles
   Surface Pattern
   Terminal Ileum

ARTIFACTS

The development of the double contrast enema has been reviewed by several authors.[1-3] Despite the continuing controversy regarding its precise role in colonic diagnosis, the double contrast enema is our routine procedure in all patients referred for radiologic examination of the colon. The contraindications to the study are basically the same as those for the conventional barium enema. In patients with suspected colonic perforation, a water-soluble contrast material is used. Toxic megacolon is also a contraindication to barium study of the colon, although in patients in whom the clinical diagnosis is not clear a small amount of dilute barium may be introduced. It has also been our custom to perform conventional single contrast enemas in patients with suspected Hirschsprung's disease, acute diverticulitis, or high grade colonic obstruction. All other patients are examined by the double contrast enema.

PATIENT PREPARATION

Adequate cleansing of the colon is equally critical for all types of colonic examination — barium enema, colonoscopy, and double contrast enema. In principle the patient should start on a low residue diet 48 hours

495

before the examination. However, in hospitalized patients a 24-hour preparation is more practical and we recommend a clear liquid diet for 24 hours. A laxative should be taken on the afternoon prior to the examination. Although we have not carried out a controlled study, we have had satisfactory results with 2 ounces of castor oil. Dodds and coworkers[4] found that the combination of magnesium citrate and bisacodyl was preferable to castor oil. The addition of calcium bisdioctyl sulfosuccinate decreased the incidence of abdominal cramping. A cleansing enema[5] should be administered at least 1 hour prior to the examination. We have used 2 liters of tap water with 2 packets of Clysodrast (Barnes-Hind Co., Sunnyvale, Cal.). Clysodrast contains a combination of tannic acid and bisacodyl which acts as a colonic irritant to insure evacuation of the cleansing enema.[6, 7] Clysodrast should not be used in children or in patients with liver disease or active inflammatory bowel disease.[8] Approximately 1 hour after administration of the cleansing enema a preliminary film of the abdomen is obtained. If the colon does not appear to be well prepared, an additional cleansing enema can be administered.

Alternatively, a preliminary film may be obtained prior to the cleansing enema. If the colon appears to be clean, no cleansing enema is administered. If there is abundant fecal residue, the examination is rescheduled for the following day after further preparation. If there is a small amount of fecal residue or if the preliminary film is indeterminate, a cleansing enema is administered and the study is performed 1 to 2 hours later. This approach results in less congestion and fewer delays, and there are fewer patients with residual fluid in the colon. On the other hand, there are some patients who will have significant fecal residue that was not apparent on the preliminary film.

We have given atropine 0.6 mg sublingually prior to the cleansing enema. This is to counteract the vasovagal syncope which some patients experience with colonic distension. Atropine also tends to dry the colon, and there may be some residual relaxant effect during the radiologic study. We have not used a relaxant drug such as glucagon routinely, although its use would result in less patient discomfort and better quality examinations.[9-11] We inject 1 mg intravenously during the examination if the patient becomes very uncomfortable; if there is spasm resulting in pain, expulsion of the contrast material, or poor colonic distension; or if an area of persistent narrowing is encountered.

There are several exceptions to the foregoing preparation. Patients who are suspected of having small bowel obstruction receive no laxative. In patients with active inflammatory bowel disease a milder laxative, such as mineral oil, may be administered. In patients with severe inflammatory bowel disease an "instant enema" may be undertaken with no preparation. (Chapter 16).[12] The purpose of such a study is to document the presence of inflammatory bowel disease and to gain a general impression of its overall extent and severity.

Recently whole gut irrigation has been used as a method of colonic cleansing. The patient consumes a large volume of fluid over a short time, either by forced drinking or by infusion through a nasogastric tube. While a clear colon can be achieved over a short period using this technique,[13] there is an increase in residual water in the colon which tends to deteriorate the quality of mucosal coating.[14]

MATERIALS

In recent years several products and devices that have greatly facilitated and simplified the double contrast enema have become available.[15-18] A barium suspension with good mucosal coating properties is essential. It has been shown by Schwartz and coworkers[19] that there is no simple relationship between the physical properties of the barium suspension and its coating ability. We have had good results with liquid Polibar (E-Z-EM Co., Westbury, N.Y.), HD-85 (Lafayette Pharmacal, Lafayette, Ind.), and Barotrast (Barnes-Hind Co., Sunnyvale, Cal.). The concentration of the barium suspension used depends on the viscosity, but good coating is achieved with 80 to 95% W/V concentration. These barium suspensions are relatively viscous. Therefore, extra-large-bore tubing is desirable for more rapid flow and drainage. Recently, tubing with ½-inch diameter has become available and has given excellent results.[18] We also use the Miller air tip routinely.[16] Its large bore allows for more rapid instillation and drainage of the barium suspension. In addition, it has a small polyethylene tube that terminates at the distal end of the enema tip (Fig. 12–1). Thus air can be insufflated directly into the rectum without pushing barium ahead of it. This is particularly valuable for obtaining double contrast views of the rectum.

PROCEDURE

1. A preliminary film of the abdomen is obtained to insure that adequate colonic cleansing has been achieved.
2. With the patient lying in the left lateral position, the enema tip is inserted and taped to the buttocks with one or two pieces of tape. This is particularly important, since the ½-inch tubing filled with high density barium becomes very heavy and tends to pull out of the rectum if not secured.
3. With the patient in the prone position, barium is introduced until it is just seen to round the splenic flexure.
4. Air is insufflated immediately until the head of the barium column crosses the spine.
5. The patient is turned onto the right side, and additional air is insufflated until the head of the column rounds the hepatic flexure. The patient is turned onto the back and onto the left side, and additional air is

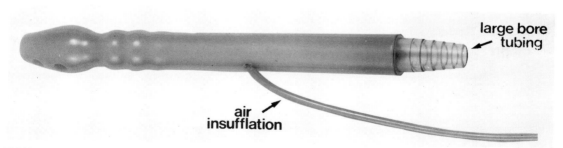

FIGURE 12–1 The Miller air tip. The catheter for air insufflation emerges at the distal end of the enema tip. The enema tip is also available with a retention cuff. (Courtesy of E-Z-EM Company, Westbury, N.Y.).

insufflated. A spot film of the sigmoid is obtained in the LPO position (Fig. 12–2A). At this time the cecum and terminal ileum have usually not filled, and therefore an unobscured view of the sigmoid is obtained.

6. The patient turns to the right and returns to the prone position while additional air is insufflated. The enema bag is dropped on the floor for drainage of barium from the rectum. Drainage may be facilitated by insufflation of air and by angulation of the enema tip.

7. When drainage is complete, the clamp is closed and additional air is insufflated to distend the rectum. A spot film of the rectosigmoid is exposed in the prone position (Fig. 12–2B).

8. Additional air is now insufflated until the entire colon is adequately distended.

9. The enema tip is removed. A spot film of the rectum is obtained with the patient in the left lateral position (Fig. 12–2C).

10. The patient returns to the supine position, and if the cecum and terminal ileum are filled a spot film may be obtained with compression (Fig. 12–2D).

11. The table is brought to the upright position for upright spot films of the flexures (Fig. 12–2E and F) and rectosigmoid (Fig. 12–2G). In this position, barium will fill the cecum.

12. The table is returned to the horizontal position, and additional views of the cecum and terminal ileum are obtained if necessary. The head of the table may be lowered further, and the patient turned from side to side to drain the cecum of barium and to distend it with air.

13. Routine overhead radiographs are obtained in the anteroposterior (AP), posteroanterior (PA), and right and left lateral decubitus positions (Fig. 12–2H to K). In all patients over the age of 35 we also include a prone view film of the rectosigmoid with the tube angled 35 degrees toward the feet (Fig. 12–2L),[20] and a prone cross-table lateral film of the rectum (Fig. 12–2M).[21]

14. A postevacuation film is not obtained routinely. However, if we are interested in the terminal ileum, and it has not filled, it will frequently be seen on the postevacuation film. In addition, if mucosal coating is not optimal and there is clinical suspicion of inflammatory bowel disease, a postevacuation film may be helpful.[2]

The procedure described is our routine complete examination of the colon. It requires seven spot films and six overhead radiographs. In some instances the study can be shortened considerably, while in problem patients additional time will have to be spent. The average normal study can be completed by the fluoroscopist in 5 minutes with 2 to 3 minutes of fluoroscopy time. The overhead radiographs can be completed in an additional 10 to 15 minutes. At this time we routinely perform 12 to 20 and sometimes as many as 25 such studies daily as well as an equal number of upper gastrointestinal studies in three fluoroscopic rooms.

Although we have not used remote control equipment for this type of examination, Hamelin and Hurtubise[22] have examined large numbers of patients with such equipment with excellent results. The use of fluoroscopy in the double contrast enema is mainly for monitoring the flow of barium and air and for positioning and timing spot films. Diagnostic fluoroscopy is minimized. Therefore, this examination is ideally suited for performance by a trained technologist.[23] Recently we have been evaluating technician performance of the double contrast enema. Although all of the data have not yet been collected, it appears that technician performance under radiologist supervision and interpretation results in no loss of diagnostic accuracy.

A double contrast enema can be performed in patients with a colostomy. This is facilitated by the colostomy device described by Goldstein.[24] This consists basically of a Foley catheter which is passed through a feeding nipple. The catheter is then advanced into the colon until the nipple occludes the colostomy. Accurate examination of the residual colon following colostomy may be particularly important because of the increased incidence of synchronous and metachronous carcinomas in patients with previous resection of a colorectal carcinoma.[25]

Text continued on page 506

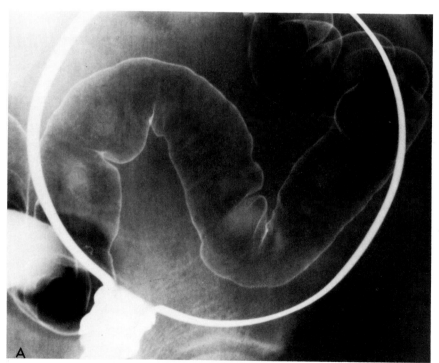

FIGURE 12–2 The normal routine double contrast enema (films from various patients).

A. Initial oblique spot film of the sigmoid in LPO projection.

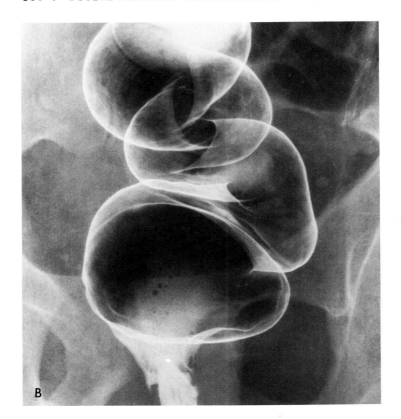

B. Prone spot film of the rectum after drainage of barium.

C. Left lateral spot film of the rectum with enema tip removed.

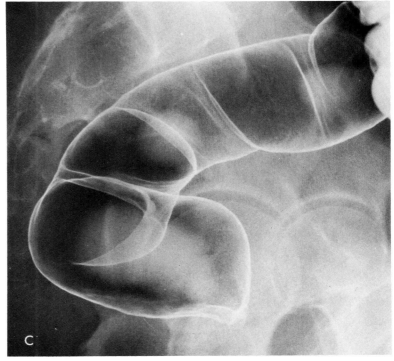

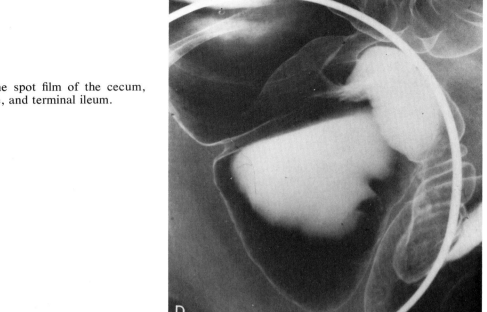

D. Supine spot film of the cecum, ileocecal valve, and terminal ileum.

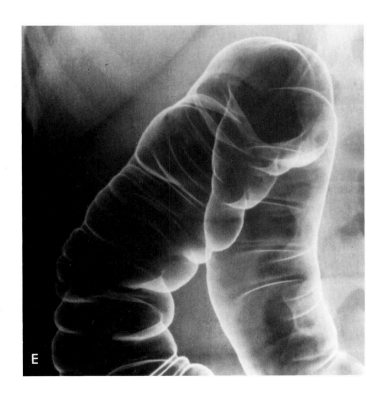

E. Upright spot film, hepatic flexure.

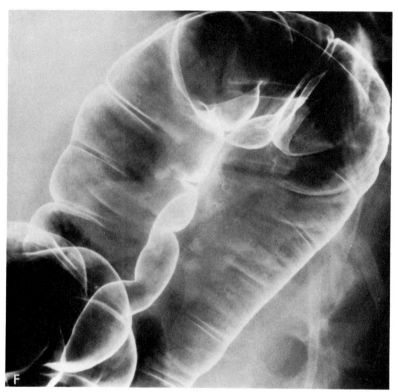

F. Upright spot film, splenic flexure.

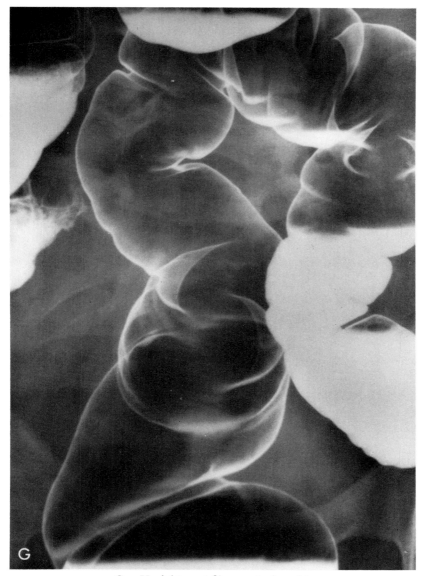

G. Upright spot film, rectosigmoid.

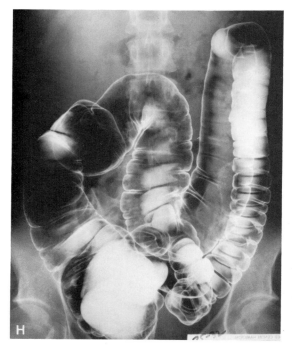

H. Supine overhead film.

I. Prone overhead film. Note the difference in distribution of the barium and air between the supine and prone views.

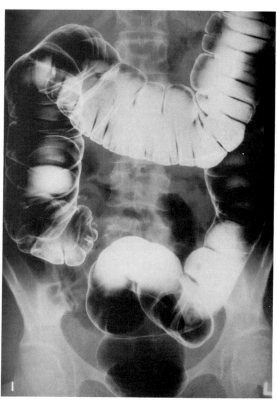

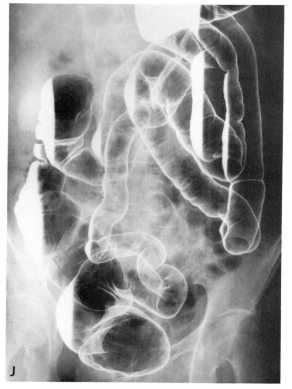

J. Right lateral decubitus.

K. Left lateral decubitus.

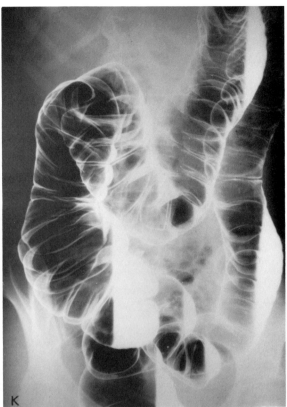

L. Prone, angled view of the rectosigmoid.

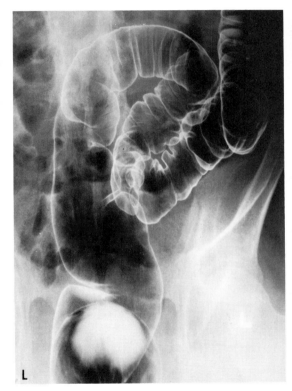

M. Prone, cross-table lateral view of the rectosigmoid.

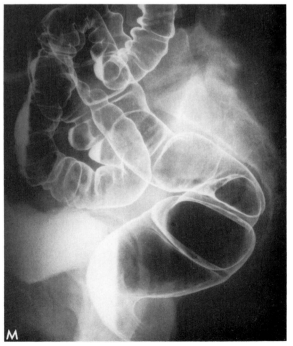

PERORAL PNEUMOCOLON (PNC)

In some patients an adequate examination of the right colon is not achieved either because of poor patient cooperation, retained fluid or fecal residue, or because of technical reasons. In these patients as well as in those in whom the radiologic findings in the right colon and terminal ileum require further study, the PNC can be used.

This examination is basically designed to examine the distal small bowel and right colon following a small bowel study.[26] It is important that the colon be cleansed. We use the same preparation as for the colonic examination. A small bowel follow-through study is performed in the usual fashion, using Barotrast. When the terminal ileum and right colon are opacified to the mid-transverse colon a small rectal catheter is inserted, and air is insufflated to obtain double contrast views. Glucagon in a dose of 1 mg may also be injected intravenously. Surprisingly good views of the right colon and terminal ileum can be obtained in this way (Figs. 12–3 and 12–4). It must be emphasized that it is important to use a barium suspension that does not flocculate or otherwise lose its coating properties during its passage through the small bowel.

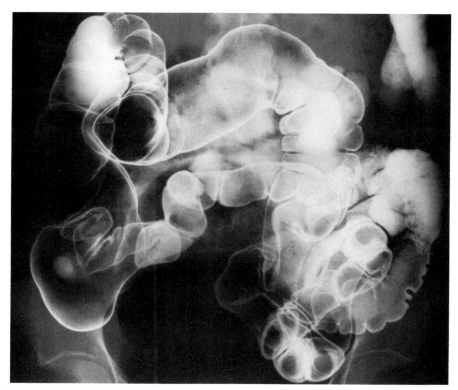

FIGURE 12–3 Peroral pneumocolon with excellent visualization of the right colon and distal small bowel.

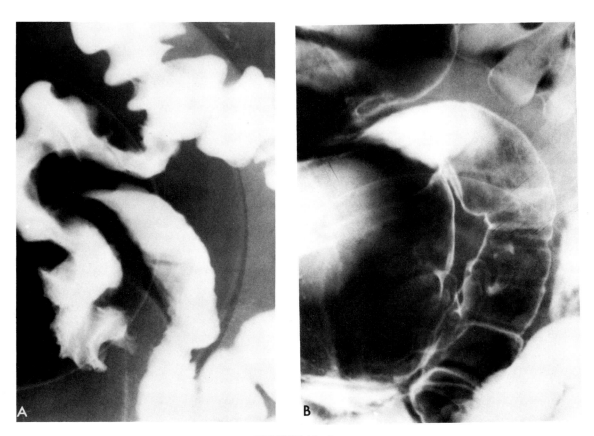

FIGURE 12-4
A. Suspicion of an abnormal cecum and terminal ileum on barium study.
B. Peroral pneumocolon technique shows a normal cecum and terminal ileum.

NORMAL APPEARANCES

Transverse Folds

In evaluating a double contrast enema examination one must assess the mucosal line as seen in profile as well as the en face appearance of the colonic mucosa. In profile the mucosal line should be thin, smooth, and straight. When viewed en face the normal mucosa is flat and featureless except for the haustral markings (Fig. 12–2). In some patients a series of tightly spaced circular folds may be seen as a transient phenomenon (Fig. 12–5). This most likely represents intermittent contraction of the muscularis mucosae and is of no pathologic significance.

Lymph Follicles

In some patients the mucosa may be studded with tiny nodules measuring 1 to 2 mm in diameter. This is seen particularly frequently in children under the age of 5 years and has been termed lymphoid hyperplasia (Fig. 12–6).[27-29] This pattern corresponds precisely to the anatomic description of the distribution of lymphoid follicles in the human colon,[30] and we believe this represents a normal feature of the pediatric colon, although in some patients these lymph follicles may become hyperplastic in response to infection, allergy, or immunologic deficiency states.[31] In such cases the lymph follicles may be larger, and the typical umbilicated appearance is more easily seen.[27] The normal lymphoid follicular pattern is seen regularly in children, but we have seen it only occasionally in adults (Fig. 12–7). It is easier to appreciate on good quality double contrast radiographs than on endoscopic examination of the colon. Burbige and associates[32] recently described the endoscopic appearance of colonic

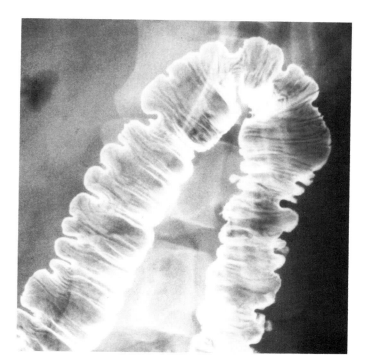

FIGURE 12–5 Fine transverse fold in the colon as a normal variant. Such folds may be caused by contraction of the muscularis mucosae.

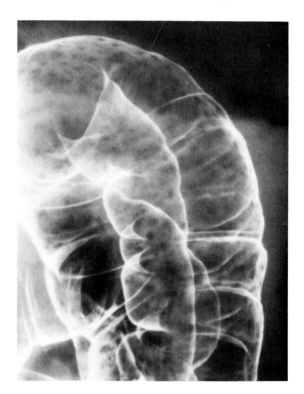

FIGURE 12–6 Multiple tiny filling defects in the colon, representing the lymphoid follicular pattern in a child.

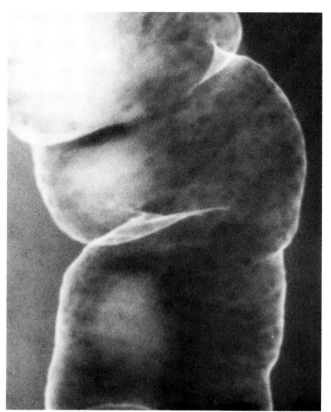

FIGURE 12–7 Lymphoid follicular pattern in an adult. (*From*: Laufer, I., and de-Sa, D., J. Roentgenology, *130*:51, 1978. Reproduced by permission.

lymphoid nodules as a normal variant. In their case they postulated that the follicles were visible as 1 mm white spots because their patient had melanosis coli. (Plate 59)

Surface Pattern

The colon has a fine surface pattern consisting of innominate lines (Fig. 12–8) analogous to the areae gastricae (Chapter 5). Several patterns have been described by Matsuura and coworkers.[33] These include linear, network, and mixed patterns (Plate 58). These appearances are rarely demonstrated on our double contrast enemas because of the high density and viscosity of our barium suspensions.

These innominate lines may result in spiculation of the contour of the colon. Occasionally pinpoint collections of barium are seen en face (Fig. 12–9). These probably represent points of intersection of innominate lines[34] and should not be mistaken for ulceration.[35]

Terminal Ileum

Depending on the degree of distension, the terminal ileum may have either a smooth surface (Figs. 12–3 and 12–4B) or prominent circular folds (Fig. 12–10A). Lymph follicles are frequently seen in the terminal ileum (Fig. 12–10B), particularly in young patients, but they may occasionally be seen in older patients and are probably of no pathologic significance.

ARTIFACTS[36]

The artifacts related to poor barium suspension have been discussed in Chapter 2. The artifacts produced by precipitation or flaking of the barium may closely simulate the appearances of inflammatory bowel disease.

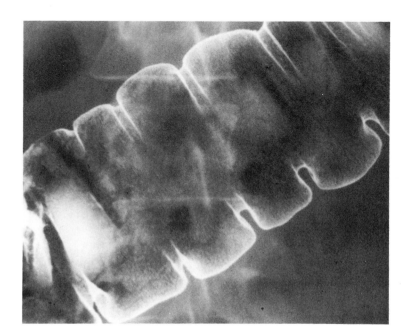

FIGURE 12–8 The innominate lines representing the surface pattern of the colon.

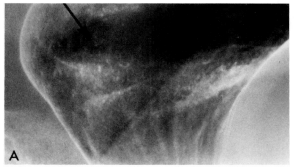

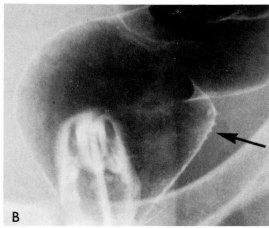

FIGURE 12–9

A. Multiple pinpoint densities in the rectum due to intersection of the innominate lines.

B. Same appearance seen in profile as fine spiculation. (*From:* Laufer, I.: J. Can. Assoc. Radiol., *26*:116, 1975. Reproduced by permission).

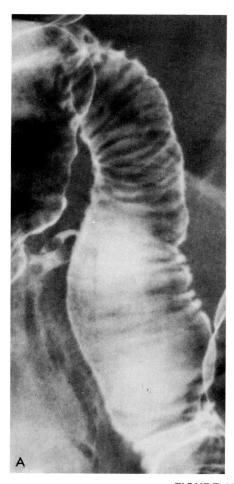

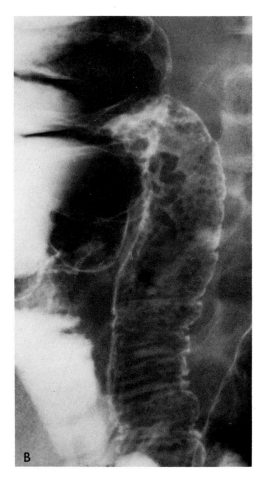

FIGURE 12–10 Normal terminal ileum.

A. Normal transverse folds in the terminal ileum. (*From:* Laufer, I., and Costopoulos, L.: Am. J. Roentgenol., *130*:307, 1978. Reproduced by permission).

B. Normal terminal ileum with tiny filling defects due to lymph follicles. (*From:* Laufer, I., Gastrointest. Radiol., *1*:19, 1976.[38] Reproduced by permission).

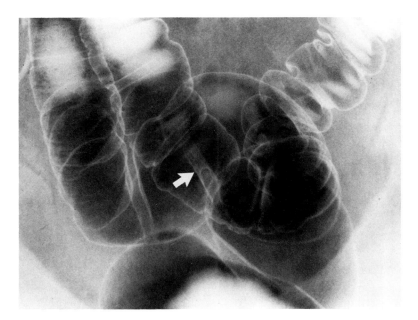

FIGURE 12-11 Folding of the colon, producing a linear filling defect (*arrow*) which could be mistaken for the stalk of a polyp.

FIGURE 12-12 Mucus strand.

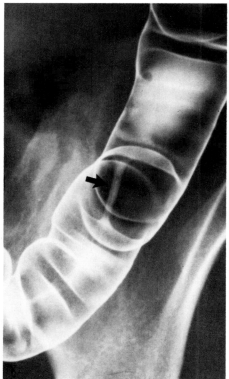

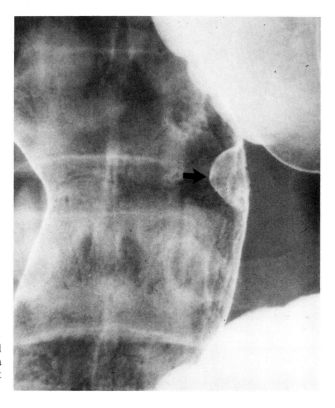

FIGURE 12-13 Tenacious mucus resembling a polypoid lesion. Colonoscopy showed only tenacious mucus and no evidence of a polypoid lesion. A repeat double contrast enema showed no abnormality.

Sharp angulation of the bowel may result in a long filling defect which may resemble the stalk of a polyp (Fig. 12–11). A similar appearance is often produced by a strand of mucus (Fig. 12–12). In other patients thick tenacious mucus may form a relatively solid, constant, polypoid mass. The case illustrated in Figure 12–13 was highly suggestive of polypoid carcinoma, but colonoscopy showed only tenacious mucus. A repeat double contrast enema showed no abnormality in this region. Although it is generally considered that a meticulously clean colon is a prerequisite for performing a double contrast enema, our experience has been that the double contrast technique is even more valuable in patients whose colon is imperfectly prepared.[38] Solid fecal material and other extraneous material will frequently be definitively diagnosed by virtue of their mobility on horizontal beam films (Fig. 12–14). Although solid fecal material is easily differentiated from polyps, smaller fecal residue and debris may adhere to the colonic mucosa and produce an appearance indistinguishable from that seen in familial polyposis or inflammatory bowel disease.

A variety of other shadows may overlap the colon and produce polypoid appearances on the double contrast enema. These include the greater trochanter projected over the rectum, hemorrhoids, an inverted appendiceal stump, the tip of the appendix projected over the rectosigmoid, renal calculi, phleboliths, and calcified lymph nodes. Most of these potential errors can be avoided by reference to a preliminary film and by careful study of the radiographs.

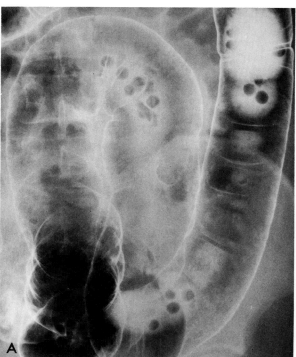 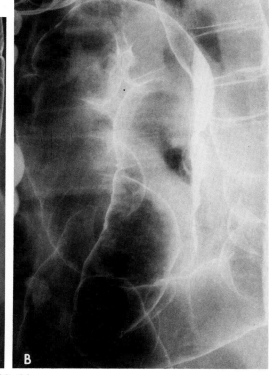

FIGURE 12–14

A.   Multiple filling defects in the colon due to undigested peas.

B.   In the lateral decubitus view the peas settle into the barium puddle, and the colonic mucosa can be seen to good advantage. (*From*: Laufer, I., Gastrointest. Radiol., *1*:19, 1976.[38] Reproduced by permission.)

REFERENCES

1. Stevenson, C. A.: The development of the colon examination. Am. J. Roentgenol., *71*:385, 1954.
2. Welin, S., and Welin, G.: The Double Contrast Examination of the Colon. Experiences with the Welin Modification. Stuttgart, Georg Thieme Verlag, 1976.
3. Maruyama, M.: Radiologic Diagnosis of Polyps and Carcinoma of the Large Bowel. Tokyo, Igaku-Shoin, 1978.
4. Dodds, W. J., Scanlon, G. T., Shaw, D. K., et al.: An evaluation of colon cleansing regimens. Am. J. Roentgenol., *128*:57, 1977.
5. Miller, R. E.: The cleansing enema. Radiology, *117*:483, 1975.
6. Christie, C. A., Coe, F. O., Hampton, A. O., et al.: The value of tannic acid enema and post evacuation roentgenograms in examination of the colon. Am. J. Roentgenol., *63*:657, 1950.
7. Janower, M. L., Robbins, L. L., Tomchik, F. S., et al.: Tannic acid and the barium enema. Radiology *85*:887, 1965.
8. Eschar, J., and Friedman, G.: Acute hepatotoxicity of tannic acid added to barium enemas. Am. J. Dig. Dis., *19*:825, 1974.
9. Miller, R. E., Chernish, S. M., Skucas, J., et al.: Hypotonic colon examination with glucagon. Radiology, *113*:555, 1974.
10. Gohel, V. K., Dalinka, M. K., and Coren, G. S.: Hypotonic examination of the colon with glucagon. Radiology, *115*:1. 1975.
11. Meeroff, J. C., Jorgens, J., and Isenberg, J. I.: The effect of glucagon on barium enema examination. Radiology, *115*:5, 1975.
12. Young, A. C.: The instant barium enema in proctocolitis. Proc. R. Soc. Med. *56*:491, 1963.
13. Skucas, J., Cutcliff, W., and Fischer, H. W.: Whole-gut irrigation as a means of cleansing the colon. Radiology, *121*:303, 1976.
14. Bakran, A., Bradley, J. A., Breshnihan, E., et al.: Whole gut irrigation. An inadequate preparation for double contrast barium enema examination. Gastroenterology, *73*:28, 1977.
15. Miller, R. E.: Barium enema examination with large-bore tubing and drainage. Radiology, *82*:905, 1964.
16. Miller, R. E.: A new enema tip. Radiology, *92*:1492, 1969.
17. Miller, R. E.: Simple apparatus for decubitus films with horizontal beam. Radiology, *97*:682, 1970.
18. Miller, R. E.: Faster-flow enema equipment. Radiology, *123*:229, 1977.
19. Schwartz, S. C., Fischer, H. W., and House, A. J.: Studies in adherence of contrast media to mucosal surfaces. Radiology, *112*:727, 1974.
20. Dysart, D. N., and Stewart, D. R.: Special angled roentgenography for lesions of the rectosigmoid. Am. J. Roentgenol., *96*:285, 1966.
21. Niizuma, S., and Kobayashi, S.: Rectosigmoid double contrast examination in the prone position with a horizontal beam. Am. J. Roentgenol., *128*:519, 1977.
22. Hamelin, L., and Hurtubise, M.: Remote control technique in double contrast study of the colon. Am. J. Roentgenol., *119*:382, 1973.
23. Campbell, J. A., Lieberman, M., Miller, R. E., et al.: Experience with technician performance of gastrointestinal examinations. Radiology, *92*:65, 1969.
24. Goldstein, H. M., and Miller, M. H.: Air contrast colon examination in patients with colostomies. Am. J. Roentgenol., *127*:607, 1976.
25. Enker, W. E., and Dragacevic, S.: Multiple carcinomas of large bowel — natural experiment in etiology and pathogenesis. Ann. Surg., *187*:8, 1978.
26. Kellett, M. J., Zboralske, F. F., and Margulis, A. R.: Per oral pneumocolon examination of the ileocecal region. Gastrointest. Radiol., *1*:361, 1977.
27. Capitanio, M. A., and Kirkpatrick, J. A.: Lymphoid hyperplasia of the colon in children. Radiology, *94*:323, 1970.
28. Franken, E. A., Jr.: Lymphoid hyperplasia of the colon. Radiology, *94*:329, 1970.
29. Theander, G., and Tragardh, B.: Lymphoid hyperplasia of the colon in childhood. Acta Radiol. (Diagn.), *17*:631, 1976.
30. Dukes, C., and Bussey, H. J. R.: The number of lymphoid follicles of the human large intestine. J. Pathol. Bacteriol., *29*:111, 1926.
31. Laufer, I., and deSa, D.: The lymphoid follicular pattern: a normal feature of the pediatric colon. Am. J. Roentgenol., *130*:51, 1978.
32. Burbige, E. J., and Sobyk, R. Z. F.: Endoscopic appearance of colonic lymphoid nodules: a normal variant. Gastroenterology, *72*:524, 1977.
33. Matsuura, K., Nakata, H., Takeda, N., et al.: Innominate lines of the colon. Radiology, *123*:581, 1977.
34. Williams, I.: Innominate grooves in the surface of the mucosa. Radiology, *84*:877, 1975.

35. Frank, D. F., Berk, R. N., and Goldstein, H. M.: Pseudoulcerations of the colon on barium enema examination. Gastrointest. Radiol., 2:129, 1977.
36. Gohel, V. K., Kressel, H. Y., and Laufer, I.: Double contrast artifacts. Gastrointest. Radiol., 3:139, 1978.
37. Laufer, I.: Air contrast studies of the colon in inflammatory bowel disease. CRC Crit. Rev. Diagnost. Imaging, 9:421, 1977.
38. Laufer, I.: Double contrast enema: Myths and misconceptions. Gastrointest. Radiol., 1:19, 1976.
39. Laufer, I.: The radiologic demonstration of early changes in ulcerative colitis by double contrast technique. J. Can Assoc. Radiol., 26:116, 1975.
40. Laufer, I., and Costopoulos, L.: Early lesions of Crohn's disease. Am. J. Roentgenol., 130:307, 1978.

13

TUMORS OF THE COLON

INTRODUCTION

BENIGN TUMORS
    Epithelial Polyps
    Other Benign Lesions
    Polypoid Artifacts

MALIGNANT TUMORS
    Advanced Cancer
    Early Cancer
    Other Malignant Tumors
        Submucosal Tumors
        Metastatic Tumors

THE POSTOPERATIVE COLON

INTRODUCTION

Carcinoma of the colon affects approximately 100,000 people in the United States every year, and approximately 50,000 die of this disease every year. It accounts for 2.4 per cent of all deaths. Stated in other terms, 1 person in 40 eventually dies of this disease.

Although the evidence is not conclusive, it is widely believed that most colonic carcinomas arise in benign polyps.[1-4] This belief is based on the frequent coexistence of benign and malignant lesions in the same colon, the frequency of malignant change in benign polyps, the invariable development of carcinoma in patients with familial polyposis, and the increasing frequency of cellular atypia as polyps increase in size.[5] There is also evidence that the systematic removal of benign polyps during routine proctosigmoidoscopy will result in a lower incidence of rectal carcinoma.[6, 7]

It is now clear that improvements in diagnosis and treatment over the past 25 years have not resulted in significantly increased survival in patients with colonic carcinoma. Thus it is apparent that a decrease in mortality from this disease will depend on the detection and treatment of early carcinoma or premalignant lesions in asymptomatic patients. For

517

practical purposes, almost all of these will be small polypoid lesions. Some will be established carcinomas, many of them Dukes' A which carries an excellent prognosis.[8] The majority will be benign polyps that can be removed endoscopically, and it is to be hoped that the systematic removal of these benign polyps will decrease the likelihood of subsequent development of colorectal cancer.

Asymptomatic lesions may be discovered in patients who present for radiologic examinations of the colon because of symptoms due to other conditions, such as diverticular disease, abdominal or pelvic masses, or functional disorders. Other patients with asymptomatic lesions may present for radiologic study because of positive findings in mass screening programs. Greegor[9] has advocated a mass screening program for the detection of early colon cancer or premalignant lesions of the colon and rectum. This is a program of multiple stool testing for occult blood, and is based on the finding that early tumors in the large bowel tend to bleed intermittently. The incidence of false positive tests[10] for occult blood is decreased by removing meat from the diet while adding roughage in order to irritate the tumor and cause it to bleed. Multiple stool samples are tested for occult blood, and all patients with positive reactions are followed up by x-ray study and appropriate endoscopy.

Hastings[11] was able to examine 3450 patients in one program and found 5 asymptomatic carcinomas. This was equivalent to 1 carcinoma in 450 patients over the age of 40. It has been found that patients with asymptomatic carcinoma frequently have a Dukes' A tumor and that a cure rate of 80 to 90 per cent can be anticipated.[5]

In addition to mass screening, regular survey of patients at high risk for the development of colonic carcinoma may result in detection of early lesions. These include patients with ulcerative colitis,[12] previous polyps or carcinomas,[13] a family history of colon cancer,[14] and Peutz-Jeghers syndrome.[15] Of course patients with conditions such as familial polyposis or Gardner's syndrome are not included. In those conditions, total colectomy is usually carried out as soon as the diagnosis is established, and therefore there is no opportunity for follow-up studies. Some patients will have a subtotal colectomy with ileorectal anastomosis. In those patients early lesions may be detected on follow-up studies of the residual rectum.

In summary, it seems likely that most colorectal carcinomas begin as benign polypoid lesions. The best hope for decreasing mortality from this disease lies in the detection of early carcinoma or the precursors of carcinoma, i.e., benign polyps, in asymptomatic patients. These may be detected by serendipity, by regular survey of high risk patients, or by a mass screening program.

BENIGN TUMORS

Epithelial Polyps

Benign tumors of the colon are extremely common, and in most patients do not produce symptoms. Several authors have reported polyp detection rates ranging from 10 to 12.5 per cent, using the double contrast enema.[16-20] There is a dramatic rise in polyp incidence with increasing age,[19, 21] as illustrated in Figure 13–1. Polyps are most frequently detected in the rectosigmoid and left colon. Figure 13–2 illustrates the distribution of 108 consecutive polyps detected by double contrast enema.

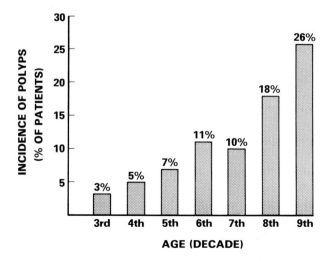

FIGURE 13-1 The incidence of colonic polyps related to age (based on 800 consecutive double contrast enemas). There is an increasing incidence of colonic polyps, ranging from 3 per cent in the third decade of life to 26 per cent in the ninth decade. (*From:* Laufer, I.; Gastrointest Radiol., *1*:19, 1976.[19] Reproduced by permission).

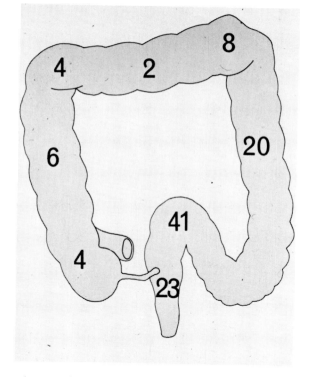

FIGURE 13-2 The distribution of colorectal polyps (based on 108 consecutive polyps). Approximately 60 per cent of the polyps are in the rectum and sigmoid.

It is obvious that a clean colon is essential for the detection of polyps. However, good mucosal coating is equally important. It has been amply demonstrated that in the presence of poor coating even large tumors can be missed.[22] An adequate number of projections must be obtained, since it is not unusual for a lesion to be demonstrated on only one of the entire series of films (Fig. 13–3). Another important prerequisite is adequate colonic distension. The collapsed colon can hide sizeable lesions (Fig. 13–4). Unraveling loops of bowel are not as important in the double contrast enema as in single contrast, since even small lesions may be seen through overlapping loops. However, in some cases very careful study of the films may be necessary to detect these lesions (Fig. 13–5). Because of this see-through effect it may be difficult to determine which of the over-lapping loops contains the polyp (Fig. 13–6).

The majority of colorectal polyps are inflammatory or metaplastic and are usually 5 mm or less in diameter (Fig. 13–7). These lesions have no malignant potential. The majority of larger polyps are adenomatous polyps. In our experience, approximately one fourth of patients who have one polyp have multiple polyps. The number may range anywhere from two to a dozen or more (Figs. 13–8 and 13–9). In the extreme case of familial polyposis the mucosal surface may be studded with polyps of varying size (Fig. 13–10).

Villous adenomas are less common and have a much higher malig-nant potential than adenomatous polyps. Small villous adenomas may be indistinguishable roentgenographically from adenomatous polyps (Fig. 13–11). However, the larger lesions may have the typical flat appearance, with a frondlike surface (Fig. 13–12), and may be associated with symp-toms of diarrhea and hypokalemia.[23] In many cases a flat lobulated ap-pearance may be suggestive of a villous adenoma, but histologic study shows an adenomatous or villoglandular polyp (Fig. 13–13).

Other nonneoplastic polyps may also occur in the colon. These in-clude juvenile polyps which may be single or multiple, and may be found in children and adults (Fig. 14–17).[24] Hamartomatous polyps are found in the Peutz-Jeghers syndrome and inflammatory polyps in the Cronkhite-Canada syndrome.[25] The polyposis syndromes are considered in detail in Chapter 14.

In most instances small polyps can be distinguished from fecal res-idue by the mobility and irregular coating of solid fecal material. However, true polyps may exhibit several other radiologic features that are help-ful. Demonstration of a stalk is conclusive proof of the presence of a polyp. The stalk may be demonstrated in profile (Figs. 13–4B, 13–7B, 13–8A and B, and 13–9). Occasionally, mucus threads that resemble the stalk may be seen, but without a polyp at the end (Fig. 13–14). The stalk may also be seen on end through the head of the polyp, producing the appearance of a target or a "Mexican hat" (Fig. 13–15). Another sign has been called the bowler hat sign by Youker and Welin.[26] This consists of two circular shadows, one representing barium caught in the angle be-tween the polyp and the bowel wall, and the other representing the head of the polyp. When the polyp is seen in profile the combination of these two shadows resembles a bowler hat (Fig. 13–16). This sign is illustrated in detail in Chapter 2, Figure 2–13.

In most cases, when a polyp is detected radiologically, further studies consist of the appropriate endoscopic examination — either proctosig-moidoscopy or colonoscopy. Most polyps can be removed from any part of the colon, particularly if the polyp is pedunculated.[27, 28] The sequence of events is illustrated in Plates 83 and 84. If any "polyp" is not con-firmed by endoscopy, it is frequently assumed that the radiologic diagno-sis was in error. However, it must be appreciated that there are endo-scopic blind spots. These include areas where there are prominent folds, such as the rectum or cecum, or areas of sharp angulation of the bowel, such as the junction of sigmoid and descending colon and the flexures. In these areas a polyp lying against the wall or behind a fold may be difficult to detect (Fig. 13–17). In some cases the endoscope had been passed through the area of the polyp several times before the polyp was finally found. In other cases the endoscopy had been repeated two, three, or four times before the polyp was finally discovered.[20] Therefore, we suggest that if there is strong radiologic evidence of a polyp which is not confirmed on a single endoscopic examination, it should not be assumed that there was a radiologic error. Instead, we suggest a repeat radiologic study, and if the polyp is still present endoscopy should be repeated.

Text continued on page 531

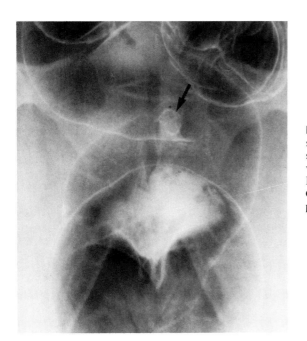

FIGURE 13–3 Small polyp (*arrow*) at the recto-sigmoid junction behind a fold. This polyp was seen only on this prone-angled view and was not visible on any of the other radiographs. (*From*: Laufer, I., Smith, N. C. W., and Mullens, J. E.: Gastroenterology, *70*:167, 1976.[20] Reproduced by permission).

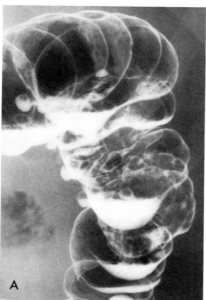

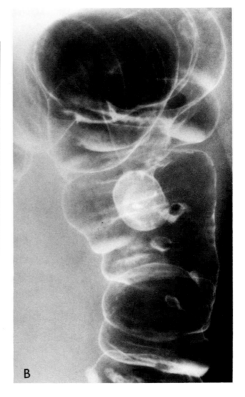

FIGURE 13–4 The importance of adequate colonic distension.

A. Poor distension of the colon. Only diverticula are seen.

B. With adequate distension a pedunculated polyp is clearly seen in addition to the diverticula.

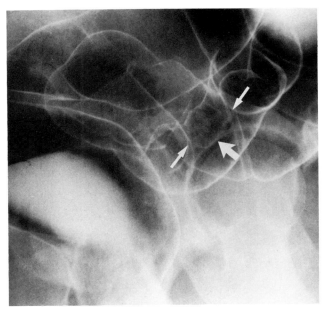

FIGURE 13–5 Sigmoid polyp (*arrow*) seen through overlapping loops of bowel.

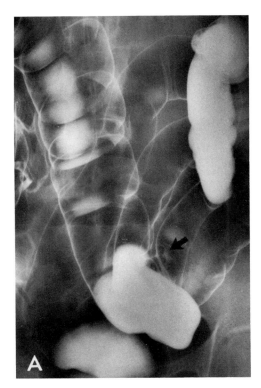

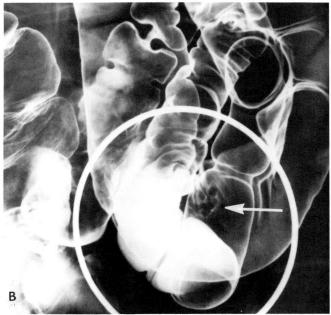

FIGURE 13–6

A. There are overlapping loops in the left lower quadrant. The lobulated polyp (*arrow*) at first was thought to be in the sigmoid colon, but was not detected at colonoscopy.

B. A repeat study showed that the polyp is actually in the descending colon. Because of the flat nature of the polyp it was removed at surgery and proved to be a benign tumor.

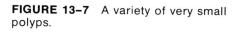
FIGURE 13-7 A variety of very small polyps.

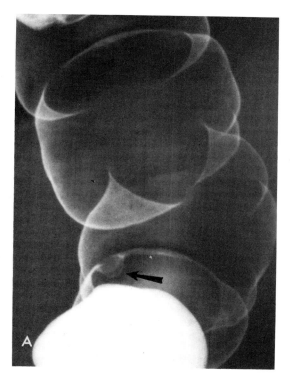

A. Sessile polyp.

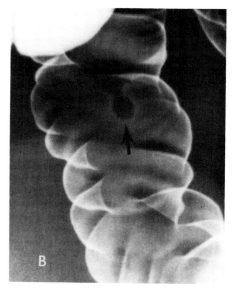

B. Pedunculated polyp.

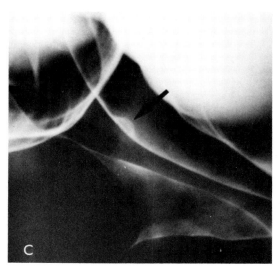

C. Flat sessile polyp.

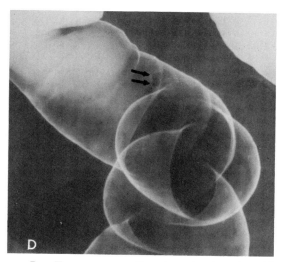

D. Two very small polyps in the sigmoid. Confirmed by endoscopy.

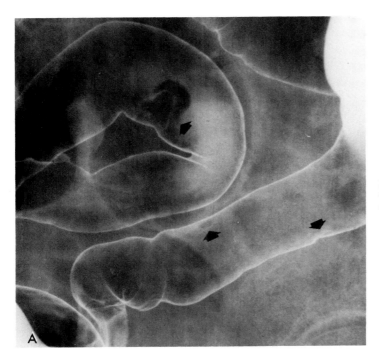

A. There is a pedunculated polyp at the apex of the sigmoid colon, and two smaller polyps in the distal descending colon.

FIGURE 13–8 Multiple polyps.

B. Four small polyps in the sigmoid colon.

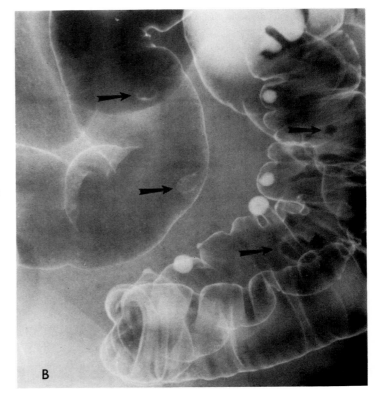

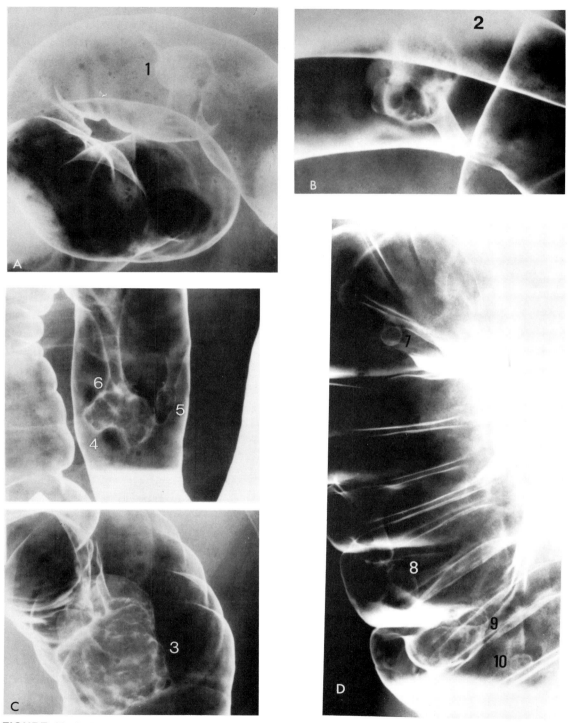

FIGURE 13–9 *A* to *D*   Ten polyps scattered throughout the colon. (B, *From*: Glass, G. B. J. (ed.): Progress in Gastroenterology. New York, Grune & Stratton, 1977. C. *From*: Laufer, I., Gastrointest. Radiol, *1*:19, 1976. Used by permission.)

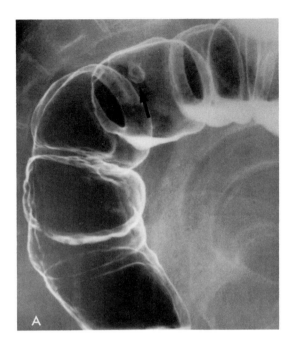

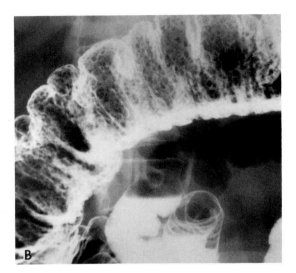

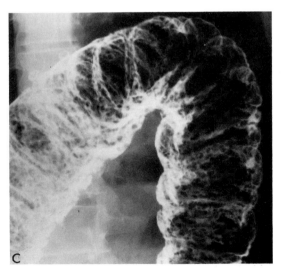

FIGURE 13–10 *A* to *C* Familial polyposis. The colon is carpeted with tiny polyps, although they are relatively sparse in the rectum.

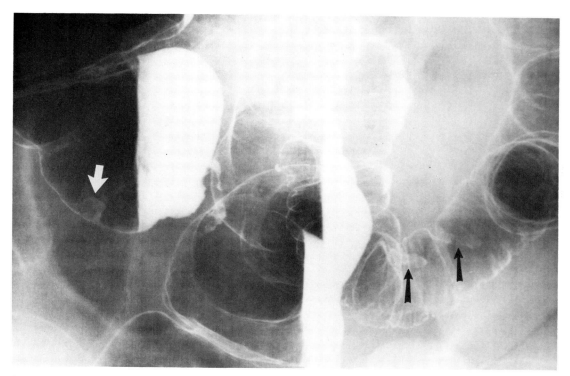

FIGURE 13–11 Small villous adenoma in the cecum (*white arrow*). It shows none of the characteristic features of a villous adenoma. There are also two small pedunculated polyps in the sigmoid (*black arrows*).

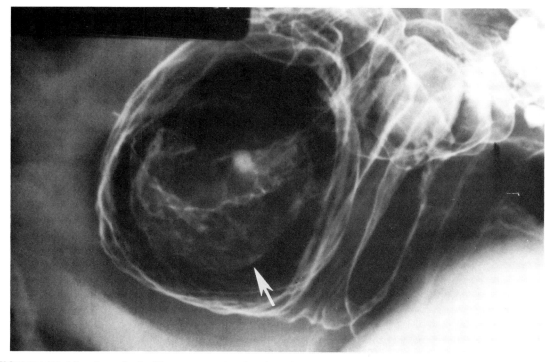

FIGURE 13–12 A typical villous tumor in the sigmoid. This exhibits the typical, irregular, frondlike surface of a villous tumor. This was a malignant villous adenoma.

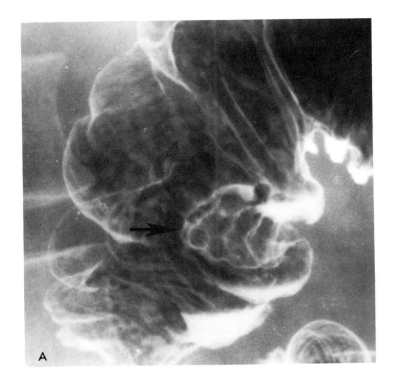

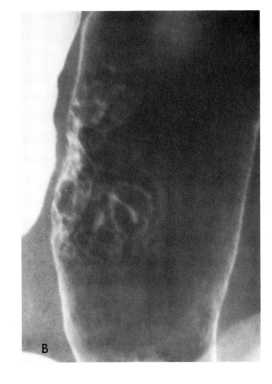

FIGURE 13–13

A. A flat, lobulated tumor at the hepatic flexure. This was an adenomatous polyp.

B. A flat tumor in the descending colon, with an irregular surface suggestive of a villous adenoma. This was a villoglandular polyp (see also Plate 87).

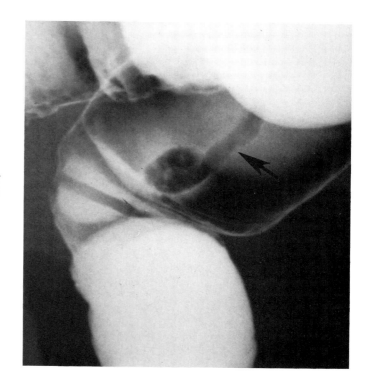

FIGURE 13–14 A coiled strand of mucus resembling a pedunculated polyp.

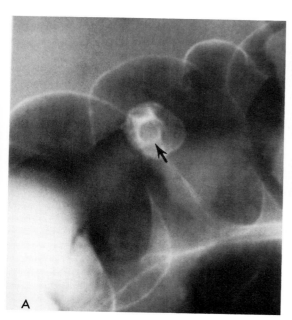

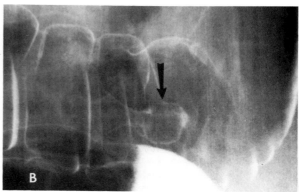

FIGURE 13–15

A. A pedunculated polyp with the stalk (*arrow*) seen through the head of the polyp, giving rise to the "Mexican hat sign."

B. A decubitus view shows the polyp and its stalk. This was a juvenile polyp in a 23-year-old male with rectal bleeding.

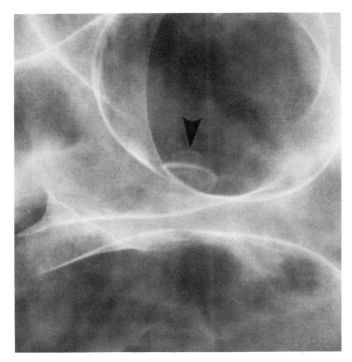

FIGURE 13–16 The "bowler hat" sign due to a sessile polyp.

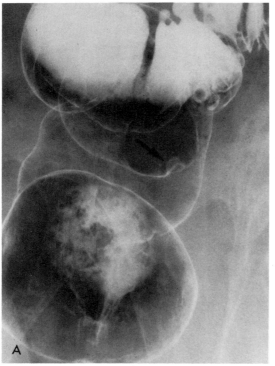

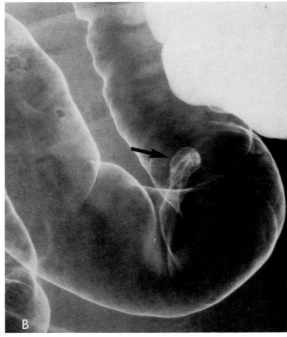

FIGURE 13–17 Polyps missed at endoscopy.

A. There is a small sessile polyp behind a fold at the rectosigmoid junction. This lesion was missed twice on sigmoidoscopy and was finally detected at the third sigmoidoscopy.

B. A small polyp situated behind a fold at an area of angulation at the junction of sigmoid and descending colon. This polyp was missed on two colonoscopic examinations and was found on the third. See Plate 86. (*From:* Laufer, I., Smith, N. C. W., and Mullens, J. E., Gastroenterology, *70:*167, 1976. Reproduced by permission.)

Other Benign Lesions

Lipomas are the most common submucosal tumors in the colon.[29, 30] They are found most frequently in the cecum and ascending colon (Fig. 13–18*A*), and must be differentiated from a prominent ileocecal valve (Fig. 13–18*B*). They frequently exhibit the characteristic findings of a submucosal mass. In addition, when seen en face they may have a typically elliptic shape (Fig. 13–19). They are also characterized by their pliability and ability to change in shape with change in position. As lipomas grow larger and extend intraluminally, they appear to develop a pedicle and may be seen to move freely at fluoroscopy (Fig. 13–18*A*).

Other submucosal tumors, such as leiomyomas, may be indistinguishable from other polyps when they are small (Fig. 13–20). When they become larger they exhibit the typical features of a submucosal tumor, and they may form the leading point of an intussusception (Fig. 13–21).

Polypoid Artifacts

As discussed and illustrated in Chapters 2 and 11, a variety of artifactual appearances may simulate a colonic polypoid lesion.[31] These include normal variants, such as a prominent ileocecal valve, folding of the intestinal wall, and lymphoid hyperplasia; nonpolypoid lesions, such as diverticula or an inverted appendiceal stump; extraneous material, including stool, air bubbles, oil droplets, pills, and undigested vegetables;[32] and calcified and skeletal structures seen through the colon.[33]

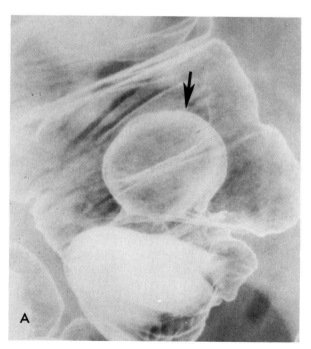

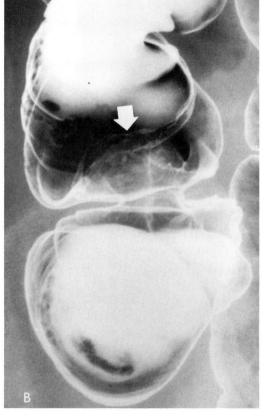

FIGURE 13–18 *A* and *B*   A lipoma arising from the superior lip of the ileocecal valve *(A)*. This is to be distinguished from fatty infiltration causing diffuse enlargement of the ileocecal valve (*B*).

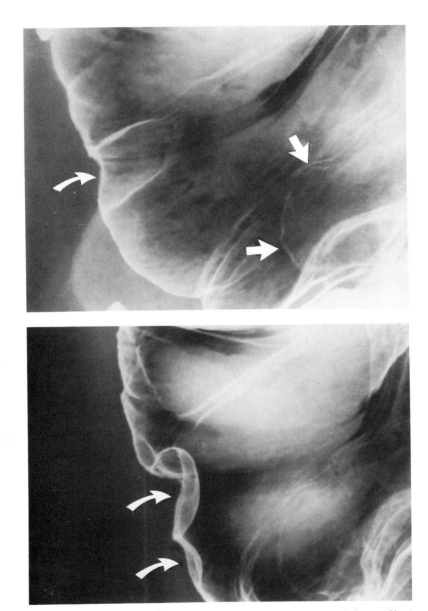

FIGURE 13–19 Bilobed lipoma of the ascending colon seen en face and in profile (*curved arrows*). There is also a polypoid carcinoma of the cecum (*straight arrows*). See also Plate 90. (Reproduced by permission. From Laufer, I.: Gastrointest, Radiol., *1*:19, 1976.)

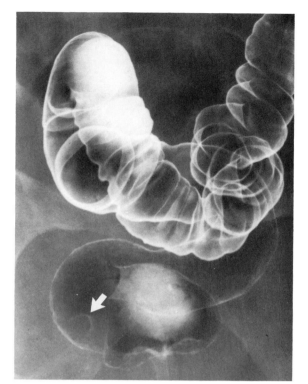

FIGURE 13–20 Leiomyoma of the rectum, presenting as a polypoid tumor (*arrow*) indistinguishable from other rectal polyps.

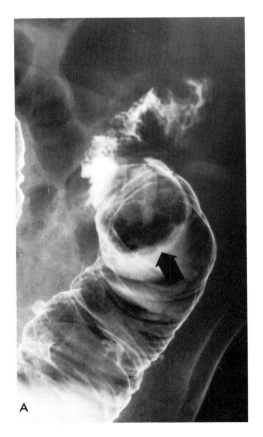

A

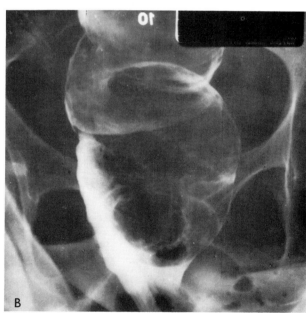

B

FIGURE 13–21

A. Leiomyoma causing colocolic intussusception, which was reduced spontaneously.

B. At a later date the patient was readmitted with large bowel obstruction, with the intussusception presenting in the rectum.

MALIGNANT TUMORS

Advanced Cancer

The majority of patients who present with symptomatic colorectal carcinoma have advanced lesions. These are generally large annular (Fig. 13–22A) or polypoid (Fig. 13–22B) lesions that present no diagnostic problem, provided the colon is reasonably clean and an adequate number of projections are obtained. The particular advantage of the double contrast technique in these lesions lies in the ability to see through overlapping loops of bowel. Thus these lesions may be seen not only in profile, but also en face (Figs. 13–23 and 13–24). However, as illustrated in these figures, it may take some experience to recognize these tumors en face or through overlapping loops. Advanced cancers are frequently associated with "sentinel" polyps (Figs. 13–24 and 13–25). In addition, approximately 5 per cent of patients have multiple synchronous carcinomas of the colon (Fig. 13–26).[34] Therefore, an attempt should be made to examine the entire colon whenever possible.

Plaque-like carcinomas are also difficult to demonstrate and recognize (Fig. 13–27). Occasionally, advanced lesions are very difficult to detect. Figure 13–28A to C illustrates three views of a normal-appearing cecum with filling of the appendix. However, Figure 13–28D, which was obtained with the patient prone and the table tilted head-down, shows the annular carcinoma. Occasionally, when the double contrast study is inconclusive we ask the patient to evacuate, and we perform a single contrast study immediately thereafter.

In some cases advanced carcinoma may have atypical appearances. These include the linitis plastica type of carcinoma with predominant submucosal infiltration.[35] The radiologic picture may be suggestive of an inflammatory stricture due to Crohn's disease, diverticulitis, or ischemia. This type of carcinoma is particularly likely to develop in patients with ulcerative colitis.[36] A similar picture may be produced by a perforated carcinoma, in which the radiologic picture is dominated by the pericolic inflammatory reaction.[37]

Text continued on page 541

FIGURE 13-22 Typical advanced colonic carcinoma.

A. Annular, apple-core lesion.

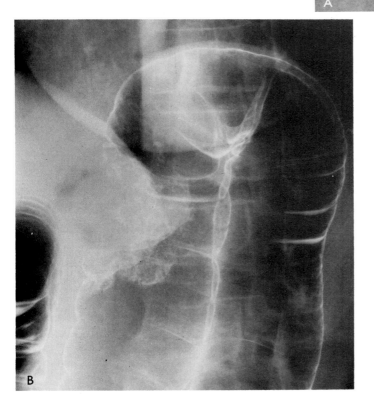

B. Large polypoid carcinoma at the splenic flexure.

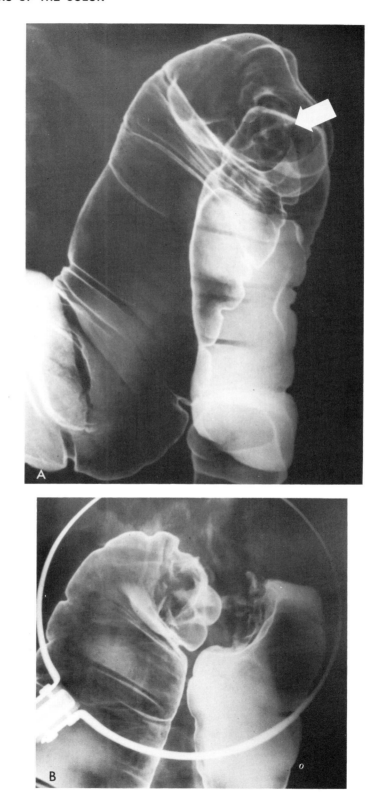

FIGURE 13–23*A* and *B*   Annular carcinoma of the splenic flexure seen en face (*A*) and in profile (*B*).

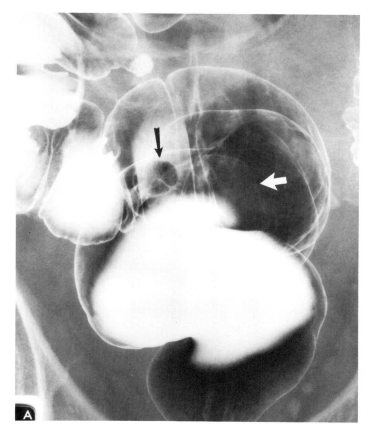

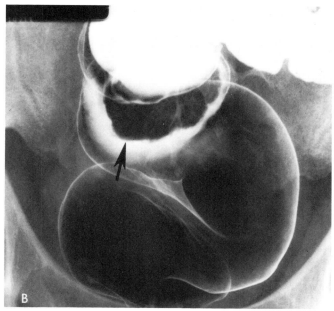

FIGURE 13–24

  A.   On this prone view, the white etching representing the outline of a polypoid carcinoma (*white arrow*) is faintly seen. Therefore, the lesion must be on the posterior wall. There is also an adjacent small benign polyp (*black arrow*).

  B.   The film in the supine position shows the polypoid carcinoma as a filling defect in the barium pool, confirming the posterior wall location of the tumor.

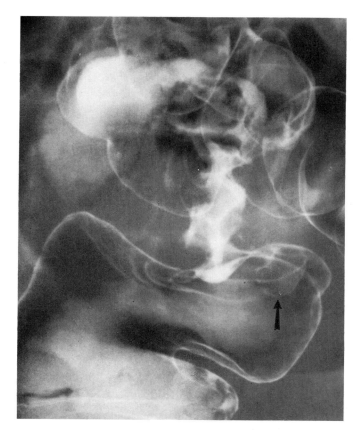

FIGURE 13–25 Annular carcinoma of the rectosigmoid junction with a sentinel polyp (*arrow*).

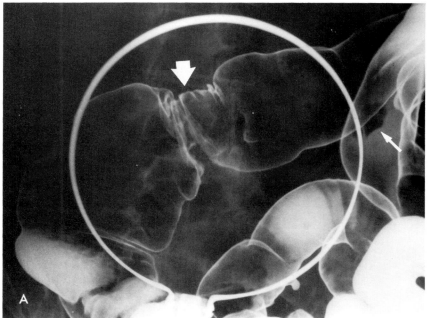

FIGURE 13–26 Multiple synchronous carcinomas.

A. There is a polypoid tumor at the hepatic flexure with circumferential extension (*large arrow*). There is a smaller polypoid carcinoma in the descending colon (*small arrow*).

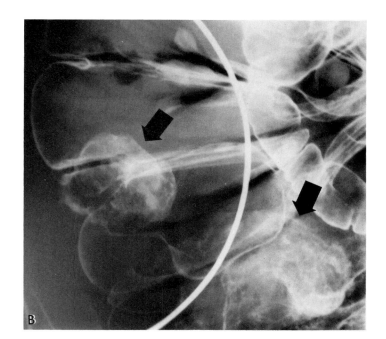

B. Multiple polypoid carcinomas in the ascending colon.

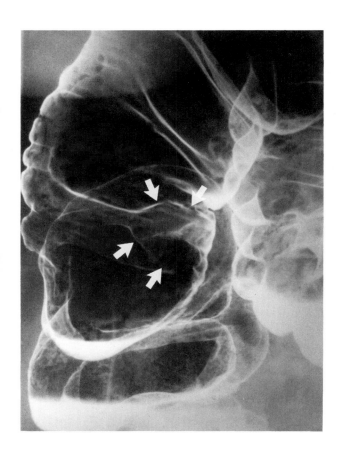

FIGURE 13–27 Plaque-like carcinoma of the ascending colon.

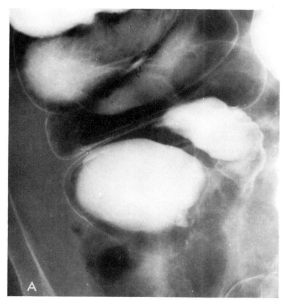

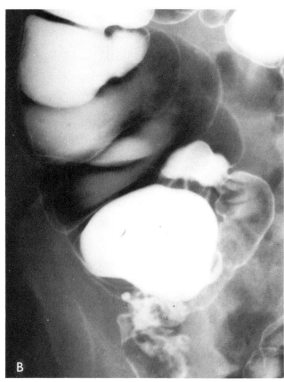

FIGURE 13–28_A_ and _B_   Apparently normal cecum with a small barium pool.

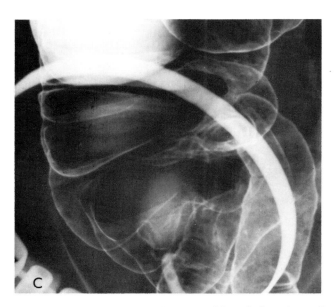

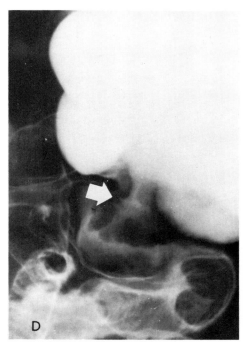

_C._   Apparently normal cecum, although there is small
bowel overlapping the tip of the cecum.

_D._   With the patient in the prone position and tilted
head-down to drain barium from the cecum, the annular
carcinoma _(arrow)_ is seen. This case illustrates the
difficulty in demonstrating some advanced carcinomas.

Early Cancer

There is little doubt that advanced cancers start as small polypoid lesions (Fig. 13–29).[38] Thus the radiologic detection of early colorectal cancer is basically an exercise in the detection of small polyps. Occasionally an early plaque-like carcinoma may be found, and even more rarely carcinoma may start as a flat ulcer with no surrounding mass.[39] Shinya and Wolff[40] found an overall 6.5 per cent rate of malignancy in polyps greater than 5 mm in size removed at colonoscopy. The incidence of malignancy depended to a large extent on the pathologic nature of the benign polyp. There was no malignancy in hyperplastic polyps. Adenomatous polyps had malignancy in 3.3 per cent of cases, while villous adenomas had a 12.6 per cent incidence of malignancy (Fig. 9–30).

A number of radiologic criteria for the diagnosis of malignancy in polyps have been suggested.[41]

Size of the Polyp. Carcinoma is virtually nonexistent in polyps under 5 mm. In polyps measuring 5 to 10 mm there is approximately a 1 per cent incidence of carcinoma, while polyps over 2 cm in size have an incidence of malignancy approaching 50 per cent.[1]

Rate of Growth. Malignant polyps tend to grow more quickly than benign polyps, although there is considerable overlap between the two groups.[42] For practical purposes, if there is definite evidence of growth on serial follow-up examinations of a polyp, malignancy should be suspected.

Pedicle. A long, thin pedicle is highly suggestive of a benign polyp. Nevertheless, Smith[43] has reported on several polypoid lesions with long, thin pedicles that turned out to harbor a malignancy. As a rule, these are early carcinomas with no invasion of the stalk.[44] However, we have seen one case in which there was carcinoma in the head of the polyp, with invasion of the stalk (Fig. 13–31A). As a rule, the stalk associated with carcinoma is short and thick (Fig. 13–31B).

Irregularity of the Head of the Polyp. If the head of the polyp is irregular or lobulated the frequency of malignancy is increased (Fig. 13–32). This is certainly not invariable, since some benign polyps have very irregular and lobulated heads (Fig. 13–9).

Indentation of the Base. Indentation or puckering of the base of the polyp is a reliable sign of malignancy (Fig. 13–33). Nevertheless, we have seen this sign in several polyps that proved to be benign (Figs. 13–34 and 13–35). This appearance in benign polyps may be due to traction by a stalk, or it may be caused by the head of the polyp resting against the mucosal surface. In other patients the stalk may lie crumpled against the mucosal surface, producing the appearance of a very irregular base.

Thus, although there are several signs that suggest malignancy in polypoid lesions, a definitive diagnosis of malignancy in small lesions can rarely be made. In addition, some small carcinomas have none of the features of malignancy described.[38] Therefore, we recommend for most patients in whom there is no contraindication to endoscopy that all polyps measuring more than 5 mm in diameter be inspected and removed endoscopically. This is based on the observation that the incidence of malignancy even in small polyps is greater than the frequency of serious complications from endoscopy.[45, 46] This is particularly true when the colonoscopic polypectomy is performed by an experienced endoscopist.

Text continued on page 549

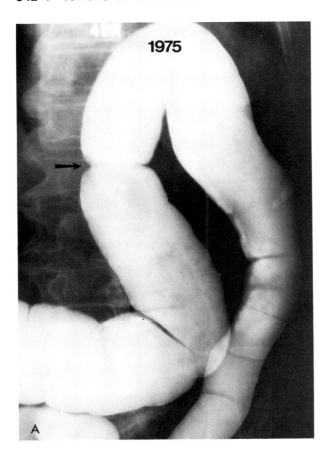

A. Barium enema in 1975 in which a small polypoid lesion (*arrow*) was not appreciated.

FIGURE 13–29 Annular carcinoma starting as a small polypoid lesion.

B. Three years later there is a typical annular carcinoma at this site.

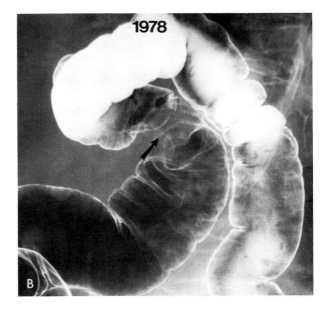

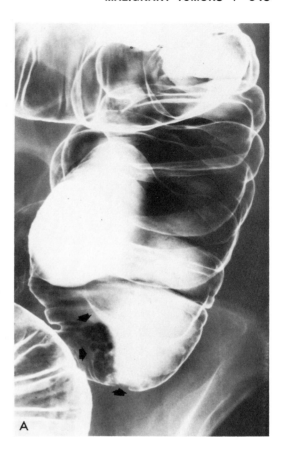

A. Film of the prone view shows a finely nodular lesion as radiolucent filling defects in the barium puddle. Therefore, the lesion must be on the anterior wall of the cecum.

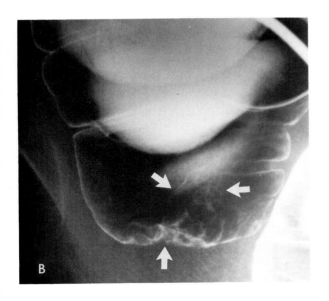

FIGURE 13–30 Villous tumor of the cecum with mucosal carcinoma.

B. This is confirmed in the supine projection, in which the lesion is etched in white, and must therefore lie on the nondependent surface, i.e., the anterior wall.

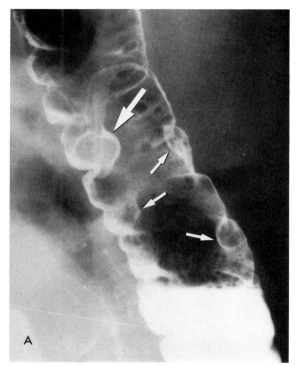

A. Polypoid carcinoma with a pedicle in a 29-year-old male with rectal bleeding. There is a pedunculated polyp in the descending colon (*large arrow*), with a typically benign appearance. This was removed at colonoscopy and was a carcinoma with invasion of the stalk. The smaller lesions (*small arrows*) were hyperplastic polyps. (*From*: Laufer, I., Gastrointest. Radiol. *1*:19, 1976.[19] Reproduced by permission.)

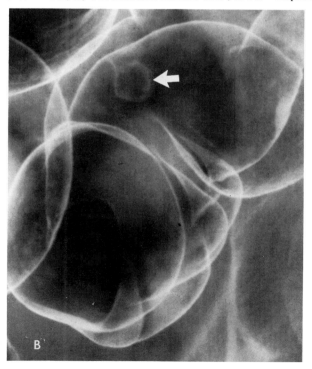

B. Early carcinoma with a short, thick stalk.

FIGURE 13–31

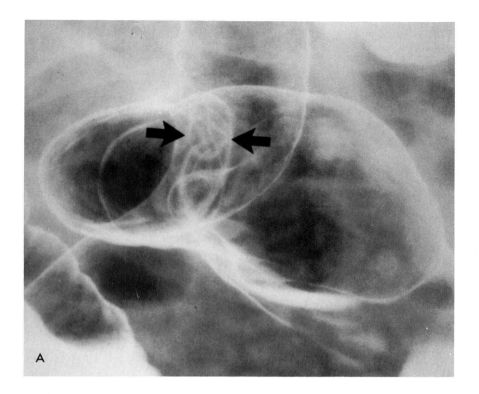

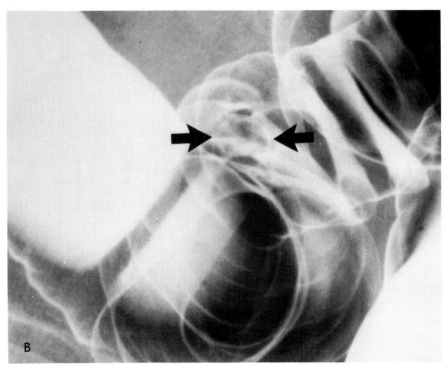

FIGURE 13–32*A* and *B*   Two examples of early polypoid carcinomas seen through overlapping loops. The surface of the tumors is slightly irregular. (*B. From*: Laufer, I.: Gastrointest. Radiol., *1*:19, 1976.[19] Reproduced by permission.)

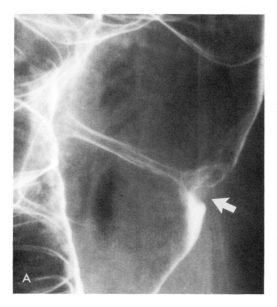

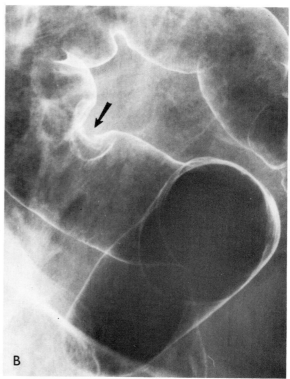

FIGURE 13–33 *A* to *C*   Three examples of early polypoid carcinomas with indentation of the base.

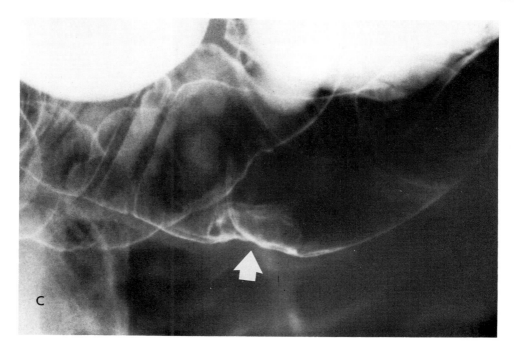

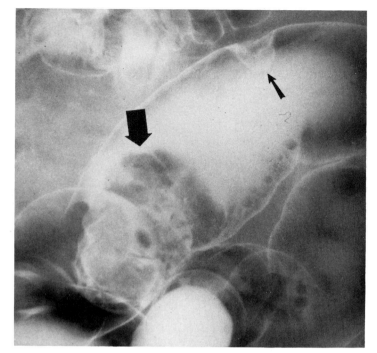

FIGURE 13–34 There are two polypoid tumors in the sigmoid. The distal lesion *(large arrow)* measures 4 cm in diameter, while the proximal lesion measures 1 cm in diameter and has an irregular puckered base. The patient had a segmental resection of the sigmoid, and both lesions were benign adenomatous polyps (Plate 88).

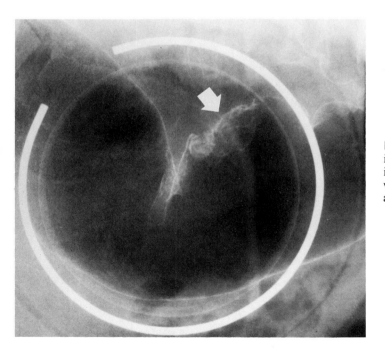

FIGURE 13–35 Polypoid lesion in the descending colon with an irregular indented base. The lesion was resected and was a benign adenomatous polyp.

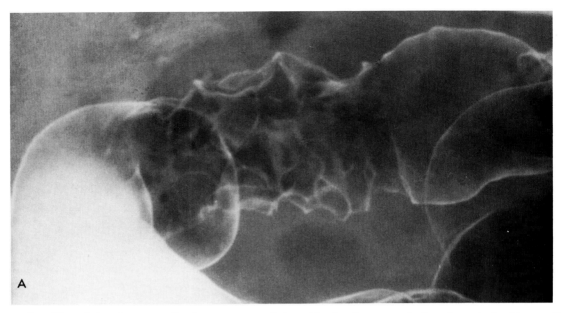

A. There is involvement of a short segment of sigmoid colon by a mass lesion characterized by small nodules. This was due to colonic involvement by disseminated lymphosarcoma.

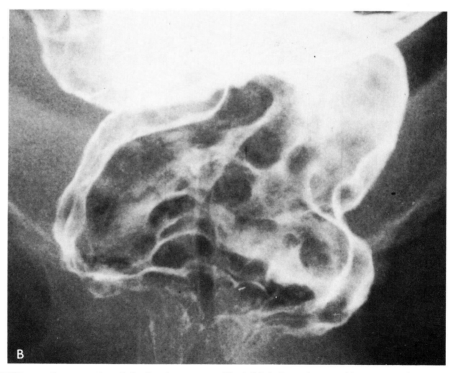

B. Diffuse submucosal nodularity due to non-Hodgkin's lymphoma. (Courtesy of J. O. Op den Orth, M.D., Haarlem, Holland.)

FIGURE 13–36 Colonic lymphoma.

Other Malignant Tumors

SUBMUCOSAL TUMORS

Other types of malignant tumors involving the colon are relatively uncommon. Primary colonic lymphoma most often involves the cecum or rectosigmoid and may produce either large ulcerated lesions or diffuse submucosal nodularity (Fig. 13–36).[47] Leiomyosarcoma of the colon is a rare lesion. Two thirds of the cases involve the rectum. The lesion usually grows as a bulky exophytic mass (Fig. 17–14).[48] It may be impossible to distinguish radiologically between leiomyoma and leiomyosarcoma.

METASTATIC TUMORS

Metastatic lesions of the colon are being seen with increasing frequency as more aggressive treatment with radiotherapy and chemotherapy prolongs the life of patients with disseminated carcinoma. The most common lesions that metastasize to the colon are carcinomas of the breast, stomach, lung, pancreas, kidney, and female genital tract.[49] The colon may be involved by extension of an extracolonic mass. This results in stretching of the loop of bowel, followed by spiculation and nodularity (Fig. 13–37), and may progress to ulceration and obstruction (Fig. 13–38). Hematogenous metastases start as intramural filling defects (Fig. 13–39), which may progress to infiltrate the entire circumference of the colonic wall. In some cases the radiologic appearance very closely mimics an inflammatory condition, particularly granulomatous colitis (Fig. 13–40).[50] Peritoneal carcinomatosis may also be detected radiographically by extrinsic pressure defects on the colon. These metastases are particularly apt to drop into the pouch of Douglas and are seen as extrinsic or intramural filling defects on the anterior wall of the rectosigmoid junction (Fig. 13–41).[51] A similar appearance may be produced by a pelvic abscess (Fig. 13–42).

Text continued on page 554

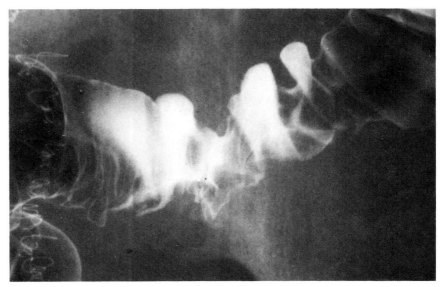

FIGURE 13–37 Carcinoma of the cervix with involvement of the inferior aspect of the sigmoid colon.

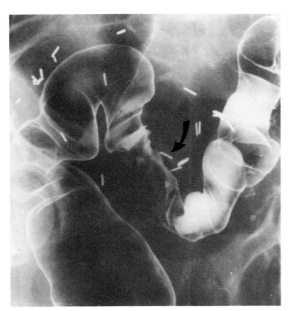

FIGURE 13–38 Carcinoma of the cervix with involvement of the sigmoid colon by an annular lesion.

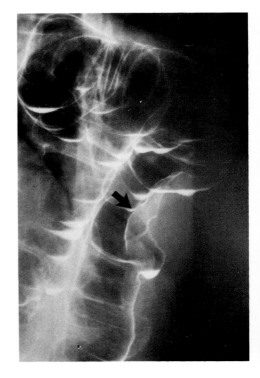

FIGURE 13–39 Submucosal mass involving the proximal descending colon due to a metastatic lesion from carcinoma of the ovary.

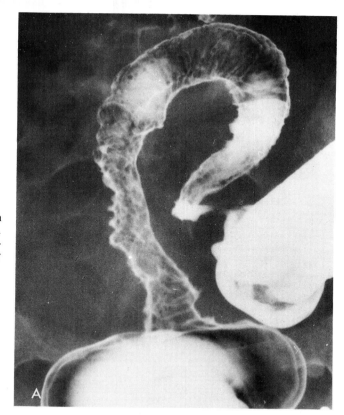

A. There is marked narrowing, with mucosal irregularity of the sigmoid colon. The appearance of the mucosa is suggestive of an inflammatory lesion, particularly granulomatous colitis.

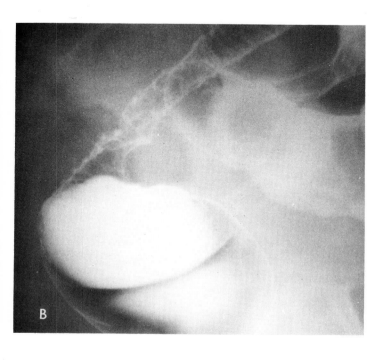

FIGURE 13–40 Metastatic disease to the colon from carcinoma of the breast, simulating inflammatory bowel disease.

B. The lateral view shows the narrowing of the sigmoid, with an increase in the retrorectal soft tissues.

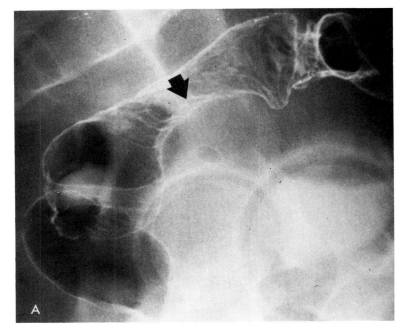

A. Metastasis to the pouch of Douglas from carcinoma of the colon. There is an intramural filling defect on the anterior wall at the rectosigmoid junction. This is characteristic of peritoneal carcinomatosis involving the pouch of Douglas.

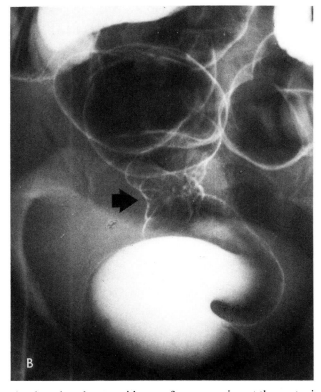

B. Frontal projection also shows evidence of compression at the rectosigmoid junction.

FIGURE 13–41

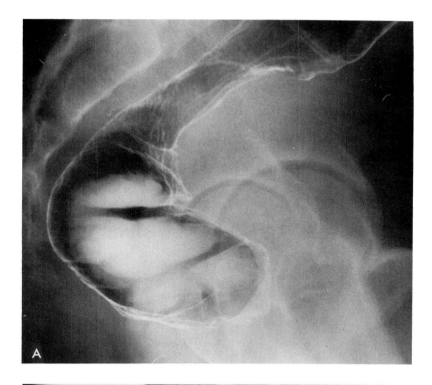

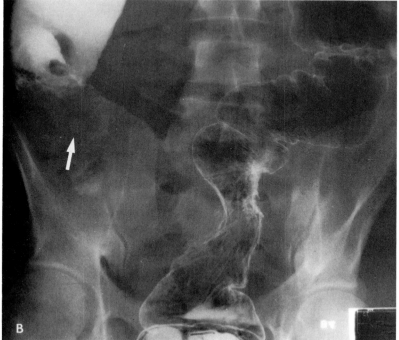

FIGURE 13–42 *A* and *B*   An identical appearance due to pelvic abscess in a patient with a ruptured appendix. Note the soft tissue mass in the region of the cecum and the appendicolith (*arrow*).

THE POSTOPERATIVE COLON

Patients who have had previous surgery for colorectal carcinoma undergo frequent postoperative examinations because of the relatively high risk of development of a second metachronous carcinoma and for the assessment of postoperative symptoms. Ileocolic (Fig. 13–43) and colocolic (Fig. 13–44) anastomoses can be demonstrated in great detail with the double contrast enema, particularly with the use of intravenous glucagon. Plication defects are frequently identified. In some patients a filling defect due to a stitch granuloma may be seen in the early postoperative period (Fig. 13–44). However, this will regress and become less prominent on follow-up studies.[52] Particular attention must be paid to the anastomotic site,[53] since metastatic deposits tend to implant at the anastomosis.[54] Occasionally tumors recur near to but not at the anastomotic site (Fig. 13–45).

When the anastomotic site appears eccentric (Fig. 13–46A) or irregular (Fig. 13–46B), or has nodular filling defects (Fig. 13–47), recurrent tumor should be suspected. Colonoscopy may be helpful in such patients, although in some instances it may be misleading, since recurrent tumor may be submucosal and biopsy findings may be negative for malignancy. Repeated follow-up studies may be necessary in these patients to document the progression of radiologic changes.

Patients who have undergone abdominoperineal resection with colostomy must also undergo regular examination because of the possibility of developing a second tumor. Double contrast examination of the residual colon can usually be performed through the colostomy. This is greatly facilitated by a device described by Goldstein.[55] This consists basically of an infant's feeding nipple through which a catheter is introduced to project about 6 inches into the colon. This is introduced by the patient into the stoma, and the nipple is held against the stoma while barium and air are injected.

Text continued on page 559

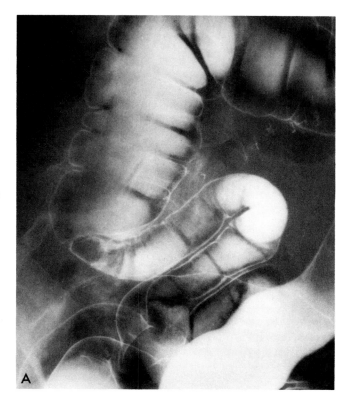

FIGURE 13–43

A. Normal ileocolic anastomosis in the ascending colon.

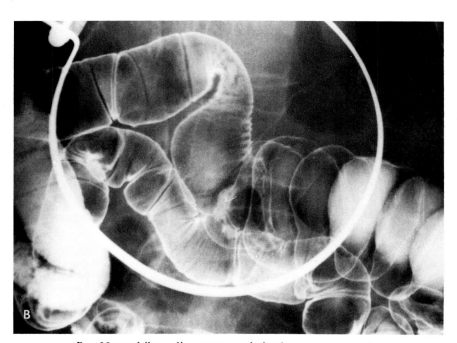

B. Normal ileocolic anastomosis in the transverse colon.

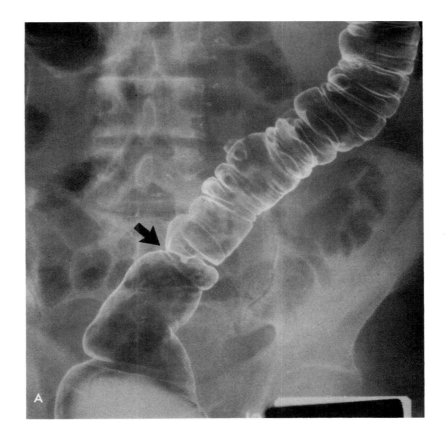

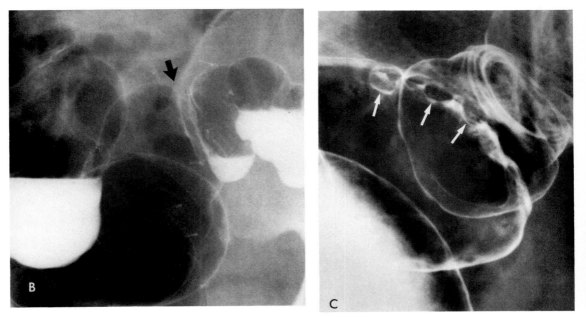

A and *B*. Two examples of a colocolic anastomosis.
C. Colocolic anastomosis with identifiable plication defects due to sutures (*arrows*).

FIGURE 13–44

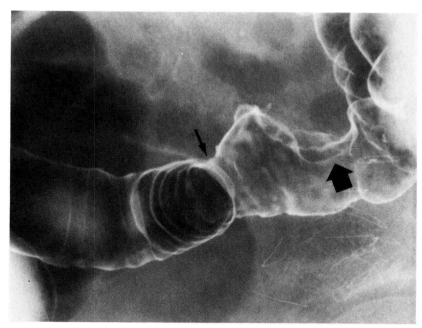

FIGURE 13–45   Recurrent carcinoma (*large arrow*) proximal to the anastomosis (*small arrow*).

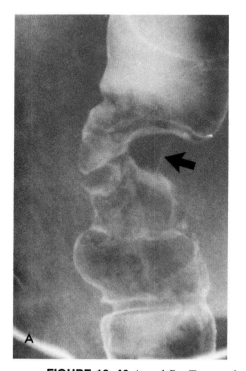

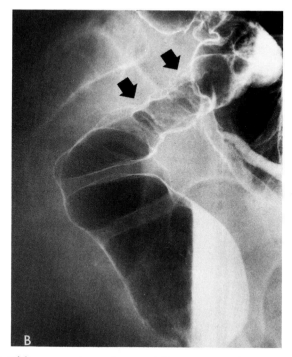

FIGURE 13–46 *A* and *B*   Two patients with recurrent carcinoma at the anastomosis.

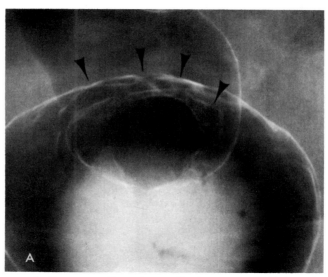

A.   Frontal view shows the anastomosis en face with the villous adenomas (*arrows*) arranged along the superior aspect.

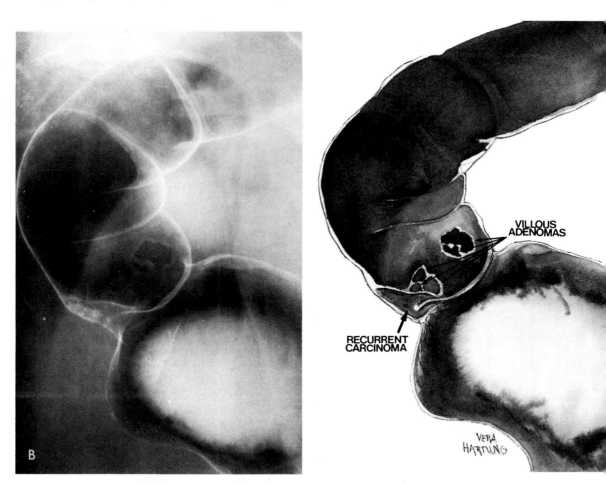

B.   Lateral view shows the recurrent carcinoma and the villous adenomas. Confirmed at surgery.

FIGURE 13–47   Recurrent carcinoma and five villous adenomas at a colorectal anastomosis.

REFERENCES

1. Morson, B. C.: The polyp-cancer sequence in the large bowel. Proc. R. Soc. Med., *67*:451, 1974.
2. Lane, N., and Fenoglio, C. M.: The adenoma-carcinoma sequence in the stomach and colon. I. Observations on the adenoma as precursor to ordinary large bowel carcinoma. Gastrointest. Radiol., *1*:111, 1976.
3. Waye, J. D.: The development of carcinoma of the colon. Am. J. Gastroenterol., *67*:427, 1977.
4. Enterline, H. T., Evans, G. W., Mercado-Lugo, R., et al.: Malignant potential of adenomas of colon and rectum. JAMA, *179*:322, 1962.
5. Winawer, S. J., Sherlock, P., Schottenfeld, D., et al.: Screening for colon cancer. Gastroenterology, *70*:783, 1976.
6. Dales, L. G., Friedman, G. D., Ramcharan, S., et al.: Multiphasic checkup evaluation study. 3. Outpatient clinic utilization, hospitalization and mortality experience after seven years. Prevent. Med., *2*:221, 1973.
7. Gilbertsen, V. A.: Procto-sigmoidoscopy and polypectomy in reducing the incidence of rectal cancer. Cancer, *34*:936, 1974.
8. Berge, T., Ekelund, G., Mellner, C., et al.: Carcinoma of the colon and rectum in a defined population. Acta Chir. Scand. (Suppl.), 438, 1973.
9. Greegor, D. H.: Occult blood testing for detection of asymptomatic colon cancer. Cancer, *28*:131, 1971.
10. Ostrow, J. D., Mulvaney, C. A., Hansel, J. R., et al.: Sensitivity and reproducibility of chemical tests for fecal occult blood with an emphasis on false-positive reactions. Am. J. Dig. Dis., *18*:930, 1973.
11. Hastings, J. B.: Mass screening for colorectal cancer. Am. J. Surg., *127*:228, 1974.
12. Devroede, G. J., Taylor, W. F., Sauer, W. G., et al.: Cancer risk and life expectancy of children with ulcerative colitis. N. Engl. J. Med., *285*:17, 1971.
13. Schottenfeld, D., Berg, J. W., and Vitsky, B.: Incidence of multiple primary cancers. II. Index cancers arising in the stomach and lower digestive systems. J. Nat. Cancer Inst., *43*:77, 1969.
14. Dodd, G. D.: Genetics and cancer of the gastrointestinal system. Radiology, *123*:263, 1977.
15. Dodds, W. J., Schulte, W. J., Hensley, G. T., et al.: Peutz-Jeghers syndrome and gastrointestinal malignancy. Am. J. Roentgenol., *115*:374, 1972.
16. Young, A. C.: Radiology of the colon and rectum. *In:* Irvine, W. I. (ed.): Modern Trends in Surgery. London, Butterworth, 1966, pp. 32–53.
17. Welin, S.: Results of the Malmö technique of colon examination. JAMA, *199*:119, 1967.
18. Hamelin, L., and Hurtubise, M.: Remote control technique in double contrast study of the colon. Am. J. Roentgenol., *119*:382, 1973.
19. Laufer, I.: The double contrast enema: Myths and misconceptions. Gastrointest. Radiol., *1*:19, 1976.
20. Laufer, I., Smith, N. C. W., and Mullens, J. E.: The radiologic demonstration of colorectal polyps undetected by endoscopy. Gastroenterology, *70*:167, 1976.
21. Andren, L., and Frieberg, S.: Frequency of polyps of rectum and colon according to age and relation to cancer. Gastroenterology, *36*:631, 1959.
22. Hartzell, H. V.: To err with air. JAMA, *187*:455, 1964.
23. Wolf, B. S.: Roentgen diagnosis of villous tumors of the colon. Am. J. Roentgenol., *84*:1093, 1960.
24. Franken, E. A., Bixler, D., Fitzgerald, J., et al.: Juvenile polyposis of the colon. Ann. Radiol., *18*:499, 1975.
25. Dodds, W. J.: Clinical and roentgen features of the intestinal polyposis syndromes. Gastrointest. Radiol., *1*:127, 1976.
26. Youker, J. E., and Welin, S.: Differentiation of true polypoid tumors of the colon from extraneous material. A new roentgen sign. Radiology, *84*:610, 1965.
27. Williams, C. B., Hunt, R. D., and Loose, H.: Colonoscopy in the management of colon polyps. Br. J. Surg., *61*:673, 1974.
28. Wolff, W. I., and Shinya, H.: Endoscopic polypectomy: therapeutic and clinicopathologic aspects. Cancer, *36*:683, 1975.
29. Margulis, A. R., and Jovanovich, A.: The roentgen diagnosis of submucous lipomas of the colon. Am. J. Roentgenol., *84*:1114, 1960.
30. Berk, R. N., and Lasser, E. C.: Radiology of the Ileocecal Area. Philadelphia, W. B. Saunders, 1975.
31. Gohel, V. K., Kressel, H. Y., and Laufer, I.: Double contrast artifacts. Gastrointest. Radiol., *3*:139, 1978.
32. Press, H. C., and Davis, T. W.: Ingested foreign bodies simulating polyposis: Report of six cases. Am. J. Roentgenol., *127*:1040, 1976.

33. Welin, S., and Welin, G.: The Double Contrast Examination of the Colon. Experiences with the Welin modification. Stuttgart, Georg Thieme Verlag, 1976.
34. Fischel, R. E., and Dermer, R.: Multifocal carcinoma of the large intestine. Clin. Radiol., *26*:495, 1975.
35. Raskin, M. M., Viamonte, M., and Viamonte, M., Jr.: Primary linitis plastica carcinoma of the colon. Radiology, *113*:17, 1974.
36. Hodgson, J. R., and Sauer, W. G.: The roentgenologic features of carcinoma in chronic ulcerative colitis. Am. J. Roentgenol., *86*:91, 1961.
37. Laufer, I., and Joffe, N.: Roentgen aspects of chronic perforating carcinoma of the colon. Dis. Colon Rectum, *16*:127, 1973.
38. Ekelund, G., Lindstrom, C., and Rosengren, J. E.: Appearance and growth of early carcinomas of the colon-rectum. Acta Radiol., *15*:670, 1974.
39. Spratt, J. S., and Ackerman, L. V.: Small primary adenocarcinomas of the colon and rectum. JAMA, *179*:337, 1962.
40. Shinya, H., and Wolff, W.: Flexible colonoscopy. Cancer, *37*:416, 1976.
41. Youker, J. E., Welin, S., and Main, G.: Computer analysis in the differentiation of benign and malignant polypoid lesions of the colon. Radiology, *90*:794, 1968.
42. Welin, S., Youker, J., and Spratt, J. S.: The rates and patterns of growth of 375 tumors of the large intestine and rectum observed serially by double contrast enema study (Malmö technique). Am. J. Roentgenol., *90*:673, 1963.
43. Smith, T. R.: Pedunculated malignant colonic polyps with superficial invasion of the stalk. Radiology, *115*:593, 1975.
44. Maruyama, M.: Radiologic Diagnosis of Polyps and Carcinoma of the Large Bowel. Tokyo, Igaku-Shoin, 1978.
45. Meyers, M. A., and Ghahremani, G. G.: Complications of fiber-optic endoscopy. II. Colonoscopy. Radiology, *115*:301, 1975.
46. Rogers, B. H. G., Silvis, S. E., Nebel, O. T., et al.: Complications of flexible fiber-optic colonoscopy and polypectomy. Gastrointest. Endosc., *22*:73, 1976.
47. Messinger, N. H., Bobroff, L. M., and Beneventano, T. C.: Lymphosarcoma of the colon. Am. J. Roentgenol., *117*:281, 1973.
48. Marshak, R. H., and Lindner, A. E.: Leiomyosarcoma of the colon. Am. J. Gastroenterol., *54*:155, 1970.
49. Khilnani, M. T., Marshak, R. H., Eliasaph, J., et al.: Roentgen features of metastases to the colon. Am. J. Roentgenol., *96*:302, 1966.
50. Meyers, M. A., Oliphant, N., Teixidor, H., et al.: Metastatic carcinoma simulating inflammatory colitis. Am. J. Roentgenol., *123*:74, 1975.
51. Meyers, M. A.: Distribution of intra-abdominal malignant seeding. Dependency on dynamics of flow of ascitic fluid. Am. J. Roentgenol., *119*:198, 1973.
52. Shauffer, I. A., and Sequeira, J.: Suture granuloma simulating recurrent carcinoma. Am. J. Roentgenol., *128*:856, 1977.
53. Sharpe, M., and Golden, R.: End-to-end anastomosis of the colon following resection: A roentgen study of 42 cases. Am. J. Roentgenol., *64*:769, 1950.
54. Fleischner, F. G., and Berenberg, A. L.: Recurrent carcinoma of the colon at the site of anastomosis. Radiology, *66*:540, 1956.
55. Goldstein, H. M., and Miller, M. H.: Air contrast colon examination in patients with colostomies. Am. J. Roentgenol., *127*:607, 1976.
56. Laufer, I.: Double contrast radiology in the diagnosis of gastrointestinal cancer. *In*: Glass, G. B. J. (ed.): Progress in Gastroenterology. Vol. 3. Grune & Stratton, 1977, pp. 643–669.

14

POLYPOSIS SYNDROMES

CLIVE I. BARTRAM, M.D.,
and IGOR LAUFER, M.D.

INTRODUCTION

Gastrointestinal polyposis refers to the presence of multiple polyps in part or all of the gastrointestinal tract. The large bowel is most often involved. A histologic classification is given in Table 14–1. Most of the polyposis syndromes have a solitary counterpart. Although determination of the exact nature of the polyposis must rely on histologic examination of one or more polyps,[1] radiologic examination is vital to show the distribution of the polyps as well as any gastrointestinal complication or extraintestinal manifestations that are important in the management and differential diagnosis.

As a generalization, the polyposis syndromes may be classified by their distribution in the GI tract into those involving mainly the stomach, the colon and rectum, or the entire GI tract.[2]

TABLE 14–1 HISTOLOGIC CLASSIFICATION OF POLYPOSIS SYNDROMES

Histologic Type of Polyp	Solitary	Multiple
Neoplastic	Adenoma	Familial adenomatous polyposis Minor adenomatous polyposis Gardner's syndrome
Hamartomatous	Juvenile	Juvenile polyposis Peutz-Jeghers syndrome
Inflammatory	Benign lymphoid	Benign lymphoid Inflammatory polyposis in colitis
Miscellaneous	Hyperplastic	Hyperplastic polyposis Cronkhite-Canada syndrome

GASTRIC POLYPOSIS

In the stomach, hyperplastic polyps are smooth, less than 1 cm in size, and randomly distributed (Fig. 14–1). Multiple hyperplastic polyps may result from excessive regeneration of the epithelium in an area of chronic gastritis.[3] These polyps are not premalignant, but a high incidence of malignancy in the surrounding mucosa has been reported, secondary to chronic gastritis.[4]

Gastric adenomas are rare. They are usually large solitary antral lesions (Fig. 14–2), but they may be multiple in patients with pernicious anemia.[5] Adenomas are liable to malignant change.

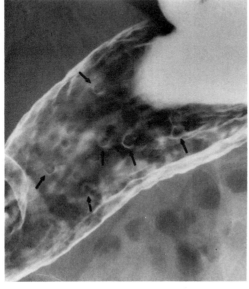

FIGURE 14–1 Multiple small hyperplastic polyps in the body of the stomach.

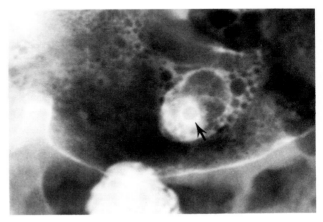

FIGURE 14–2 Pedunculated adenomatous polyp in the gastric antrum. The thin pedicle (*arrow*) is seen through the head of the polyp.

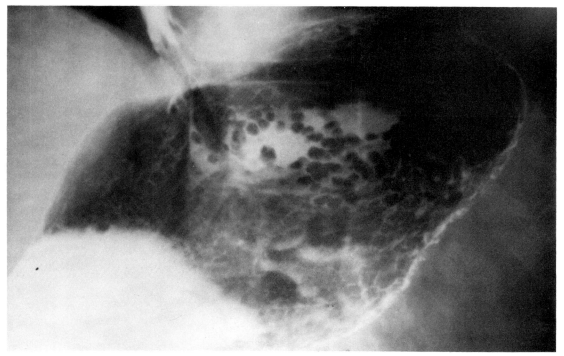

FIGURE 14–3 Multiple hamartomatous gastric polyps around the cardia and fundus in a patient with familial adenomatous polyposis.

Numerous small hamartomatous polyps have been found in the body and fundus in patients with familial polyposis of the large bowel (Fig. 14–3).[6]

COLONIC POLYPOSIS

Inflammatory Polyposis

The development of inflammatory polyps in colitis is discussed in Chapter 16. They are found in 10 to 20 per cent of patients with ulcerative colitis. Invariably there is a history of a severe previous attack with remission. The lesions may be sessile, but usually show a frondlike appearance and are adherent in parts (Fig. 14–4). Some patients who have had a severe episode of colitis develop multiple fingerlike postinflammatory polyps, a condition that has been termed filiform polyposis.[7] These polyps have been seen in the colon in patients with either ulcerative or granulomatous colitis (Fig. 14–5A and B), and in the stomach in a patient with Crohn's disease (Fig. 14–6).

Adenomatous polyps can be distinguished because they are usually sessile, but never adherent. The distribution of the polyps is also different. Inflammatory polyps may occur in any part of the colon, but are commonest in the left hemicolon, as this is the area most often affected in an acute attack. In familial adenomatous polyposis the polyps are found throughout the colon and rectum. The double contrast enema allows these

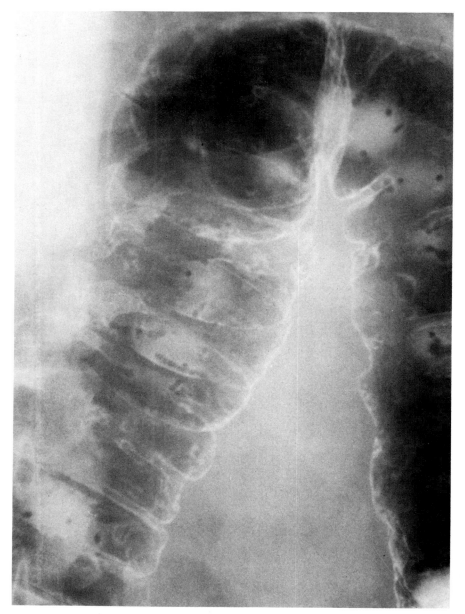

FIGURE 14–4 Postinflammatory polyposis in a patient with ulcerative colitis, showing sessile and frondlike lesions.

two conditions to be differentiated. This is important, as they may be confused on sigmoidoscopy. In all patients, histologic examination is indicated.

Inflammatory polyps are found less frequently in Crohn's colitis. In many areas where schistosomiasis is endemic, bilharzial polyposis occurs.[8] Occasionally inflammatory polyps may be associated with amebic colitis.[9]

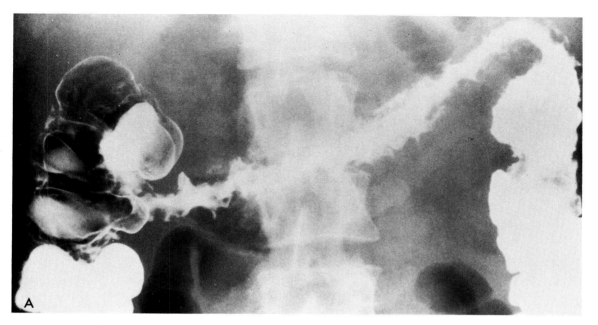

A. During the acute attack of colitis there is extensive ulceration in the transverse colon.

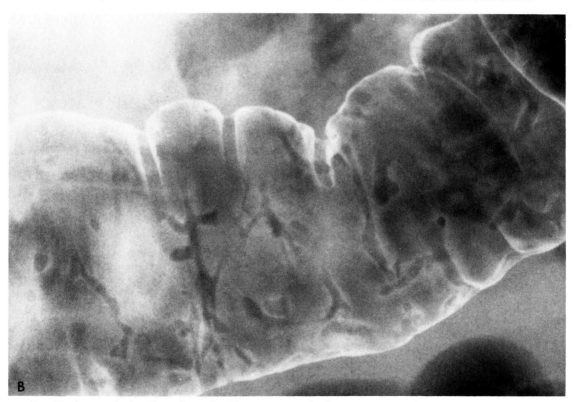

B. During remission there is marked improvement in the appearance of the transverse colon with a few linear filling defects representing filiform polyps. (*From*: Zegel, H. G., and Laufer, I.: Radiology, *127*:615, 1978.[7] Reproduced by permission.)

FIGURE 14–5 Filiform polyposis developing in a patient with granulomatous colitis.

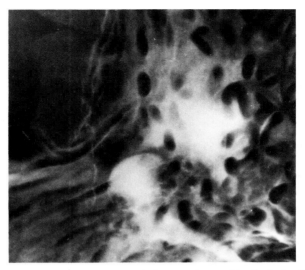

FIGURE 14–6 Filiform polyposis of the stomach in a patient with Crohn's disease. This patient had extensive involvement by Crohn's disease throughout the small bowel and in the stomach and duodenum. See also Plate 77. (*From*: Zegel, H. G., and Laufer, I.: Radiology, *127*:615, 1978.[7] Reproduced by permission.)

Adenomatous Polyposis

FAMILIAL ADENOMATOUS POLYPOSIS COLI

This is an hereditary condition of dominant character, in which numerous adenomas of the large bowel develop at an early age. The incidence lies between 1 in 24,000[10] and 1 in 7646.[11] The significance of the condition is the high risk of colonic cancer developing in early adult life.

The adenomas develop in the late teens. Symptoms of bleeding, diarrhea, pain, and mucus discharge may occur when the patient is in the early 30's. Of the patients presenting with symptoms, two thirds will have cancer (Fig. 14–7).[12] The average age at which cancer is present is 39 years. The youngest in the St. Mark's series is 19 years, but there are isolated reports of cancer appearing in the early teens.[13] Multiple cancers are found in 47.6 per cent of patients, compared with only 3.9 per cent in the general population. The distribution of the tumors is similar in the two groups.[2]

In familial adenomatous polyposis (FAP) the polyps are present throughout the colon and rectum. They may be more numerous distally, but as there are usually about 1000 adenomas present this is difficult to appreciate. The polyps are sessile and show only slight variation in size (Figs. 14–7 and 14–8). Although it is rare for any other condition to mimic this carpetlike growth of polyps, the diagnosis must always be confirmed histologically, as the diagnosis of FAP commits the patient to colectomy. If a double contrast enema (DCE) is performed in patients in early adult life, relatively few polyps may be seen (Fig. 14–9). This is because the polpys are only just developing. However, if polyps are present they can always be found in the rectum.

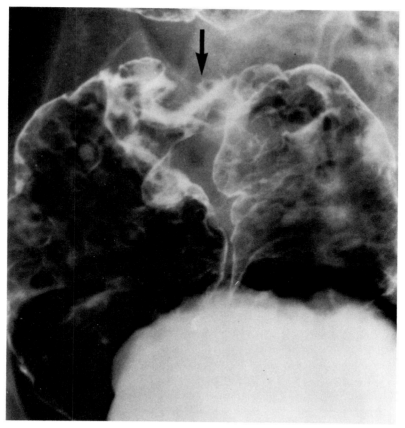

FIGURE 14–7 Typical annular carcinoma in the sigmoid colon *(arrow)* in a 32-year-old patient with familial adenomatous polyposis. Note that the mucosa proximal and distal to the carcinoma is carpeted with adenomatous polyps.

Members of an FAP family can be monitored by sigmoidoscopy and by histologic verification of the diagnosis obtained by biopsy excision of any polyp found. Sigmoidoscopic examination should start at the age of 14 years and be continued throughout life, as the development of polyps may be delayed until middle age. In patients thought to have the disease on sigmoidosocpic evidence, a DCE is indicated:

1. To demonstrate that the polyps extend throughout the colon, as is typical of FAP.

2. To show any large polyp that might be malignant or an overt carcinoma.

3. In patients who may wish to delay operation, for example, a young adult who wishes to complete higher education. The risk of developing cancer in the first 5 years after the diagnosis is established is 11.9 per cent.[14] This figure includes all ages, so that the risk would be less for a young adult. Nevertheless, it would justify an annual DCE to exclude the development of any large polyps.

4. For the same reasons, any patient who is unfit for colectomy should have a regular DCE. The risk of cancer increases appreciably with

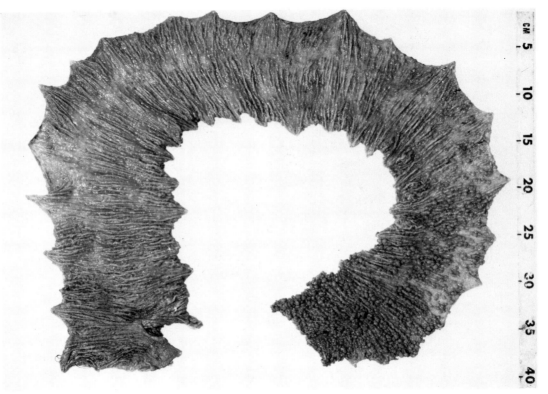

FIGURE 14–8 Colectomy specimen in a patient with familial adenomatous polyposis. There are innumerable small polyps throughout the colon. They are most prominent in the distal left colon.

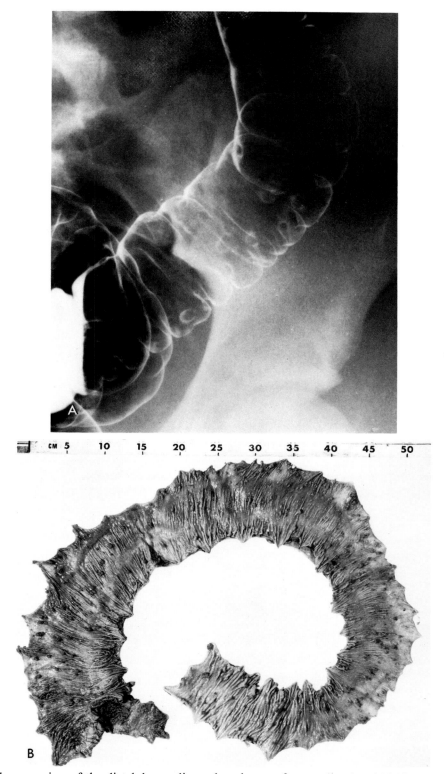

A. Close-up view of the distal descending colon shows a few small polypoid lesions.

B. The colectomy specimen shows polyps scattered throughout the colon. These polyps develop during the teens and therefore are less numerous at this age.

FIGURE 14–9   Familial adenomatous polyposis in a 17-year-old.

delay. Cancer is found in 31.6 per cent of patients after the diagnosis has been established for 10 to 15 years, and in 100 per cent of patients with a history of over 20 years.[14]

5. As a part of a general investigation of polyposis in the gastrointestinal tract.

The treatment of FAP involves colectomy and ileorectal anastomosis with fulguration of the remaining polyps in the rectum. Regular follow-up is required, as there is a risk of cancer developing in the rectum.

GARDNER'S SYNDROME

The combination of adenomatous polyps of the large bowel, multiple osteomata of the skull and mandible (Fig. 14–10A), multiple epidermoid cysts, and soft tissue tumors of the skin was described in a family of seven members by Gardner and Richards.[15] Subsequently, abnormal dentition and desmoid tumor formation were added to the syndrome.[16]

An important consideration in Gardner's syndrome is that in spite of the extracolonic lesions, the colonic polyposis is precisely similar to that in familial adenomatous polyposis and has the same cancer risk. Management of the colon is therefore similar to that in FAP

Desmoid tumors may arise 1 to 3 years after surgery for the polyposis.[17] In the St. Mark's series this complication occurred in 5.7 per cent of cases.[2] The tumors grow in the mesentery of the small bowel or in the anterior abdominal wall. Symptoms arise from obstruction to the gastrointestinal or urinary tract. The lesions are usually inoperable and are best left alone, since after a period of growth they remain static in size. Other recorded associations with the syndrome are carcinoma of the thyroid,[18] adrenal cancer,[19] adenomas of the small bowel and carcinoid tumors,[20] skin pigmentation, lymphoid polyps of the ileum,[21] and hamartomas of the stomach (Fig. 14–3).[6] However, the most important is carcinoma of the periampullary region.[22] About 40 such cases are known. The incidence in the St. Mark's series is 12 per cent,[12] indicating its seriousness (Fig. 14–10B).

Evidence is now accumulating that the adenomas of FAP are not limited to the large bowel, as has long been thought to be the case. In patients with FAP, Ushio and coworkers[23] have shown polyps to be present in the stomach in 68.2 per cent, and in the duodenum in 90 per cent of patients. Abnormalities were also noted in the skeleton in 50 per cent and in the mandible in 81.3 per cent of cases. Failure to adequately investigate the upper gastrointestinal tract with double contrast studies and endoscopy undoubtedly accounts for the belief that the polyps are limited to the large bowel. The presence of adenomatous polyps in the duodenum is probably responsible for the high incidence of periampullary cancers. Clinically about 15 to 18 per cent of the St. Mark's patients with FAP are affected by the extracolonic manifestations of Gardner's syndrome.

The lack of clear distinction between these groups increases the need for complete double contrast studies of the upper gastrointestinal tract and skull views in all patients with FAP. If polyps are found in the duodenum, the high incidence of periampullary cancer must be considered, and may justify repeat examination to detect early tumor formation.

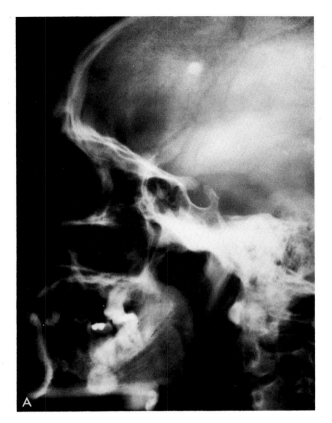

FIGURE 14-10 Gardner's syndrome.

A. Osteomata of the cranial vault and mandible.

B. Resected duodenum from a patient with Gardner's syndrome, showing small polyps (*small arrows*) and a carcinoma of the ampulla of Vater (*large arrow*) with a needle in the ampulla. The small polyps are adenomas.

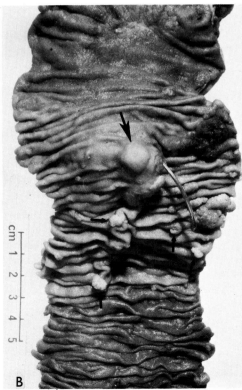

MINOR OR RECESSIVE ADENOMATOUS POLYPOSIS

Veale[10] has suggested that there are two genes controlling adenoma formation. *P* is dominant and responsible for FAP, whereas *p* is recessive, causing only a few polyps to develop. Patients with the recessive type usually have only one or a few adenomas, but can form up to 50 to 60. The minimum number found with FAP in a survey of 150 colectomies was 150, the average number being about 1000.[2] The dividing line would seem to be about 100. To the radiologist a simple rule is that if the polyps can be counted, the recessive form is present, but if the polyps are too numerous to count, FAP is present. The only exception to this is that patients with FAP examined in early adult life, when the polyps are just developing, may have only a few polyps. However, the minor form should not be present in this age group, as the adenomas develop in middle age, in keeping with the age distribution of solitary adenomas.

Although patients with the recessive form do not have such a high cancer risk as those with FAP, the risk is still appreciable. A review of 1577 patients with one or more adenomas showed that 27.5 per cent had a separate cancer either synchronously or metachronously.[14] The risk of cancer with one adenoma was 21.9 per cent, rising to 68.8 per cent when six or more adenomas were present (Fig. 14–11). Patients with a cancer who are also found to have multiple adenomas will require a more extensive resection and possibly total colectomy. They will also require careful follow-up, as the incidence of metachronous cancer rises from 4 per cent when no adenoma is present to 10 per cent when an adenoma is associated with the cancer at the original operation.

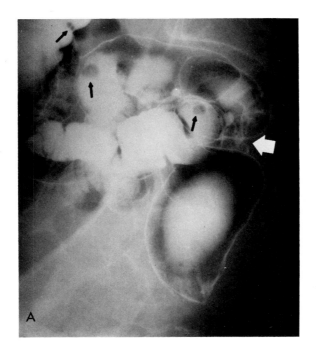

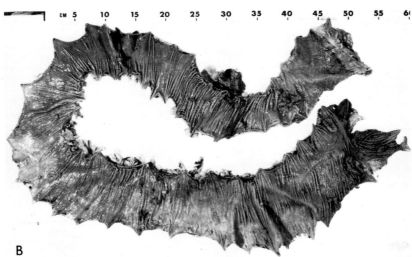

FIGURE 14–11 Minor adenomatous polyposis with carcinoma.

A. A lateral view shows a rectal carcinoma (*white arrow*) with several smaller polyps (*black arrows*).

B. The resected specimen shows approximately 30 adenomas scattered throughout the colon. The carcinoma is not included in this specimen.

Hyperplastic Polyposis

A hyperplastic polyp is a common finding. Usually small and smooth and located in the rectum, one or two such polyps are of no significance. However, occasionally they are found in large numbers and may be confused with adenomatous polyposis (Fig. 14–12). The distinction is made by histologic examination.

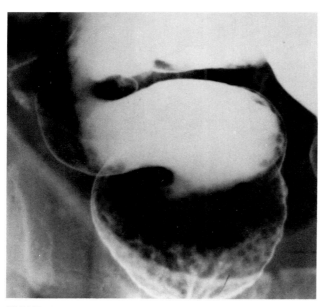

FIGURE 14–12 Hyperplastic polyposis. There are multiple hyperplastic polyps in the rectum in a 31-year-old male.

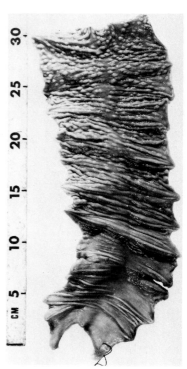

FIGURE 14–14 The resected specimen in a patient with benign lymphoid polyposis.

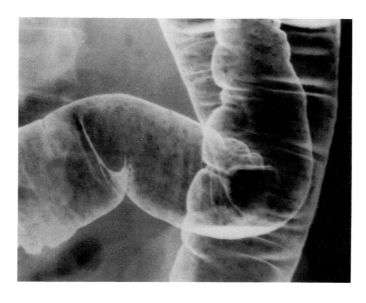

FIGURE 14–13 Lymphoid nodular hyperplasia of the colon in a 29-year-old.

The colon is rich in lymphoid follicles. Nodular hyperplasia of these follicles may be extensive and produce numerous very small filling defects of the mucosa. The condition is usually seen in children, and is self-limiting and nonspecific. Rarely, it is seen in young adults (Fig. 14–13). Occasionally, non-neoplastic hypertrophy of the lymphoid follicles produces a prominent benign lymphoid polyposis (Fig. 14–14).[24] In such circumstances, confusion with FAP must be prevented by biopsy and histologic definition of the lesions.

DIFFUSE POLYPOSIS

Peutz-Jeghers Syndrome

The association of polyposis and mucocutaneous pigmentation was first described by Peutz in 1921,[25] and the dominant inheritance by Jeghers and coworkers in 1949.[26] The polyps are hamartomatous and most common in the small bowel. Intussusception produces episodes of abdominal cramping. The large bowel is involved in about 30 per cent of patients (Fig. 14–15A) and the stomach in 25 per cent (Fig. 14–15B and C).[27] Rarely, the esophagus is affected. In the colon the polyps are macroscopically similar to adenomas.[27] Numerous polyps may be found in the small bowel, but such carpeting is not found in the colon or stomach. Surgery may be required to remove large polyps causing small bowel obstruction or repeated intussusception (Fig. 14–16). Patients with this syndrome have a higher incidence of carcinoma of the stomach and duodenum[27] and ovarian tumors.[28] The hamartomatous tumors themselves are not premalignant.

Juvenile Polyposis

Juvenile polyps are smooth rounded polyps which are often attached by a thin pedicle (Fig. 14–17A). This can rupture, autoamputating the polyp. Polyposis is rare. The condition affects children under 10 years of age.

The polyps are mainly colonic (Fig. 14–17B, Plate 89), but may also be found in the small bowel or stomach. The condition may be familial or nonfamilial.[29] The nonfamilial type is associated with congenital abnormalities. Patients with juvenile polyposis probably have a greater incidence of intestinal cancer in later life. This reflects their increased tendency to develop adenomas as adults.

Cronkhite-Canada Syndrome[30]

The main features are diarrhea, alopecia, atrophy of the nails, skin pigmentation, and diffuse gastrointestinal polyposis. The polyps are found throughout the gastrointestinal tract (Fig. 14–18) and are caused by cystic degeneration in the mucosa. The prognosis is poor.

Text continued on page 580

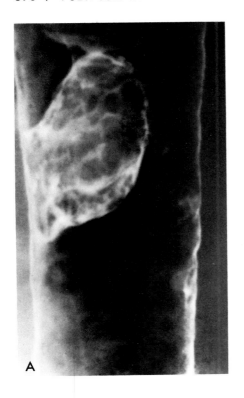

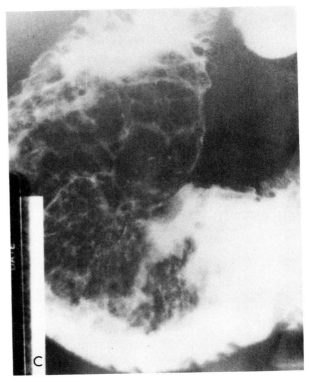

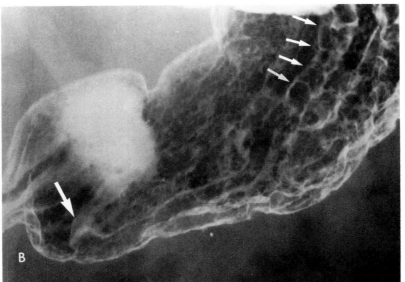

FIGURE 14–15 Peutz-Jeghers syndrome.

A. Large sessile and pedunculated polyps in the colon.

B and *C.* In another patient there are small polyps in the stomach and a large hamartomatous polyp in the duodenum.

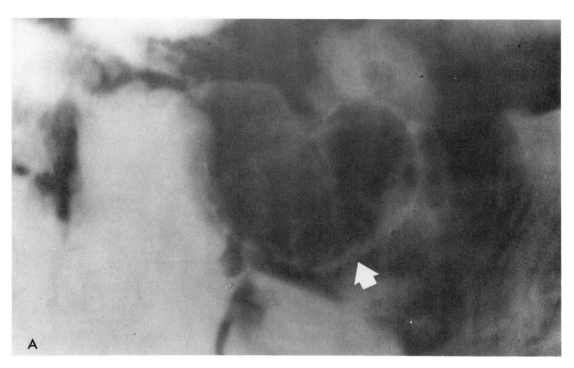

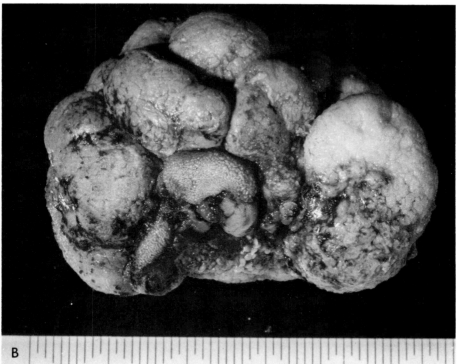

FIGURE 14–16 Hamartomatous polyp in the small bowel with repeated intussusception.
  A. There is a 4-cm lobulated polyp in the jejunum.
  B. Close-up view of the resected polyp.

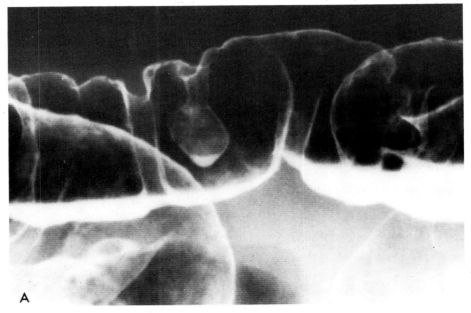

A

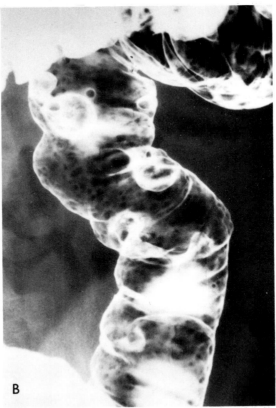

B

FIGURE 14–17 Juvenile polyps.

A. Pedunculated juvenile polyp in the colon.

B. Another patient, an 8-year-old girl with multiple colonic polyps due to juvenile polyposis. See also Plate 89.

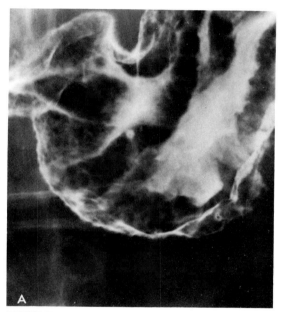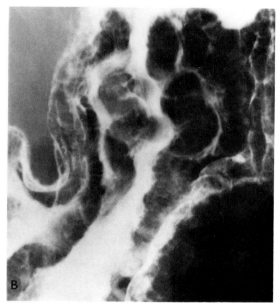

FIGURE 14–18 *A* and *B*   Cronkhite-Canada syndrome. Two views of the stomach show markedly thickened gastric folds with multiple polyps. There were also polyps in the small bowel and colon. Typical clinical features of the Cronkhite-Canada syndrome were present and open biopsy of the stomach confirmed the diagnosis.

Others

Other rare forms of gastrointestinal polyposis are nodular lymphoma (Fig. 14–19) and metastatic disease.

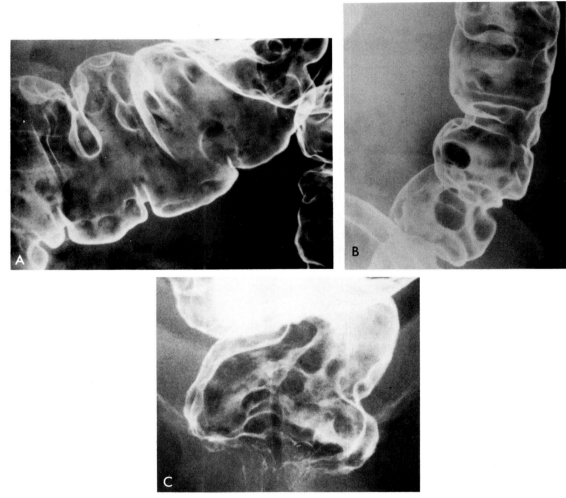

FIGURE 14–19 *A* to *C*   Polyposis due to colonic lymphoma. There are multiple polypoid lesions scattered throughout the colon owing to lymphoma. (Courtesy of J. O. Op den Orth, M.D., Haarlem, Holland.)

SUMMARY

Gastrointestinal polyposis may present by various means; clinically, as in the Peutz-Jeghers syndrome; on sigmoidoscopic examination; or fortuitously during radiologic investigation. In most patients the age, clinical features, and radiologic findings will provide a likely diagnosis. This must always be confirmed by histologic examination, as the nature of the polyposis will have a profound effect on the management of the patient. All patients should have full double contrast studies of the upper and lower gastrointestinal tract. Those with adenomatous polyposis coli should also have skeletal and skull films. Special consideration should be given to associated malignancies, notably periampullary carcinoma in Gardner's syndrome.

ACKNOWLEDGMENT

We would like to acknowledge the advice received from H. J. R. Bussey, Ph.D., in the preparation of this manuscript.

REFERENCES

1. Morson, B. C., Some peculiarities in the histology of intestinal polyps. Dis. Colon Rectum, *5*:337, 1962.
2. Bussey, H. J. R.: Gastrointestinal polyposis. Gut, *11*:970, 1970.
3. Morson, B. C.: Intestinal metaplasia of the gastric mucosa. Br. J. Cancer, *9*:365, 1955.
4. Ming, S. C., and Goldman, H.: Gastric polyps; a histogenetic classification and its relation to carcinoma. Cancer, *18*:721, 1965.
5. Jorgensen, J.: The mortality among patients with pernicious anaemia in Denmark and the incidence of gastric cancer among the same. Acta Med. Scand., *139*:472, 1951.
6. Parks, T. G., Bussey, H. J. R., and Lockhart-Mummery, H. E.: Familial polyposis coli associated with extra-colonic abnormalities. Gut, *11*:323, 1970.
7. Zegel, H. G., and Laufer, I.: Filiform polyposis. Radiology, *127*:615, 1978.
8. Medina, J. T., Seaman, W. B., Guzman-Acosta, C., et al.: The roentgen appearances of *Schistosomiasis mansoni* involving the colon. Radiology, *85*:682, 1965.
9. Berkowitz, D., and Bernstein, L. H.: Colonic pseudopolyps in association with amoebic colitis. Gastroenterology, *68*:786, 1975.
10. Veale, A. M. O.: Intestinal Polyposis. (Eugenics Laboratory memoirs, series 40.) London, Cambridge University Press, 1965.
11. Alm, T., and Licznerski, G.: The intestinal polyposis. Clin. Gastroenterol., *2–3*:577, 1973.
12. Bussey, H. J. R.: Familial Polyposis Coli: Family Studies, Histopathology. Differential Diagnosis and Results of Treatment. Baltimore, Johns Hopkins Press, 1975.
13. Coleman, S. T., and Eckert, C.: Preservation of rectum in familial polyposis of the colon and rectum. Arch. Surg., *73*:635, 1956.
14. Muto, T., Bussey, H. J. R., and Morson, B. C.: The evolution of cancer of the colon and rectum. Cancer, *36*:2251, 1975.
15. Gardner, E. J., and Richards, R. C.: Multiple cutaneous and subcutaneous lesions occurring simultaneously with hereditary polyposis and osteomatosis. Am. J. Hum. Genet., *5*:139, 1953.
16. Gardner, E. J.: Follow-up study of a family exhibiting dominant inheritance for a syndrome including intestinal polyps, osteomas, fibromas and epidermal cysts. Am. J. Hum. Genet., *14*:376, 1962.
17. Simpson, R. D., Harrison, E. G., and Mayo, C. W.: Mesenteric fibromatosis in familial polyposis. A variant of Gardner's syndrome. Cancer, *17*:526, 1964.
18. Camiel, M. R., Mulé, J. E., Alexander, L. L., et al.: Association of thyroid carcinoma with Gardner's syndrome in siblings. N. Engl. J. Med., *278*:1056, 1968.
19. Marshall, W. H., Martin, F. I. R., and Mackay, I. R.: Gardner's syndrome with adrenal carcinoma. Aust. Ann. Med., *16*:242, 1967.

20. Heald, R. J.: Gardner's syndrome in association with two tumors in the ileum. Proc. R. Soc. Med., *60*:914, 1967.

21. Thomford, N. R., and Greenberger, N. J.: Lymphoid polyps of the ileum associated with Gardner's syndrome. Arch. Surg., *96*:289, 1968.

22. MacDonald, J. M., Davis, W. C., Crago, H. R., et al.: Gardner's syndrome and periampullary malignancy. Am. J. Surg., *113*:425, 1967.

23. Ushio, K., Sasagawa, M., Doi, H., et al.: Lesions associated with familial polyposis coli. Studies of lesions of the stomach, duodenum, bones and teeth. Gastrointest. Radiol., *1*:67, 1976.

24. Collins, J. O., Falk, M., and Gilbone, R.: Benign lymphoid polyposis of the colon. Pediatrics, *38*:897, 1966.

25. Peutz, J. L. A.: Over een zeer merkwaardige gecombineerde familiaire polyposis van des slijmvliezen van den tractus intestinalis met die van de neuskeenlholte en gepaard met eigenaardige pigmentaties van huid en slijmvliezen. Ned. Maandschr. Geneeskd., *2*:134, 1921.

26. Jeghers, H., McKusick, V. A., and Katz, K. H.: Generalized intestinal polyposis and melanin spots of the oral mucosa, lips and digits. N. Engl. J. Med., *241*:993, 1949.

27. Dodds, W. J.: Clinical and roentgen features of the intestinal polyposis syndromes. Gastrointest. Radiol., *1*:127, 1976.

28. Christian, C. D., McLoughlin, T. G., Cathcart, E. R., et al.: Peutz-Jeghers syndrome associated with functioning ovarian tumour. J.A.M.A., *190*:935, 1964.

29. Veale, A. M. O., McColl, I., Bussey, H. J. R., et al.: Juvenile polyposis coli. J. Med. Genet., *3*:5, 1966.

30. Cronkhite, L. W., and Canada, W. J.: Generalized gastrointestinal polyposis. An unusual syndrome of polyposis, pigmentation, alopecia and onychotrophia. N. Engl. J. Med., *252*:1011, 1955.

15

DIVERTICULAR DISEASE

CLIVE I. BARTRAM, M.D.

INTRODUCTION

This is a common disease of the elderly in Western countries, affecting between 33 and 48 per cent[1,2] of the population over the age of 50. About 1 in 70 will require hospital treatment, and 1 in 200 will need an operation.[3]

The term diverticular disease implies the presence of a characteristic muscle abnormality. Diverticula are often present, and there may be associated inflammatory changes.[4] Diverticulosis refers only to the presence of diverticula, with or without a muscle abnormality. Diverticulitis indicates either macroscopic or microscopic inflammation affecting one or more diverticula, and it is often accompanied by pericolic abscess formation.

583

RADIOLOGIC PATHOLOGY

The most consistent abnormality involves the muscle of the sigmoid colon.[4] The teniae and circular muscle are thickened, and marked shortening causes corrugation of the circular muscle with redundant mucosal folds (Fig. 15–1). The muscle change is thought not to be due to hypertrophy or hyperplasia, but has been likened to a myostatic contracture.[5] The circular muscle thickening is commonly localized to two semicircular arcs between the mesenteric and antimesenteric teniae (Fig. 15–2), but may show uniform thickening.

The diverticula, composed of mucosa and muscularis mucosae, are of the false, pulsion type. They develop as small outpouches through defects in the circular muscle at the sites of small penetrating arteries. Lateral diverticula arise between the mesenteric and antimesenteric teniae. They emerge from the convexity of the folded circular muscle, often in two lateral rows, their openings alternating with the opposite side (Fig. 15–2).

Small diverticula are found in the antimesenteric intertenial area. They are usually associated with lateral diverticula and are of the small saccular, ridge, or intramural type.[6] Diverticula are commonest in the sigmoid colon. In about 17 per cent of cases they are distributed throughout the colon.[7] Isolated diverticula in the cecum and ascending colon are found in 4 to 12 per cent of patients.[2, 7, 8]

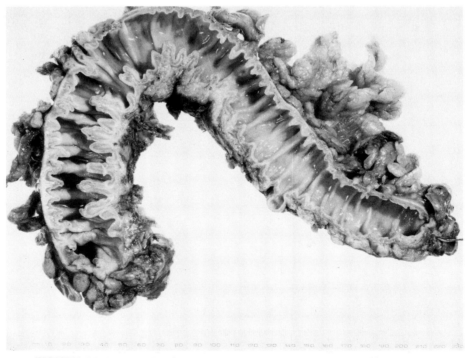

FIGURE 15–1 Muscle changes in diverticular disease. No inflammation.

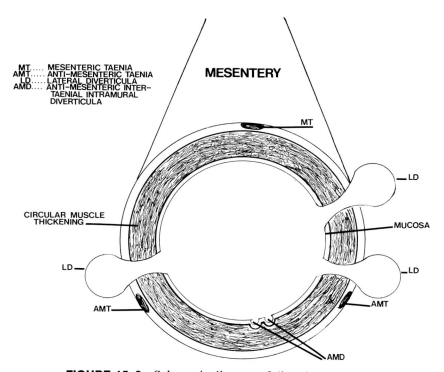

MT..... MESENTERIC TAENIA
AMT..... ANTI-MESENTERIC TAENIA
LD..... LATERAL DIVERTICULA
AMD.... ANTI-MESENTERIC INTER-
          TAENIAL INTRAMURAL
          DIVERTICULA

MESENTERY

MT

LD

CIRCULAR MUSCLE
THICKENING

MUCOSA

LD

LD

AMT

AMT

AMD

FIGURE 15–2   Schematic diagram of diverticular anatomy.

ROENTGEN CHANGES

Plain Film

This is of little value in the primary assessment of disease. A bubbly appearance due to air in the diverticula has been described.[9] Plain films are mostly used in the evaluation of diverticular disease complicated by an inflammatory mass, with or without intestinal obstruction.

Contrast Examinations

A double contrast enema (DCE) will show both the muscular and the diverticular components of the disease. The interdigitating clefts of the mucosal surface reflect the muscle change (Fig. 15–3).[10] As this is not circumferentially uniform, the appearances may vary with the angle at which the surface is viewed. The muscle clefts and diverticula may be more apparent in the prone-angled view, which is nearer the plane of the mesentery, than in the supine oblique view, which is more at right angles to the mesentery.

The diverticula will vary in appearance with the angle at which they are viewed, and also with the amount of air and barium they contain (Fig. 15–4). In about 20 per cent of patients a spiky, irregular outline along one side of the bowel wall is seen (Fig. 15–5). This is caused by diverticula in the antimesenteric intertenial ridge.[6] This appearance has been referred to as prediverticular,[11] but this is incorrect, as it has been shown to be the result of small diverticula. The usual large lateral diverticula may develop later, as shown by Welin,[12] but such a progression is not established. The appearance is perhaps best considered as a minor change of diverticular disease.

Muscle change is usually associated with diverticula, but in about 8 per cent of cases only the muscle abnormality is present, and in 19 per cent only diverticula.[2] It should be noted that diverticula do not always fill, as contraction of the longitudinal muscle will close the necks of the diverticula. This may be apparent during filling when the bowel has a palisade configuration. When the longitudinal muscle relaxes the palisading disappears, and the diverticula fill.[13]

COMPLICATIONS OF DIVERTICULAR DISEASE

Inflammation

Inspissated feces cause abrasion and chronic inflammation, which may lead to the development of lymphoid hyperplasia at the apex of a diverticulum.[4] Such changes cannot be distinguished radiologically from retained residue in the diverticulum.

The diagnosis of diverticulitis can be made radiologically only by the recognition of a perforated diverticulum or its sequela, a pericolic abscess. Barium may track through the perforated diverticulum into the abscess. The abscess itself will cause an extrinsic deformity of the lumen

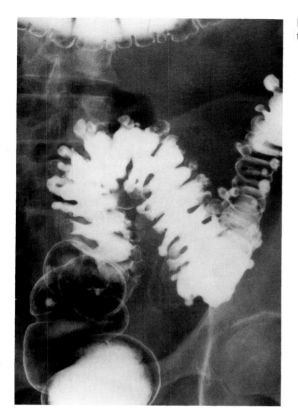

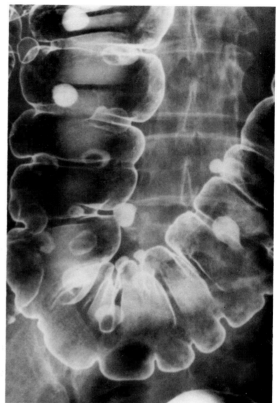

FIGURE 15–3 Diverticular disease with interdigitating muscle clefts and diverticula.

FIGURE 15–4 Diverticula containing varying amounts of air and barium.

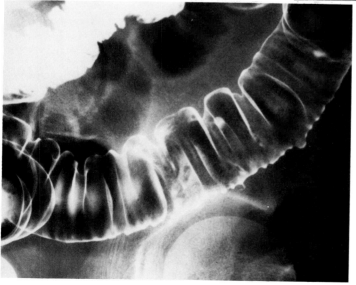

FIGURE 15–5 Small diverticula in the antimesenteric intertenial ridge.

(Fig. 15–6). Initially this should be on the mesenteric side, but it may spread to encircle the lumen. Any extrinsic defect originating on the lateral border between the antimesenteric teniae should be the result of other disease,[14] as only the lateral diverticula perforate. The abscess lies outside the muscle, and suppuration spreads easily within the pericolic fat, forming a dissecting abscess. The fat may outline the abscess mass on plain films.[15]

Further manifestations of pericolic abscess formation are:

1. Localized small bowel ileus.
2. Less commonly, complete small bowel obstruction from kinking or edema of the bowel adjacent to the abscess.
3. A degree of large bowel obstruction. This is quite common, but complete obstruction is rare.
4. Free intraperitoneal air from the perforated diverticulum (rare).
5. Fistula formation.

Fistulae

Spontaneous fistulae may result from spread of inflammation from a pericolic abscess adjacent to other organs, notably the bladder, vagina, or small bowel. Sometimes the rupture of a diverticulum that has become adherent to an adjacent organ leads to a fistula. In such circumstances the underlying disease may be minimal.

The bladder is most commonly involved. The communication is shown on barium enema in about 30 per cent of patients (Fig. 15–7), and by air in the bladder on a plain film in about another 30 per cent. Taken in conjunction, radiology can show a colovesical fistula in about 40 per cent of cases.[16]

Hemorrhage

Classically the affected patient is elderly, obese, and hypertensive. Slight hypogastric pain is experienced, and a large volume of bright red blood is passed rectally. Angiography has shown that hemorrhage is twice as likely to arise in the right colon as in the left.[17] The vascular architecture has been studied by Meyers.[18] The intramural branches of the marginal artery, the vasa recta, penetrate the colonic wall from serosa to submucosa, and course over the domes of the diverticula in the serosa. Intimal thickening, with weakening of the wall, can lead to eccentric rupture and massive bleeding.[14] Why this should be more common in the right colon is unknown, but possibly the wider necks of the diverticula may lead to greater exposure to noxious agents in the colon.

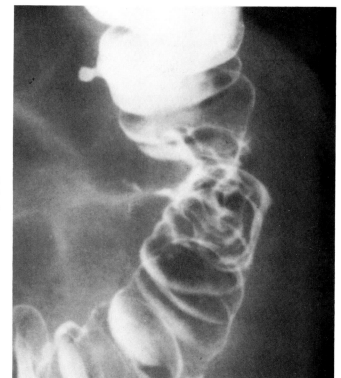

FIGURE 15–6 Pericolic abscess with barium track into the abscess and extrinsic deformity on the mesenteric side.

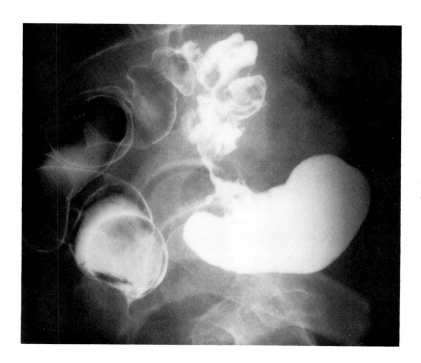

FIGURE 15–7 Colovesical fistula due to diverticular disease.

UNUSUAL PRESENTATIONS

Cecal Diverticula

Isolated cecal diverticula may be seen in 4 to 12 per cent of patients found to have diverticula on radiologic examination.[2, 7] Often thought to be congenital, these have been shown to be pulsion, false diverticula similar to those in the sigmoid.[2] An association with solitary ulcers of the cecum has been suggested,[8] but a recent study showed no such relationship.[19]

Rectal Diverticula

Such diverticula are extremely rare (Fig. 15–8A), as the teniae fuse to completely ensheath the rectum. When found, they tend to be large and in continuity with sigmoid diverticular disease (Fig. 15–8B).[20]

Giant Sigmoid Diverticula

Also rare, these may present as large, smooth-walled, air-containing cavities arising from the left iliac fossa (Fig. 15–8B). A ball valve mechanism may be responsible for their development. The cyst is lined by a thin membrane.[21] If the wall contains mucosa and smooth muscle, the cyst may represent a communicating intestinal duplication. The cyst may also undergo torsion or perforation. Barium enema will show the communication with the bowel and the presence of other diverticula.

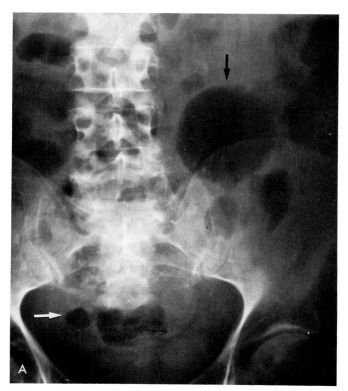

A. Plain abdominal film of the patient shown in *B*. Air is present in the giant sigmoid and rectal diverticula (*arrows*).

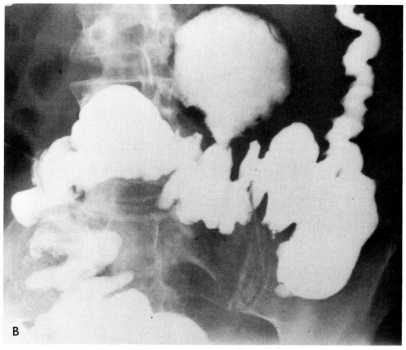

B. Giant sigmoid diverticulum (*arrow*) filled with barium.

FIGURE 15–8

COEXISTENT LESIONS

Polyps

The presence of diverticular disease adds to the difficulty of detecting polyps in the sigmoid. Colonoscopy has shown that this is the situation in which polyps are most likely to be missed on double contrast barium enema.[22]

If a diverticulum is shown by double contrast en face, the appearance may simulate the ring shadow around a polyp. The meniscus in a diverticulum fades centrally, whereas around a polyp it fades peripherally.[23] A polyp may be seen as a negative shadow lying in a pool of barium. With any suspicious lesion a stalk should always be looked for, as its presence will indicate a pedunculated polyp. The stalk may be recognized when seen in profile, or when seen end-on through the head of the polyp as a target or Mexican hat sign (Figs. 2–14 and 13–15).[23] Some of these distinguishing features are shown in Figure 15–9.

Often with marked muscle thickening, a double contrast view of the lumen is not obtained, and polyps cannot be excluded. Antispasmodics are useful to provide relaxation and to enable a reasonable double contrast view to be obtained.[24]

Carcinoma

Approximately 10 per cent of sigmoid carcinomas will be associated with diverticular disease. However, the differentiation between a benign and a malignant stricture may be difficult.

Strictures in diverticular disease may result from a combination of inflammatory change, muscle thickening, and redundant mucosal folds narrowing the lumen. Such lesions have tapered ends with an intact mucosa. Within the strictured segment a few diverticula may fill, or barium may enter the closed necks of diverticula, causing a spiky outline (Fig. 15–10). Carcinoma tends to cause a shorter stricture, with irregular, shouldered ends (Fig. 15–11). The lumen of the stricture is irregular, and no normal mucosal folds are present.[25] Inflammatory changes superimposed on malignancy may obscure such distinguishing features. Relaxants are useful in obtaining some dilatation in benign strictures and a better definition of the ends of the stricture. In a series of patients with strictures in diverticular disease the distinction between benignity and malignancy was impossible in 16 per cent with diverticular disease and in 4 per cent with carcinoma.[26]

Inflammatory Bowel Disease

Both ulcerative and Crohn's colitis have a second peak of frequency of presentation in the older age group. It is therefore likely that diverticular disease will also be present in some of these patients.

ULCERATIVE COLITIS

The diagnosis of distal ulcerative colitis in the presence of diverticular disease has been considered difficult.[27] However, provided a double contrast view is obtained, the finding of a granular mucosa is sufficient radiologic evidence to establish the diagnosis of colitis. The smooth muscle changes and mucosal edema that accompany active colitis may modify the radiologic appearances of the diverticular disease. The mouths of the diverticula may be occluded, so that they do not fill on barium enema. Inflammatory involvement of the diverticula can alter their shape, so that they are conical or pointed.[27] This can cause confusion with deep ulceration (Fig. 15–12). The muscle abnormality may not be so apparent, as deep interdigitating folds are not seen. Muscle changes have been considered partly responsible for fecal stasis.[28] However, with regression of the colitis, the underlying diverticula and muscle changes may revert to a typical appearance.

Complications from diverticulitis in the presence of ulcerative colitis are said to have a grave prognosis,[29] possibly because the diagnosis is difficult to establish until the condition is advanced, and in the meantime the symptoms may have been wrongly attributed to colitis.

CROHN'S DISEASE

Occasionally the deep fissuring in Crohn's disease may suggest the muscle abnormality of diverticular disease. The ulceration of Crohn's disease is spiky and haphazard compared with the smooth interdigitating folds of the muscle abnormality.[30] Usually other stigmata of Crohn's disease are present. Multiple anal fistulae are common, and the characteristic aphthous ulceration may be seen in the rectal or sigmoid colonic mucosa.[31] However, this may be technically difficult to detect in the sigmoid with muscle changes, multiple diverticula, and a poor double contrast view. The aphthous ulceration is also seen in the mucosa of the diverticula. The domes of the diverticula are in the pericolic tissue outside the muscle barrier, so that ulceration and inflammation are not impeded. A higher incidence of peridiverticulitis and dissecting abscess formation is found than would be expected in diverticular disease alone (Fig. 15–13).[32] Although long fissuring tracts of 10 cm or more are usually associated with Crohn's disease,[33] they may occasionally occur in its absence.[34, 35]

Text continued on page 599

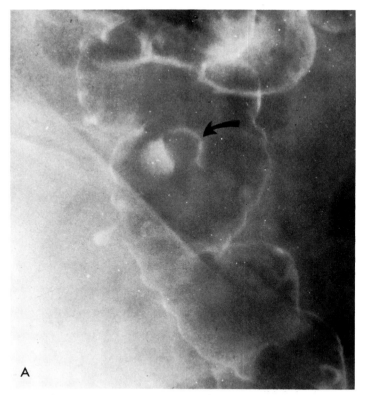

A. Polyp causing a filling defect in a pool of barium. Note the sharp inner margin with peripheral fade-off.

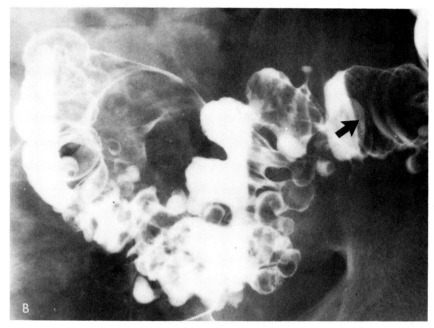

B. Polyp showing the increased density sign (*arrow*).

FIGURE 15–9 Colonic polyps.

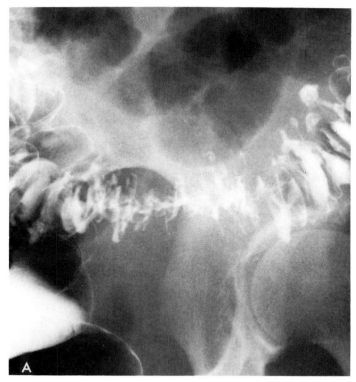

A. Stricture due to inflammatory changes.

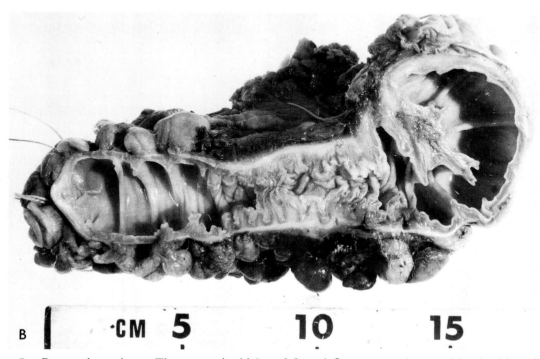

B. Resected specimen. The serosa is thickened from inflammatory changes. Muscle thickening and redundant mucosal folds contribute to the stricture.

FIGURE 15–10

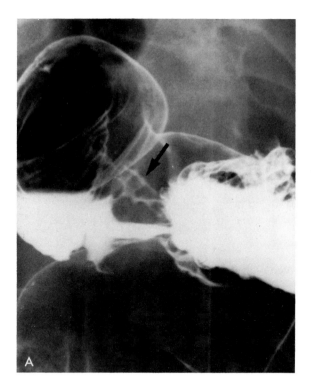

FIGURE 15–11 Carcinoma.

A. Carcinomatous stricture in diverticular disease showing shouldered ends. The lesion is seen through overlapping loops of sigmoid.

B. Same examination after relaxants, showing the lumen of the strictured segment in double contrast. Irregular pools of barium reflect the mucosal destruction due to malignancy.

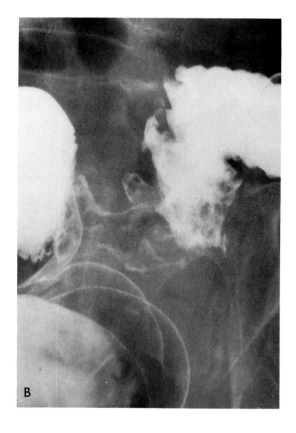

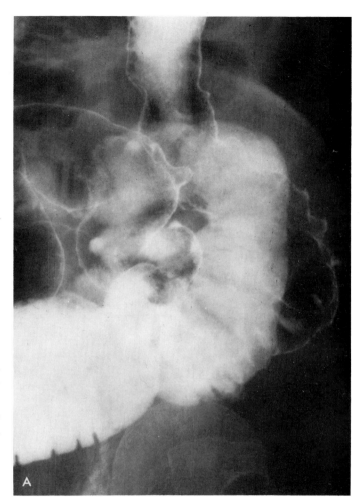

FIGURE **15–12** Ulcerative colitis with diverticular disease.

A. Granular sigmoid mucosa with some interdigitating folds and several conical diverticula.

B. Part of resected specimen confirming muscle change of diverticular disease, with thickened folds and only a few patent ostia to diverticula.

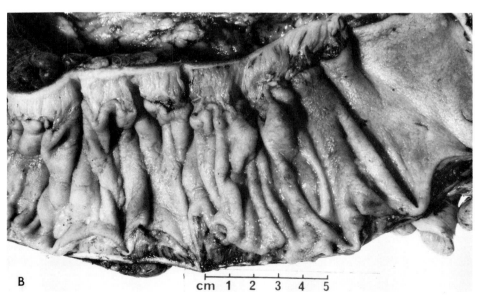

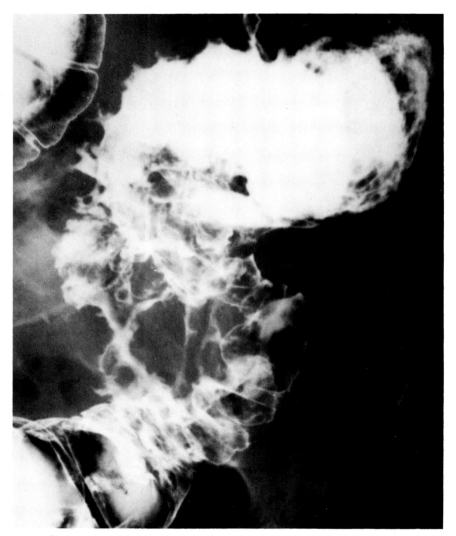

FIGURE 15–13 Crohn's colitis complicating diverticular disease. Multiple dissecting fistulous tracts are present in the sigmoid. Many of the diverticula show ulcers and tracks owing to involvement of their mucosa by Crohn's disease.

REFERENCES

1. Manousos, O. N., Truelove, S. C., and Lumsden, K.: Prevalence of colonic diverticulosis in the general population of Oxford area. Br. Med. J., *3*:762, 1967.
2. Hughes, L. E.: Postmortem survey of diverticular disease of the colon. Gut, *10*:336, 1969.
3. Hughes, L. E.: Complications of diverticular disease: Inflammation, obstruction and bleeding. Clin. Gastroenterol., *4*:147, 1975.
4. Morson, B. C.: The muscle abnormality in diverticular disease of the sigmoid colon. Br. J. Radiol., *36*:385, 1963.
5. Williams, I.: Diverticular disease of the colon, a 1968 view. Gut, *9*:498, 1968.
6. Marcus, R., and Watt, J.: The radiological appearances of diverticula in the anti-mesenteric intertaenial area of the pelvic colon. Clin. Radiol., *16*:87, 1965.
7. Zollinger, R. W.: The prognosis of diverticulitis of the colon. Arch. Surg., *97*:418, 1968.
8. Lloyd-Williams, K.: Acute solitary ulcers and acute diverticulitis of the cecum and ascending colon. Br. J. Surg., *47*:351, 1960.
9. Massik, P., and Wheatley, F. E.: The recognition of air in diverticula of the colon as a diagnostic aid. Radiology, *64*:417, 1955.
10. Williams, I: Changing emphasis in diverticular disease of the colon. Br. J. Radiol., *36*:393, 1963.
11. Spriggs, E. I., and Marter, O. A.: Intestinal diverticula. Quart. J. Med., *19*:1, 1925.
12. Welin, S., and Welin, G.: The Double Contrast Examination of the Colon. Experiences with the Welin Modification. Stuttgart, Georg Thieme Verlag, 1976.
13. Williams, I.: Diverticular disease of the colon without diverticula. Radiology, *89*:401, 1967.
14. Meyers, M. A., Alonso, D. R., Gray, G. F., et al.: Pathogenesis of bleeding colonic diverticulosis. Gastroenterology, *71*:577, 1976.
15. Fleischner, F. G., and Ming, S. C.: Revised concepts on diverticular disease of the colon. II. So-called diverticulitis; diverticular sigmoiditis and perisigmoiditis; diverticular abscess, fistula, and frank peritonitis. Radiology, *84*:599, 1965.
16. Small, W. P., and Smith, A. N.: Fistula and conditions associated with diverticular disease of the colon. Clin. Gastroenterol., *4*(1):176, 1975.
17. Casarella, W. J., Kantor, I. E., and Seaman, W. B.: Right-sided colonic diverticula as a cause of acute rectal hemorrhage. N. Engl. J. Med., *286*:450, 1972.
18. Meyers, M. A., Volberg, F., and Katzen, B.: Angioarchitecture of colonic diverticula; significance in bleeding diverticulosis. Radiology, *108*:249, 1973.
19. Brodey, P. A., Hill, R. P., and Baron, S.: Benign ulceration of the cecum. Radiology, *122*:323, 1977.
20. Dawson, J. R., Lieber, A., and Simmons, T.: Rectal diverticula. Radiology, *84*:610, 1976.
21. Kempczinski, R. F., and Ferrucci, J. T.: Giant sigmoid diverticula. Ann. Surg., *180*:864, 1974.
22. Williams, C. B., Hunt, R. H., and Loose, H.: Colonoscopy in the management of colon polyps. Br. J. Surg., *61*:673, 1974.
23. Youker, J. E., and Welin, S.: Differentiation of true polypoid lesions of the colon from extraneous material, a new roentgen sign. Radiology, *84*:610, 1965.
24. Htoo, M. M., and Bartram, C. I.: The radiological detection of polyps in diverticular disease. In preparation.
25. Schatzki, R.: The roentgenologic differential diagnosis between cancer and diverticulitis. Radiology, *34*:651, 1940.
26. Colcock, B. P., and Sass, R. E.: Diverticulitis and carcinoma of the colon; differential diagnosis. Surg. Gynecol. Obstet., *99*:627, 1954.
27. Beranbaum, S. L., Yaghmai, M., and Beranbaum, E. R.: Ulcerative colitis in association with diverticular disease of the colon. Radiology, *85*:880, 1965.
28. Jalan, K. N., Walker, R. J., Prescott, R. J., et al.: Fecal stasis and diverticular disease in ulcerative colitis. Gut, *11*:688, 1970.
29. Bates, T., and Kaminsky, V.: Diverticulitis and ulcerative colitis. Br. J. Surg., *61*:293, 1974.
30. Schmidt, G. T., Lennard-Jones, J. E., and Morson, B. C.: Crohn's disease of the colon and its distinction from diverticulitis. Gut, *9*:7, 1968.
31. Laufer, I., and Costopoulos, L.: Early lesions of Crohn's disease. Am. J. Roentgenol., *130*:307, 1978.
32. Meyers, M. A., Alonso, D. R., Morson, B. C., et al.: Pathogenesis of diverticulitis complicating granulomatous colitis. Gastroenterology, *74*:24, 1978.
33. Marshak, R. H., Janowitz, H. D., and Present, D. H.: Granulomatous colitis in association with diverticula. N. Engl. J. Med., *283*:1080, 1970.
34. Loeb, P. M., Berk, R. N., and Saltzstein, S. L.: Longitudinal fistula of the colon in diverticulitis. Gastroenterology, *67*:720, 1974.
35. Ferrucci, J. T., Ragsdale, B. D., and Barrett, P. J.: Double tracking of the sigmoid colon. Radiology, *120*:307, 1976.

16

INFLAMMATORY BOWEL DISEASE

CLIVE I. BARTRAM, M.D., and IGOR LAUFER, M.D.

TECHNIQUE

Many radiologists and gastroenterologists have been reluctant to use the double contrast enema in patients with inflammatory bowel disease, believing that there is a higher risk of perforation or toxic megacolon with the use of air. No data have been published to support this prejudice. Nevertheless, it is clear that any type of contrast study performed in patients with active inflammatory bowel disease must be undertaken only after due consideration of the clinical condition of the patient, the severity of the disease, the nature of the information to be gained from the contrast study, and the clinical relevance of this information. The examination must be performed gently and with regard for patient discomfort. It should not be pursued beyond what is necessary to obtain the desired information.

In general the purpose of contrast examinations in patients with known or suspected inflammatory bowel disease is to answer the following questions.

1. Does the patient have inflammatory bowel disease?
2. If there is inflammatory bowel disease, what is its extent?
3. Can a specific radiologic diagnosis be made?
4. Is there any evidence of complications of inflammatory bowel disease and, in particular of epithelial dysplasia or carcinoma?

Double Contrast Enema (DCE)

In many cases the answers to these questions are found in very subtle radiologic abnormalities that are best demonstrated by the double contrast enema. In most patients with inflammatory bowel disease the examination can be performed as a modification of the routine technique described in Chapter 12.

The following modifications should be incorporated into the examination of patients with active inflammatory bowel disease. A mild laxative, such as mineral oil or bisacodyl, should be used. In patients who have Crohn's disease with evidence of partial small bowel obstruction, no laxative should be used. The cleansing enema should not contain Clysodrast. In many patients the preparation may consist only of a clear liquid diet for 24 hours and a cleansing enema with no additives.

Instant Enema

The instant enema was developed as a modification of the double contrast enema by Young.[1] A double contrast study of the diseased colon is obtained without bowel preparation. This is possible for two reasons: Residue does not accumulate adjacent to inflamed mucosa because of exudate from the mucosa, and at least in ulcerative disease, colitis starts distally and remains in continuity to its proximal extent. The affected colon will therefore be internally cleansed to its proximal limit and can be shown in double contrast.

Indications

The instant enema may be used for the following purposes:

1. To show the extent and severity of the mucosal lesions in patients found to have proctitis sigmoidoscopically.

2. In follow-up of the patient, to monitor the extension or regression of the disease and the severity of the mucosal changes.

3. To accurately assess patients in an acute attack.

Contraindications

Contraindications to the use of the instant enema are as follows:

1. Toxic megacolon or perforation.

2. In long-standing, relatively quiescent disease when there is a risk of carcinoma. A full DCE with complete bowel preparation should be performed so that the entire mucosal surface of the colon is examined.

3. Immediately following rectal biopsy. A delay of 10 days is advised to allow any perforation to become sealed.

4. In Crohn's colitis the instant enema may not be successful. A residue can accumulate adjacent to patchy ulceration, and proximal skip lesions may be missed. However, the examination is useful in patients in an acute attack and in those with severe anal lesions in whom bowel preparation would be difficult. Provided that it is understood that aphthous ulceration may be obscured and the proximal colon may not be well shown, the instant enema may be performed. If fecal residue prevents an adequate examination, that is easily remedied by proceeding to the standard DCE with full bowel preparation.

TECHNIQUE

The patient receives no bowel preparation and continues on a normal diet and therapeutic regime. A preliminary plain film is taken to exclude toxic megacolon and to show the fecal residue. The barium suspension used is similar to that for a standard DCE and is administered in the prone position. Barium is injected until the splenic flexure is reached or residue is encountered. The rectum is then drained and air is insufflated, with the patient rotated from left lateral, to prone, to right lateral, until adequate double contrast views of the affected colon are obtained. Overhead radiographs are taken in the prone, erect, and left lateral projections (Fig. 16–1).

With experience, the examination may be modified. For example, with a distal colitis, the extent of the residue may prevent filling of the transverse colon. There is then little value in taking an erect view, as this is needed only to show the flexures and transverse colon in double contrast. If the colitis is extensive and follow-up examinations are performed frequently, the examination may be limited to a single prone double contrast view without significant loss of information.

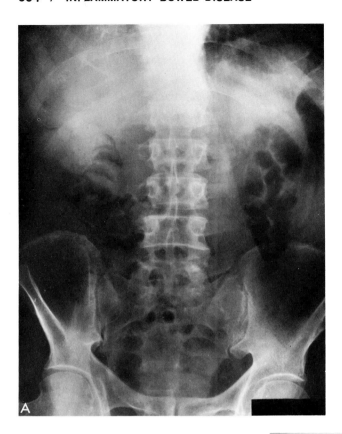

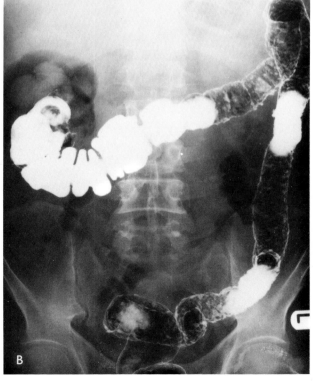

FIGURE 16–1 The instant enema.

A. The preliminary film shows fecal residue to the proximal transverse colon, suggesting that the colitis involves the distal half of the colon.

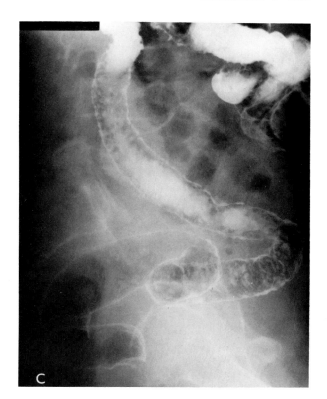

B, C, D. Overhead radiographs in the prone, lateral, and upright positions show extensive ulceration caused by ulcerative colitis involving the left half of the colon, extending to the mid-transverse colon.

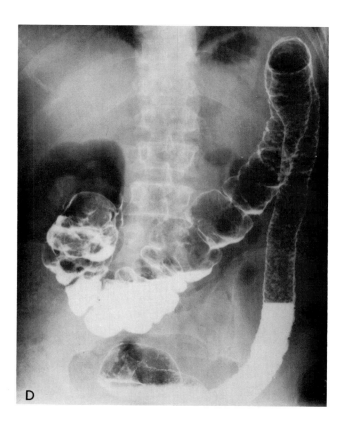

RISKS

The barium enema has been considered a predisposing factor in toxic megacolon.[2] A number of factors other than the barium examination may be relevant. For example, the use of purgatives for bowel preparation or antispasmodics during the examination are also likely to affect the bowel. The instant enema obviates such risks, as bowel preparation and relaxants are not used. Even if they are, there is no definite evidence of a harmful effect. Welin[3] recommends the use of atropine, and Fraser and Findlay[4] advocate bowel preparation in patients with active disease.

The technique of the instant enema has been in regular use for 13 years at St. Mark's Hospital. It is the firm opinion of the clinical and radiologic staff that the examination is safe to use in acute colitis, and that there is no basis for suggesting that double contrast techniques are contraindicated.[5]

It is possible that bacteremia may occur following a barium enema. A recent study[6] suggests that this does not occur, but other studies[7] have shown bacteremia following barium enema in 12 per cent of patients with lower gastrointestinal lesions. This has also been shown following sigmoidoscopy, so that distension of the colon by any medium may be the cause. However, the evidence is conflicting, and there are no grounds for believing that this represents a hazard.

ULCERATIVE COLITIS

Introduction

In the uncomplicated state the inflammatory changes of ulcerative colitis are limited to the mucosa and are accompanied by a considerable increase in vascularity.[8] The disease invariably starts in the rectum where it may remain as a proctitis, or it may spread proximally to involve the colon. The extent and severity are variable. In an acute attack the majority of the colon may be ulcerated, but with remission it can return to normal. Such attacks may come and go, or the disease may remain at a lower level of chronic activity. The radiologist is required to address the following issues:

1. The extent and severity of the mucosal lesions.
2. The presence of complications.
3. The extent to which the radiologic changes are compatible with the clinical diagnosis.

The routine examinations employed are plain films and contrast examinations, which may be either single or double contrast barium enemas with or without bowel preparation.

Plain Films

Correct interpretation of the plain films is of considerable importance in the acute attack. Failure to recognize grave complications, such as toxic megacolon, is the commonest cause of mortality in ulcerative colitis.[9]

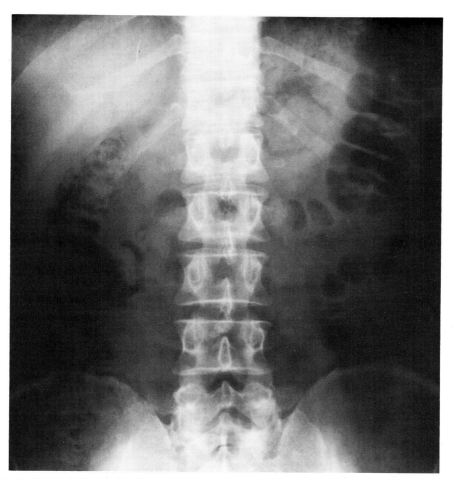

FIGURE 16-2   Plain abdominal radiograph in a normal unprepared patient. There is fecal residue in the cecum and ascending colon. Air in the traverse colon shows a smooth mucosal margin and sharp haustral clefts.

The extent of disease can be assessed in part from the fecal residue. A residue does not accumulate adjacent to inflamed mucosa,[10] so that the presence of a residue suggests that the mucosa is normal or relatively inactive. However, the extent of the residue can show considerable variation in noncolitic patients. In approximately one third of noncolitic patients the residue extends throughout the colon, in one third to the splenic flexure, and in the remaining third to the hepatic flexure. A residue should always be present in the cecum (Fig. 16–2).[11] The complete absence of any residue therefore suggests a total colitis (Fig. 16–3). Owing to the variability of the residue its distal extent cannot always be equated with the proximal extent of active disease. Further evidence of the extent and activity of the colitis is obtained from the presence of air in the lumen, revealing the mucosal outline and haustral pattern.[11, 12]

The diagnosis of toxic megacolon implies that the inflammation has become transmural with neuromuscular degeneration. It is based both on the clinical state of the patient and on the radiologic evidence of dilatation and severe mucosal disease. Rigorous criteria cannot be applied. The upper limit of normal for the diameter of the transverse colon is 5.5 cm.[12] A mean of 8.5 cm has been reported with toxic megacolon, and dilatation

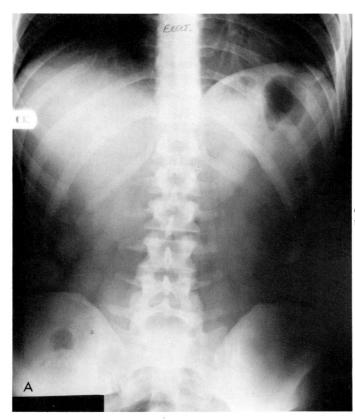

A. On the plain film there is no evidence of fecal residue, suggesting that there is a total colitis.

FIGURE 16–3 Total colitis.

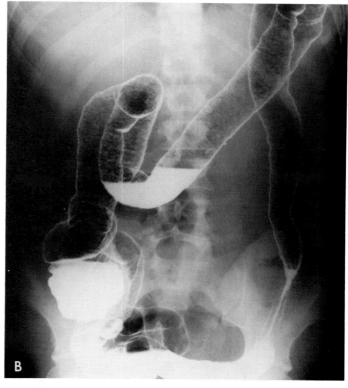

B. This is confirmed on the instant enema which shows diffuse granularity and ulceration throughout the entire colon.

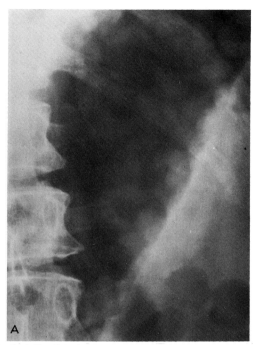

FIGURE 16–4 Toxic megacolon.

A. The plain film shows a dilated transverse colon with mucosal islands.

B. The resected specimen shows dilatation localized to a short segment. Most of the mucosa has been sloughed, and a few polypoid mucosal remnants form the mucosal islands.

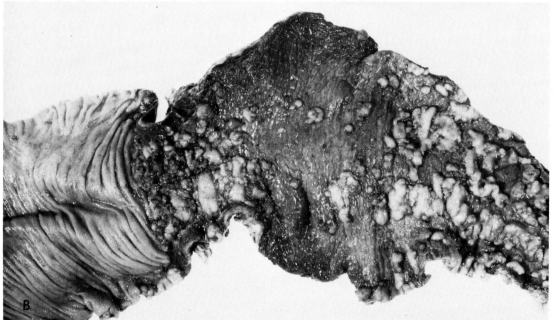

in excess of 6.5 cm indicates severe disease.[11] Destruction of the mucosa may be very extensive, leaving only small areas of edematous mucosa, the so-called mucosal islands.[14] The presence of mucosal islands always indicates very severe mucosal disease (Fig. 16–4).

Perforation is a complication that tends to occur in the sigmoid in an initial severe attack.[15] It may be free, when the intraperitoneal air is apparent on erect or decubitus view films, or sealed, which may be impossible to diagnose radiologically. Air tracking in the bowel wall is a sign of deep ulceration and suggests that perforation is imminent (Fig. 16–5).

609

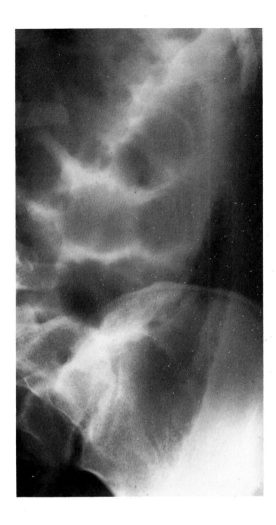

FIGURE 16–5 Air tracking in the bowel wall. A close-up view of the descending colon shows deep longitudinal ulceration containing air. Within 24 hours there was perforation with free intraperitoneal air. (*From*: Bartram, C. I.: Gastrointest. Radiol., *1*:383, 1977.[12] Reproduced by permission.)

Mucosal Changes

Ulcerative colitis being a mucosal disease, the radiologic changes are observed primarily in the mucosa, but secondary changes in the configuration of the bowel occur because of alteration in the smooth muscle tone.[8] The latter are readily apparent in both single and double contrast examinations. The detailed topography of the mucosal surface is more accurately shown in double contrast, as the mucosa is viewed en face and tangentially. The spectrum of mucosal abnormalities as seen by radiology and endoscopy in ulcerative colitis is illustrated in Plates 60 to 64.

GRANULARITY

This term was introduced by Welin and Brahme[16] to describe the earliest mucosal abnormality that can be detected. The smooth, even texture of the barium coating is lost, becoming amorphous or finely stippled. Seen tangentially, the fine, even mucosal line is slightly thickened and indistinct. The texture of granularity can vary considerably. Fine granularity is seen in the earliest stages of ulcerative colitis before the development of ulceration or erosion and is the result of mucosal edema and hyperemia

(Fig. 16–6). As the disease progresses, superficial erosions develop. The high density barium adheres to these erosions, producing a stippled appearance (Fig. 16–7).[17, 18] In the chronic stage the mucosa is replaced by granulation tissue and has a coarse granular appearance (Fig. 16–8). In patients having chronic disease with an acute exacerbation, there may be ill-defined barium collections representing superficial ulcerations superimposed on a diffusely granular background (Fig. 16–9).

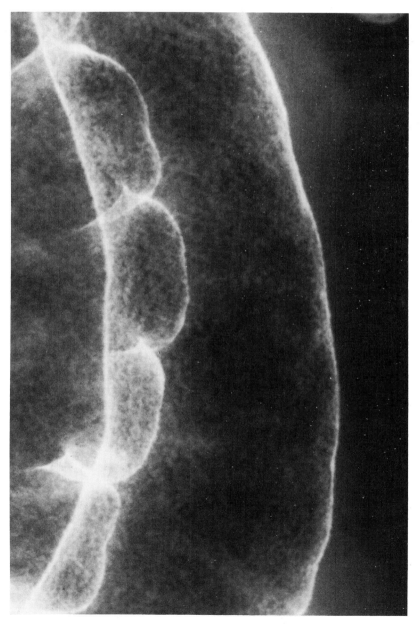

FIGURE 16–6   Early ulcerative colitis with fine mucosal granularity due to mucosal edema and hyperemia. (*From*:Laufer, I., Mullens, J. E., and Hamilton, J.: Radiology, *118*:1, 1976.[18] Reproduced by permission.)

In the filled single contrast examination the profile view of the mucosa is often normal, or if irregular the appearance may be confused with filling of the innominate grooves.[19] The earliest change of colitis on the single contrast barium enema (SCBE) is an abnormal mucosal fold pattern on the postevacuation film.[20] However, as evacuation is often incomplete, this is an unreliable sign.[21] A recent study comparing the radiologic changes on SCBE and DCE to sigmoidoscopy has shown that the SCBE is normal when early sigmoidoscopic abnormalities are present and the DCE demonstrates a granular change.[4]

Recognition of granularity on DCE enables the radiologist to detect colitis with more confidence and at an earlier stage than is possible using single contrast techniques.

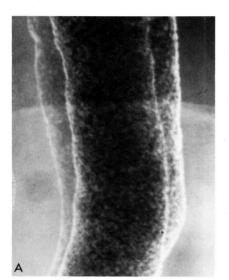
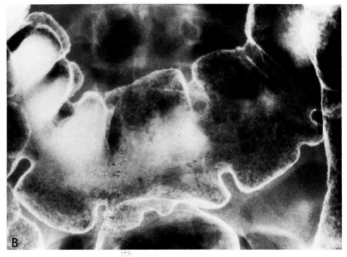

FIGURE 16–7

A and *B*. Diffuse granularity with stippling due to superficial ulceration or erosion.

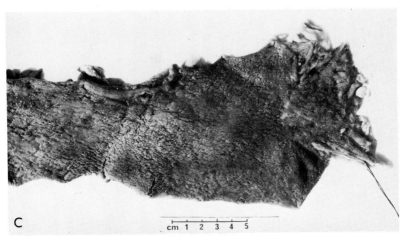

C. The resected colon in a patient with chronic ulcerative colitis shows the granular surface with small defects which account for the stippled appearance on radiographs.

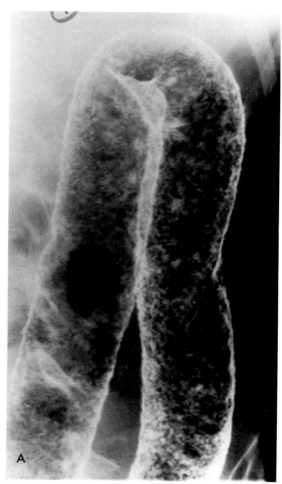

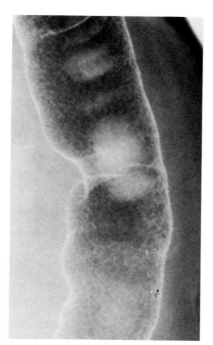

FIGURE 16–8 Coarse granular appearance in chronic ulcerative colitis. (*From* Laufer, I.: CRC Crit. Rev. Diagnost. Imaging, 9:421, 1977.[36] Reproduced by permission.)

FIGURE 16–9 *A* to *C* Three examples of ulceration superimposed on a background of diffuse granularity. Ulcers are seen en face as blotchy collections of barium.

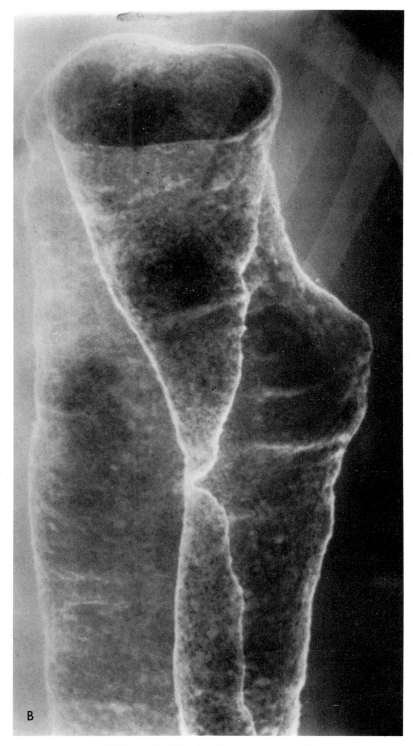

FIGURE 16–9 *B See legend on page 613.*

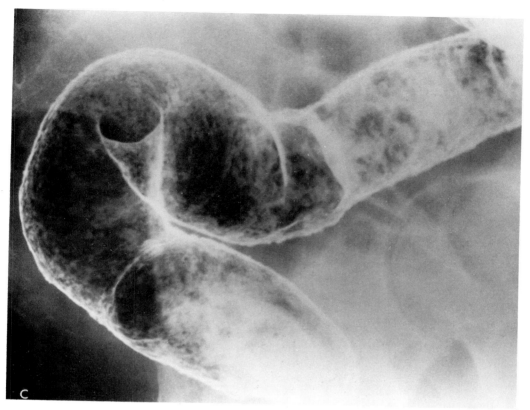

FIGURE 16–9C *See legend on page 613.*

ULCERATION

This develops as the result of patchy sloughing of the mucous membrane. The ulceration is often linear in relation to the attachment of the teniae, and may undermine adjacent mucosa. Unlike granularity, this is clearly defined in profile (Fig. 16–10). Disruption of the mucosal line is the key to the presence of ulceration, and allows distinction from the en face view of coarse granularity.[17] Small T-shaped projections are common. Sometimes the ulceration may extend longitudinally under the mucosa for several centimeters, the so-called double-tracking sign (Fig. 16–11). The important point is that ulceration on a background of diffuse granularity is characteristic of ulcerative colitis (Fig. 16–12). The presence of ulceration is important, as it implies a severe attack both clinically and pathologically.

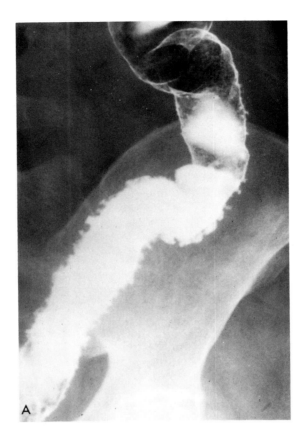

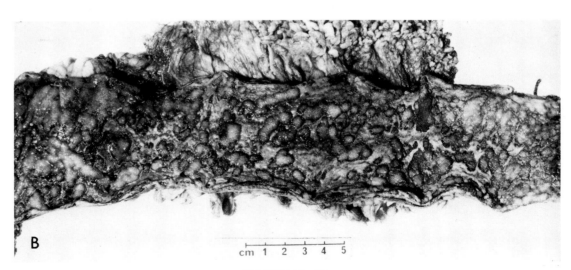

FIGURE 16–10

A. Deep ulceration in ulcerative colitis.

B. The resected specimen shows extensive serpiginous ulceration with nodular mucosal remnants.

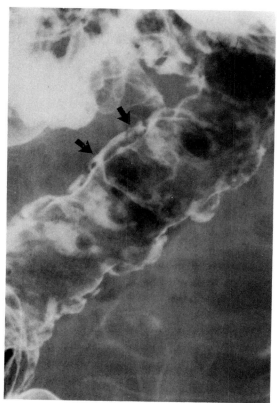

FIGURE 16–11 Double contrast view of deep ulcers, with double tracking (*arrows*) formed by submucosal extension of the ulcers.

FIGURE 16–12*A* and *B*   Two examples of deep ulceration on a background of granular mucosa. Although the ulcers are nonspecific, the background granularity is characteristic of ulcerative as opposed to granulomatous colitis.

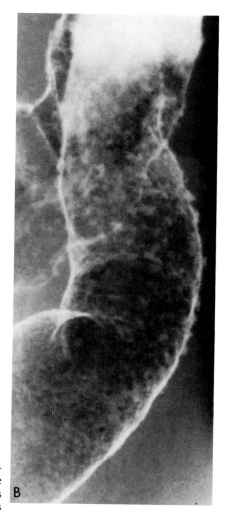

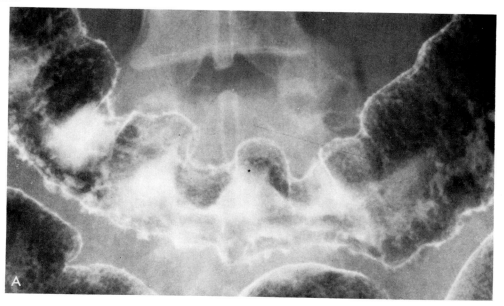

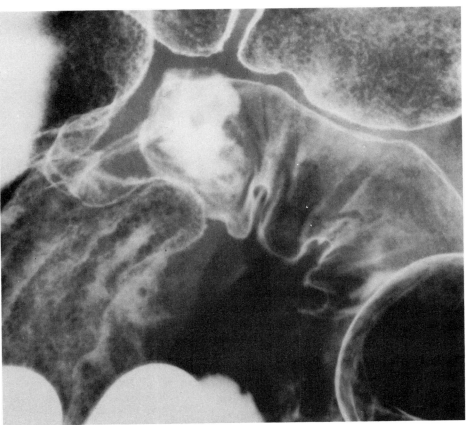

FIGURE 16–13 Normal terminal ileum in a patient with extensive involvement of the entire colon by ulcerative colitis.

TERMINAL ILEUM

The terminal ileum is normal in the large majority of patients with ulcerative colitis (Fig. 16–13). However, involvement of the terminal ileum has been found in 10 per cent of colectomies in ulcerative colitis.[22, 23] Involvement is confined to between 5 and 25 cm of terminal ileum. Characteristic features are dilatation, absent peristalsis, and a granular mucosa (Fig. 16–14). Discrete ulceration is not seen in "backwash ileitis" that is due to ulcerative colitis. When present it usually indicates that the abnormalities are the result of Crohn's disease.

The ileocecal valve is usually dilated and incompetent. The exact reason for this change is unknown. It may be due to backwash of colonic contents through an incompetent valve. However, pathologic changes in the ileum have been found to precede incompetence of the valve.[23] Reflux ileitis is always associated with a total colitis, usually of long-standing low-grade activity. Radiologically, it is of little significance except that it confirms the presence of a total colitis.

There is probably a tendency to overdiagnose reflux ileitis utilizing the single contrast enema. Reflux of colonic contents into the terminal ileum may produce an indistinct mucosal outline which may be mistaken for mucosal inflammation. Sellink[24] has shown that with the small bowel enteroclysis technique the terminal ileum can be washed out and a normal appearance produced.

618

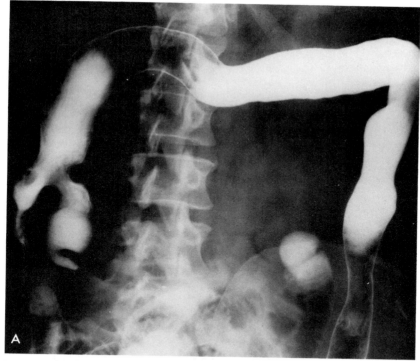

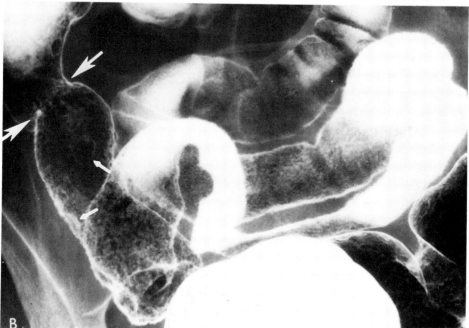

FIGURE 16–14 Backwash ileitis.

A. The colon exhibits changes of long-standing total colitis with a granular mucosa and loss of haustration. There are a few inflammatory polyps in the distal descending colon. The ileocecal valve is patulous, and the terminal ileum is dilated.

B. In another patient there is marked contraction of the cecum. The ileocecal valve *(arrows)* is patulous, and the mucosa of the distal small bowel has the granular appearance characteristic of the colon in ulcerative colitis. In addition there are inflammatory polyps *(arrows)* in the terminal ileum.[116]

POLYPOID CHANGE

Polypoid appearances may be seen during all stages of activity in ulcerative colitis. The terms pseudopolyp and inflammatory polyp have been used interchangeably and inconsistently.

In the acute, severe attack of ulcerative colitis with deep ulceration, the inflamed mucosal remnants between ulcers produce a polypoid appearance (Fig. 16–15A). These apparent filling defects are properly called *pseudopolyps,* since they represent the actual mucosal surface and do not represent polypoid protuberances. With partial healing the mucosal line is undulating, and en face the crisscross pattern of residual ulceration is seen in between the pseudopolypoid regenerative mucosa (Fig. 16–15B).

In patients with low-grade activity manifest by a granular mucosal surface, localized polypoid lesions can be seen. These may be sessile, frondlike, or rarely, pedunculated (Fig. 16–16). These are most properly called *inflammatory polyps,* since they consist of localized mucosal inflammation resulting in a polypoid protuberance on a background of actively inflamed mucosa.

In patients with quiescent disease a variety of polypoid lesions may be found. Histologically, they may be composed of either inflamed or normal mucosa. They may be termed *postinflammatory polyps,* because their pathogenesis involves a previous attack of severe ulceration with healing. They are found in 10 to 20 per cent of patients.[25] They may be single or multiple, segmental or diffuse. The postinflammatory polyps may be small sessile nodules (Fig. 16–17A), or they may be long, wormlike outgrowths from the mucosa, which branch and adhere to each other (Figs. 16–17B, 16–18, and 16–19). This particular appearance has also been termed filiform polyposis[26] and is a nonspecific sequela of severe mucosal ulceration.

The occurrence of inflammatory and postinflammatory polyps is related to a previous severe attack of extensive colitis (Fig. 16–20 A and B), but not to the length of clinical history. A positive association with toxic megacolon has been noted.[27] The probable pathogenesis is the undermining, during a severe episode, of the remaining mucosa by extensive full-thickness ulceration, which raises up strips of mucosa. Epithelialization occurs beneath, so that the mucosal tags are prevented from rejoining with the mucosal surface, although they may rejoin other parts of the mucosa to form bridges (Fig. 16–19 B).[28]

Inflammatory and postinflammatory polyps have no malignant potential.[29] Once formed they remain, even though the colitis may be in complete remission. The colon may appear otherwise normal. This can cause problems if localized areas of polyps are present, as the lesions can simulate a neoplasm, particularly a villous adenoma.[30] A careful examination of the lesion should reveal the fronds and normal background mucosa, but endoscopic biopsy may be required. Rarely, a seaweedlike mass of inflammatory polyps can cause obstruction to filling on barium enema (Fig. 16–21).

These are uncommon problems. In the majority of cases a confident diagnosis of inflammatory or postinflammatory polyposis can be made on DCE findings. The commonest diagnostic problem occurs when only solitary or multiple sessile polyps are present in a patient with quiescent colitis and a background of normal mucosa. The majority of these will be postinflammatory polyps, but they are difficult to distinguish radiologically from adenomas or carcinoma, particularly when they are solitary. Inflammatory lesions tend to have a rough surface when associated with an active mucosa. This probably reflects the granulation tissue with which they are covered (Fig. 16–20). Adenomas tend to have a smooth surface. However, this distinction is not infallible, as inflammatory lesions have variable epithelization and so can also have a smooth surface, as indeed is the case with most of the frondlike lesions. Inflammatory polyps are usually not pedunculated, so that any lesion with a stalk should be considered an adenoma. Adenomas and polypoid carcinomas are uncommon in ulcerative colitis, but their exclusion will usually require endoscopic excision.

Text continued on page 628

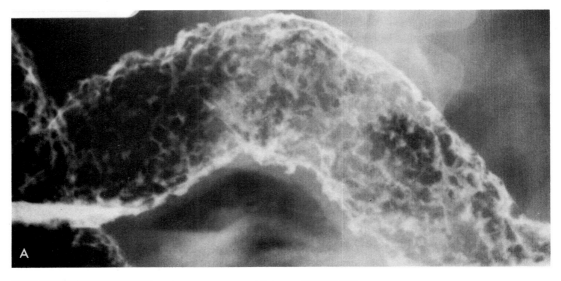

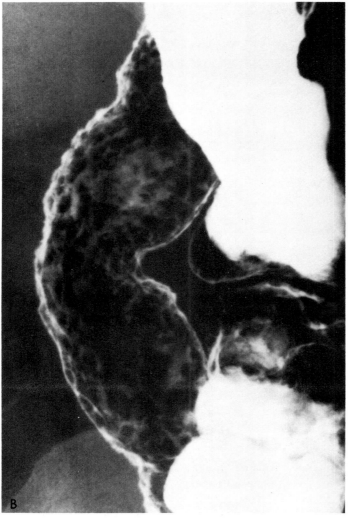

FIGURE 16–15 *A* and *B* Extensive mucosal ulceration with inflamed mucosal remnants resulting in pseudopolyposis. (*B* from: Bartram, C. I.: Gastrointest. Radiol., *1*:383, 1977.[12] Reproduced by permission.

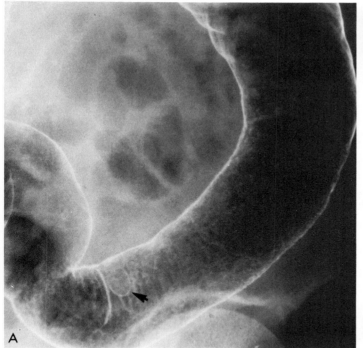

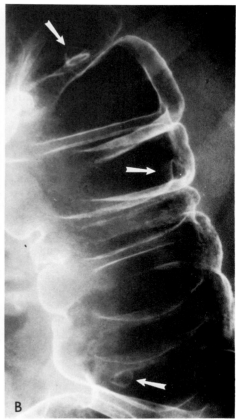

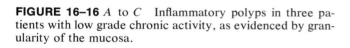

FIGURE 16–16 *A* to *C* Inflammatory polyps in three patients with low grade chronic activity, as evidenced by granularity of the mucosa.

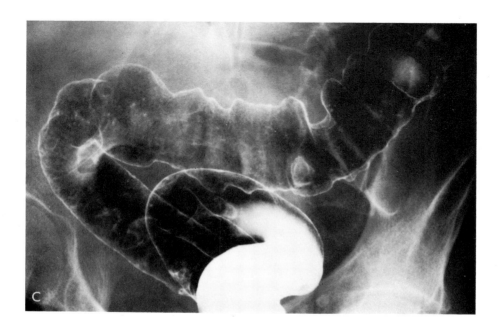

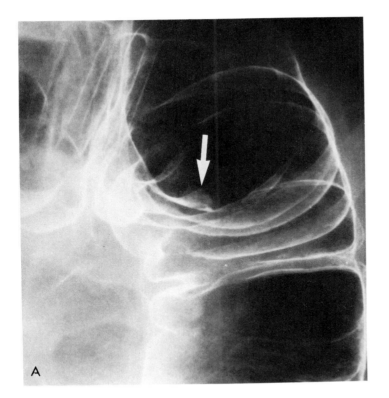

A. A small sessile polyp at the splenic flexure in a patient with a past history of actue ulcerative colitis. Note that the mucosa now has a smooth appearance, indicating that the disease is quiescent.

FIGURE 16–17 Postinflammatory polyps.

B. Filiform polyposis in a patient with a past history of acute ulcerative colitis. (*From*: Bartram, C. I.: Gastrointest. Radiol. *1*:383, 1977.[12] Reproduced by permission.)

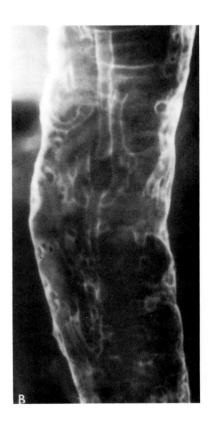

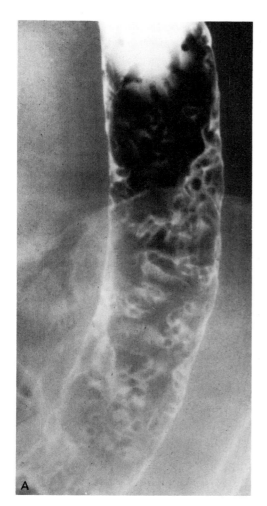

A. The mucosal line is intact, but there are multiple sessile and frondlike postinflammatory polyps.

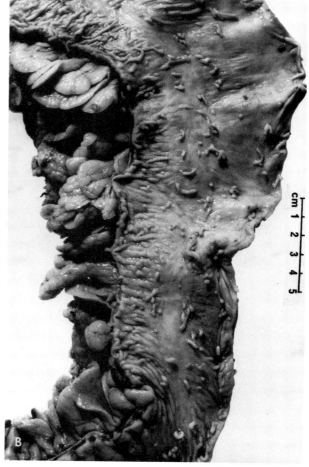

FIGURE 16–18 Postinflammatory polyposis.

B. The resected specimen shows a normal mucosa with postinflammatory polyps.

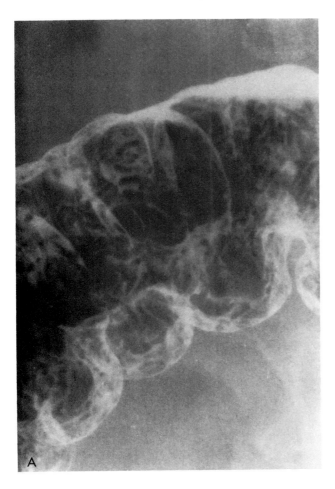

FIGURE 16–19 Postinflammatory polyposis.

A. There is a mass of frondlike inflammatory polyps on a background of normal mucosa.

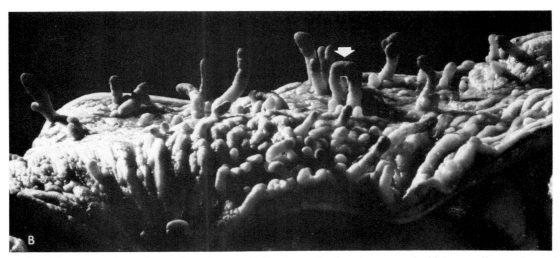

B. The resected specimen viewed tangentially shows the fronds, some of which are adherent to each other, forming mucosal bridges *(arrow)*.[28, 117] (*From*: Morson, B. C.: The Pathogenesis of Colorectal Cancer. Philadelphia, W. B. Saunders, 1978. Reproduced by permission.)

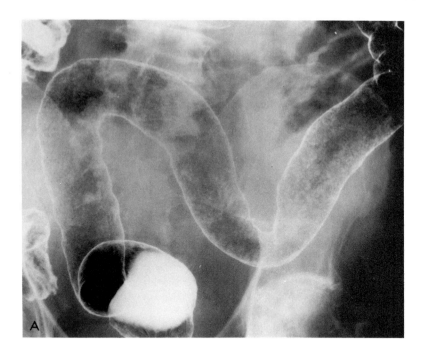

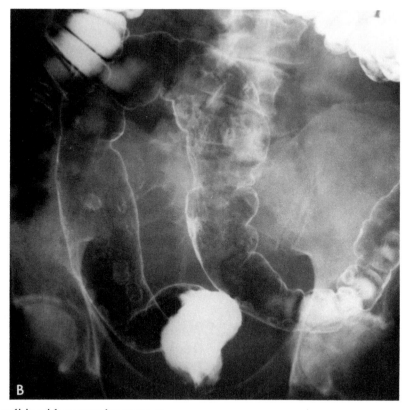

A. Active colitis with a granular mucosa.
B. Three years later the colitis is inactive, but there are multiple sessile postinflammatory polyps.

FIGURE 16–20 The development of postinflammatory polyps.

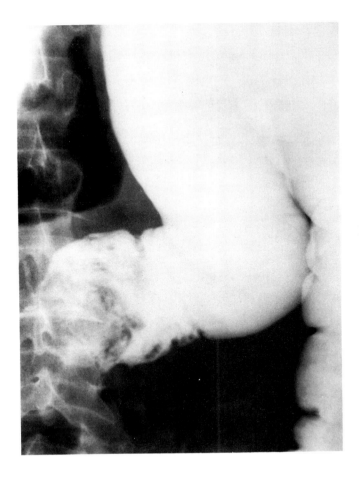

FIGURE 16–21 There is a mass of postinflammatory polyps in the transverse colon, causing obstruction to filling with barium.

Secondary Changes

These mainly reflect the smooth muscle changes that accompany active disease.[8]

Postrectal Space. Normally this is less than 1 cm as seen on the lateral pelvic view.[31] Widening is a useful indicator of active disease (Fig. 16–22), especially if the mucosal changes are minimal. An inverse relationship exists between the postrectal space and the width of the rectum, the postrectal space increasing as the rectum narrows. The width of the postrectal space appears to be related to the length of history and the age of onset of disease, being greater in those with an early age of onset of colitis and chronic active disease.[32] The postrectal space may, however, be normal with active disease. When the rectal mucosa was granular the space was found to be widened in only 3 per cent of patients.[33]

Valves of Houston. The valves of Houston, or rectal folds, are obliterated with active disease in 43 per cent of patients (Fig. 16–22).[33]

Haustration. Haustration of the colon is affected in active disease. The earliest change is widening of the haustral clefts (Fig. 16–23), followed by complete loss of haustration. The change is circumferentially symmetric and reflects the mucosal lesions, so that blunting is seen only with minimal mucosal lesions, and haustral loss is always associated with severe active disease. When interpreting haustral changes it is important to remember that the left hemicolon may be without haustration on DCE in

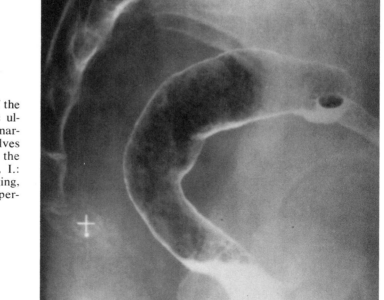

FIGURE 16–22 Lateral view of the rectum in a patient with chronic ulcerative colitis. The rectum is narrowed, with obliteration of the valves of Houston and an increase in the postrectal space. (*From*: Laufer, I.: CRC Crit. Rev. Diagnost. Imaging, 9:421, 1977.[36] Reproduced by permission.)

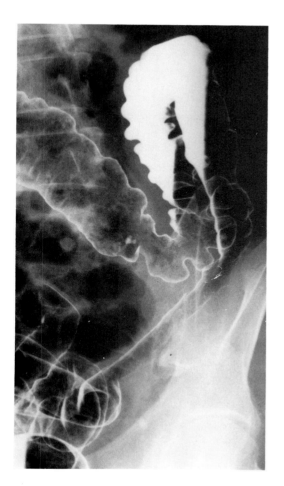

FIGURE 16–23 Ulcerative colitis with abnormal haustration and a stricture. There is a granular mucosa, with thickening of the haustral folds in the distal transverse colon, and a long benign stricture in the descending colon.

normal subjects. Therefore, if haustration alone is considered, only changes in the colon proximal to the mid-transverse colon can be considered abnormal. In practice, loss of haustration in the proximal colon is useful supplementary evidence when the mucosal changes are minimal, to confirm that the patient has a total active colitis.

Configurational Change.   There is also a generalized change in the configuration of the colon, which becomes narrowed and shortened with depression of the flexures. Typically, such a colon will also be without haustration, or will have a widened postrectal space and a minimally granular mucosa. These are the characteristic changes found in a long-standing total colitis of chronic activity (Fig. 16–14A). The secondary changes mirror the primary mucosal abnormality, so that with regression of the disease the colon can revert to an entirely normal appearance (Fig. 16–24).

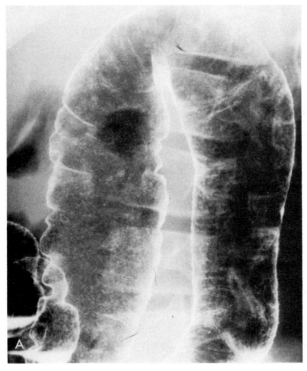

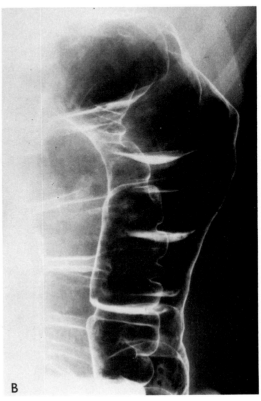

FIGURE 16–24   Reversibility of the haustral changes.

A.   Active ulcerative colitis, with stippling of the mucosa and loss of haustration.

B.   In remission the mucosa is flat and the haustra have returned.

Accuracy

The accuracy of the examination refers to its ability to show the extent and severity of the mucosal abnormality. In general, the radiologic findings have correlated closely with the gross appearance of the resected specimen. However, radiology tends to underestimate the extent of involvement as judged by histology. A total colitis was found histologically in almost every case in which the disease appeared to extend to the hepatic flexure only.[17] This supports the use of the term *extensive colitis*[34] to describe a colitis that extends radiologically to the hepatic flexure, implying that the whole colon is affected histologically. The reason for this underestimation is probably twofold. First, in the unprepared colon any residue will be pushed into the proximal colon and will obscure mucosal detail. Second, the transition from abnormal to normal is usually not abrupt but gradual.

Because of the vascular component an abnormality may be seen on direct examination when the surface irregularity is not sufficient to alter the barium covering. Hence the ability of colonoscopy to show more proximal involvement. Histologic changes may be present without visible abnormality on DCE or at colonoscopy. Occasionally an adequate DCE will be normal, but extensive colitis will be found on multiple biopsies.[35] The clinical significance of "histologic colitis" has not yet been determined.[36]

Complications

STRICTURE

The presence of strictures is associated with long-standing disease, usually having a history in excess of 5 years and extensive involvement.[25] Strictures are most common in the sigmoid; they are of variable length and may be multiple (Figs. 16–23 and 16–25).

Benign strictures once were considered rare in ulcerative colitis, but endoscopic examination has shown that this is not the case and that the majority are benign.[37] A benign stricture may contain dysplastic epithelium, but a true malignant stricture due to narrowing from the tumor mass is rare.

Typically, a benign stricture has smooth margins with a symmetric central lumen and regularly tapering ends. The mucosa throughout is similar to that on either side of the stricture (Fig. 16–25 A and B). The malignant stricture has an irregular contour with uneven narrowing or shouldering, an eccentric lumen, and irregularity of part or all of the mucosa, which differs from the mucosa outside the stricture (Fig. 16–26).[38]

Frequently the distinction between benign and malignant strictures on a purely radiologic basis is difficult, and endoscopic examination is indicated (Fig. 16–27).

Text continued on page 635

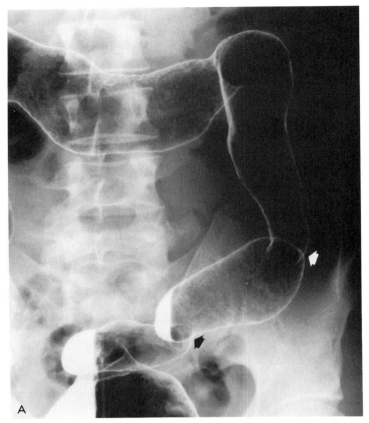

A. Total, long-standing colitis with two short, benign strictures *(arrows)* in the descending colon. (*From*: Bartram, C. I.: Gastrointest. Radiol., *1*:383, 1977.[12] Reproduced by permission.)

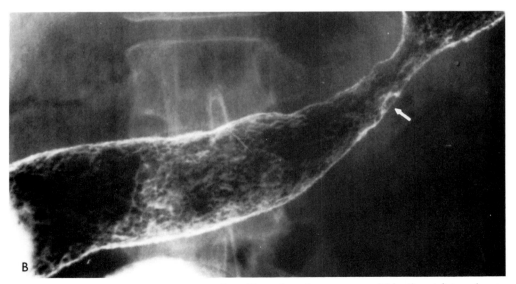

B. Stricture of the distal transverse colon. Note that the mucosa within the strictured segment is granular and is identical to the mucosa distally and proximally. There are also inflammatory polyps *(arrow)*.

FIGURE 16–25 Strictures in ulcerative colitis.

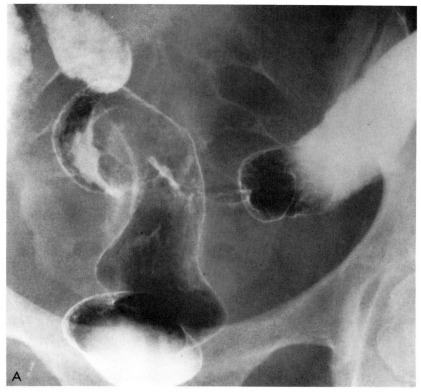

A. Annular adenocarcinoma in a patient with ulcerative colitis. There is an irregular lumen with shouldered margins.

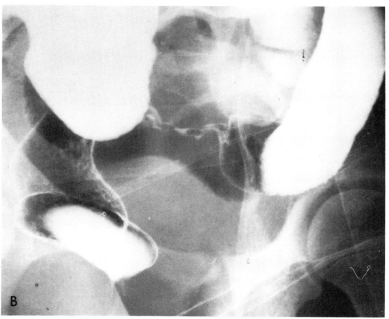

B. Another patient with a malignant stricture due to adenocarcinoma.

FIGURE 16–26 Malignant strictures.

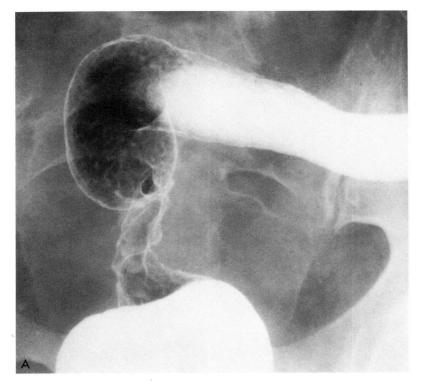

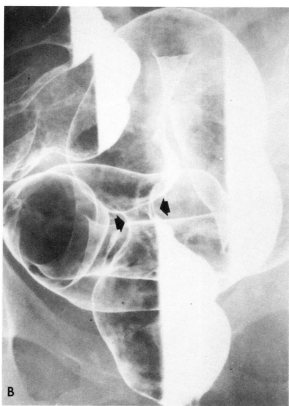

FIGURE 16–27 Difficulty in distinguishing benign from malignant strictures.

A. Asymmetric and irregular stricture suggestive of carcinoma. However, this proved to be a benign stricture.

B. Smooth, tapered stricture in the rectum, with no radiologic suggestion of malignancy. Nevertheless, this proved to be a carcinoma.

MALIGNANCY

Cancer is an uncommon complication in ulcerative colitis. However, patients with ulcerative colitis are more likely to develop a tumor than is the general population,[39] and at an earlier age. The tumors show a different distribution from those in the noncolitic bowel. Rectosigmoid tumors are less common, and the lesions are more evenly distributed around the colon.[40] Synchronous growths are more common and have been reported in 34 per cent of cases.[41] Most of the tumors are annular in shape (Fig. 16–28). Polypoid growths (Fig. 16–29A) are rare. Scirrhous carcinomas are a feature of colitic carcinoma (Fig. 16–29B), although they are still uncommon.[42]

The risk of cancer in ulcerative colitis is not uniform, and a high-risk group can be identified.[43] The factors that define this group are:

1. *The extent of disease.* Many studies have shown that cancer is associated with a total colitis.[25, 39, 44, 45]

2. *The length of history.* The increased risk of carcinoma starts approximately 10 years after the onset of the disease. Thereafter the risk of carcinoma is approximately equal to 10 per cent for every 10 years of disease.[25, 43, 46] Carcinoma frequently develops in patients with quiescent or minimally active colitis.

3. *Age of onset.* If colitis begins in childhood the risk of cancer may be greater than if it starts in adulthood.[39, 46]

4. *Epithelial dysplasia.* Severe dysplasia is usually present in the colon of patients with cancer complicating colitis.[47] Persistent severe dysplasia is considered an indication for colectomy.[43] Unfortunately, dysplasia usually cannot be recognized radiologically, as the mucosa is already abnormal. Recently it has been suggested that epithelial dysplasia can be recognized on DCE as small, flat, faceted filling defects which can be distinguished from the granularity of ulcerative colitis.[48]

The management of high-risk patients requires regular radiologic surveillance and endoscopic biopsy to determine the presence of dysplasia.[43] The role of the radiologist is to determine the extent of the colitis and the configuration of the colon in order to aid the endoscopist, and to draw attention to any area suspicious of dysplasia or carcinoma. Strictures and large polyps are not diagnostic of cancer, as most strictures are benign,[37] and even solitary polyps are commonly benign and inflammatory in nature.[49]

FECAL STASIS

This may occur when the proximal colon is relatively normal but the distal colon has severe active disease (Fig. 16–30). The patient may pass frequent liquid stools when the abdominal film shows a large residue. This is thought to develop from the severe distal disease producing a functional obstruction and the proximal colon continuing with its normal function of water reabsorption.[50] Therefore, an impacted residue gradually accumulates in the right colon, and can in itself cause diarrhea from retention with overflow.

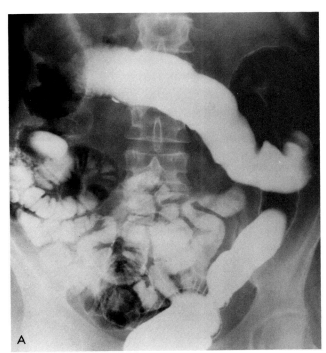

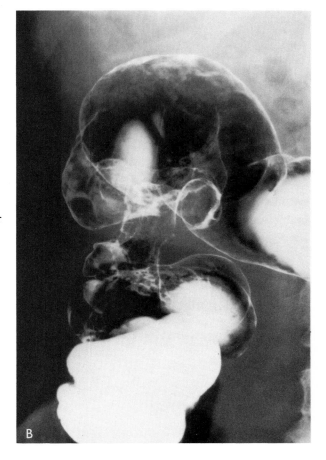

FIGURE 16–28 The development of colitic carcinoma.

A. Total active colitis for 11 years.

B. Three years later there is an annular carcinoma in the ascending colon.

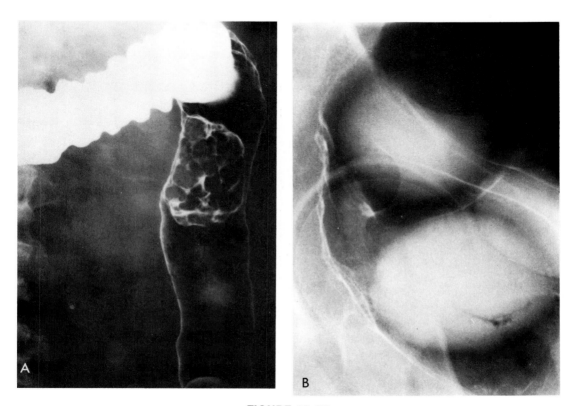

FIGURE 16–29

A.   Unusual polypoid carcinoma in ulcerative colitis.

B.   Flat infiltrating carcinoma along the lateral wall of the rectum in a patient with a long history of ulcerative colitis.

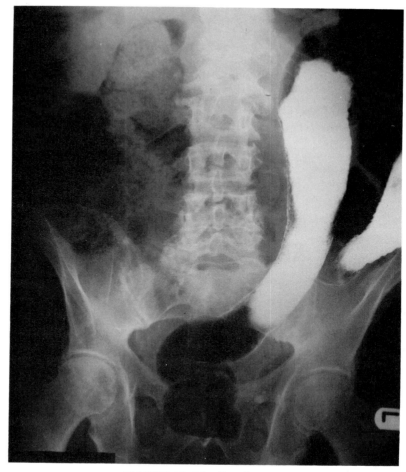

FIGURE 16-30 Fecal stasis.

Active disease in the left colon with a normal right colon containing a large fecal residue. (*From*: Bartram, C. I.: Gastrointest. Radiol. *1*:383, 1977.[12] Reproduced by permission.)

Clinical Significance

Radiologic examination is of greatest value in the acute attack. The presence of colonic dilatation and mucosal islands on a plain film establishes the diagnosis of toxic megacolon. Failure to recognize this is the main cause of death in acute colitis.[9]

Information derived from the instant enema provides useful supportive evidence in assessing an acute attack. The presence of extensive disease or ulceration is associated with an increased incidence of failure of medical treatment, necessitating surgical intervention.[34] The presence of ulceration invariably indicates that the patient is in a severe acute attack.

The extent of distal colitis has some value in predicting the future course of the disease. If the upper limit of disease is defined sigmoidoscopically, there is only a 10 per cent chance of proximal spread in 10 years, whereas if the disease extends to the left iliac crest, there is a 30 per cent chance of more proximal involvement and an increased risk of death related to the colitis.[51]

The risk of malignancy with an extensive colitis has been discussed. The discovery of postinflammatory polyps indicates the patient has had a previous severe attack with remission. The presence of strictures suggests that the disease is of at least 5 years' duration.

The state of the rectum is significant if ileorectal anastomosis is contemplated. If the rectum is narrowed with an active mucosa it is usually considered to be unsuitable for anastomosis.

CROHN'S DISEASE

Introduction

The radiologic and pathologic features of the advanced stages of Crohn's disease are well known. This disorder may affect every part of the gastrointestinal tract with transmural inflammation. It is characterized by marked thickening of the bowel wall and involvement of regional lymph nodes. There is also a tendency toward the formation of deep ulcers, abscesses, and fistulae. In most cases Crohn's disease is characterized by discontinuous involvement of the gastrointestinal tract. This may be manifest in its early stages by separated small ulcers on a background of normal mucosa. In the later stages, multiple areas of severe disease may be separated by normal mucosa. In other cases there may be severe focal disease, with minimal disease in remote portions of the gastrointestinal tract. This tendency for discontinuous disease stands in marked contrast to the continuous, symmetric, and diffuse involvement of the colon in ulcerative colitis.

The corresponding radiologic features have been described extensively and in great detail over the past 20 years. The findings on single contrast barium enemas correspond reasonably well to the pathologic features in advanced cases of Crohn's disease. Marshak[52, 53] has minimized the diagnostic difficulties in the distinction between ulcerative and granulomatous colitis, except in advanced cases of total colitis when there may be no distinguishing features. Other authors[54-56] have indicated that diagnostic difficulties may exist in 20 to 25 per cent of cases, and that some of this difficulty can be ascribed to inconclusive radiologic studies.

Early Changes

Marshak[52] has described the earliest roentgen features of Crohn's disease as small irregular nodules along the contour of the bowel. From his illustrations it appears that these are usually of the order of 5 mm in diameter. Some of them are associated with central ulcerations or with rigidity and thickening of haustral markings. However, the earliest pathologic features of Crohn's disease consist of focal granulomatous inflammation, which may be most prominent in the submucosa but also involves the mucosa and serosa. These focal areas of inflammation may go on to form the "aphthous" ulcers described by Lockhart-Mummery and Morson.[57, 58]

These abnormalities may be detected by careful radiologic study of the mucosal surface of the colon. Focal granulomatous inflammation may be manifest as a mamillated surface due to tiny nodular filling defects measuring 1 to 2 mm in diameter (Fig. 16–31A). The appearance is very similar to that of lymphoid hyperplasia in the pediatric colon,[59] and indeed this is probably due to exaggeration of the normal lymphoid follicular pattern. Some of these nodules may go on to ulcerate (Fig. 16–31 B and C). The aphthous ulcers of Crohn's disease can be demonstrated radiologically as small central collections of barium surrounded by a radiolucent halo.[60, 61] These produce a very typical "bull's-eye" or "target" lesion (Fig. 16–32). These lesions may be seen in any portion of the colon or rectum (Fig. 16–33) and are frequently found on a background of normal mucosa, either adjacent to an area of more severe involvement or in a remote portion of the gastrointestinal tract (Fig. 16–34).

These aphthous ulcers have a similar appearance in the stomach, small bowel, and colon. They have never been convincingly shown on a single contrast barium study, although several authors have demonstrated their appearance using double contrast techniques.[18, 36, 60-63] Brahme has pointed out that these are unstable lesions which change quickly.[64] Usually they progress to more extensive ulceration, but in some cases they may regress (Fig. 16–35), although invariably the disease will recur at a later date.

Aphthous ulcers may be seen in other conditions, such as Yersinia enterocolitis, Behçet's syndrome, and amebic colitis. These conditions are rarely encountered in most Western countries. Therefore, the finding of aphthous ulcers is highly suggestive of Crohn's disease.

Text continued on page 647

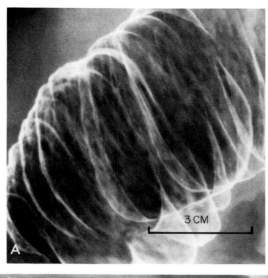

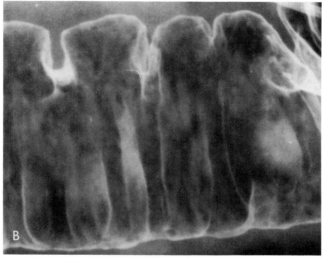

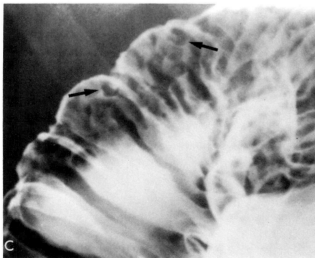

FIGURE 16–31 *A* to *C*   Lymphoid hyperplasia in the early stages of Crohn's disease.

There is very fine nodularity of the colon owing to enlargement of the lymph follicles. Some of the follicles have small central collections of barium which probably represent superficial ulceration. (*A* from: Laufer, I., and de Sa, D.: Am J. Roentgenol., *130*:51, 1978.[59] *B* from: Laufer, I.: CRC Crit. Rev. Diagnost. Imaging, *9*:421, 1977.[36] Reproduced by permission.)

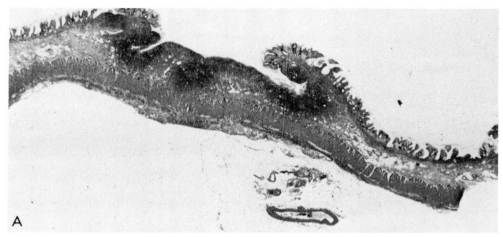

A. This histologic section shows a superficial ulcer with transmural inflammation. The ulcer has elevated margins and is surrounded by normal mucosa. (*From*: Laufer, I., and Costopoulos, L.: Am. J. Roentgenol., *130*:307, 1978.[60] Reproduced by permission.)

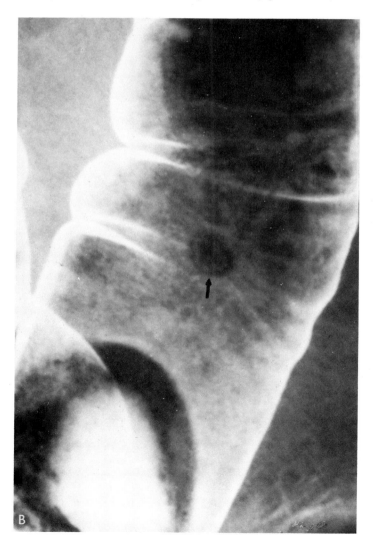

FIGURE 16–32 Aphthous ulcers in Crohn's disease.

B. The radiologic appearance of an aphthous ulcer with a superficial central ulcer surrounded by a radiolucent halo *(arrow)*. In this case there is also a suggestion of radiating folds and slight retraction.

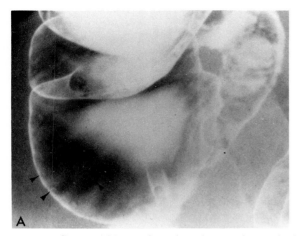

A. Cecum. Note also the abnormal terminal ileum.

FIGURE 16–33 Examples of aphthous ulcers throughout the colon.

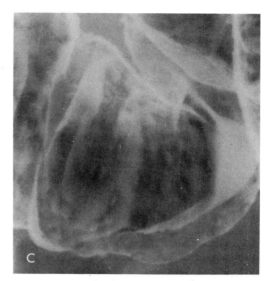

C. Distal transverse colon.

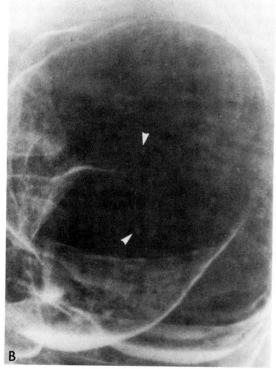

B. The hepatic flexure is studded with tiny target lesions owing to diffuse aphthous ulceration. *From*: Laufer, I.: CRC Crit. Rev. Diagnost. Imaging, *9*:421, 1977.[36] Reproduced by permission.

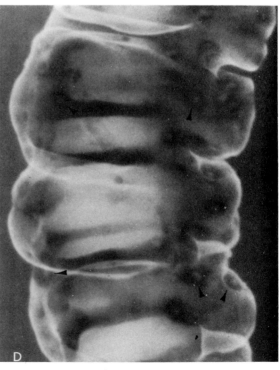

D. Descending colon. (*From*: Laufer, I., and Costopoulos, L.: Am. J. Roentgenol., *130*:307, 1978.[60] Reproduced by permission.)

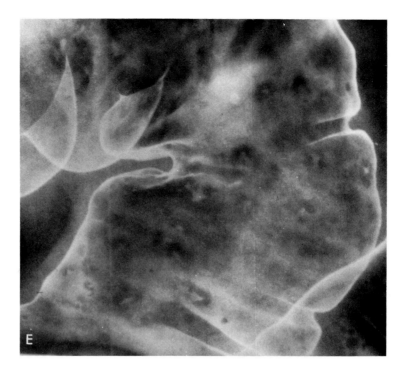

E. Sigmoid.

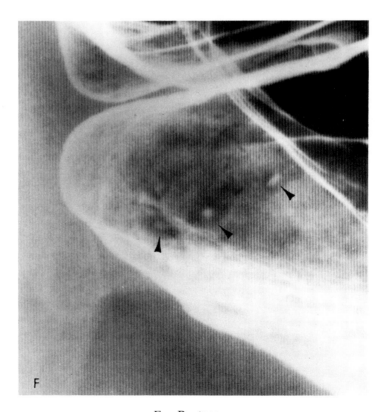

F. Rectum.

FIGURE 6–33 *Continued*

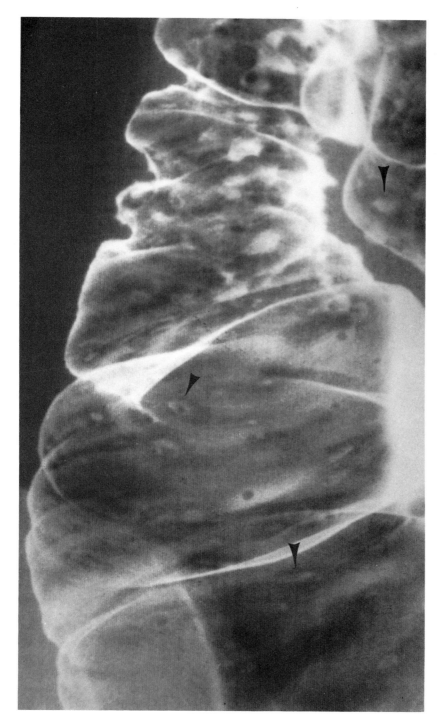

FIGURE 16–34 Aphthous ulcers in association with more severe disease.

There is obvious involvement by Crohn's disease of the distal ascending colon and hepatic flexure. Multiple aphthous ulcers are seen in the proximal ascending colon and in the proximal transverse colon. Note the normal appearance of the mucosa between the aphthous ulcers (*From*: Laufer, I., and Costopoulos, L.: Am. J. Roentgenol., *130*:307, 1978. Reproduced by permission.)

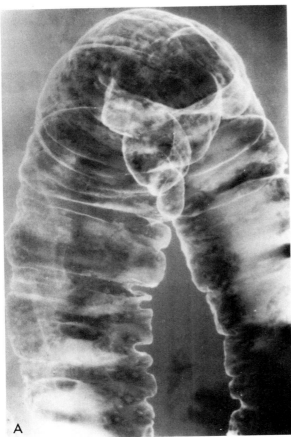

A

FIGURE 16–35 Reversibility in the early stages of Crohn's disease.

A. Diffuse aphthous ulceration at the splenic flexure.

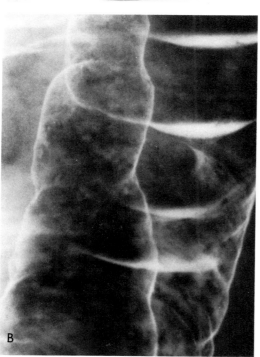

B

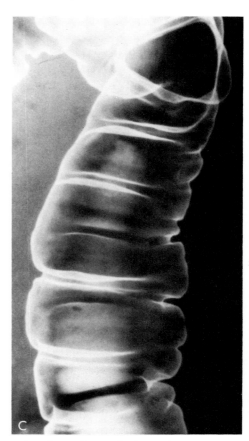

C

B. Several months later there is marked improvement, although a few superficial ulcers remain.

C. Several months later the appearance of the colon has returned entirely to normal.

Advanced Disease

DISCONTINUOUS ULCERATION

As previously mentioned, the tendency for discontinuity of ulceration is one of the main hallmarks of Crohn's disease. Even in the earliest stages the aphthous ulcers are separated by a normal mucosa. As the ulcers enlarge, large patches of normal mucosa can still be identified in between them (Fig. 16–36). With further progression, larger segments of colon become involved (Fig. 16–37), but discontinuous involvement has been demonstrated in 90 per cent of our patients with Crohn's disease.[65] The tendency toward discontinuity may be manifest only by a few aphthous ulcers at a distance from a segment of severe disease, or by a few aphthous ulcers in the colon of a patient with extensive small bowel disease.

The large ulcers may be indistinguishable from the ulcers in ulcerative colitis, but in Crohn's disease the intervening mucosa tends to be normal and is not granular.

ASYMMETRY

In addition to discontinuity, asymmetric involvement is a major hallmark of Crohn's disease. In the early stages this may be manifest by involvement of one wall of the bowel, while the opposite wall remains completely normal (Fig. 16–38). In more advanced disease with fibrous scarring, it may be manifest as sacculation of the bowel wall as the involved segment contracts and causes the remaining uninvolved portion to balloon out (Fig. 16–39A).[66] This sacculation may resemble the sacculation seen in the small and large bowel in patients with scleroderma (Fig. 16–39B). However, in scleroderma the intervening mucosa has a normal appearance, while in sacculation due to Crohn's disease there is mucosal thickening and nodularity.

Text continued on page 651

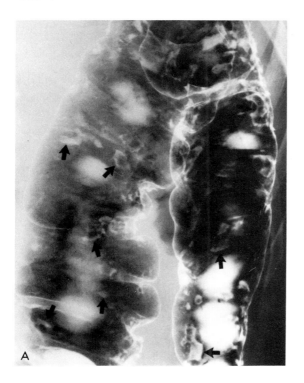

FIGURE 16–36

A. Crohn's disease with large ulcers (*arrows*) with normal intervening mucosa. Note also the discontinuous nature of the ulceration along the inferior aspect of the transverse colon.

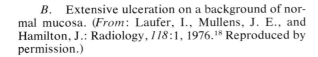

B. Extensive ulceration on a background of normal mucosa. (*From*: Laufer, I., Mullens, J. E., and Hamilton, J.: Radiology, *118*:1, 1976.[18] Reproduced by permission.)

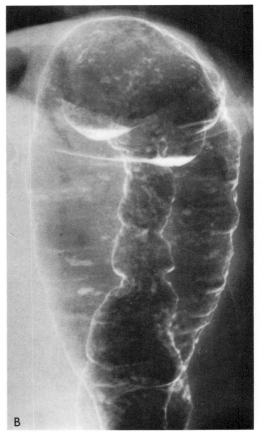

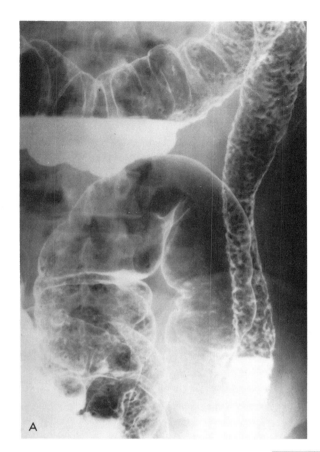

FIGURE 16–37

A. Variability of the lesions in Crohn's disease. There are postinflammatory polyps in the splenic flexure, confluent ulceration in the descending colon, and separated discrete ulcers in the sigmoid.

B. Typical skip lesions *(arrows)* separated by intervening normal mucosa. (*From*: Laufer, I., and Hamilton, J. E.: Am. J. Gastroenterol., 66:259, 1976.[65] Reproduced by permission.)

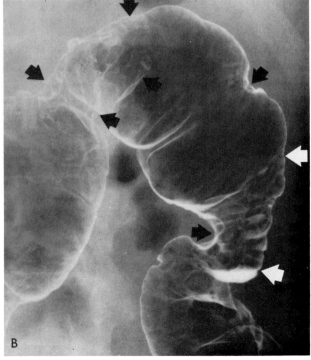

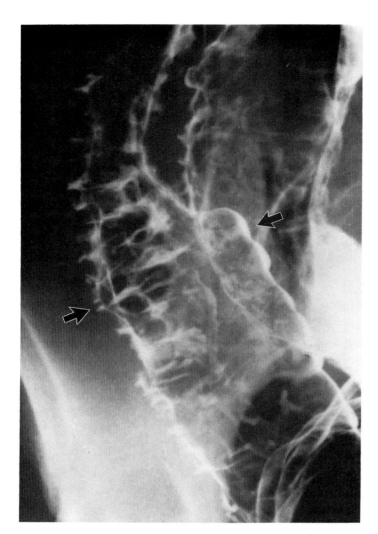

FIGURE 16–38 Deep ulceration in Crohn's colitis with asymmetric lesions. The arrows indicate a segment that is ulcerated on the lateral aspect, but is unaffected on the medial side.

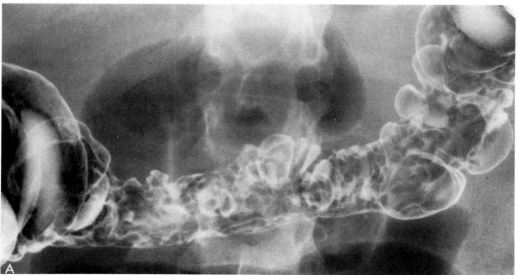

FIGURE 16–39 Sacculation in Crohn's disease.

A. There is extensive sacculation of the transverse colon owing to asymmetric fibrosis. The intervening mucosa has a nodular appearance.

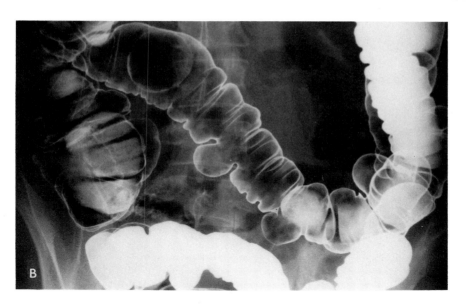

B. Sacculation in scleroderma. This is the result of atrophy and fibrosis of the smooth muscle. However, note that the intervening mucosa is smooth.

OTHER MANIFESTATIONS

There are numerous other manifestations of Crohn's disease, particularly in its more advanced stages. Serpiginous longitudinal and transverse ulcers are a frequent finding and produce the typical cobblestone mucosa (Fig. 16–40). A stricture is a frequent development in Crohn's disease. However, the possibility of carcinoma need rarely be considered in the presence of colonic strictures in Crohn's disease. There is probably a slight increase in the incidence of carcinoma in Crohn's disease, but certainly this is a much lower incidence than in ulcerative colitis.[67, 68]

Fistulae and abscesses are well-recognized features of Crohn's disease. Fistulae may be better demonstrated by the thin barium used in a single contrast enema. Therefore, when a study is done primarily to demonstrate a fistula, we usually prefer the single contrast study.

Welin[69] described a transverse stripe as being characteristic of colonic Crohn's disease (Fig. 16–41). In some cases this was a manifestation of transverse ulceration; in others it was caused by a stripe of contrast material being caught between two transverse folds. Intramural or paracolonic sinus tracts are also a feature of Crohn's disease, particularly in patients with diverticulosis (Fig. 15–13).[70] Meyers and coworkers[71] have shown that these sinus tracts develop because of granulomatous inflammation involving the base of the diverticula. However, these sinus tracts are not specific for Crohn's disease, since they are also found in patients with acute diverticulitis (Fig. 16–42), and rarely in patients with carcinoma.[72]

Some patients with chronic disease due to granulomatous colitis may have total involvement of the colon manifest only as slight narrowing of the colon and mucosal thickening (Fig. 16–43). These cases may be particularly difficult to distinguish from ulcerative colitis, although careful double contrast study may show some patches of uninvolved colon.

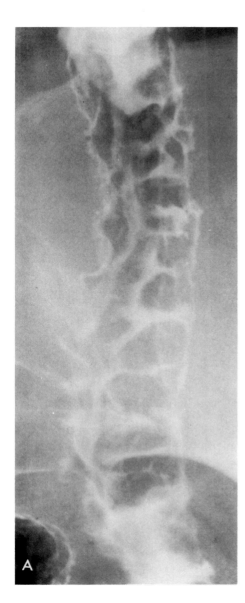

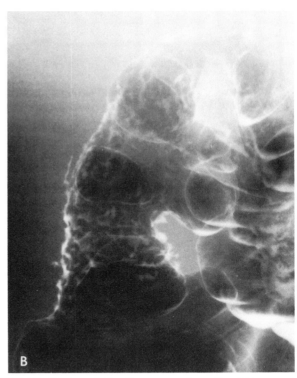

FIGURE 16–40 *A* and *B* Two examples of cobblestoned mucosa in Crohn's colitis.

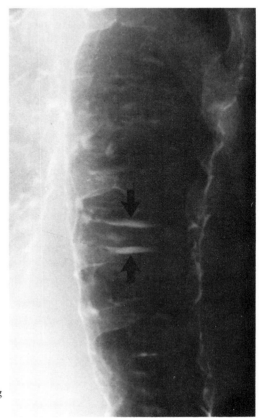

FIGURE 16–41 The transverse stripe, which according to Welin[69] is pathognomonic of Crohn's disease.

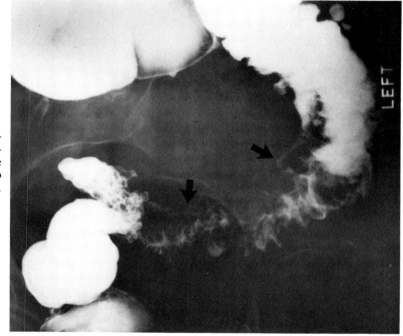

FIGURE 16–42 An intramural sinus tract *(arrows)* in a patient with diverticulitis. The resected specimen showed no evidence of Crohn's disease.

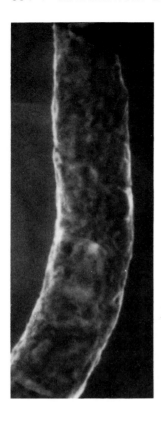

FIGURE 16–43 Diffuse mucosal thickening with loss of haustration in a patient with chronic granulomatous colitis.

RECTAL DISEASE

Endoscopically and histologically, rectal disease is found in approximately 50 per cent of patients with colonic Crohn's disease.[73] However, it may be difficult to demonstrate this condition radiologically because it tends to be patchy and asymmetric. We have been able to demonstrate rectal disease in 37 per cent of patients with granulomatous colitis. This represented 75 per cent of those with endoscopic or histologic evidence of rectal involvement.[65]

Rectal involvement in Crohn's disease differs from rectal involvement in ulcerative colitis. Deep or collar-button ulcers are seen in Crohn's disease (Fig. 17–16*A*); they are rarely seen in the rectum in ulcerative colitis, although they may be seen in the more proximal portions of the colon.[74] In addition, rectal sinus tracts are a characteristic feature of Crohn's disease (Fig. 17–16*B*).

POLYPOID LESIONS

Polypoid lesions in Crohn's disease are similar to those in ulcerative colitis and include pseudopolyps due to extensive ulceration, inflammatory polypoid masses (Fig. 16–44*A*), and postinflammatory polyps, which may be sessile (Fig. 17–16*B*), pedunculated (Fig. 16–44*B*), or filiform (Fig. 16–45). Neoplastic polyps are rare in Crohn's disease.

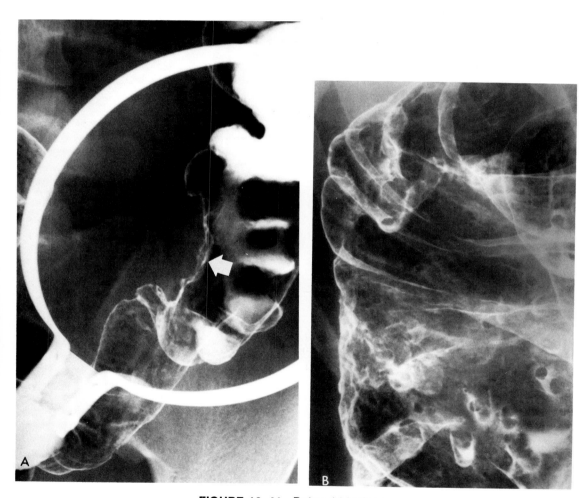

FIGURE 16–44 Polypoid lesions.

A.   Inflammatory, sessile, polypoid mass in a patient with granulomatous colitis.
B.   Multiple sessile and pedunculated postinflammatory polyps in a patient with a previous history of severe granulomatous colitis.

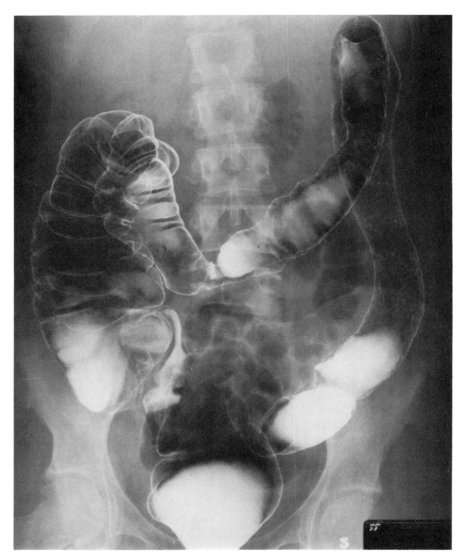

FIGURE 16–45 Filiform polyposis in the descending colon in a patient with granulomatous colitis. There is a skip lesion in the transverse colon.

Reversibility

Reversibility of lesions is a much more frequent occurrence in the colon than in the small bowel. As mentioned previously, the aphthous ulcers of Crohn's disease are unstable lesions which most commonly progress to more extensive disease, but not infrequently regress (Fig. 16–35). Even the more advanced lesions of Crohn's disease may regress either spontaneously or after medical treatment (Fig. 16–46). Hywel-Jones and coworkers[75] reported on 11 patients in whom radiographic regression of the colonic lesions occurred. Brahme and associates[64] found temporary regression in only 7 per cent of 86 patients with Crohn's disease. Definitive permanent healing after medical treatment was not observed in their series.

When the lesions of Crohn's disease regress, the colon may rarely heal completely with no radiologic evidence of scarring (Fig. 16–46). However, this is uncommon, and more frequently there will be some evidence of scarring (Fig. 16–47). The sacculation described previously is also a manifestation of a focal colonic scarring. This scarring is understandable in view of the transmural inflammation that is characteristic of Crohn's disease. It stands in marked contrast to the mucosal involvement in ulcerative colitis, which frequently heals completely without residual scarring even when there has been extensive and deep ulceration.

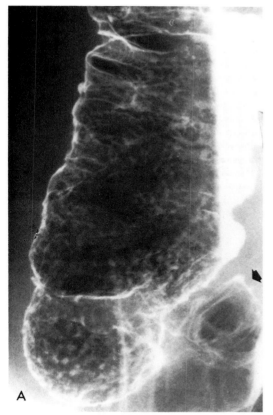

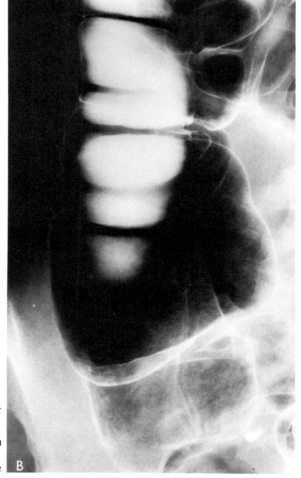

FIGURE 16–46 Reversibility in Crohn's disease.

A. Extensive involvement of the right colon and terminal ileum *(arrow)* by Crohn's disease.

B. Six months later the appearance of the colon has returned to normal.

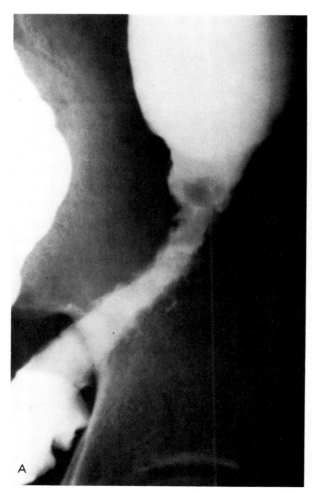 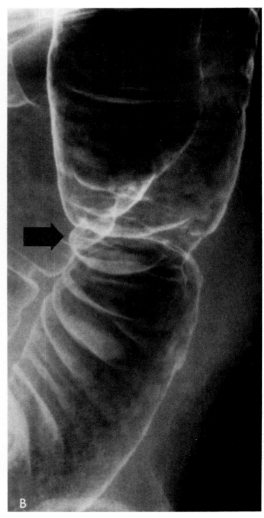

FIGURE 16–47

A. Segmental disease in the distal descending colon, with narrowing and deep ulceration.

B. Two years later the patient was asymptomatic, and there was marked regression with minimal narrowing and shortening along the medial aspect *(arrow)*, resulting in retraction and convergence of the folds.

Terminal Ileum

Double contrast views of the terminal ileum can frequently be obtained during the course of the routine double contrast enema. When the terminal ileum is not visualized during the routine examination, it will often be filled on a postevacuation film. Alternatively, the terminal ileum can be examined by the small bowel enema technique with rectal insufflation of air as the terminal ileum is filled (Figs. 12–3 and 12–4). Double contrast views will show the normal circular folds, which are thin, delicate, and straight (Fig. 12–10). Using these techniques the early lesions of Crohn's disease involving the small bowel can be demonstrated. In some patients, mucosal and submucosal inflammation may be manifest as thickening and slight nodularity of the circular folds (Fig. 16–48A). In others the typical aphthous ulcers of Crohn's disease can be seen (Fig. 16–48B). In more advanced cases the typical features of ulceration, cobblestone mucosa, and stricture are demonstrated (Fig. 16–49).

Patients with previous ileocolic anastomoses are particularly easy to examine with the double contrast technique (Fig 16–50). The absence of the ileocecal valve facilitates the visualization of the neoterminal ileum.

The early lesions must be differentiated from lymphoid hyperplasia in the terminal ileum (Fig. 16–51). This is probably a normal variant which results in tiny nodular filling defects best seen in the terminal ileum. There is no associated ulceration. Inflammation of the terminal ileum is also a feature of Yersinia enterocolitis.[76, 77] This is manifest as swelling of the mucosa of the terminal ileum, which returns to normal within a 2 month period (Fig. 16–52). Inflammatory changes in the terminal ileum can also be caused by a periappendiceal abscess. This is characterized by a soft tissue mass in the ileocecal area, with swelling of ileal mucosa. However, the mucosal abnormalities in the small bowel are relatively minor compared to the soft tissue mass. Patients with Crohn's disease frequently have a mass in the right lower quadrant, but this is invariably accompanied by extensive mucosal ulceration, frequently with fistula formation. (Figs. 11–45 to 11–47).

Disease of the terminal ileum may also have a number of indirect manifestations on the colon. Berridge[66] has described a medial cecal defect that appears to be characteristic of Crohn's disease (Fig. 16–53). This is due not to intrinsic cecal involvement, but rather to small bowel disease, with thickening of the bowel wall and mesentery compressing the medial aspect of the cecum. Similar effects may be produced in other parts of the colon, and appear to be particularly common in the sigmoid, which is frequently affected by disease in the small bowel (Fig. 16–54). Presumably, this is the pathogenesis of ileosigmoid fistulae which are so common in this condition.

Text continued on page 664

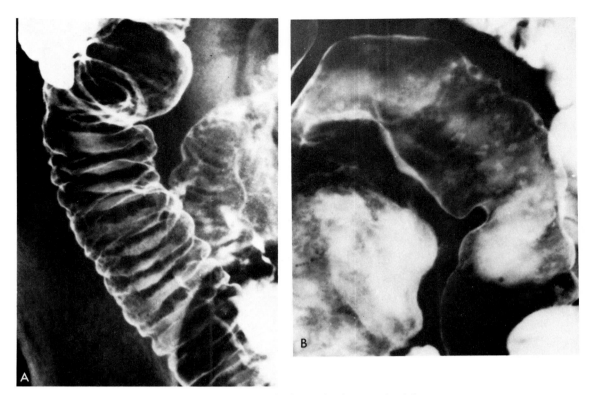

FIGURE 16–48 Early lesions in the terminal ileum.

A. Enlargement and nodularity of the valvulae conniventes due to granulomatous inflammation.
B. Aphthous ulcers in the terminal ileum. (Courtesy of L. Costopoulos, M. D., Edmonton, Alberta. *From:* Laufer, I., and Costopoulos, L.: Am. J. Roentgenol. *130*:307, 1978.[60] Reproduced by permission.)

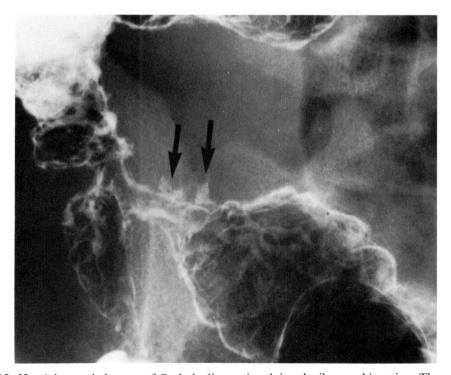

FIGURE 16–49 Advanced changes of Crohn's disease involving the ileocecal junction. There is marked contraction of the cecum, with stricture and ulceration in the terminal ileum *(arrows)*. The terminal ileum is moderately dilated. (*From:* Laufer, I.: CRC Crit. Rev. Diagnost. Imaging, *9*:421, 1977.[36] Reproduced by permission.)

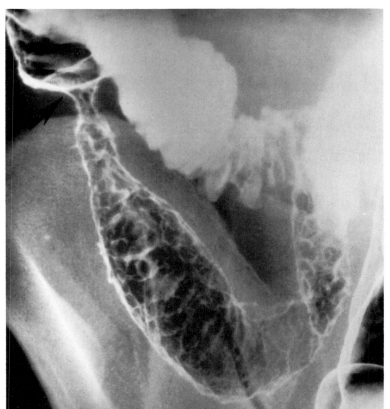

FIGURE 16–50 Recurrent Crohn's disease following ileocolic anastomosis.

Typical cobblestoning is seen involving the neoterminal ileum to the anastomosis with the ascending colon *(arrow)*.

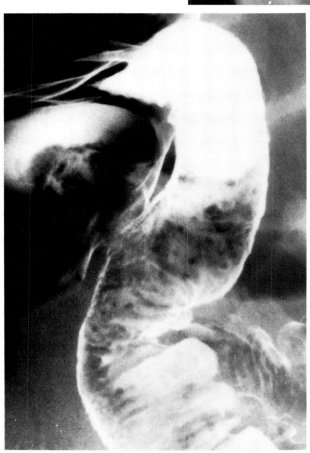

FIGURE 16–51 Lymphoid hyperplasia in the terminal ileum.

There are tiny nodular filling defects owing to lymph follicles. There is no associated enlargement of the folds, ulceration, or spasm.

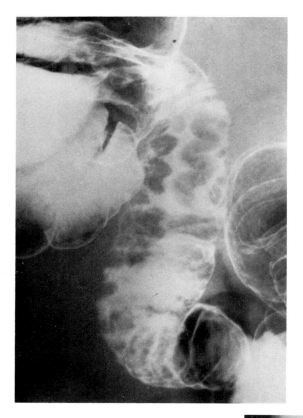

FIGURE 16–52 Yersinia enteritis.

There is marked swelling and tortuosity of the folds in the terminal ileum in this patient with proven Yersinia enteritis. The appearance returned to normal within 2 months.

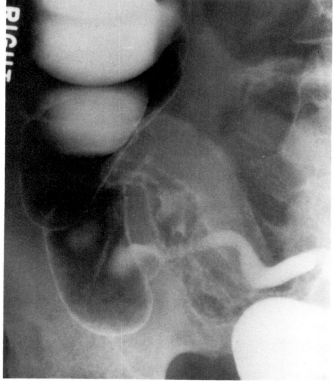

FIGURE 16–53 Medial cecal defect in Crohn's disease.

There is compression on the medial aspect of the cecum by the diseased terminal ileum and its affected mesentery.

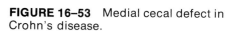

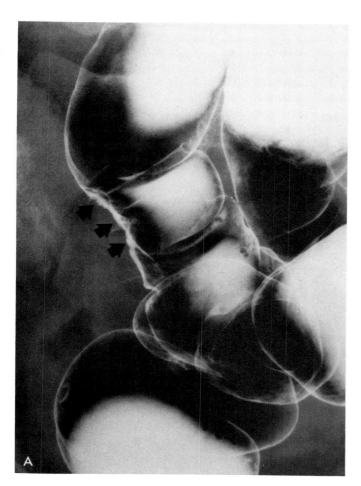

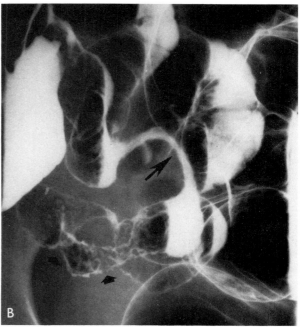

FIGURE 16–54 *A* and *B*   Involvement of the lateral aspect of the sigmoid colon (*A*) by extensive disease in the terminal ileum, (*B*), characterized by stricture *(arrow)* and cobblestoned mucosa *(arrows)*.

Gastroduodenal Crohn's Disease

Involvement of the stomach and duodenum in Crohn's disease has been illustrated in Chapter 6 (Fig. 6–16) and Chapter 9 (Figs. 9–25 to 9–28). Previous series have reported gastroduodenal involvement in 2 to 3 per cent of patients with Crohn's disease.[78, 79] However, these invariably represent advanced disease, characterized clinically by gastric outlet obstruction and radiologically by deformity and narrowing of the antrum and proximal duodenum (Fig. 16–55).[80]

The early lesions of Crohn's disease are the same in the upper gastrointestinal tract as elsewhere. These consist of mild thickening of the folds due to granulomatous inflammation (Fig. 16–56) and aphthous ulceration (Figs. 9–27 and 16–57).[81] The aphthous ulcers are indistinguishable from gastric or duodenal erosions of other etiologies.[82]

These subtle gastroduodenal abnormalities were found in 40 per cent of patients with Crohn's disease involving the small or large bowel. In half of these there was histologic confirmation that the radiologic findings were due to Crohn's disease.[83] Since some of the patients without histologic confirmation undoubtedly had gastroduodenal Crohn's disease, it appears that the stomach and duodenum were involved in 20 to 40 per cent of cases.

Esophageal involvement has been noted in isolated case reports and appears to be rare.[84]

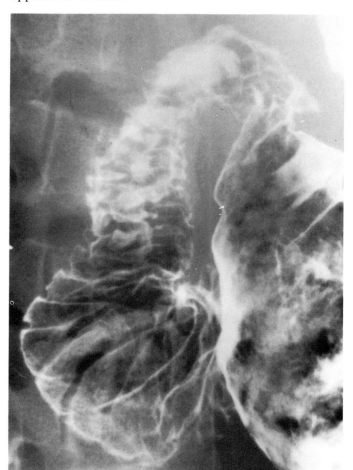

FIGURE 16–55 Advanced gastroduodenal Crohn's disease.

This presents the typical appearance, with deformity and narrowing of the distal antrum extending to involve the duodenal cap and proximal portion of the descending duodenum. Note the normal distensibility of the distal duodenum.

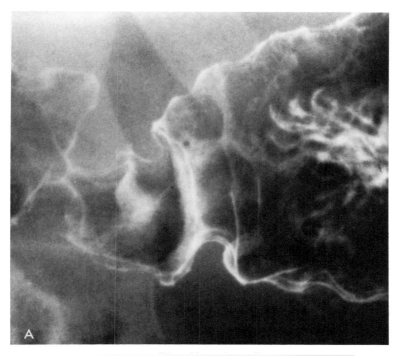

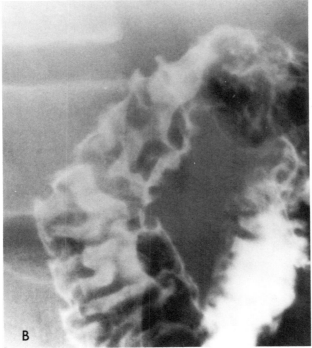

FIGURE 16–56 *A* and *B*   Thickening of the folds as a result of Crohn's disease involving the stomach (*A*) and duodenum (*B*).

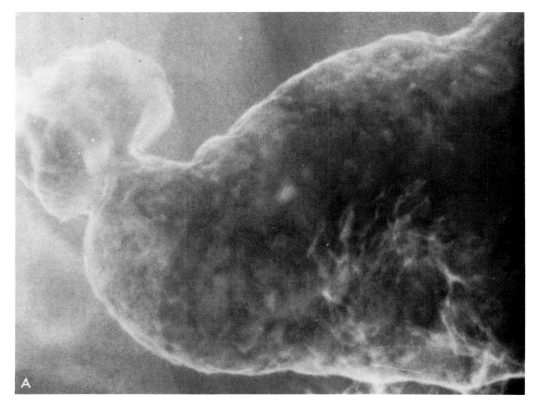

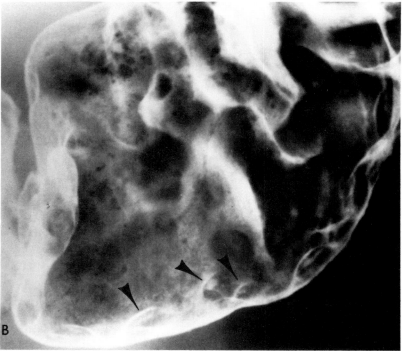

FIGURE 16–57 *A* and *B*   Two examples of erosive gastritis due to Crohn's disease (see Plates 75 and 76) (*From*: Laufer, I., Trueman, T., and de Sa, D.: Br. J. Radiol. *49*:726, 1976.[81] Reproduced by permission.)

DIFFERENTIAL DIAGNOSIS OF COLITIS

Colitis may have no known cause or may be due to a variety of specific agents. The colon is limited in its ability to respond, and therefore it is not surprising that there may be some overlap in the radiologic findings in various types of colitis.

In North America and Europe the vast majority of cases of colitis are idiopathic. On the basis of a number of clinical, radiologic, and pathologic features these may be subdivided into ulcerative and granulomatous colitis. However, before relegating a patient with colitis into the idiopathic group, the various specific types of colitis must be excluded by the appropriate bacteriologic and histologic studies.

Ulcerative versus Granulomatous Colitis

In the majority of cases the differential diagnosis is narrowed down to the distinction between ulcerative and granulomatous colitis. This is of clinical significance since it affects the treatment of the disease, the approach to surgery, and the prognosis with respect to recurrent disease and development of carcinoma.

The specific features of the two diseases have been described in detail. In general terms, ulcerative colitis can be described as a disease with mucosal inflammation starting in the rectum and extending proximally to a variable extent. The involvement is confluent and symmetric, and the terminal ileum is normal. The major complications are toxic megacolon and the markedly increased incidence of carcinoma in patients who have had the disease for 10 years or more. By comparison, granulomatous colitis can be described as a transmural inflammatory process that involves the entire

TABLE 16–1 RADIOLOGIC FEATURES OF ULCERATIVE AND GRANULOMATOUS COLITIS*

Radiologic Finding		Ulcerative Colitis (23 patients)	Granulomatous Colitis (27 Patients)
Granular Mucosa		20	0
	Normal	4†(17%)	19(70%)
Rectum	Diffuse disease	19(18%)	0
	Patchy disease	0	3(11%)
	Punched-out ulcers	0	5(19%)
Continuity	Continuous	22(96%)	5(19%)
	Discontinuous	1(4%)	22(81%)
Ulcers	On granular mucosa	4(17%)	0
	On normal mucosa	0	19(70%)
	Normal	17(74%)	12(44%)
Terminal Ileum	Abnormal	0	15(55%)
	Intermediate	6	0

*From: Laufer, I., and Hamilton, J. D.: Am. J. Gastroenterol., 66:259, 1976. Reproduced by permission.

†In two patients rectal disease has never been documented radiologically or endoscopically. The two other patients had had rectal disease in the past, but were examined during remission when the rectum appeared normal radiologically and endoscopically.

gastrointestinal tract in a discontinuous distribution. The discontinuity is manifest by discrete ulceration with intervening normal mucosa, or by skip lesions consisting of larger diseased segments separated by normal segments. There is a particular tendency to involve the terminal ileum and right colon. The complications are fistula and abscess formation.

Table 16–1 lists the incidence of various radiologic findings in a group of patients with either ulcerative or granulomatous colitis. From this table it is apparent that there are a number of radiologic findings that are relatively specific for each condition. In ulcerative colitis these are a granular mucosa, diffuse rectal disease, continuous inflammation, ulcers on a granular mucosa, and a normal terminal ileum. In granulomatous colitis these are patchy rectal disease with punched-out ulcers, discontinuous disease, ulcers on a normal mucosa, and involvement of the terminal ileum. Utilizing these criteria, it has been possible to distinguish between these two diseases in at least 95 per cent of patients. We have found the differentiation easier to make in the early stages of disease, since the early manifestations are particularly distinctive. In the later stages, when the disease is chronic or when there have been numerous exacerbations and remissions, the distinction may be more difficult. For instance, ulcerative colitis in remission may become discontinuous, while chronic granulomatous colitis may involve the entire colon. Nevertheless, in most cases the distinction can still be made by careful examination of the mucosal surface.

Infections and Infestations

AMEBIASIS

Entamoeba histolytica may exist in the intestine as a commensal in a cyst form which can transmit the disease. However, for reasons not understood it may change into the trophozoite form which is invasive. Four clinical forms of invasive amebiasis are recognized:[85] ulcerative rectocolitis, typhloappendicitis, ameboma, and fulminating colitis.

Ulcerative Rectocolitis. This is the most common form. It presents with diarrhea with blood and mucus, and colicky abdominal pain. On barium enema, ulceration of the sawtooth or collar-button type may be seen. Ulceration is commonest in the rectosigmoid, cecum, and ascending colon. Skip lesions are present, so that Crohn's colitis may be simulated.

Typhloappendicitis. Primary involvement of the appendix may occur, but more commonly the cecum is involved as well. Plain radiographs may show a soft tissue mass in the right iliac fossa, with a dilated cecum containing an air fluid level.

Ameboma. Segmental stricturing lesions can result from necrosis and edema in the intestinal wall, with secondary bacterial infection causing an inflammatory granuloma. The cecum and flexures are commonly involved (Fig. 16–58A).[86] The incidence of ameboma in invasive amebiasis is 1.5 per cent to 8.4 per cent.[85] In about half the cases the lesions are multiple. The distinction from carcinoma may be difficult (Fig. 16–58B). A rapid improvement following antiamebic therapy is diagnostic. Compared with neoplastic strictures, amebomas usually are longer and more concentric, with tapering ends.

Fulminating Colitis. Colonic distension and irregularity of the wall indicate extensive ulceration. Thumbprinting has been reported,[87] and toxic megacolon may develop. Single or multiple perforations can result from the ulceration. The perforations usually form a sealed abscess in the paracolic gutter.

Amebiasis must always be considered in patients from an endemic area who present with colitis. The radiologic features usually simulate Crohn's disease. Confirmation of the disease is obtained by finding trophozoites in fresh swabs of mucus, or by indirect hemagglutination tests. The response to treatment is rapid, and within a few weeks the colon should return to normal. Stenoses secondary to fibrotic strictures are an uncommon complication in properly treated cases, and only a few are reported.[88]

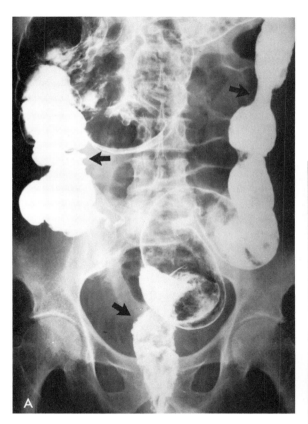

FIGURE 16–58 Amebiasis with amebomas.

A. There are multiple areas of narrowing and ulceration *(arrows)* compatible with amebomas. A repeat barium enema after 3 weeks of chemotherapy was normal, confirming the diagnosis of amebiasis.

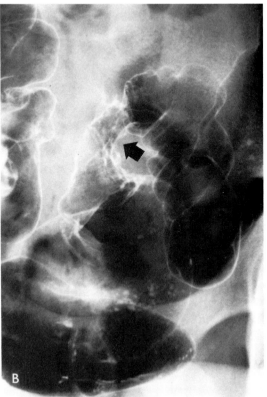

B. Ameboma in the sigmoid *(arrow)*, with narrowing and an irregular surface suggestive of carcinoma.

TUBERCULOSIS

In contrast to Asia, the diagnosis of abdominal tuberculosis in the Western hemisphere is uncommon. It is, however, an important therapeutic distinction and should always be borne in mind when ileocecal lesions are present. Infection most commonly comes from milk infected with *Mycobacterium bovis,* but can also occur by hematogenous spread to submucosal lymphatic structures from a distant primary infection. Although the latter mode of infection is associated with pulmonary disease,[89] less than 50 per cent of patients with intestinal tuberculosis will have radiographic evidence of pulmonary tuberculosis.[90] Any part of the bowel may be involved, but by far the most common site is the ileocecal region (Fig. 16–59 and 60).[91] Ulcerative hypertrophic, and mixed types are described.

Typically, the ulcers are circumferential, but they may also be longitudinal or stellate. The hypertrophic form presents as an abdominal mass, usually affecting the ileocecal region. The bowel is narrowed with a pipe-stem lumen, and deformed by involvement of the adjacent mesentery. The mixed type combines both features. Tuberculosis and Crohn's disease may present with similar changes. Hypertrophic changes with a large mesenteric mass and relatively little change in the bowel is more suggestive of tuberculosis.[92] A thickened, patulous ileocecal valve with deformity of the adjacent ileum is also characteristic.[93] The cecum is often deformed and contracted (Fig. 16–60). Short hourglass strictures in the small bowel or colon are typical of the hypertrophic form (Fig. 16–61).[94] Perforation of the bowel from tuberculosis is a rare complication.[95] Figures 16–61 and 16–62 show additional examples of tuberculous involvement of the right colon[96] and illustrate the difficulty in differentiation from Crohn's disease.

Text continued on page 676

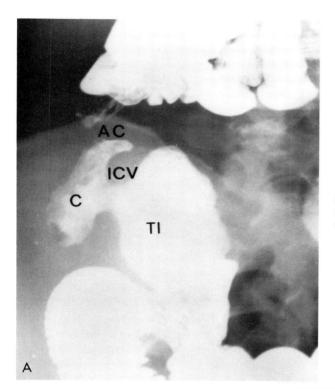

FIGURE 16–59 Ileocecal tuberculosis.

A. Deformity of the cecum, a patulous ileocecal valve, dilated terminal ileum, and stricture in the ascending colon shown on a small bowel follow-through examination.

B. Double contrast enema in the same patient shows the abrupt narrow stricture in the ascending colon (*arrow*).

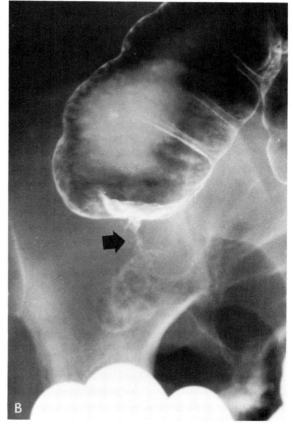

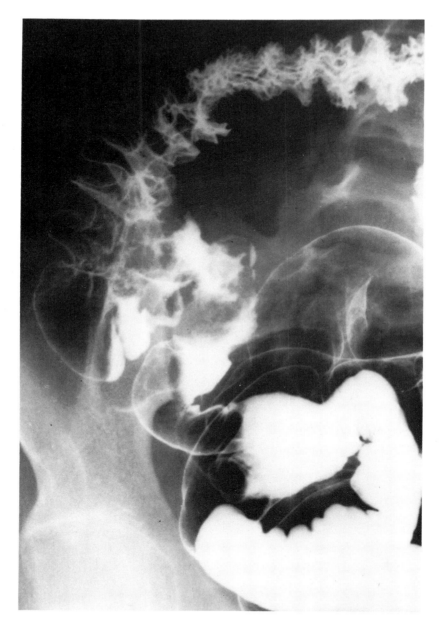

FIGURE 16–60 Ileocecal tuberculosis with florid irregular ulceration and thickening of the bowel wall.

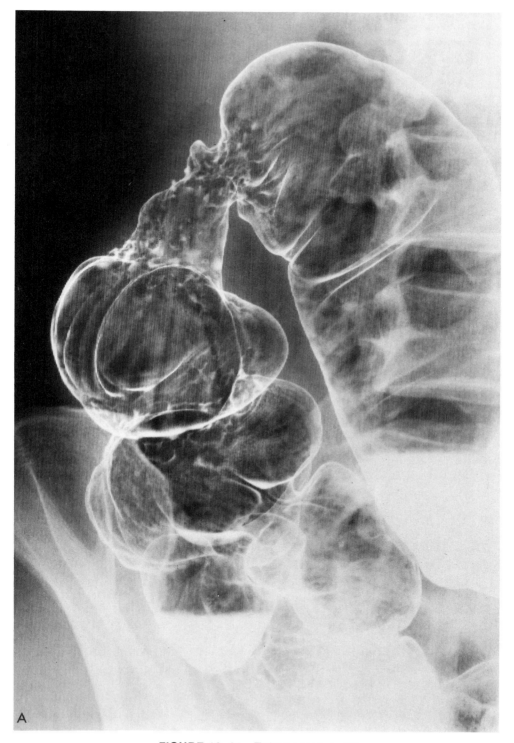

FIGURE 16–61   Tuberculous colitis.
 A.   There are multiple short strictures and superficial ulcers in the ascending colon. At the hepatic flexure there is a longer stricture with deeper ulceration.

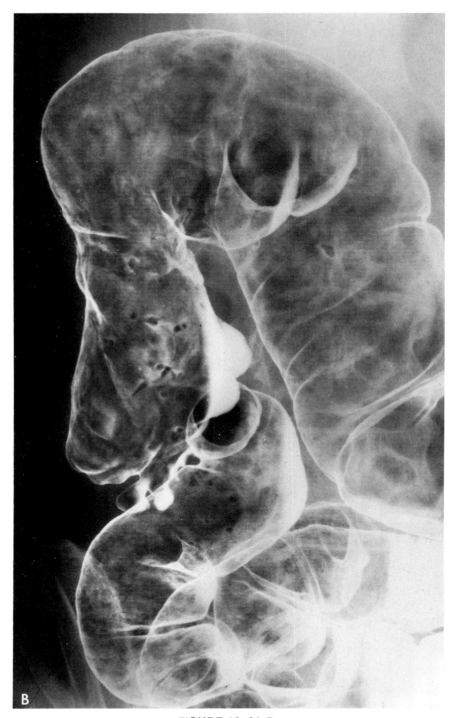

FIGURE 16–61 *B*

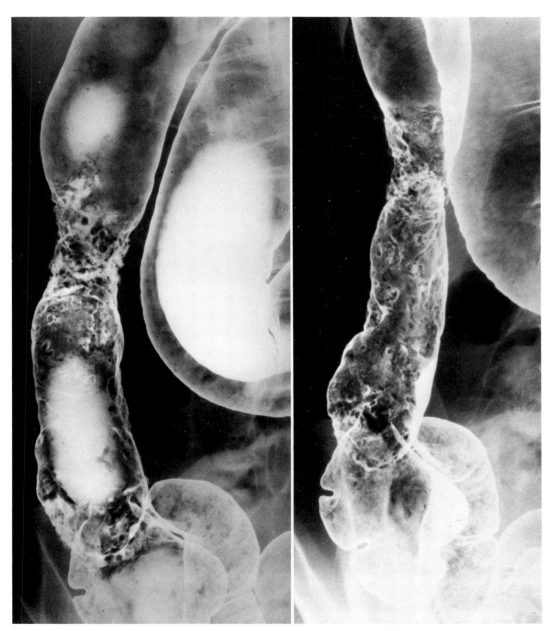

FIGURE 16–62   Tuberculous colitis with ulceration and narrowing affecting the right colon. (Figures 16–61 and 16–62 courtesy of M. Maruyama, M.D., Tokyo. *From*: Maruyama, M.: Stom. Intest. *9*:865, 1974.[96] Reproduced by permission.)

LYMPHOGRANULOMA VENEREUM (LGV)

This is a disease found in the West Indies and caused by a venereally transmitted virus. The primary lesion is a very small papule. This is followed in a few weeks by enlargement of the inguinal lymph nodes. The barium enema appearances are characteristic.[97] There is a long narrow stricture with a smooth surface and loss of haustration. The upper end is cone-shaped as it merges with normal bowel (Fig. 16–63A). The rectum is always involved. The stricture may extend upward into the descending colon, and rarely into the transverse colon. Occasionally a skip lesion is present, with a normal segment of colon between the diseased rectal area and a more proximal stricture. The sigmoid loop often becomes shortened and straightened, so that in severe cases it disappears. Paracolic abscesses and rectovaginal fistulae are common (Fig. 16–63B), and cause problems in management. The pathologic changes in LGV are nonspecific chronic inflammations. Extensive submucosal fibrosis is characteristic. The diagnosis is usually established on the clinical and radiologic findings.

OTHERS

Yersinia Enterocolitis. Yersinia enterocolitis affects mainly the terminal ileum with thickened folds and ulceration (Fig. 16–52). Lymphoid nodular hyperplasia may remain for some months after the infection has been treated

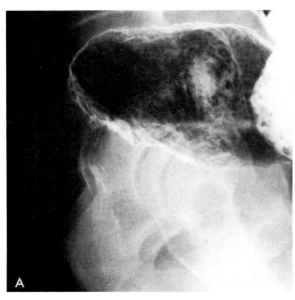
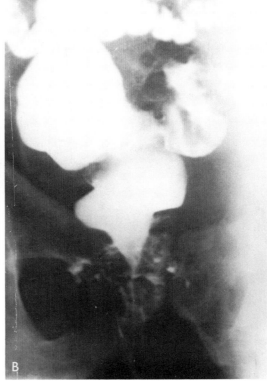

FIGURE 16–63 Lymphogranuloma venereum.

.*A.* A lateral view showing a narrow anorectal stricture.

B. Multiple anorectal fistulae.

(Fig. 16–64). The barium enema has been reported as normal, but ulceration over hypertrophied lymphoid tissue has been found endoscopically, indicating that enterocolitis is also present.[76] Endoscopically, the aphthoid ulceration is considered different from that found in Crohn's disease.[98] Unfortunately, there is no report of double contrast barium enemas in this condition to determine whether the ulceration can be distinguished radiologically.

Schistosomiasis. Colonic involvement in schistosomiasis is most common in the rectum and sigmoid, although the entire colon may be involved.[86] The radiologic abnormalities are characterized by edema, thickened folds, and inflammatory polyps. The granulation tissue may produce diffuse infiltration,[99] which sometimes results in strictures that may resemble carcinoma. Portal hypertension is produced by obliteration of the mesenteric venules.

Strongyloides Stercoralis Colitis. Strongyloides colitis has been reported by Drasin and coworkers.[100] The radiologic features include mucosal edema and ulceration. Strictures may also develop.

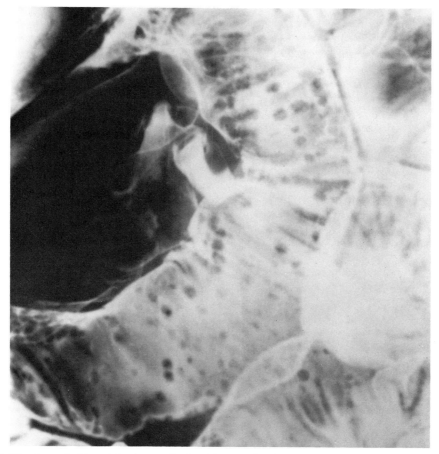

FIGURE 16–64 Lymphoid nodular hyperplasia of the terminal ileum in a patient resolving yersinial enterocolitis.

Ischemia

Three stages may be recognized: transient, gangrene, and stricture.[101] The clinical presentation of ischemia is sudden onset of abdominal pain, with marked tenderness over the affected part of the colon, and melena. Thumbprinting, due to submucosal edema and hemorrhage, is the earliest radiologic change, and is seen on plain films and contrast examinations. The affected segment is narrowed and exhibits marked spasm. There is a short transitional zone where the colon widens to merge into normal bowel. The term funneling has been applied to this appearance (Fig. 16–66A).[102] The splenic flexure region is most commonly affected, possibly owing to the inadequacy of the anastomosis between the mesenteric systems.[103] In 20 per cent of patients, other areas of the colon are affected.[104] Rarely, the rectum may be involved (Fig. 17–17C).[105] Thumbprinting may be seen on the DCE (Fig. 16–65), although in some patients there may be sufficient distension to obliterate the thumbprints (Fig. 16–66 B).[106] Since this may be a disadvantage when trying to diagnose ischemic colitis, in such cases we tend to use the single contrast barium enema. However, thumbprinting is seen in other conditions, such as Crohn's disease, ulcerative colitis,[107] amebiasis,[87] and schistosomiasis.[108] The DCE may be helpful in showing the underlying mucosa to aid in the differential diagnosis.

Thumbprinting in ischemic colitis may disappear after 48 hours, but can persist for several weeks.[102] If a repeat barium enema after a month shows a normal colon, the ischemia is confirmed as transient. However, if the bowel is sufficiently compromised, more extensive infarction will develop (Fig. 16–67). This may go on to perforation or may heal with stricture.

FIGURE 16–65 Ischemic colitis with "thumbprinting" in the proximal descending colon.

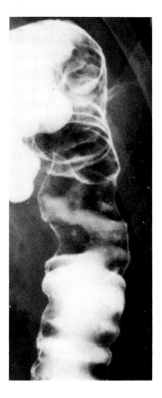

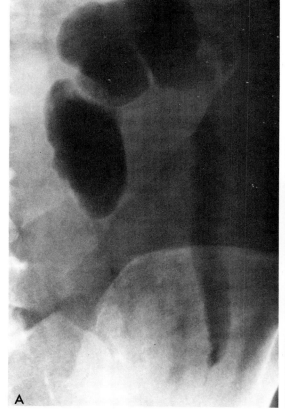

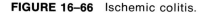

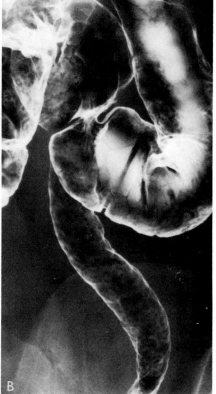

FIGURE 16–66 Ischemic colitis.

A. The plain film shows a narrowed descending colon with small thumbprints.

B. An instant enema performed immediately after the plain film shows a narrowed, spastic descending colon, but the thumbprinting has been obliterated. (*From*: Bartram, C. I.: Gastrointest. Radiol., in press.[106] Reproduced by permission.)

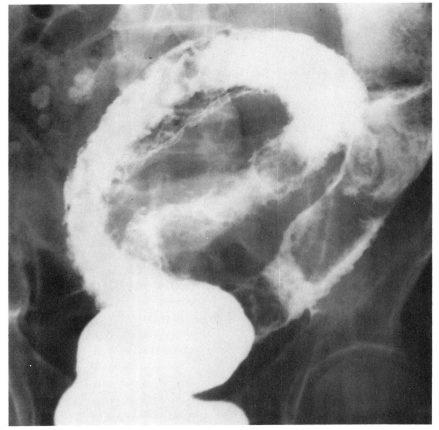

FIGURE 16–67 Severe ischemic colitis in the sigmoid with extensive mucosal ulceration. Toxic mega-colon developed within 48 hours.

Pseudomembranous Enterocolitis

This is related to the use of broad spectrum antibiotics. The sigmoidoscopic findings are typical. The pseudomembrane forms slightly raised yellowish plaques, which may be scattered or confluent. Where the membrane has become separated the underlying mucosa is ulcerated. These changes are reflected in the DCE. The plaques are seen as small elevated lesions (Fig. 16–68).[109] Where the membrane is confluent the surface is shaggy, and the plaques cannot be defined. The appearance of the colon in some areas may simulate ulcerative colitis (Fig. 16–69). The whole colon is involved, and plain film changes of dilated, air-filled small bowel loops with thickened walls indicate small bowel involvement.

FIGURE 16–68 Pseudomembranous colitis due to carbenicillin. There are multiple plaque-like filling defects, representing the pseudomembrane, in the descending colon.

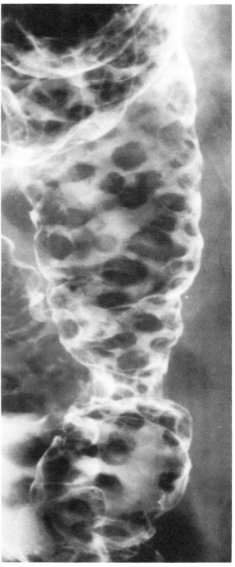

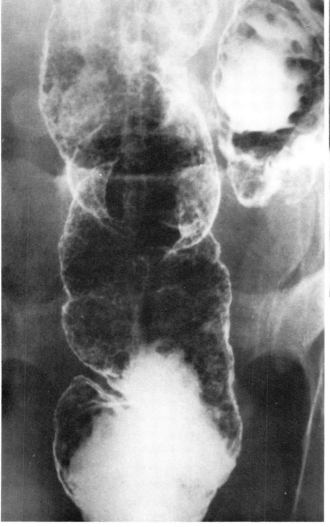

FIGURE 16–69 Psuedomembranous colitis with plaques in the proximal sigmoid colon. The distal rectosigmoid has a somewhat granular appearance, suggestive of ulcerative colitis. (Courtesy of Dr. L. Berger, Royal Free Hospital, London, England.)

Miscellaneous Forms of Colitis

BEHÇET'S DISEASE

The syndrome of recurrent oral and genital ulceration with ocular manifestations was first described by Behçet in 1937. It is now recognized as a multisystem disease in which colitis can occur.[110] Radiologically, involvement of the colon is characterized by deep ulcers which are discrete, multiple, and set in a normal mucosa with intact haustration. The ulcers are more common in the ileocecal region. Perhaps because of their depth and lack of surrounding inflammatory or fibrotic change, the ulcers tend to perforate more easily than the ulcers of Crohn's disease.[111]

Ulceration is common to many forms of colitis. Although the possibility of coincidental inflammatory bowel disease with Behçet's syndrome has been discussed,[112] it has been concluded that primary Behçet's disease of the colon is a genuine entity. Radiologically, the ulceration of Behçet's disease is distinguished from ulcerative colitis by the ulcers being deep and surrounded by a normal mucosa, and from Crohn's disease by the absence of fibrosis and stricture formation.

COLITIS CYSTICA PROFUNDA

This is a rare benign condition in which submucosal mucus-filled cysts are found in the rectum and sigmoid. These may result in the passage of blood or mucus per rectum. The cysts form nodular masses usually less than 2 cm in size. These could be confused with carcinoma, adenomatous polyps, inflammatory polyps, or pneumatosis cystoides intestinalis.[113] A more diffuse form of the condition may be associated with ulcerative colitis or dysentery.[114] Precise diagnosis will depend on endoscopic biopsy and histologic findings.

COLONIC URTICARIA

This is a rare condition due to a severe allergic reaction resulting in focal submucosal edema in the colon. It produces a characteristic mosaic pattern[115] caused by barium lying between irregular elevated plaques of mucosa (Fig. 16–70). The crazy-paving appearance of these channels is unlikely to cause confusion with ulceration or inflammatory polyposis, provided that the examiner is familiar with the condition.

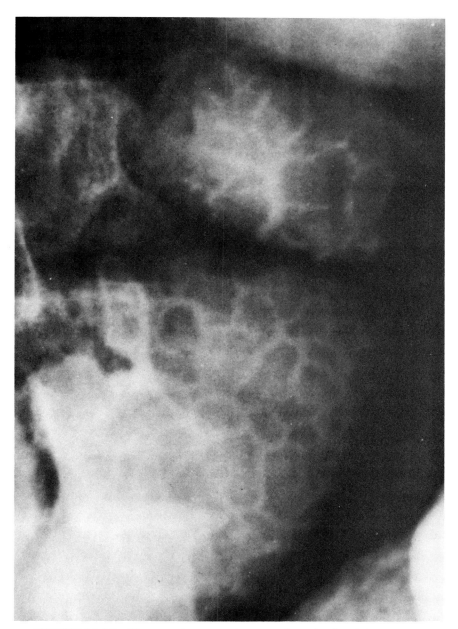

FIGURE 16–70   The mosaic mucosal pattern in urticaria of the colon.[115]

SUMMARY

Table 16–2 lists the major radiologic features of colitis and the conditions in which they are commonly found as well as those conditions in which they are occasionally found.

TABLE 16–2 SUMMARY OF THE PREDOMINANT RADIOLOGIC FEATURES IN COLITIS

Radiologic Feature	Commonly Found In	May Be Found In
Granular Mucosa	Ulcerative colitis	
Ulceration		
Discrete	Crohn's disease	Amebiasis
	Yersinia enterocolitis	Ischemia
	Behçet's disease	Tuberculosis
Confluent shallow	Ulcerative colitis	Crohn's disease
		Amebiasis
Confluent deep	Crohn's disease	Ischemia
		Amebiasis
		Tuberculosis
		Strongyloides colitis
Stricture Formation		
Symmetric	Ulcerative colitis	Tuberculosis
	Lymphogranuloma venereum	
Asymmetric	Crohn's disease	
	Ischemia	
	Tuberculosis	
Fistula	Crohn's disease	Tuberculosis
	Lymphogranuloma venereum	
Inflammatory Polyps	Ulcerative colitis	Ischemia (rare)
	Crohn's disease	
	Schistosomiasis	
	(Colitis cystica profunda)	
Small Bowel Involvement	Yersinia enterocolitis	Ulcerative colitis (backwash)
	Tuberculosis	Behçet's disease
	Pseudomembranous enterocolitis	Ischemia
	Crohn's disease	
Skip Lesions	Crohn's disease	Lymphogranuloma venereum
	Tuberculosis	
	Amebiasis	
Toxic Megacolon	Ulcerative colitis	Crohn's disease
		Ischemia
		Amebiasis

ACKNOWLEDGMENT

We are grateful to Dr. Basil C. Morson of the Department of Pathology. St. Mark's Hospital, London, for supplying the specimen photographs for Chapters 14, 15, and 16.

REFERENCES

1. Young, A. C.: The instant barium enema in procto-colitis. Proc. R. Soc. Med., 56:491, 1963.
2. Roth, J. L. A., Valdes-Dapena, A., Stein, G. N., et al.: Toxic megacolon in ulcerative colitis. Gastroenterology, 37:239, 1959.
3. Welin, S., and Welin, G.: The Double Contrast Examination of the Colon. Experiences with the Welin Modification. Stuttgart, Georg Thieme Verlag, 1976.
4. Fraser, G. M., and Findlay, J. M.: The double contrast enema in ulcerative colitis and Crohn's disease. Clin. Radiol., 27:103, 1976.
5. Apsimon, H. T.: The single phase double contrast enema, a technique for the average department. Clin. Radiol., 21:188, 1970.
6. Schimmel, D. H., Havelin, L. G., Cohen, S., et al.: Bacteraemia and the barium enema. Am. J. Roentgenol., 128:207, 1977.
7. Le Frock, T., Ellis, C. A., Klainer, A. B., et al.: Transient bacteraemia associated with barium enema. Arch. Intern. Med., 135:835, 1975.
8. Morson, B. C., and Dawson, I. M. P.: Gastrointestinal Pathology. Oxford, Blackwell Scientific Publications, 1972, pp. 458–470.
9. Ritchie, J. K.: Results of surgery for inflammatory bowel disease, a further survey of one hospital region. Br. Med. J., 1:264, 1974.
10. Halls, J., and Young, A. C.: Plain abdominal films in colonic disease. Proc. R. Soc. Med., 58:859, 1964.
11. Bartram, C. I.: the plain abdominal x-ray in acute colitis. Proc. R. Soc. Med., 69:617, 1976.
12. Bartram, C. I.: Radiology in the current assessment of ulcerative colitis. Gastrointest. Radiol., 1:383, 1977.
13. Hywel-Jones, J., and Chapman, M.: Definition of megacolon in colitis. Gut, 10:562, 1969.
14. Brooke, B. N., and Sampson, P. A.: An indication for surgery in acute ulcerative colitis. Lancet, 2:1272, 1964.
15. de Dombal, F. T., Watts, J. M. K., Watkinson, G., et al.: Intraperitoneal perforation of the colon in ulcerative colitis. Proc. R. Soc. Med., 58:713, 1965.
16. Welin, S., and Brahme, F.: The double contrast method in ulcerative colitis. Acta Radiol., 55:257, 1961.
17. Bartram, C. I., and Walmesley, K.: A pathological and radiological correlation of the mucosal changes in ulcerative colitis. Clin. Radiol., 29:323, 1978.
18. Laufer, I., Mullens, J. E., and Hamilton, J.: Correlation of endoscopy and double contrast radiography in the early stages of ulcerative and granulomatous colitis. Radiology, 118:1, 1976.
19. Dassell, P. M.: Innocuous filling of the intestinal glands of the colon during barium enema (spiculation) simulating organic disease. Radiology, 78:799, 1962.
20. Marshak, R. H., and Lindner, A. E.: Ulcerative and granulomatous colitis. In: Margulis, A. R., and Burhenne, H. J. (eds.): Alimentary Tract Roentgenology, Vol. 2. St. Louis, C. V. Mosby, 1973, pp. 963–1013.
21. Beranbaum, S. L.: Roentgenologic diagnosis of idiopathic nonspecific ulcerative colitis with special reference to early manifestations. Dis. Colon Rectum, 7:135, 1964.
22. Golligher, J. C.: Primary excisional surgery in the treatment of ulcerative colitis. Ann. R. Coll. Surg. (Engl.), 15:316, 1954.
23. Counsell, B.: Lesions of the ileum associated with ulcerative colitis. Br. J. Surg., 185:276, 1956.
24. Sellink, J. L.: Radiological Atlas of Common Disease of the Small Bowel. Leiden, Stenfert Kroese, 1976.
25. de Dombal, F. T., Watts, J., Watkins, G., et al.: Local complications of ulcerative colitis, strictures, pseudopolyps, and carcinoma of colon and rectum. Br. Med. J., 1:1442, 1966.
26. Zegel, H., and Laufer, I.: Filiform polyposis. Radiology, 127:615, 1978.
27. Jalan, K. N., Walker, R. J., Sircus, W., et al.: Pseudopolyposis in ulcerative colitis. Lancet, 11:555, 1969.
28. Goldberger, L. E., Neely, H. R., and Stammer, J. L.: Large mucosal bridges. An unusual roentgenographic manifestation of ulcerative colitis. Gastrointest. Radiol., 3:81, 1978.
29. Dawson, I. M. P., and Pryse-Davies, J.: The development of carcinoma of the large intestine in ulcerative colitis. Br. J. Surg., 47:113, 1959.
30. Martinez, C. R., Siegelman, S. S., Saba, G. P., et al.: Localized tumor-like lesions in ulcerative colitis and Crohn's disease of the colon. Johns Hopkins Med. J., 140:249, 1977.
31. Edling, N. P. G., and Eklof, O.: The retrorectal soft tissue space in ulcerative colitis. A roentgen diagnostic study. Radiology, 80:949, 1963.

32. Farthing, M. J. G., and Lennard-Jones, J. E.: The recto-sacral distance and rectal size in ulcerative colitis. Submitted for publication.
33. Simpkins, K. C., and Stevenson, G. W.: The modified Malmö double contrast barium enema in colitis: An assessment of its accuracy in reflecting sigmoidoscopic findings. Br. J. Radiol., 45:486, 1972.
34. Lennard-Jones, J. F., Misiewicz, J. J., Parish, J. A., et al.: Prospective study of outpatients with extensive colitis. Lancet, 1:1065, 1974.
35. Williams, C. B., and Teague, R.: Colonoscopy. Gut, 14:990, 1973.
36. Laufer, I.: Air contrast studies of the colon in inflammatory bowel disease. CRC Crit. Rev. Diagnost. Imaging, 9:421, 1977.
37. Hunt, R. H., Teague, R. H., Swartbrick, E. T., et al.: Colonoscopy in the management of colonic strictures. Br. Med. J., 3:360, 1975.
38. Simpkins, K. C., and Young, A. C.: The differential diagnosis of large bowel strictures. Clin. Radiol., 22:449, 1971.
39. Edwards, F. C., and Truelove, S. C.: The course and prognosis of ulcerative colitis. IV. Carcinoma of the colon. Gut, 5:15, 1964.
40. Edling, N. P. G., Lagercrantz, R., and Rosenquist, H.: Roentgenologic findings in ulcerative colitis with malignant degeneration. Acta Radiol., 52:123, 1959.
41. Fennessey, J. J., Sparberg, M. B., and Kirsner, J. B.: Radiological findings in carcinoma of the colon complicating chronic ulcerative colitis. Gut, 9:388, 1968.
42. Hodgson, J. R., and Sauer, W. G.: The roentgenologic features of carcinoma in chronic ulcerative colitis. Am. J. Roentgenol., 86:91, 1961.
43. Lennard-Jones, J. E., Morson, B. C., Ritchie, J. K., et al.: Cancer in colitis; assessment of the individual risk by clinical and histological criteria. Gastroenterology, 73:1280, 1977.
44. MacDougall, I. P. M.: Clinical identification of those cases of ulcerative colitis most likely to develop cancer of the bowel. Dis. Colon Rectum, 7:447, 1964.
45. Hinton, J. M.: Risk of malignant change in ulcerative colitis. Gut, 7:427, 1966.
46. Devroede, G., and Taylor, W. F.: On calculating cancer risk and survival of ulcerative colitis patients with the life table method. Gastroenterology, 71:505, 1976.
47. Morson, B. C., and Pang, L. S. C.: Rectal biopsy as an aid to cancer control in ulcerative colitis. Gut, 8:423, 1967.
48. Frank, P. H., Riddell, R. H., Feczko, P. J., et al.: Radiological detection of colonic dysplasia (precarcinoma) in chronic ulcerative colitis. Gastrointest. Radiol., 3:209, 1978.
49. Teague, R. H., and Read, A. E.: Polyposis in ulcerative colitis. Gut, 16:792, 1975.
50. Lennard-Jones, J. E., Langman, M. J. S., and Avery Jones, F.: Fecal stasis in proctocolitis. Gut, 3:301, 1962.
51. Powell-Tuck, J., Ritchie, J. K., and Lennard-Jones, J. E.: The prognosis of idiopathic proctitis and distal colitis. Gut, 17:392, 1976.
52. Marshak, R. H.: Granulomatous disease of the intestinal tract (Crohn's disease). Radiology, 114:3, 1975.
53. Marshak, R. H., and Lindner, A. E.: Granulomatous colitis and ileocolitis with emphasis on the radiologic features. In Glass, G. B. J. (ed.): Progress in Gastroenterology, 1:357, 1968.
54. Margulis, A. R., Goldberg, H. I., Lawson, T. L., et al.: The overlapping spectrum of ulcerative and granulomatous colitis: A roentgenographic pathologic study. Am. J. Roentgenol., 113:325, 1971.
55. Nelson, J. A., Margulis, A. R., Goldberg, H. I., et al.: Ulcerative and granulomatous colitis: Variation in observer interpretation and in roentgenographic appearance as related to time. Am. J. Roentgenol., 119:369, 1973.
56. Kirsner, J. B.: Problems in the differential diagnosis of ulcerative colitis and Crohn's disease of the colon. Gastroenterology, 68:187, 1975.
57. Lockhart-Mummery, H. E., and Morson, B. C.: Crohn's disease of the large intestine. Gut, 5:493, 1964.
58. Lockhart-Mummery, H. E., and Morson, B. C.: Crohn's disease (regional enteritis) of the large intestine and its distinction from ulcerative colitis. Gut, 1:87, 1960.
59. Laufer, I., and deSa, D.: The lymphoid follicular pattern: A normal feature of the pediatric colon. Am. J. Roentgenol., 130:51, 1978.
60. Laufer, I., and Costopoulos, L.: Early lesions of Crohn's disease. Am. J. Roentgenol., 130:307, 1978.
61. Simpkins, K. C.: Aphthoid ulcers in Crohn's colitis. Clin. Radiol., 28:601, 1978.
62. Brahme, F.: Granulomatous colitis: Roentgenologic appearance and course of the lesion. Am. J. Roentgenol., 97:35, 1967.
63. Brahme, F.: Radiology. In: Engel, A., and Larsson, T. (eds.): Regional Enteritis (Crohn's Disease). Stockholm, Nordiska Bokhandelns, Forlag., 1971, pp. 81–101.
64. Brahme, F., and Fork, F. T.: Dynamic aspects of colonic Crohn's disease. Radiologe, 15:463, 1975.

65. Laufer, I., and Hamilton, J. D.: The radiologic differentiation between ulcerative and granulomatous colitis by double contrast radiology. Am. J. Gastroenterol., 66:259, 1976.
66. Berridge, F. R.: Two unusual radiological signs of Crohn's disease of the colon. Clin. Radiol., 22:444, 1971.
67. Darke, S. G., Parks, A. G., Grogono, J. L., et al.: Adenocarcinoma and Crohn's disease. Br. J. Surg., 60:169, 1973.
68. Greenstein, A. J., and Janowitz, H. D.: Cancer in Crohn's disease. Am. J. Gastroenterol., 64:122, 1976.
69. Welin, S., and Welin, G.: A pathognomonic roentgenologic sign of regional ileitis (Crohn's disease). Dis. Colon Rectum, 16:473, 1973.
70. Marshak, R. H., Janowitz, H. D., and Present, D. H.: Granulomatous colitis in association with diverticula. N. Engl. J. Med., 283:1080, 1970.
71. Meyers, M. A., Alonso, D. R., Morson, B. C., et al.: Pathogenesis of diverticulitis complicating granulomatous colitis. Gastroenterology, 74:24, 1978.
72. Ferrucci, J. T., Jr., Ragsdale, B. D., Barrett, P. J., et al.: Double tracking in the sigmoid colon. Radiology, 120:307, 1976.
73. Korelitz, B. I., and Sommers, S. C.: Differential diagnosis of ulcerative and granulomatous colitis by sigmoidoscopy, rectal biopsy and cell counts of rectal mucosa. Am. J. Gastroenterol., 61:460, 1974.
74. Deveroede, G. J.: The differential diagnosis of colitis. Can. J. Surg., 17:369, 1974.
75. Hywel-Jones, J., Lennard-Jones, J. E., and Young, A. C.: Reversibility of radiological appearances during clinical improvement in colonic Crohn's disease. Gut, 10:738, 1969.
76. Vantrappen, G., Ayg, H. O., Ponette, E., et al.: Yersinial enteritis and enterocolitis; gastroenterological aspects. Gastroenterology, 72:220, 1977.
77. Ekberg, O., Sjostrom, B., and Brahme, F. J.: Radiological findings in Yersinia ileitis. Radiology, 123:15, 1977.
78. Kusakeioglu, O., and Norton, R. A.: Granulomatous duodenitis, clubbed digits and psoriasis; report of a case. Lahey Clin. Found. Bull., 16:191, 1967.
79. Wilder, W. M., and Davis, W. D.: Duodenal enteritis. South. Med. J., 59:884, 1966.
80. Legge, D. A., Carlson, H. C., and Judd, E. S.: Roentgenologic features of regional enteritis of the upper gastrointestinal tract. Am. J. Roentgenol., 110:355, 1970.
81. Laufer, I., Trueman, T., and deSa, D.: Multiple superficial gastric erosions due to Crohn's disease of the stomach. Radiologic and endoscopic diagnosis. Br. J. Radiol., 49:726, 1976.
82. Laufer, I., Hamilton, J., and Mullens, J. E.: Demonstration of superficial gastric erosions by double contrast radiology. Gastroenterology, 68:387, 1975.
83. Stevenson, G. W., Hyland, J., Laufer, I., et al.: Gastroduodenal lesions in Crohn's disease. In press.
84. Cynn, W. S., Chon, H. K., Gureghian, P. A., et al.: Crohn's disease of the esophagus. Am. J. Roentgenol., 125:359, 1975.
85. Cardosa, J. M., Kimura, K., Stoopen, M., et al.: Radiology of invasive amebiasis of the colon. Am. J. Roentgenol., 128:935, 1977.
86. Middlemiss, H.: Tropical Radiology. London, William Heineman, 1961, pp. 128–132.
87. Hardy, R., and Scullin, D.: Thumbprinting in a case of amebiasis. Radiology, 98:147, 1971.
88. Kolawole, T. M., and Lewis, E. A.: Radiologic observations on intestinal amebiasis. Am. J. Roentgenol., 122:257, 1974.
89. Mitchell, R. S.: The prognosis of bilateral symmetrical diffuse nodular tuberculosis and its possible relation to intestinal tuberculosis. Ann. Intern. Med., 74:559, 1956.
90. Werbeloff, L., Novis, B. H., Banks, S., et al.: The radiology of tuberculosis of the gastrointestinal tract. Br. J. Radiol., 46:329, 1973.
91. Abscombe, A. R., Keddie, N. C., and Schofield, P. F.: Cecal tuberculosis. Gut, 8:337, 1967.
92. Brombart, M., and Massions, J.: Radiologic differences between ileocecal tuberculosis and Crohn's disease. Am. J. Dig. Dis., 6:589, 1961.
93. Boles, R. S., and Gershon-Cohen, J.: Intestinal tuberculosis; pathologic and roentgenologic observations. JAMA, 103:1841, 1934.
94. Carrera, F., Young, S., and Lewick, A. M.: Intestinal tuberculosis. Gastrointest. Radiol., 1:147, 1976.
95. Porter, J. M., Snowe, R. J., and Silver, D.: Tuberculous enteritis with perforation and abscess formation in childhood. Surgery, 71:254, 1972.
96. Maruyama, M.: Diagnosis of ileocecal tuberculosis — A clinico-pathological study on 12 operated cases (in Japanese). Stom. Intest., 9:865, 1974.
97. Annamunthodo, H., and Marryatt, J.: Barium studies in intestinal lymphogranuloma venereum. Br. J. Radiol., 34:53, 1961.

98. Williams, C. B., and Waye, J. D.: Endoscopy in inflammatory bowel disease. Clin. Gastroenterol., 7:701, 1978.

99. Medina, J. T., Seaman, W. B., Gazman-Acosta, C., et al.: The roentgen appearance of *Schistosomiasis mansoni*. Radiology, 85:628, 1978.

100. Drasin, G. F., Moss, J. P., and Cheng, S. H.: *Strongyloides stercoralis* colitis. Findings in four cases. Radiology, 126:619, 1978.

101. Marston, A., Pheils, M. Y., Lea-Thomas, M., et al.: Ischemic colitis. Gut, 7:1, 1966.

102. Lea-Thomas, M.: Further observations on ischemic colitis. Proc. R. Soc. Med., 61:341, 1968.

103. Griffiths, J. D.: Surgical anatomy of the distal colon. Ann. R. Coll. Surg. Engl., 19:241, 1956.

104. Tomchik, F. S., Wittenberg, J., and Ottinger, L. W.: The roentgenographic spectrum of bowel infarction. Radiology, 96:249, 1970.

105. Kilpatrick, Z. M.: Ischemic proctitis. JAMA, 205:78, 1968.

106. Bartram, C. I.: Loss of thumbprinting with double contrast barium enemas in acute ischemic colitis. Gastrointest. Radiol., in press.

107. Marshak, R. H., and Lindner, A. E.: Vascular disease. *In:* Margulis, A. R., and Burhenne, H. J. (eds.): Alimentary Tract Roentgenology. Vol. 2. St. Louis, C. V. Mosby, 1973, pp. 1608–1635.

108. Boley, S. J., Schwartz, S., Lash, J., et al.: Reversible vascular occlusion of the colon. Surg. Gynecol. Obstet., 116:53, 1963.

109. Stanley, R. J., Melson, G. L., and Tedesco, F. J.: The spectrum of radiographic findings in antibiotic-related pseudomembranous colitis. Radiology, 111:519, 1974.

110. Boe, J., Dalgaard, J. B., and Scott, D.: Mucocutaneous-ocular syndrome with intestinal involvement. A clinical and pathological study of four fatal cases. Am. J. Med., 25:857, 1958.

111. Baba, S., Maruto, M., Ando, K., et al.: Intestinal Behçet's disease. Dis. Colon Rectum, 19:428, 1976.

112. Smith, G. E., Kime, L. R., and Pitcher, J. L.: The colitis of Behçet's disease; a separate entity? Colonoscopic findings and literature review. Am. J. Dig. Dis., 18:987, 1973.

113. Epstein, S. E., Ascari, W. O., Ablow, R. C., et al.: Colitis cystica profunda. Am. J. Clin. Pathol., 45:186, 1966.

114. Wayte, D. M., and Helwig, E. B.: Colitis cystica profunda. Am. J. Clin. Pathol., 48:159, 1967.

115. Berk, R. N., and Millman, S. J.: Urticaria of the colon. Radiology, 99:539, 1971.

116. Gardiner, G. A.:"Backwash ileitis" with pseudo-polyposis. Am. J. Roentgenol., 129:506, 1977.

117. Hammerman, A. M., Shatz, B. A., and Sussman, N.: Radiographic characteristics of colonic "mucosal bridges": Sequelae of inflammatory bowel disease. Radiology, 127:611, 1978.

17

RADIOLOGY OF THE RECTUM

INTRODUCTION

Several studies have shown that the conventional barium enema is ineffective in demonstrating neoplastic or inflammatory conditions in the rectum.[1] Because of this many radiologists feel that the rectum is not the province of radiology and that this area should be left to the endoscopist. This is unfortunate, since a large proportion of disease in the large bowel either is limited to or involves the rectum. In addition, it is now becoming appreciated that endoscopic examination of this area may be difficult and that significant abnormalities may remain undetected.[2-4]

Rectal lesions may be missed at endoscopy for several reasons. Proctosigmoidoscopy is frequently performed by examiners who are not expert in the procedure or in the interpretation of findings.[5] Even an experienced examiner may miss abnormalities that lie hidden behind the valves of Houston or at any area of sharp angulation of the colon (Fig. 17–4).
In some cases, anatomic configuration or patient discomfort may preclude complete insertion of the sigmoidoscope, and lesions may be missed for this reason (Fig. 17–7). In others, anatomic distortion due to disease may rule out endoscopic visualization of rectal pathology (Fig. 17–7).

For all of these reasons, radiologic examination of the colon should include a careful assessment of the rectum, even in the patients who have been or who are about to be examined by endoscopy. In addition, asymptomatic lesions in the rectum will be found even in patients for whom proctosigmoidoscopy was not being planned (Fig. 17–10).

ANATOMY

The anatomy of the rectum has been well described.[6, 7] There are usually three prominent folds, which are called the valves of Houston. The most prominent of these has been termed the fold of Kohlrausch (Fig. 17–1). Small lesions may often be hidden behind these valves or folds. Occasionally, with the rectum partially collapsed, the columns of Morgagni may be seen in the distal portion of the rectum (Fig. 17–2). In the lateral projection the rectum lies close to (usually within 1 cm of) the curve of the sacrum. At the rectosigmoid junction there is a sharp angulation as the rectosigmoid heads anteriorly and inferiorly (Fig. 17–1A).

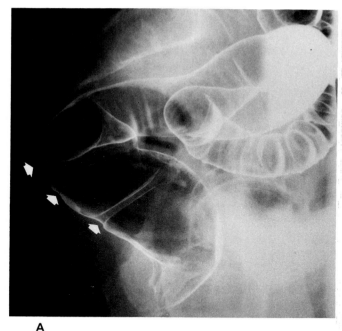

A

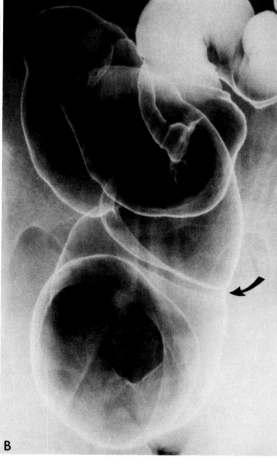

B

FIGURE 17–1 Anatomy of the rectum.

A. Lateral view showing the valves of Houston *(arrows).*

B. Angled view showing the prominent valve of Kohlrausch *(arrow).*

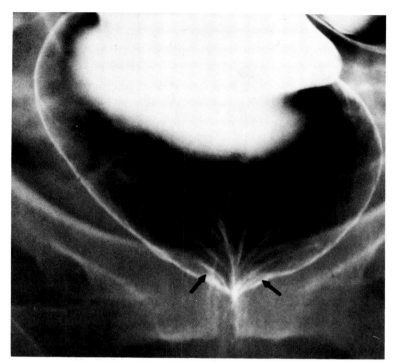

FIGURE 17–2 The rectal columns of Morgagni.

TECHNIQUE

A complete study of the rectum is included in the routine double contrast enema. The important elements of a high quality examination of the rectum include drainage of barium followed by insufflation without introduction of additional barium.[8] The frontal view will often give better mucosal detail because of diminished scatter. At least one film of the rectum should be obtained after the enema tip has been removed, so that the distal portion of the rectum is not obscured. We have routinely included a prone, angled view of the rectosigmoid in all patients over the age of 35 as well as in all patients being examined for the possibility of polyps.[9] Some small lesions have been visible only on this view, while other larger lesions have been suspected on other views, but could only be demonstrated conclusively on the angled view (Fig. 17–12A).

In any patient with a particular suspicion of rectal disease, additional spot films in appropriate projections may be obtained. We have also used a prone, cross-table, lateral film of the rectum in such cases.[10] In this position almost the entire rectum can usually be visualized free of barium. This is also particularly useful for the detection of perirectal disease (Figs. 17–19B and 17–20A).

RECTAL ABNORMALITIES

Intrinsic Abnormalities

HEMORRHOIDS

Hemorrhoids can frequently be recognized on the double contrast enema after the enema tip has been removed. They may appear as polypoid, grapelike filling defects at the very distal extent of the rectum or as tortuous filling defects similar to esophageal varices (Fig. 17–3). Hemorrhoids may also become large enough to be mistaken for a polypoid lesion (Fig. 17–3*C*).

POLYPS

Benign rectal polyps are particularly common. They are apt to be overlooked on sigmoidoscopy if they lie behind one of the valves of Houston (Fig. 17–4).[2, 11] Small villous tumors may be indistinguishable from adenomatous polyps (Fig. 17–5). The radiologic aspects of rectal polyps are as described in Chapter 13 under colonic polyps.

There are frequently calcifications in the pelvis which are projected over the rectum and may simulate a rectal polyp. This condition may be due to a calcified uterine fibroid (Fig. 17–6*A*) or to a phlebolith (Fig. 17–6*B*). A similar effect can be pronounced by lymphangiographic contrast in pelvic lymph nodes.

Text continued on page 696

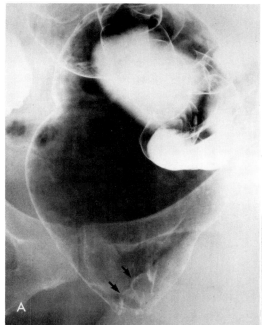

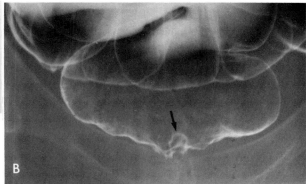

FIGURE 17–3 Internal hemorrhoids.

A. Grapelike filling defects due to internal hemorrhoids.

B. Smaller filling defect.

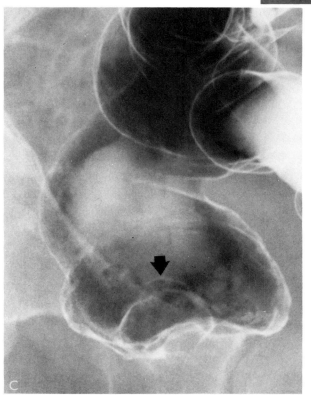

C. A polypoid mass due to hemorrhoids.

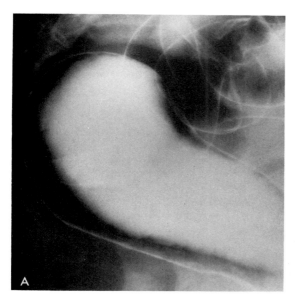

FIGURE 17–4 Rectal polyp missed at endoscopy.

    A. Lateral view of the rectum with a small amount of barium. No polyp is seen.

    B. With barium drained from the rectum the pedunculated polyp is clearly seen.

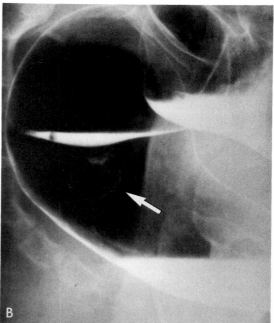

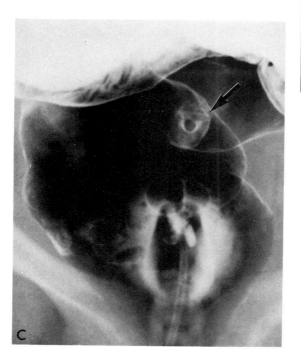

    C. In the prone position the polyp and its stalk are seen lying behind the valve of Houston. Polyps in this location are frequently missed at proctosigmoidoscopy.

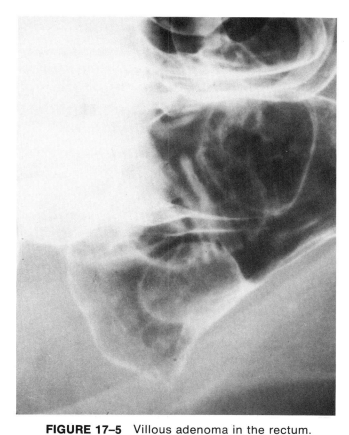

FIGURE 17–5 Villous adenoma in the rectum.

The polyp has a smooth surface and none of the radiologic characteristics of a villous tumor.

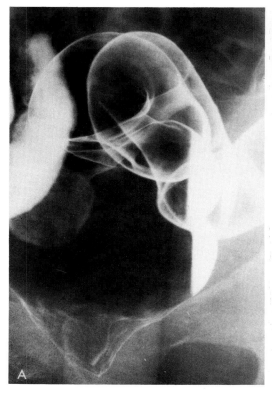

FIGURE 17–6 Pelvic calcifications simulating a rectal polyp.

A. Calcified uterine fibroid.
B. Phlebolith.

MALIGNANT TUMORS

Rectal carcinoma may be either annular (Fig. 17–7) or polypoid. (Fig. 17–8), although early carcinomas are virtually all polypoid in nature (Figs. 17–9 to 17–11). Many rectal lesions are seen exclusively or to best advantage on the prone-angled projection (Fig. 17–12). Posterior wall lesions are seen particularly well on the prone, cross-table, lateral view (Fig. 17–13).

A large proportion of large bowel carcinomas lie within reach of the sigmoidoscope. Some of these lesions may be missed if the sigmoidoscope is not advanced to its full extent. In other patients an annular constricting lesion may preclude visualization of the entire rectum. The patient illustrated in Figure 17–7 had been examined sigmoidoscopically twice in the preceding 1½ years, and the lesion had not been found. The patient illustrated in Figure 17–10 had a double contrast enema because of right lower quadrant pain. The sessile, polypoid lesion in the rectum was an asymptomatic unrelated finding. This proved to be a localized polypoid carcinoma.

Other types of malignant tumors are rare in the rectum. Lymphoma (Fig. 14–19) and leiomyosarcoma may occasionally be seen (Fig. 17–14).[12]

Text continued on page 704

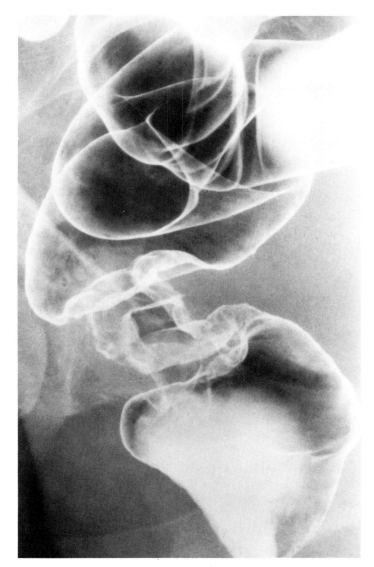

FIGURE 17–7   Annular carcinoma of the rectum.

This tumor was missed on two preceding barium enemas and sigmoidoscopies. Angulation caused by the tumor prevented the sigmoidoscope from reaching the carcinoma.

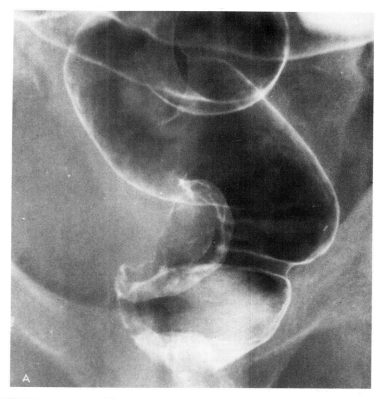

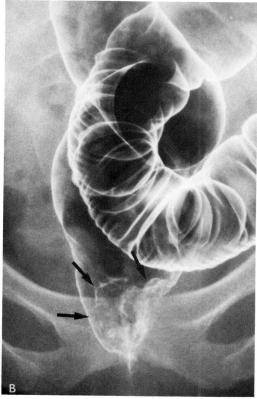

FIGURE 17–8 *A* and *B*   Two examples of polypoid carcinomas of the rectum.

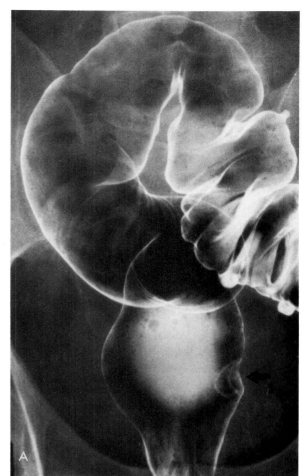

FIGURE **17–9** Early carcinoma of the rectum.

A. Frontal view showing slight retraction of the base of the polyp.

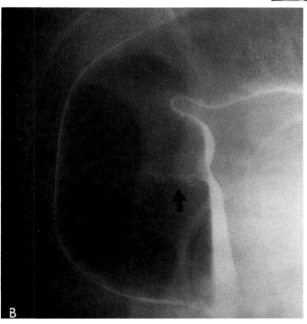

B. Lateral view in which the polyp is seen only with difficulty.

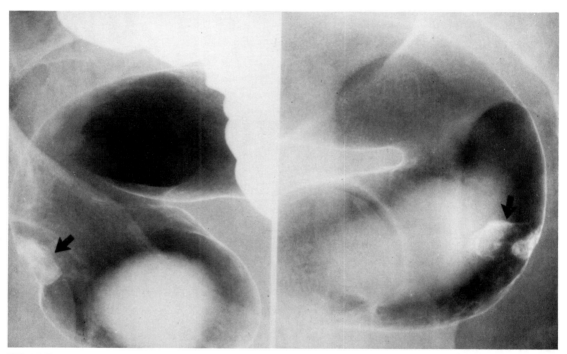

FIGURE 17–10 Early asymptomatic carcinoma of the rectum presenting as a sessile polypoid lesion. This patient presented with right lower quadrant pain. The rectal tumor was an incidental finding. (See also Plate 91.)

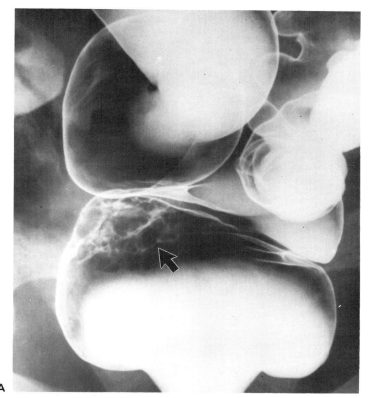

A. Frontal projection.

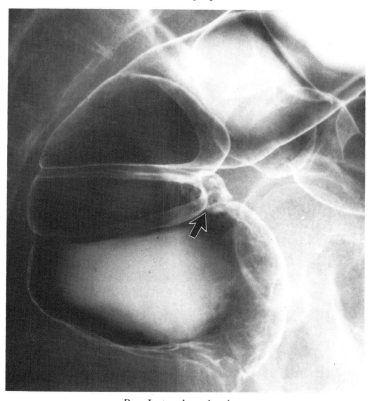

B. Lateral projection.

FIGURE 17–11 Villous carcinoma of the rectum.

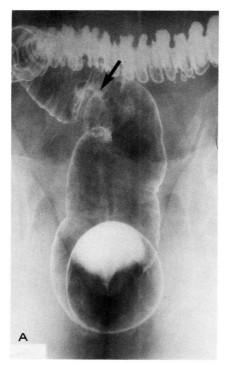 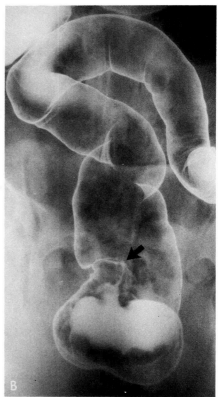

FIGURE 17–12

A. Polypoid carcinoma at the rectosigmoid junction, best seen on the prone-angled view.
B. Polypoid carcinoma of the distal portion of the rectum.

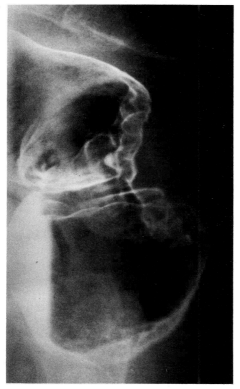

FIGURE 17–13 Carcinoma of the posterior wall of the rectum, best demonstrated on the prone, cross-table lateral projection.

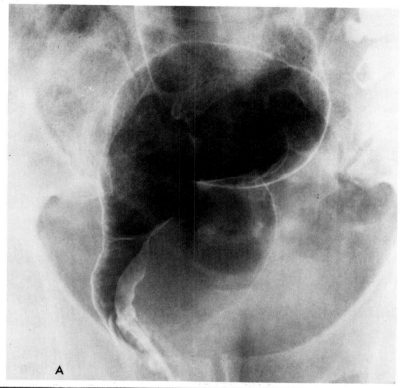

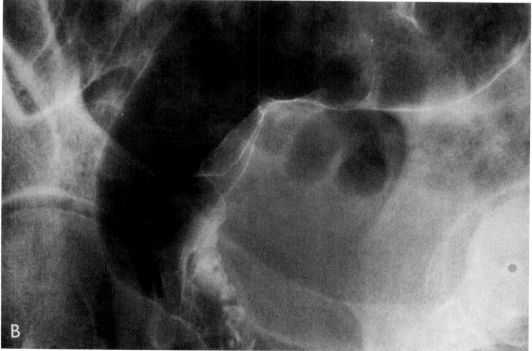

FIGURE 17–14 *A* and *B*   Leiomyosarcoma of the rectum.

ULCERATIVE PROCTITIS

Ulcerative proctitis is a mild variant of ulcerative colitis, in which involvement is limited to the rectum. In the majority of such cases the conventional barium enema reveals no abnormality.[13] However, utilizing double contrast technique, inflammatory changes can be demonstrated regularly in the rectum, even in its most distal portion (Fig. 17–15).[14]

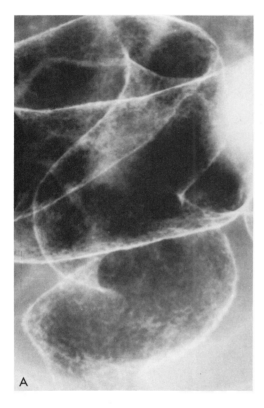

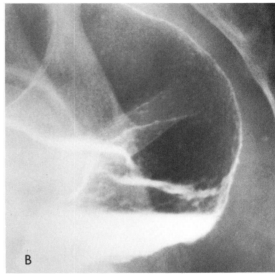

FIGURE 17–15 Ulcerative proctosigmoiditis.

A. The mucosa of the rectum and sigmoid has a granular, shaggy appearance owing to chronic inflammation and ulceration.

B. Ulcerative proctitis limited to the distal portion of the rectum. Stippling of the distal rectal mucosa is due to superficial ulceration.

CROHN'S DISEASE

The rectum is involved endoscopically in approximately 50 per cent of patients with granulomatous colitis.[15, 16] However, the involvement tends to be patchy, as opposed to the diffuse involvement in ulcerative colitis. In addition, discrete, deep ulcers may be seen (Fig. 17–16*A*). Such ulcers are rarely encountered in the rectum in ulcerative colitis.[17] Sinus tracts are another feature of rectal disease in granulomatous colitis (Fig. 17–16*B*)

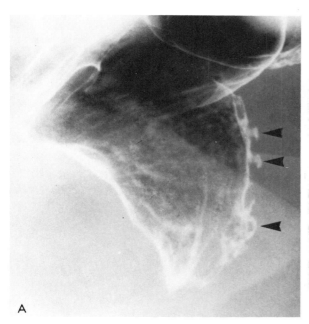
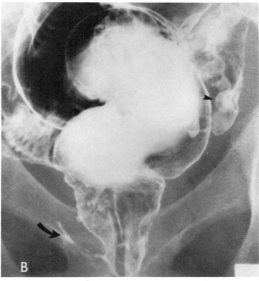

FIGURE 17–16 The rectum in Crohn's disease.

A. Collar button ulcers *(arrows)* in the rectum. When found in the rectum, these are characteristic of Crohn's disease as opposed to ulcerative colitis.

B. Ulcers and a sinus tract *(arrow)* in the rectum. There are also inflammatory polyps *(arrowheads)*.

OTHER FORMS OF PROCTITIS

The rectum is frequently involved by radiation damage. In the acute phase[18] the mucosa may have a granular or ulcerated appearance indistinguishable from that of ulcerative proctitis (Fig. 17–17A). In the late stage[19] the rectum is narrowed, with a smooth surface (Fig. 17–17B). The rectum is usually spared in ischemic colitis. However, when it is affected,[20] the appearance is similar to that of ulcerative proctitis (Fig. 17–17C). Rectal involvement in other forms of inflammatory bowel disease is considered in Chapter 16.

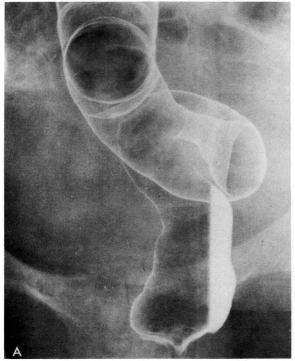

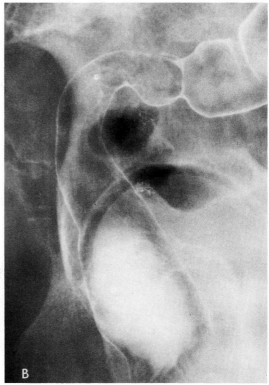

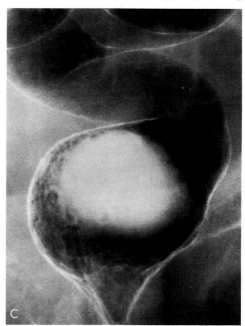

FIGURE 17–17

A. Acute radiation proctitis with minimal granularity of the rectal mucosa.

B. Chronic radiation proctitis with diffuse narrowing of the rectum and loss of the valves of Houston.

C. Ischemic proctitis with coarse granularity of the rectal mucosa.

Extrinsic Abnormalities

Various types of perirectal disease are well demonstrated with the double contrast technique. They include compression of the rectosigmoid by pelvic masses, such as ovarian or uterine tumors. These are usually quite obvious and are readily recognized on the lateral view (Fig. 17–18). Occasionally the findings are more subtle (Fig. 17–19A) and may be easiest to appreciate on the prone, cross-table view (Fig. 17–19B).

Endometriosis may produce a nonspecific pelvic mass. However, several other appearances are very suggestive of endometriosis.[21,22] An intramural lesion on the anterior wall at the rectosigmoid junction is frequently seen with crinkling of the mucosa, presumably due to the associated desmoplastic reaction (Fig. 17–20).[21] Additional intramural lesions may be found in the sigmoid (Fig. 17–21) or cecum.

Malignant pelvic tumors may involve the rectum by direct extension. In females this is usually due to carcinoma of the cervix or endometrium (Fig. 17–22), while in males it is usually the result of prostatic carcinoma (Fig. 17–23).

The rectum and sigmoid may also be affected by pelvic (Figs. 17–13 to 17–24) and tubo-ovarian abscesses (Fig. 17–24). There is usually evidence of a pelvic mass and mucosal thickening or nodularity caused by spread of inflammation to the serosa.

Text continued on page 713

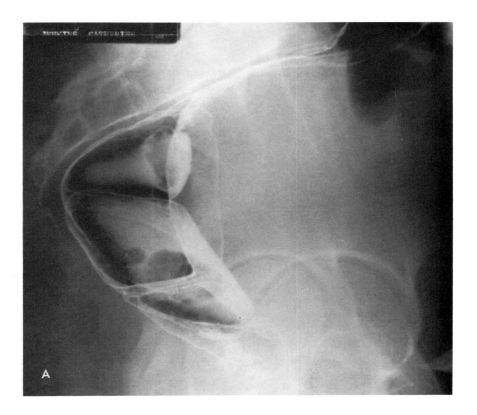

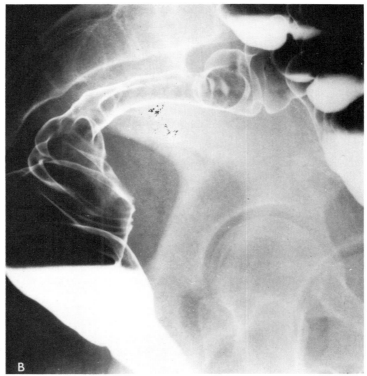

FIGURE 17–18 *A* and *B*   Two examples of a pelvic mass with compression of the rectosigmoid.

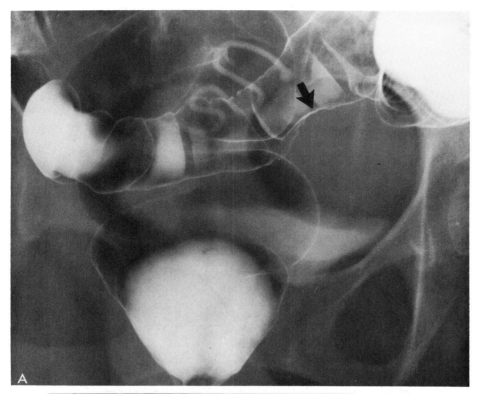

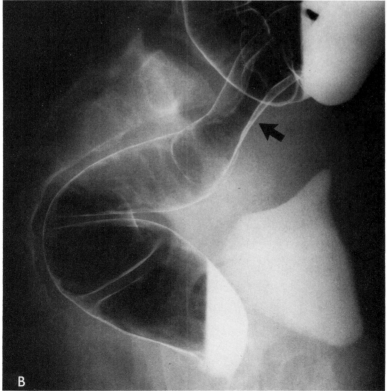

FIGURE 17–19

A. Slight displacement of the sigmoid colon by a small pelvic mass.

B. Cross-table lateral view showing displacement of the sigmoid colon by a pelvic mass.

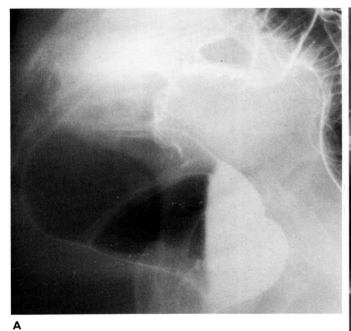

A

FIGURE 17–20 Pelvic endometriosis.

A. Lateral view, showing the typical intramural lesion at the rectosigmoid junction.

B. Frontal view, showing crinkling of the mucosa in pelvic endometriosis.

B

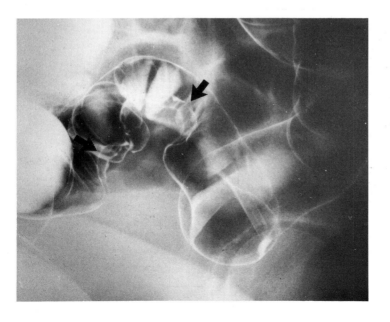

FIGURE 17–21 Multiple submucosal masses in the sigmoid as a result of pelvic endometriosis. (Courtesy of Giles W. Stevenson, M.D., and Sat Somers, M.D., Hamilton, Ontario.)

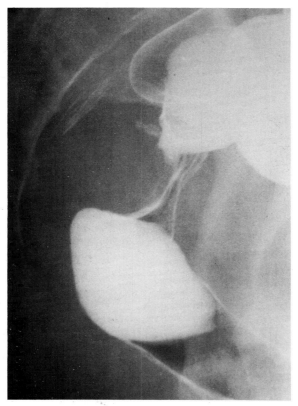

FIGURE 17–22   Carcinoma of the cervix, encircling the rectum.

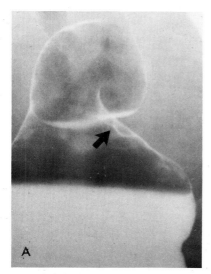

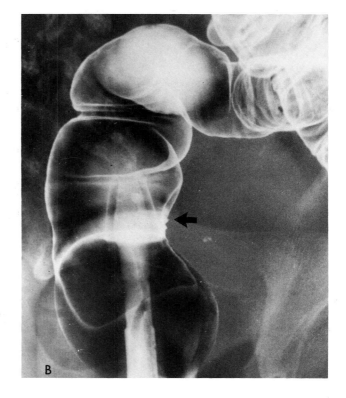

FIGURE 17–23A and B   Involvement of the rectum by carcinoma of the prostate.

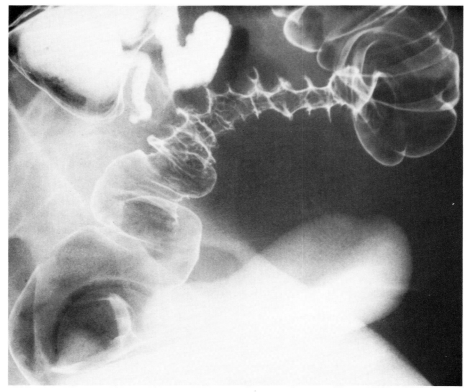

FIGURE 17–24 Tuberculous tubo-ovarian abscess with involvement of the sigmoid colon.

REFERENCES

1. Cooley, R. N.: The diagnostic accuracy of radiologic studies of the biliary tract, small intestine and colon. Am. J. Med. Sci., *246*:610, 1963.
2. Laufer, I., Smith, N. C. W., and Mullens, J. E.: The radiologic demonstration of colorectal polyps undetected by endoscopy. Gastroenterology, *70*:167, 1976.
3. Laufer, I.: The double-contrast enema: myths and misconceptions. Gastrointest. Radiol., *1*:19, 1976.
4. Simpkins, K. C., and Young, A. C.: The radiology of colonic and rectal polyps. Br. J. Surg., *55*:731, 1968.
5. Kirsner, J. B.: Problems in the differentiation of ulcerative colitis and Crohn's disease of the colon: the need for repeated diagnostic evaluation. Gastroenterology *68*:187, 1975.
6. Netter, F. H.: The CIBA Collection of Medical Illustrations. Vol. 3. Digestive System. Part II. Lower Digestive Tract. New York, CIBA, pp. 57–59.
7. Cohen, W. N.: Roentgenographic evaluation of the rectal valves of Houston in the normal and ulcerative colitis. Am. J. Roentgenol., *104*:580, 1968.
8. Miller, R. E.: Barium enema examination with large bore tubing and drainage. Radiology, *82*:905, 1964.
9. Dysart, D. N., and Stewart, H. R.: Special angled roentgenography for lesions of the rectosigmoid. Am. J. Roentgenol., *96*:285, 1966.
10. Niizuma, S., and Kobayashi, S.: Rectosigmoid double contrast examination in the prone position with a horizontal beam. Am. J. Roentgenol., *128*:519, 1977.
11. Oppenheimer, A.: Roentgen diagnosis of incipient carcinoma of the rectum. Am. J. Roentgenol., *52*:637, 1944.
12. Marshak, R. H., and Lindner, A. E.: Leiomyosarcoma of the colon. Am. J. Gastroenterol., *54*:155, 1970.
13. Fennessey, J. J., Sparberg, M., and Kirsner, J. B.: Early roentgen manifestations of mild ulcerative colitis and proctitis. Radiology, *87*:848, 1966.
14. Laufer, I.: The radiologic demonstration of early changes in ulcerative colitis by double contrast technique. J. Can. Assoc. Radiol., *26*:116, 1975.
15. Laufer, I., and Hamilton, J. D.: The radiologic differentiation between ulcerative and granulomatous colitis by double contrast radiology. Am. J. Gastroenterol., *66*:259, 1976.
16. Korelitz, B. I., and Sommers, S. C.: Differential diagnosis of ulcerative and granulomatous colitis by sigmoidoscopy, rectal biopsy and cell counts of rectal mucosa. Am. J. Gastroenterol., *61*:460, 1974.
17. Devroede, G. J.: Differential diagnosis of colitis. Can. J. Surg., *17*:369, 1974.
18. Gelfand, M. D., Tepper, M., Katz, L. A., et al.: Acute irradiation proctitis in man. Gastroenterology, *54*:401, 1968.
19. DeCrosse, J. J., Rhodes, R. S., Wentz, W. B., et al.: The natural history and management of radiation-induced injury of the gastrointestinal tract. Ann. Surg., *170*:369, 1969.
20. Kilpatrick, Z. M., Farman, J., Yesner, R., et al.: Ischemic proctitis. JAMA, *205*:74, 1968.
21. Theander, G., and Whelin, L.: Deformation of the rectosigmoid junction in pelvic endometriosis. Acta Radiol., *55*:241, 1961.
22. Fagan, C. J.: Endometriosis. Clinical and roentgenographic manifestations. Radiol. Clin. North Am., *12*:109, 1974.

INDEX

Page numbers in *italics* refer to illustrations; (t) indicates tables.

715